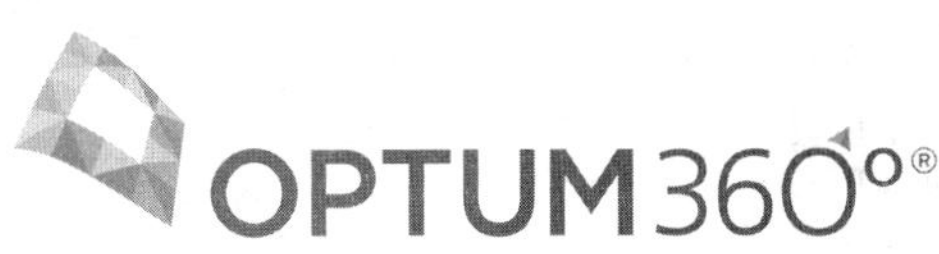

CODING & PAYMENT GUIDE

# Dental Services

## An essential coding, billing and reimbursement resource for dental services

**2022** **optum360coding.com**

## Optum360 Notice



Optum360
2525 Lake Park Blvd.
West Valley City, UT 84120

## American Medical Association Notice



## American Dental Association Notice



## Our Commitment to Accuracy

Optum360 is committed to producing accurate and reliable materials.

To report corrections, please email accuracy@optum.com. You can also reach customer service by calling 1.800.464.3649, option 1.

## Copyright



Made in the USA

ISBN 978-1-62254-724-1

## Acknowledgments

Marianne Randall, CPC, *Product Manager*
Stacy Perry, *Desktop Publishing Manager*
Nannette Orme, CPC, CCS-P, CPMA, CEMC, *Subject Matter Expert*
Jacqueline Petersen, RHIA, CHDA, CPC, *Subject Matter Expert*
Tracy Betzler, *Senior Desktop Publishing Specialist*
Hope M. Dunn, *Senior Desktop Publishing Specialist*
Katie Russell, *Desktop Publishing Specialist*
Kimberli Turner, *Editor*

## Subject Matter Experts

***Nannette Orme, CPC, CCS-P, CPMA, CEMC***

Ms. Orme has more than 20 years of experience in the health care profession. She has extensive background in CPT/HCPCS and ICD-9-CM coding and has completed comprehensive ICD-10-CM and PCS training. Her prior experience includes physician clinics and health care consulting. Her areas of expertise include physician audits and education, compliance and HIPAA legislation, litigation support for Medicare self-disclosure cases, hospital chargemaster maintenance, workers' compensation, and emergency department coding. Ms. Orme has presented at national professional conferences and contributed articles for several professional publications. She is a member of the American Academy of Professional Coders (AAPC), American Health Information Management Association (AHIMA), and on the advisory board of a local college.

***Jacqueline Petersen, RHIA, CHDA, CPC***

Ms. Petersen is a Clinical/Technical editor with Optum360. She has served as Senior Clinical Product Research Analyst with Optum360 developing business requirements for edits to support correct coding and reimbursement for claims processing applications. Her experience includes development of data-driven and system rules for both professional and facility claims and in-depth analysis of claims data inclusive of ICD-10-CM, CPT, HCPCS, and modifiers. Her background also includes consulting work for Optum, serving as an SME, providing coding, and reimbursement education to internal and external clients. Ms. Petersen is a member of the American Academy of Professional Coders (AAPC), and the American Health Information Management Association (AHIMA).

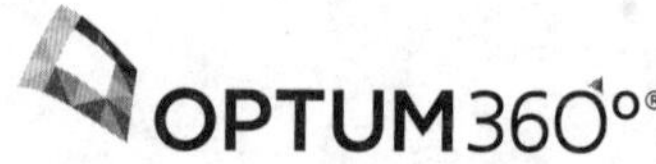
OPTUM360°

# Contents

**Getting Started with Coding and Payment Guide** .......... **1**
- Resequencing of CDT and CPT Codes .......... 1
- ICD-10-CM .......... 1
- Detailed Code Information .......... 1
- Appendix Codes and Descriptions .......... 1
- CCI Edit Updates .......... 1
- Index .......... 1
- General Guidelines .......... 1
- Sample Page and Key .......... 2
- Reimbursement Issues .......... 5
- Fee Schedules .......... 5
- Relative Value Scale .......... 5
- Documentation .......... 5

**Procedure Codes** .......... **9**
- HCPCS Level I or CPT Codes .......... 9
- HCPCS Level II Codes .......... 9

**HCPCS Level II D Codes** .......... **11**
- Diagnostic .......... 11
- Preventive .......... 73
- Restoration .......... 85
- Endodontics .......... 117
- Periodontics .......... 138
- Removable Prosthodontics .......... 163
- Maxillofacial Prosthetics .......... 184
- Implant Services .......... 186
- Fixed Prosthodontics .......... 219
- Oral and Maxillofacial Surgery .......... 245
- Orthodontics .......... 280
- Adjunctive Services .......... 286

**Appendix** .......... **309**

**CPT Codes** .......... **314**
- E/M Services .......... 314
- Integumentary .......... 323
- Musculoskeletal .......... 324
- Digestive .......... 325
- Medicine .......... 346

**Correct Coding Intiative Update 27.3** .......... **347**

**CDT Index** .......... **361**

**CPT Index** .......... **365**

**Medicare Official Regulatory Information** .......... **367**
- The CMS Online Manual System .......... 367
- Pub. 100 References .......... 368

# Getting Started with Coding and Payment Guide

The *Coding and Payment Guide for Dental Services* is designed to be a guide to the specialty procedures classified in the CDT® and CPT® books. It is structured to help coders understand procedures and translate physician narrative into correct CPT codes by combining many clinical resources into one, easy-to-use source book. The book also allows coders to validate the intended code selection by providing an easy-to-understand explanation of the procedure and associated conditions or indications for performing the various procedures. As a result, data quality and reimbursement will be improved by providing code-specific clinical information and helpful tips regarding the coding of procedures.

## Resequencing of CDT and CPT Codes

The American Dental Association (ADA) and the American Medical Association (AMA) employ a resequenced numbering methodology. According to the associations, there are instances where a new code is needed within an existing grouping of codes, but an unused code number is not available to keep the range sequential. In the instance where the existing codes were not changed or had only minimal changes, the ADA and AMA have assigned a code out of numeric sequence with the other related codes being grouped together. The resequenced codes and their descriptions have been placed with their related codes, out of numeric sequence. Codes within the Optum360 *Coding and Payment Guide* series display in their resequenced order. Resequenced codes are enclosed in brackets for easy identification.

## ICD-10-CM

Overall, in the 10th revision of the ICD-10-CM codes, conditions are grouped with general epidemiological purposes and the evaluation of health care in mind. Features include icons to identify newborn, pediatric, adult, male only, female only, and laterality. Refer to the ICD-10-CM book for more ICD-10-CM coding information.

## Detailed Code Information

One or more columns are dedicated to each procedure or service to a series of similar procedures/services. Following the specific CDT and CPT code and its narrative, is a combination of features. A sample is shown on page 2. The black boxes with numbers in them correspond to the information on the page following the example.

## Appendix Codes and Descriptions

Some procedure codes are presented in a less comprehensive format in the appendix. The CDT and CPT codes appropriate to the specialty are included the appendix with the official code description. The codes are presented in numeric order, and each code is followed by an easy-to-understand lay description of the procedure.

## CCI Edits and Other Coding Updates

This *Coding and Payment Guide* includes the a list of codes from the official Centers for Medicare and Medicaid Services' *National Correct Coding Policy Manual for Part B Medicare Contractors* that are considered to be an integral part of the comprehensive code or mutually exclusive of it and should not be reported separately. The codes in the Correct Coding Initiative (CCI) section are from version 27.3, the most current version available at press time. CCI edits are updated quarterly and will be posted on the product updates page listed below. The CCI edits are located in a section at the back of the book. As other CPT (including COVID-related vaccine and administration codes), CDT, and ICD-10-CM codes relevant to your specialty are released, updates will be posted to the Optum360 website. The website address is http://www.optum360coding.com/ProductUpdates/. The 2022 edition password is: **CODING22.** Log in frequently to ensure you receive the most current updates.

## Index

Comprehensive indexes for both the CPT and the CDT coding systems are provided for easy access to the codes. The indexes have several axes. A code can be looked up by its procedure name or by the anatomical site associated with it. For example:

**Debridement**
- endodontic, D3221
- periodontal, D4355
  - implant
    - peri, D6101-D6102
    - single, D6081

## General Guidelines

### Providers

The ADA and AMA advises coders that while a particular service or procedure may be assigned to a specific section, the service or procedure itself is not limited to use only by that specialty group. Additionally, the procedures and services listed throughout the book are for use by any qualified dentist, physician, or other qualified healthcare professional or entity (e.g., hospitals, laboratories, or home health agencies). Keep in mind that there may be other policies or guidance that can affect who may report a specific service.

### Supplies

Some payers may allow providers to separately report drugs and other supplies when reporting the place of service as office or other nonfacility setting. Drugs and supplies are to be reported by the facility only when performed in a facility setting.

### Professional and Technical Component

Radiology and some pathology codes have a technical and a professional component. When providers do not own their own equipment and send their patients to outside testing facilities, they should append modifier 26 to the procedural code to indicate they performed only the professional component.

## Sample Page and Key

On the following pages are a sample page from the book displaying the new format of *Coding and Payment Guide for Dental Services* with each element identified and explained on the opposite page.

# D1206-D1208 1

**D1206** topical application of fluoride varnish
**D1208** topical application of fluoride - excluding varnish

## Explanation 2

Topically applied fluoride treatments are done in the office with a variety of solutions or gels and different application protocols, excluding rinsing or "swish." The fluoride may be applied with trays or specifically to a few, isolated teeth at a time to prevent a high systemic dose from occurring. Fluoride varnish is painted directly on certain areas to help prevent further decay. The fluoride treatment reported here must be applied separately from any prophylaxis paste. Report D1206 for therapeutic application of varnish or D1208 for topical application of fluoride other than varnish.

## Coding Tips 3

These services must be provided under direct supervision of the dental provider. Appropriate code selection is determined method used. Code D1206 should be used for the application of topical fluoride varnish only. Report D1208 for other topical applications. Any evaluation, radiograph, restorative, or extraction service is reported separately. Removal of coronal plaque is reported separately using D1110 or D1120. Report D9910 if the varnish is applied solely to desensitize the tooth. To report application of interim caries arresting medicament, see D1354.

## Documentation Tips 4

The following information can be documented on a tooth chart: treatment/location of caries, endodontic procedures, prosthetic services, preventive services, treatment of lesions and dental disease, or other special procedures. A tooth chart may also be used to identify structure and rationale of disease process and the type of service performed on intraoral structures other than teeth.

## Reimbursement Tips 5

When selecting the procedure or service that accurately identifies the service performed, dentists must use the most accurate code. If the CDT code more accurately identifies the service, this should be used rather than the CPT codes. When an oral health assessment is performed by someone other than the dentist, for example, a licensed dental hygienist, some third-party payers may require that modifier DA Oral health assessment by a licensed health professional other than a dentist, be appended to the code. Check with third-party payers for their specific requirements.

## Associated CPT Codes 6

| | |
|---|---|
| 99188 | Application of topical fluoride varnish by a physician or other qualified health care professional |

## ICD-10-CM Diagnostic Codes 7

| | |
|---|---|
| Z01.20 | Encounter for dental examination and cleaning without abnormal findings |
| Z01.21 | Encounter for dental examination and cleaning with abnormal findings |
| Z41.8 | Encounter for other procedures for purposes other than remedying health state |
| Z46.4 | Encounter for fitting and adjustment of orthodontic device |
| Z91.120 | Patient's intentional underdosing of medication regimen due to financial hardship |
| Z91.128 | Patient's intentional underdosing of medication regimen for other reason |
| Z91.14 | Patient's other noncompliance with medication regimen |
| Z91.841 | Risk for dental caries, low |
| Z91.842 | Risk for dental caries, moderate |
| Z91.843 | Risk for dental caries, high |
| Z98.810 | Dental sealant status |
| Z98.811 | Dental restoration status |
| Z98.818 | Other dental procedure status |

## Relative Value Units/Medicare Edits 8

| Non-Facility RVU | Work | PE | MP | Total |
|---|---|---|---|---|
| **D1206** | 0.20 | 0.39 | 0.02 | 0.61 |
| **D1208** | 0.10 | 0.19 | 0.01 | 0.30 |
| **Facility RVU** | **Work** | **PE** | **MP** | **Total** |
| **D1206** | 0.20 | 0.39 | 0.02 | 0.61 |
| **D1208** | 0.10 | 0.19 | 0.01 | 0.30 |

| | FUD | Status | MUE | Modifiers | | | | IOM Reference |
|---|---|---|---|---|---|---|---|---|
| **D1206** | N/A | N | - | N/A | N/A | N/A | N/A | None |
| **D1208** | N/A | N | - | N/A | N/A | N/A | N/A | |

* with documentation

## Terms To Know 9

**fluoride.** Compound of the gaseous element fluorine that can be incorporated into bone and teeth and provides some protection in reducing dental decay.

**plaque.** Accumulation of a soft sticky substance on the teeth largely composed of bacteria and its byproducts.

**prophylaxis.** Intervention or protective therapy intended to prevent a disease.

**scaling.** Removal of plaque, calculus, and stains from teeth.

## 1. CDT/CPT Codes and Descriptions

This edition of *Coding and Payment Guide for Dental Services* is updated with CDT and CPT codes for year 2022. The following icons are used in the *Coding and Payment Guide*:

- ● This CDT/CPT code is new for 2022.
- ▲ This CDT/CPT code description is revised for 2022.
- + This CDT/CPT code is an add-on code.
- ★ This CPT code is identified by CPT as appropriate for telemedicine services
- [ ] CPT codes enclosed in brackets are resequenced and may not appear in numerical order.

Add-on codes are not subject to bilateral or multiple procedure rules, reimbursement reduction, or appending modifier 50 or 51. Add-on codes describe additional intraservice work associated with the primary procedure performed by the same practitioner on the same date of service and are not reported as stand-alone procedures. Add-on codes for procedures performed on bilateral structures are reported by listing the add-on code twice.

## 2. Explanation

Every CDT or CPT code or series of similar codes is presented with its official CDT code description and nomenclature or CPT code description. However, sometimes these descriptions do not provide the coder with sufficient information to make a proper code selection. In *Coding and Payment Guide for Dental Services*, a step-by-step clinical description of the procedure is provided, in simple terms. Technical language that might be used by the dentist is included and defined. *Coding and Payment Guide for Dental Services* describes the most common method of performing each procedure.

## 3. Coding Tips

Coding and reimbursement tips provide information on how the code should be used, provides related procedure codes, and offers help concerning common billing errors, modifier usage, and anesthesia. This information comes from consultants and subject matter experts at Optum360 and from the coding guidelines provided in the CDT or CPT book.

## 4. Documentation Tips

Documentation tips provide code-specific tips to the coder regarding the information that should be noted in the medical record to support code assignment. Documentation should be complete and support the CDT, CPT, or ICD-10-CM codes reported.

## 5. Reimbursement Tips

Medicare and other payer guidelines that could affect the reimbursement of this service or procedure are included in the Reimbursement Tips section.

## 6. Associated CPT Codes

The 2022 edition of the *Coding and Payment Guide for Dental Services* contains a crosswalk from the driver CDT or CPT code to its corresponding CPT or CDT code. CDT codes should be reported for the majority of dental services. On occasion, coverage of trauma, injury, or neoplasm may be covered by the health care insurer. In the rare instance when reporting a medical claim, CPT codes should be reported. This heading will not appear if there is no valid crosswalk.

## 7. ICD-10-CM Diagnostic Codes

ICD-10-CM diagnostic codes listed are common diagnoses or reasons the procedure may be necessary. This list in most cases is inclusive to the specialty. Some ICD-10-CM codes are further identified with the following icons:

- N Newborn: 0
- P Pediatric: 0-17
- M Maternity: 9-64
- A Adult: 15-124
- ♂ Male only
- ♀ Female Only
- ☑ Laterality

Please note that in some instances the ICD-10-CM codes for only one side of the body (right) have been listed with the CPT code. The associated ICD-10-CM codes for the other side and/or bilateral may also be appropriate. Codes that refer to the right or left are identified with the ☑ icon to alert the user to check for laterality. In some cases, not every possible code is listed and the ICD-10-CM book should be referenced for other valid codes.

## 8. Relative Value Units/Medicare Edits

The 2022 Medicare edits and gap filled relative values (RVU) were not available at the time this book went to press. Updated 2022 values will be posted at https://www.optum360coding.com/ProductUpdates/. The 2022 edition password is **CODING22**.

### *Gap Filled Relative Value Units*

Included in this edition are 2021 gap filled relative value units (RVU) for the CDT codes. These are useful in assisting with establishing fee schedules for your practice.

The gap relative value units are created by Optum360 using various methodologies depending on the code. For most codes, gap relative values are calculated by using relative value information from the Optum360 Relative Value Scale and adjusted to a scale similar to the Medicare physician fee schedule (MPFS) relative values (RBRVS). The Optum360 relative values are developed by and are proprietary to Optum360, Inc. The Optum360 relative values are assigned when Optum360 has an understanding of how the procedure is typically billed by the industry and how it relates to other procedures. Relative values are based on difficulty, time, work, risk, and resources. Relative values are established by Optum360 employees, including an Optum360 medical director, clinicians, certified procedural coders, and analysts. Optum360 also consults with a panel of outside physicians and dentists during the relative value development process for certain codes.

Because the Optum360 relative values are on a different scale than RBRVS relative values, ratios are developed relating the RBRVS and Optum360 scales for approximately 250 code ranges within the CPT, HCPCS, and CDT coding systems. These ratios are multiplied by the Optum360 relative value to create the gap value. If Optum360 does not assign a relative value to a code, a gap value is not calculated.

### *Relative Value Units*

In a resource based relative value scale (RBRVS), services are ranked based on the relative costs of the resources required to provide those services as opposed to the average fee for the service, or average prevailing Medicare charge. The Medicare RBRVS defines three distinct components affecting the value of each service or procedure:

- Physician work component, reflecting the physician's time and skill
- Practice expense (PE) component, reflecting the physician's rent, staff, supplies, equipment, and other overhead

- Malpractice (MP) component, reflecting the relative risk or liability associated with the service

There are two RVU groups listed for each CPT code. The first RVU group is for nonfacilities, which includes provider services performed in offices, patients' homes, or other nonhospital settings. The second RVU group is for facilities, which represents provider services performed by the practitioner in hospitals, ambulatory surgical centers, or skilled nursing facilities.

#### *Medicare Follow-Up Days (FUD)*

Information on the Medicare global period is provided here. The global period is the time following a surgery during which routine care by the practitioner is considered postoperative and included in the surgical fee. Office visits or other routine care related to the original surgery cannot be separately reported if they occur during the global period.

#### *Status*

The Medicare status indicates if the service is separately payable by Medicare. The Medicare RBRVS includes:

A Active code—separate payment may be made

B Bundled code—payment is bundled into other service

C Carrier priced—individual carrier will price the code

I Not valid—Medicare uses another code for this service

N Non-covered—service is not covered by Medicare

R Restricted—special coverage instructions apply

T Injections—separately payable if no other services on same date

X Statutory exclusion—no RVUs or payment

#### *Medically Unlikely Edits*

This column provides the maximum number of units allowed by Medicare. However, it is also important to note that not every code has a Medically unlikely edit (MUE) available. Medicare has assigned some MUE values that are not available. If there is no information in the MUE column for a particular code, this does not mean that there is no MUE. It may simply mean that CMS has not released information on that MUE. Watch the remittance advice for possible details on MUE denials related to those codes. If there is no published MUE, a dash will display in the field.

An additional component of the MUE edit is the MUE adjudication indicator (MAI). This edit is the result of an audit by the Office of the Inspector General (OIG) that identified inappropriate billing practices that bypassed the MUEs. These included inappropriate reporting of bilateral services and split billing.

There are three MUE adjudication indicators.

1 Line Edit

2 Date of Service Edit: Policy

3 Date of Service Edit: Clinical

The MAI will be listed following the MUE value. For example code 41870 has an MUE value of 2 and a MAI value of 3. This will display in the MUE field as "2(3)."

#### *Modifiers*

Medicare identifies some modifiers that are required or appropriate to report with the CPT code. When the modifiers are not appropriate, they will be indicated with N/A. Four modifiers are included.

50 Bilateral Procedures

This modifier is used to identify when the same procedure is performed bilaterally. Medicare requires one line with modifier 50 and the reimbursement is 50 percent of the allowable. Other payers may require two lines and will reduce the second procedure.

51 Multiple Procedures

Medicare and other payers reduce the reimbursement of second and subsequent procedures performed at the same session to 50 percent of the allowable. For endoscopic procedures, the reimbursement is reduced by the value of the endoscopic base code.

62* Two Surgeons

Medicare identifies procedures that may be performed by co-surgeons. The reimbursement is split between both providers. Both surgeons must report the same code when using this modifier.

80* Assistant Surgeon

An assistant surgeon is allowed if modifier 80 is listed. Reimbursement is usually 20 percent of the allowable. For Medicare, it is 16 percent to account for the patient's co-pay amount.

* with documentation

Modifiers 62 and 80 may require supporting documentation to justify the co- or assistant surgeon.

#### *Medicare Official Regulatory Information*

Medicare official regulatory information provides official regulatory guidelines. Also known as the CMS Online Manual System, the Internet-only Manuals (IOM) contain official CMS information pertaining to program issuances, instructions, policies, and procedures based on statutes, regulations, guidelines, models, and directives. Optum360 has provided the reference for the surgery codes. The full text of guidelines can be found online at https://www.cms.gov/Regulations-and-Guidance/Guidance/Manuals/.

Medicare edits are provided for most codes. These 2022 Medicare edits were current as of November 2021.

### 9. Terms to Know

Some codes are accompanied by general information pertinent to the procedure, labeled "Terms to Know." This information is not critical to code selection, but is a useful supplement to coders hoping to expand their knowledge of the specialty.

## AMA References

The AMA references for *CPT Assistant* are listed by CPT the code, with the most recent reference listed first. Generally only the last six years of references are listed.

## Telehealth Services

Telehealth/Telemedicine services are identified by CPT with the ★ icon at the code level. The Centers for Medicare and Medicaid Services (CMS) identify additional services that may be performed via telehealth. Due to the COVID-19 public health emergency (PHE) some services have been designated as temporarily appropriate for telehealth. These CMS-approved services are identified in the coding tips where appropriate. Payers may require telehealth/telemedicine to be reported with place of service 02 Telehealth Provided Other than the Patient's Home or 10 Telehealth Provided in Patient's Home and modifier 95 appended. If specialized equipment is used at the originating site code Q3014 may be reported. Individual payers should be contacted for additional or different guidelines regarding telehealth/telemedicine services.

Documentation should include the type of technology used for the treatment in addition to the patient evaluation, treatment, and consents.

**Modifier**

95 Synchronous Telemedicine Service Rendered Via a Real-Time Interactive Audio and Video Telecommunications System

# Reimbursement Issues

## Reporting Dental versus Medical Claims

When selecting the name of the procedure or service that accurately identifies the service performed, dentists must use the most accurate code. Common dental terminology (CDT) codes are specific for dental procedures. As identified in the *CPT® Professional* manual, it is inappropriate to use a code that merely approximates the services provided. If the CDT code more accurately identifies the service, this should be used for third party payers rather than the CPT codes.

CPT codes are not used to report dental services including dental implants, grafts (tooth, tissue, and bone), biopsy, sutures, and radiology procedures unless they are the result of current injury or trauma. Healthcare, auto, or workers' compensation insurance do not normally cover dental procedures. Routine reporting of CPT codes by dental providers may lead to audits by healthcare insurers to evaluate the reporting practices of the practitioner. Providers should review the patients insurance and the certificate of coverage to determine the circumstances and specific services that should be reported to dental or medical insurance. Reporting of CPT codes must be linked to ICD-10-CM codes for the documented diagnosis and support the patient's injury or trauma.

## Medicaid Coverage of Dental and Maxillofacial Services

Title XIX of the Social Security Act, the Medicaid Program mandates that states provide dental services in certain specific instances.

## Dental Coverage for Children

Early and Periodic Screening, Diagnostic and Treatment (EPSDT) is Medicaid's comprehensive child health program. The program's focus is on prevention, early diagnosis, and treatment of medical conditions. EPSDT is a mandatory service required to be provided under a state's Medicaid program. Dental services are covered under this program.

All state Medicaid programs must provide coverage of dental services to children at intervals that meet reasonable standards of dental practice, as determined by the state, after consultation with recognized dental organizations involved in child health, and at such other intervals, as indicated by medical necessity, to determine the existence of a suspected illness or condition.

Recognized dental organizations may include a state's dental association, dental advisory committee, or other groups or associations that the state recognizes as being involved in child health care. A state may also choose to adopt nationally recognized dental periodicity schedules such as those developed by the American Dental Association or the Academy of Pediatric Dentistry.

Services must include at a minimum, relief of pain and infections, restoration of teeth, and maintenance of dental health. Dental services may not be limited to emergency services for EPSDT recipients.

States that provide Children's Health Insurance Program (CHIP) coverage to children through a Medicaid expansion program are required to offer the same dental benefit as that provided under the EPSDT program. Basically, dental coverage in separate CHIP programs is required to include coverage that is necessary to prevent disease and promote oral health, restore oral structures to health and function, and treat emergency conditions according to CMS.

Oral screening may be part of a physical exam performed by a medical physician, but does not substitute for a dental examination performed by a dentist as a result of a direct referral to a dentist. A direct dental referral is required for every child in accordance with the periodicity schedule set by the state.

CMS does not further define what specific dental services must be provided; however, EPSDT requires that all services coverable under the Medicaid program must be provided to EPSDT recipients if determined to be medically necessary. Under the Medicaid program, the state determines medical necessity.

If a condition requiring treatment is discovered during a screening, the state must provide the necessary services to treat that condition, whether or not such services are included in the state's Medicaid plan.

Most states require that a treatment plan be developed and approved by the state prior to the rendering of dental services.

## Adult Coverage

Individual states may elect to provide dental services to their adult Medicaid-eligible population. Remember, it is not mandatory that a state provide dental coverage to adult patients. While most states provide at least emergency dental services for adults, less than half of the states provide comprehensive dental care. There are no minimum requirements for adult dental coverage.

## Patient Cost Sharing

There are some instances where a state may require patients to be responsible for copayments of dental services. The Deficit Reduction Act of 2005 granted state Medicaid agencies the authority to impose premiums and cost sharing upon certain Medicaid recipients (section 1916A of the Act) and for certain services. Dental providers should carefully read all Medicaid communications, including Medicaid provider manuals and bulletins to determine individual state policies.

# Fee Schedules

Fee schedules are replacing the customary and reasonable payment methodology as the system of choice. Fee schedules eliminate the wide payment variation for similar services that occurs with the customary and reasonable method and allows both payers and providers to estimate the amount of reimbursement they can expect to pay and receive. Using a fee schedule to maintain a fee-for-service system was considered by many medical professionals to be critical in protecting practitioners clinical and professional autonomy.

# Relative Value Scale

A relative value scale (RVS) ranks services according to "value" where that value is defined with respect to a base value. All services are assigned a unit value, with more complex, more time-consuming services having higher unit values and vice versa. Values are then multiplied by a dollar conversion factor to become a fee schedule.

# Documentation

Documentation in the medical record should include patient evaluation, identification of missing teeth, caries, prior treatment (fillings and appliances), current treatment, ongoing plan of care, and patient instruction. Diagnoses for current treatment, including preventive services, should be clearly stated.

## Tooth Number and Surface

Dental claims are unique in that the specific tooth and often the areas of oral cavity involved in the treatment must be indicated to payers. The systems used to identify this information are similar to the modifiers used in the CPT/HCPCS systems.

## Tooth Numbering

Specific teeth are identified by a number from 1 to 32 across both arches for permanent teeth. Tooth 1 is the patient's upper right third molar; the numbering follows around sequentially to the upper left third molar (tooth 16). Numbering continues by dropping to the patient's lower left third molar (tooth 17) and moving around the lower arch to the patient's lower right third molar (tooth 32). The illustration on page 7 illustrates tooth numbering.

Deciduous teeth are identified with an uppercase letter beginning with A and ending with T. Each tooth is identified in sequential order across the upper arch and descending to and following around the lower arch. For example, tooth A is the patient's upper right second primary molar, and T is the patient's lower right second primary molar. Again, see the illustration on page 7.

## Tooth Surface

Most payers require that the dentist designate tooth surface when the procedure code reported directly involves one or more tooth surfaces. Up to five of the following codes may be entered (with spaces).

B Buccal

D Distal

F Facial

L Lingual

M Mesial

O Occlusal

Other payers may require the International Standards Organization system, which is commonly used to indicate areas of oral cavity involvement. These codes are indicated below.

00 Whole of the oral cavity
01 Maxillary area
02 Mandibular area
03 Upper right sextant
04 Upper anterior sextant
05 Upper left sextant
06 Lower left sextant
07 Lower anterior sextant
08 Lower right sextant
09 Other area of oral cavity
10 Right upper quadrant
20 Left upper quadrant
30 Left lower quadrant
40 Right lower quadrant
50 Right upper quadrant, deciduous dentition
60 Left upper quadrant, deciduous dentition
70 Right lower quadrant, deciduous dentition
80 Left lower quadrant, deciduous dentition

## Oral Cavity

Area of the oral cavity treated is indicated using two-digit code:

00 Entire oral cavity
01 Maxillary arch
02 Mandibular arch
10 Upper right quadrant
20 Upper left quadrant
30 Lower left quadrant
40 Lower right quadrant

Dental documentation varies from all other specialties in the identification of services performed on teeth and oral structures. There are also variations between the documentation required of oral and maxillofacial surgeons, dentists, and support staff such as dental hygienists and assistants.

## Medical Record Documentation

The basic information that should be readily available from the dental record includes:

- Evaluations
  - complete, periodic, or limited dental exam
  - preorthodontic visit
  - consultations, case management
  - evaluations at other locations (e.g., home, hospital)
- Anesthesia
  - local anesthesia
  - inhalation (i.e., nitrous oxide)
  - conscious sedation or general anesthesia (indication that the dentist was present) and appropriate monitoring provided
  - unusual events occurring during the anesthesia-monitoring period
  - total time
  - drugs provided to the patient including the dosage and time
  - any unusual anesthesia events or complications
  - initiation of any pain management services such as oral analgesics or patient controlled anesthesia

**Note:** The preanesthesia examination and evaluation should include a review of the patient's past medical history, medications, family history, social history, and adverse reactions to previous anesthesia.

- Radiographs
  - type of x-ray (e.g., intraoral, bitewing, panoramic)
  - results of x-ray
- Testing or diagnostic service
  - other testing or diagnostic services (e.g., pulp vitality)
- Documentation of tooth (teeth) treated
  - use standard identification of teeth as approved by ADA and CMS (alpha designation for primary teeth, numeric for permanent)
  - tooth surface treated if appropriate (See pages 7 and 8 for more information on tooth surface reporting methods.)
  - missing teeth documented in permanent record
  - record in usual manner on accepted illustration of the mouth and teeth

**Note:** This information can be illustrated on a tooth chart such as the one found below.

- Type of treatment
  - treatment of caries
  - endodontic procedures
  - prosthetic services
  - preventive services
  - treatment of lesions and dental disease
  - other special procedures
- Service on other intraoral structures
  - identify structure and rational or disease process identify type of service performed

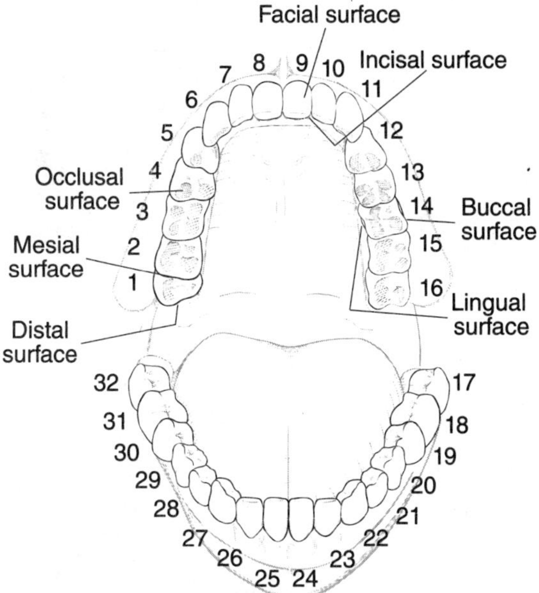


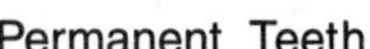

Permanent Teeth

Central and lateral incisors
Canine
First and second molars
A B C D E F G H I J
K L M N O P Q R S T

Primary Teeth

1 3rd molar (wisdom tooth)
2 2nd molar (12-yr molar)
3 1st molar (6-yr molar)
4 2nd bicuspid (2nd premolar)
5 1st bicuspid (1st premolar)
6 cuspid (canine/eye tooth)
7 lateral incisor
8 central incisor
9 central incisor
10 lateral incisor
11 cuspid (canine/eye tooth)
12 1st bicuspid (1st premolar)
13 2nd bicuspid (2nd premolar)
14 1st molar (6-yr molar)
15 2nd molar (12-yr molar)
16 3rd molar (wisdom tooth)

17 3rd molar (wisdom tooth)
18 2nd molar (12-yr molar)
19 1st molar (6-yr molar)
20 2nd bicuspid (2nd premolar)
21 1st bicuspid (1st premolar)
22 cuspid (canine/eye tooth)
23 lateral incisor
24 central incisor
25 central incisor
26 lateral incisor
27 cuspid (canine/eye tooth)
28 1st bicuspid (1st premolar)
29 2nd bicuspid (2nd premolar)
30 1st molar (6-yr molar)
31 2nd molar (12-yr molar)
32 3rd molar (wisdom tooth)

# Procedure Codes

One of the keys to gaining accurate reimbursement lies in understanding the multiple coding systems that are used to identify services. To be well versed in reimbursement practices, coders should be familiar with the CDT, HCPCS Level II, ICD-10-CM, and CPT® coding systems. The first of these, the CDT system, is increasingly important to reimbursement, as it has been extended to a wider array of dental services.

- Coding and billing should be based on the service and supplies provided. Documentation should describe the patient's problems and the service provided to enable the payer to determine reasonableness and necessity of care.
- Refer to Medicare coverage reference to determine whether the care provided is a covered service. The references are noted, when they apply, on the pages following.

## HCPCS Level I or CPT Codes

Known as HCPCS Level I, the CPT coding system is the most commonly used system to report procedures and services. Copyright of CPT codes and descriptions is held by the American Medical Association. This system reports outpatient and provider services.

CPT codes predominantly describe medical services and procedures, and are adapted to provide a common billing language that providers and payers can use for payment purposes. The codes are required for billing by both private and public insurance carriers, managed care companies, and workers' compensation programs. Dental professional may find that a third-party payer will occasionally require that a procedures be reported using a CPT code. Unless otherwise instructed, dental professional should report services using the appropriate American Dental Association (ADA) dental code when one exists.

## HCPCS Level II Codes

HCPCS Level II codes are commonly referred to as national codes or by the acronym HCPCS (pronounced "hik piks"). HCPCS codes are used for billing Medicare and Medicaid patients and have also been adopted by some third-party payers. HCPCS Level II codes published annually by CMS, are intended to supplement the CPT coding system by including codes for durable medical equipment, prosthetics, orthotics, and supplies (DMEPOS); drugs; and biologicals. These Level II codes consist of one alphabetic character (A–V) followed by four numbers. In many instances, HCPCS Level II codes are developed as precursors to CPT codes.

A complete list of the HCPCS Level II codes and the quarterly updates to this code set may be found at http://www.cms.gov/Medicare/Coding/HCPCSReleaseCodeSets/Alpha-Numeric-HCPCS.html.

The following is a list of the HCPCS Level II supply codes used to identify supplies commonly used by dentists.

### Medical and Surgical Supplies A4000–A8999

The A and E code sections of the HCPCS Level II code system cover a wide variety of medical and surgical supplies, and some durable medical equipment (DME), supplies and accessories.

**A4550** **Surgical trays**

**A4649** **Surgical supply; miscellaneous**

**E1700** **Jaw motion rehabilitation system**

**E1701** **Replacement cushions for jaw motion rehabilitation system, package of 6**

**E1702** **Replacement measuring scales for jaw motion rehabilitation system, package of 200**

***Drugs Administered Other Than Oral Method J0000–J8999***

Drugs and biologicals are usually covered by Medicare if: they are of the type that cannot be self-administered; they are not excluded by being immunizations; they are reasonable and necessary for the diagnosis or treatment of the illness or injury for which they are administered; and they have not been determined by the Food and Drug Administration (FDA) to be less than effective. In addition they must meet all the general requirements for coverage of items as incident to a physician's services. Generally, prescription and nonprescription drugs and biologicals purchased by or dispensed to a patient are not covered.

The following list of drugs can be injected either subcutaneously, intramuscularly, or intravenously. Third-party payers may wish to determine a threshold and pay up to a certain dollar limit for the drug.

J codes fall under the jurisdiction of the DME regional office for Medicare, unless incidental or otherwise noted. See Pub. 100-2, chap. 15, sec. 50.4

**J0670** **Injection, mepivacaine HCl, per 10 ml**

**J1790** **Injection, droperidol, up to 5 mg**

**J2250** **Injection, midazolam HCl, per 1 mg**

**J2400** **Injection, chloroprocaine HCl, per 30 ml**

**J2515** **Injection, pentobarbital sodium, per 50 mg**

**J2550** **Injection, promethazine HCl, up to 50 mg**

**J3010** **Injection, fentanyl citrate, 0.1 mg**

**J3360** **Injection, diazepam, up to 5 mg**

***Temporary National Codes (Non-Medicare) (S0000–S9999)***

**S0020** **Injection, bupivicaine HCl, 30 ml**

# D0120

▲ **D0120** periodic oral evaluation - established patient

*An evaluation performed on a patient of record to determine any changes in the patient's dental and medical health status since a previous comprehensive or periodic evaluation. This includes an oral cancer evaluation, periodontal screening where indicated, and may require interpretation of information acquired through additional diagnostic procedures. The findings are discussed with the patient. Report additional diagnostic procedures separately.*

## Explanation

The periodic oral evaluation is done to determine the patient's dental health status since the previous check-up. It includes screening for periodontal disease and/or oral cancer and possibly the interpretation of information acquired through additional, separately reportable diagnostic oral health tests.

## Coding Tips

When the patient is referred by another dentist for an opinion or advice regarding a particular condition, see code D9310. When a comprehensive oral examination is performed, see code D0150. When a problem-focused limited oral evaluation is performed, see codes D0140-D0145. A detailed oral evaluation that is problem focused is reported using code D0160; a limited, problem-focused exam is reported using D0170. When the provider performs a caries risk assessment using a standardized risk assessment tool, see D0601-D0603. A comprehensive periodontal evaluation, new or established patient, is reported using D0180. Code D0180 should not be reported in addition to this code as the components of D0120 are included in the comprehensive periodic evaluation. According to the ADA, codes D0120 and D4355 may be reported on the same date of service; however, it should be noted that some third-party payer policies prohibit billing these procedures concurrently. Any radiograph, prophylaxis, fluoride, restorative, or extraction service is reported separately.

## Documentation Tips

The following information can be documented on a tooth chart: treatment/location of caries, endodontic procedures, prosthetic services, preventive services, treatment of lesions and dental disease, or other special procedures. A tooth chart may also be used to identify structure and rationale of disease process and the type of service performed on intraoral structures other than teeth.

## Reimbursement Tips

When an oral health assessment is performed by someone other than the dentist, for example, a licensed dental hygienist, some third-party payers may require that modifier DA Oral health assessment by a licensed health professional other than a dentist, be appended to the this code. Check with third-party payers for their specific requirements.

## ICD-10-CM Diagnostic Codes

| | |
|---|---|
| K00.0 | Anodontia |
| K00.1 | Supernumerary teeth |
| K00.2 | Abnormalities of size and form of teeth |
| K00.3 | Mottled teeth |
| K00.4 | Disturbances in tooth formation |
| K00.5 | Hereditary disturbances in tooth structure, not elsewhere classified |
| K00.6 | Disturbances in tooth eruption |
| K00.7 | Teething syndrome |
| K00.8 | Other disorders of tooth development |
| K01.0 | Embedded teeth |
| K01.1 | Impacted teeth |
| K02.3 | Arrested dental caries |
| K02.51 | Dental caries on pit and fissure surface limited to enamel |
| K02.52 | Dental caries on pit and fissure surface penetrating into dentin |
| K02.53 | Dental caries on pit and fissure surface penetrating into pulp |
| K02.61 | Dental caries on smooth surface limited to enamel |
| K02.62 | Dental caries on smooth surface penetrating into dentin |
| K02.63 | Dental caries on smooth surface penetrating into pulp |
| K02.7 | Dental root caries |
| K03.0 | Excessive attrition of teeth |
| K03.1 | Abrasion of teeth |
| K03.2 | Erosion of teeth |
| K03.3 | Pathological resorption of teeth |
| K03.4 | Hypercementosis |
| K03.5 | Ankylosis of teeth |
| K03.6 | Deposits [accretions] on teeth |
| K03.7 | Posteruptive color changes of dental hard tissues |
| K03.81 | Cracked tooth |
| K04.01 | Reversible pulpitis |
| K04.02 | Irreversible pulpitis |
| K04.1 | Necrosis of pulp |
| K04.2 | Pulp degeneration |
| K04.3 | Abnormal hard tissue formation in pulp |
| K04.4 | Acute apical periodontitis of pulpal origin |
| K04.5 | Chronic apical periodontitis |
| K04.6 | Periapical abscess with sinus |
| K04.7 | Periapical abscess without sinus |
| K04.8 | Radicular cyst |
| K05.00 | Acute gingivitis, plaque induced |
| K05.01 | Acute gingivitis, non-plaque induced |
| K05.10 | Chronic gingivitis, plaque induced |
| K05.11 | Chronic gingivitis, non-plaque induced |
| K05.211 | Aggressive periodontitis, localized, slight |
| K05.212 | Aggressive periodontitis, localized, moderate |
| K05.213 | Aggressive periodontitis, localized, severe |
| K05.222 | Aggressive periodontitis, generalized, moderate |
| K05.223 | Aggressive periodontitis, generalized, severe |
| K05.311 | Chronic periodontitis, localized, slight |
| K05.312 | Chronic periodontitis, localized, moderate |
| K05.313 | Chronic periodontitis, localized, severe |
| K05.321 | Chronic periodontitis, generalized, slight |
| K05.322 | Chronic periodontitis, generalized, moderate |
| K05.323 | Chronic periodontitis, generalized, severe |
| K05.4 | Periodontosis |
| K05.5 | Other periodontal diseases |
| K06.011 | Localized gingival recession, minimal |
| K06.012 | Localized gingival recession, moderate |
| K06.013 | Localized gingival recession, severe |
| K06.021 | Generalized gingival recession, minimal |
| K06.022 | Generalized gingival recession, moderate |
| K06.023 | Generalized gingival recession, severe |
| K06.1 | Gingival enlargement |
| K06.2 | Gingival and edentulous alveolar ridge lesions associated with trauma |
| K08.0 | Exfoliation of teeth due to systemic causes |
| K08.111 | Complete loss of teeth due to trauma, class I |

K08.112 Complete loss of teeth due to trauma, class II
K08.113 Complete loss of teeth due to trauma, class III
K08.114 Complete loss of teeth due to trauma, class IV
K08.121 Complete loss of teeth due to periodontal diseases, class I
K08.122 Complete loss of teeth due to periodontal diseases, class II
K08.123 Complete loss of teeth due to periodontal diseases, class III
K08.124 Complete loss of teeth due to periodontal diseases, class IV
K08.131 Complete loss of teeth due to caries, class I
K08.132 Complete loss of teeth due to caries, class II
K08.133 Complete loss of teeth due to caries, class III
K08.134 Complete loss of teeth due to caries, class IV
K08.191 Complete loss of teeth due to other specified cause, class I
K08.192 Complete loss of teeth due to other specified cause, class II
K08.193 Complete loss of teeth due to other specified cause, class III
K08.194 Complete loss of teeth due to other specified cause, class IV
K08.21 Minimal atrophy of the mandible
K08.22 Moderate atrophy of the mandible
K08.23 Severe atrophy of the mandible
K08.24 Minimal atrophy of maxilla
K08.25 Moderate atrophy of the maxilla
K08.26 Severe atrophy of the maxilla
K08.3 Retained dental root
K08.411 Partial loss of teeth due to trauma, class I
K08.412 Partial loss of teeth due to trauma, class II
K08.413 Partial loss of teeth due to trauma, class III
K08.414 Partial loss of teeth due to trauma, class IV
K08.421 Partial loss of teeth due to periodontal diseases, class I
K08.422 Partial loss of teeth due to periodontal diseases, class II
K08.423 Partial loss of teeth due to periodontal diseases, class III
K08.424 Partial loss of teeth due to periodontal diseases, class IV
K08.431 Partial loss of teeth due to caries, class I
K08.432 Partial loss of teeth due to caries, class II
K08.433 Partial loss of teeth due to caries, class III
K08.434 Partial loss of teeth due to caries, class IV
K08.491 Partial loss of teeth due to other specified cause, class I
K08.492 Partial loss of teeth due to other specified cause, class II
K08.493 Partial loss of teeth due to other specified cause, class III
K08.494 Partial loss of teeth due to other specified cause, class IV
K08.51 Open restoration margins of tooth
K08.52 Unrepairable overhanging of dental restorative materials
K08.530 Fractured dental restorative material without loss of material
K08.531 Fractured dental restorative material with loss of material
K08.54 Contour of existing restoration of tooth biologically incompatible with oral health
K08.55 Allergy to existing dental restorative material
K08.56 Poor aesthetic of existing restoration of tooth
K09.0 Developmental odontogenic cysts
K09.1 Developmental (nonodontogenic) cysts of oral region
K09.8 Other cysts of oral region, not elsewhere classified
K11.0 Atrophy of salivary gland
K11.1 Hypertrophy of salivary gland
K11.21 Acute sialoadenitis
K11.22 Acute recurrent sialoadenitis
K11.23 Chronic sialoadenitis
K11.3 Abscess of salivary gland
K11.4 Fistula of salivary gland
K11.5 Sialolithiasis
K11.6 Mucocele of salivary gland
K11.7 Disturbances of salivary secretion
K11.8 Other diseases of salivary glands
K12.0 Recurrent oral aphthae
K12.1 Other forms of stomatitis
K12.2 Cellulitis and abscess of mouth
K12.31 Oral mucositis (ulcerative) due to antineoplastic therapy
K12.32 Oral mucositis (ulcerative) due to other drugs
K12.33 Oral mucositis (ulcerative) due to radiation
K12.39 Other oral mucositis (ulcerative)
K13.0 Diseases of lips
K13.1 Cheek and lip biting
K13.21 Leukoplakia of oral mucosa, including tongue
K13.22 Minimal keratinized residual ridge mucosa
K13.23 Excessive keratinized residual ridge mucosa
K13.24 Leukokeratosis nicotina palati
K13.29 Other disturbances of oral epithelium, including tongue
K13.3 Hairy leukoplakia
K13.4 Granuloma and granuloma-like lesions of oral mucosa
K13.5 Oral submucous fibrosis
K13.6 Irritative hyperplasia of oral mucosa
K13.79 Other lesions of oral mucosa
K14.0 Glossitis
K14.1 Geographic tongue
K14.2 Median rhomboid glossitis
K14.3 Hypertrophy of tongue papillae
K14.4 Atrophy of tongue papillae
K14.5 Plicated tongue
K14.6 Glossodynia
K14.8 Other diseases of tongue

## Relative Value Units/Medicare Edits

| Non-Facility RVU | Work | PE | MP | Total |
|---|---|---|---|---|
| D0120 | 0.31 | 0.17 | 0.02 | 0.50 |
| **Facility RVU** | **Work** | **PE** | **MP** | **Total** |
| D0120 | 0.31 | 0.17 | 0.02 | 0.50 |

| | FUD | Status | MUE | Modifiers | | | | IOM Reference |
|---|---|---|---|---|---|---|---|---|
| D0120 | N/A | N | - | N/A | N/A | N/A | N/A | 100-01,5,70.2 |

* with documentation

## Terms To Know

**evaluation.** Dynamic process in which the dentist makes clinical judgments based on data gathered during the examination.

# D0140-D0145

**D0140** limited oral evaluation - problem focused

*An evaluation limited to a specific oral health problem or complaint. This may require interpretation of information acquired through additional diagnostic procedures. Report additional diagnostic procedures separately. Definitive procedures may be required on the same date as the evaluation. Typically, patients receiving this type of evaluation present with a specific problem and/or dental emergencies, trauma, acute infections, etc.*

**D0145** oral evaluation for a patient under three years of age and counseling with primary caregiver

*Diagnostic services performed for a child under the age of three, preferably within the first six months of the eruption of the first primary tooth, including recording the oral and physical health history, evaluation of caries susceptibility, development of an appropriate preventive oral health regimen and communication with and counseling of the child's parent, legal guardian and/or primary caregiver.*

## Explanation

The limited evaluation is problem focused on a particular dental health problem or concern presented by the patient. It includes the interpretation of information acquired through additional, separately-reportable, diagnostic oral health tests. It may lead to the decision that other definitive procedures are also required. Report D0145 when patient is younger than three years and primary caregiver is counseled.

## Coding Tips

Code D0140 reports a type of evaluation typically provided if the patient presents with trauma, acute infection, other oral care emergency, or when the patient has been referred for a specific problem. Report code D0160 when a detailed and extensive oral evaluation is provided. When a comprehensive examination is performed, see D0150. When the provider performs a caries risk assessment using a standardized risk assessment tool, see D0601-D0603. Any radiograph, prophylaxis, fluoride, restorative, or extraction service is reported separately.

## Documentation Tips

Documentation supporting an evaluation must indicate if the evaluation was complete, periodic, or limited. Documentation for code D0145 should include oral and physical health history, evaluation of caries susceptibility, and development of appropriate oral health regimen including discussion of said regimen with a caregiver. Because of the level of care required by children under the age of 3, code D0145 may be reported for re-evaluations if all of the above components are performed and documented. Treatment plan documentation should reflect any treatment failure or change in diagnosis and/or a change in treatment plan. There should also be evidence of any initiation or reinstatement of a drug regime, which requires close and continuous skilled medical observation. Dentists should be certain that sufficient documentation is provided in the dental records to accurately verify and describe the services rendered. Additionally, records should be legible and signed with the appropriate name and title of the provider of the service. The following information can be documented on a tooth chart: treatment/location of caries, endodontic procedures, prosthetic services, preventive services, treatment of lesions and dental disease, or other special procedures. A tooth chart may also be used to identify structure and rationale of disease process and the type of service performed on intraoral structures other than teeth.

## Reimbursement Tips

When an oral health assessment is performed by someone other than the dentist for example, a licensed dental hygienist, some third-party payers may require that modifier DA Oral health assessment by a licensed health professional other than a dentist, be appended to codes D0140 and D0145. Check with third-party payers for their specific requirements.

## ICD-10-CM Diagnostic Codes

| | |
|---|---|
| K00.0 | Anodontia |
| K00.1 | Supernumerary teeth |
| K00.2 | Abnormalities of size and form of teeth |
| K00.3 | Mottled teeth |
| K00.4 | Disturbances in tooth formation |
| K00.5 | Hereditary disturbances in tooth structure, not elsewhere classified |
| K00.6 | Disturbances in tooth eruption |
| K00.7 | Teething syndrome |
| K01.0 | Embedded teeth |
| K01.1 | Impacted teeth |
| K02.3 | Arrested dental caries |
| K02.51 | Dental caries on pit and fissure surface limited to enamel |
| K02.52 | Dental caries on pit and fissure surface penetrating into dentin |
| K02.53 | Dental caries on pit and fissure surface penetrating into pulp |
| K02.61 | Dental caries on smooth surface limited to enamel |
| K02.62 | Dental caries on smooth surface penetrating into dentin |
| K02.63 | Dental caries on smooth surface penetrating into pulp |
| K02.7 | Dental root caries |
| K03.0 | Excessive attrition of teeth |
| K03.1 | Abrasion of teeth |
| K03.2 | Erosion of teeth |
| K03.3 | Pathological resorption of teeth |
| K03.4 | Hypercementosis |
| K03.5 | Ankylosis of teeth |
| K03.6 | Deposits [accretions] on teeth |
| K03.7 | Posteruptive color changes of dental hard tissues |
| K03.81 | Cracked tooth |
| K04.01 | Reversible pulpitis |
| K04.02 | Irreversible pulpitis |
| K04.1 | Necrosis of pulp |
| K04.2 | Pulp degeneration |
| K04.3 | Abnormal hard tissue formation in pulp |
| K04.4 | Acute apical periodontitis of pulpal origin |
| K04.5 | Chronic apical periodontitis |
| K04.6 | Periapical abscess with sinus |
| K04.7 | Periapical abscess without sinus |
| K04.8 | Radicular cyst |
| K05.00 | Acute gingivitis, plaque induced |
| K05.01 | Acute gingivitis, non-plaque induced |
| K05.10 | Chronic gingivitis, plaque induced |
| K05.11 | Chronic gingivitis, non-plaque induced |
| K05.211 | Aggressive periodontitis, localized, slight |
| K05.212 | Aggressive periodontitis, localized, moderate |
| K05.213 | Aggressive periodontitis, localized, severe |
| K05.221 | Aggressive periodontitis, generalized, slight |
| K05.222 | Aggressive periodontitis, generalized, moderate |
| K05.223 | Aggressive periodontitis, generalized, severe |
| K05.311 | Chronic periodontitis, localized, slight |

| | |
|---|---|
| K05.312 | Chronic periodontitis, localized, moderate |
| K05.313 | Chronic periodontitis, localized, severe |
| K05.321 | Chronic periodontitis, generalized, slight |
| K05.322 | Chronic periodontitis, generalized, moderate |
| K05.323 | Chronic periodontitis, generalized, severe |
| K05.4 | Periodontosis |
| K06.011 | Localized gingival recession, minimal |
| K06.012 | Localized gingival recession, moderate |
| K06.013 | Localized gingival recession, severe |
| K06.021 | Generalized gingival recession, minimal |
| K06.022 | Generalized gingival recession, moderate |
| K06.023 | Generalized gingival recession, severe |
| K06.1 | Gingival enlargement |
| K06.2 | Gingival and edentulous alveolar ridge lesions associated with trauma |
| K08.111 | Complete loss of teeth due to trauma, class I |
| K08.112 | Complete loss of teeth due to trauma, class II |
| K08.113 | Complete loss of teeth due to trauma, class III |
| K08.114 | Complete loss of teeth due to trauma, class IV |
| K08.121 | Complete loss of teeth due to periodontal diseases, class I |
| K08.122 | Complete loss of teeth due to periodontal diseases, class II |
| K08.123 | Complete loss of teeth due to periodontal diseases, class III |
| K08.124 | Complete loss of teeth due to periodontal diseases, class IV |
| K08.131 | Complete loss of teeth due to caries, class I |
| K08.132 | Complete loss of teeth due to caries, class II |
| K08.133 | Complete loss of teeth due to caries, class III |
| K08.134 | Complete loss of teeth due to caries, class IV |
| K08.21 | Minimal atrophy of the mandible |
| K08.22 | Moderate atrophy of the mandible |
| K08.23 | Severe atrophy of the mandible |
| K08.24 | Minimal atrophy of maxilla |
| K08.25 | Moderate atrophy of the maxilla |
| K08.26 | Severe atrophy of the maxilla |
| K08.411 | Partial loss of teeth due to trauma, class I |
| K08.412 | Partial loss of teeth due to trauma, class II |
| K08.413 | Partial loss of teeth due to trauma, class III |
| K08.414 | Partial loss of teeth due to trauma, class IV |
| K08.421 | Partial loss of teeth due to periodontal diseases, class I |
| K08.422 | Partial loss of teeth due to periodontal diseases, class II |
| K08.423 | Partial loss of teeth due to periodontal diseases, class III |
| K08.424 | Partial loss of teeth due to periodontal diseases, class IV |
| K08.431 | Partial loss of teeth due to caries, class I |
| K08.432 | Partial loss of teeth due to caries, class II |
| K08.433 | Partial loss of teeth due to caries, class III |
| K08.434 | Partial loss of teeth due to caries, class IV |
| K08.491 | Partial loss of teeth due to other specified cause, class I |
| K08.492 | Partial loss of teeth due to other specified cause, class II |
| K08.493 | Partial loss of teeth due to other specified cause, class III |
| K08.494 | Partial loss of teeth due to other specified cause, class IV |
| K08.51 | Open restoration margins of tooth |
| K08.52 | Unrepairable overhanging of dental restorative materials |
| K08.530 | Fractured dental restorative material without loss of material |
| K08.531 | Fractured dental restorative material with loss of material |
| K08.54 | Contour of existing restoration of tooth biologically incompatible with oral health |
| K08.55 | Allergy to existing dental restorative material |
| K08.56 | Poor aesthetic of existing restoration of tooth |
| K08.81 | Primary occlusal trauma |
| K08.82 | Secondary occlusal trauma |
| K09.0 | Developmental odontogenic cysts |
| K09.1 | Developmental (nonodontogenic) cysts of oral region |
| K11.0 | Atrophy of salivary gland |
| K11.1 | Hypertrophy of salivary gland |
| K11.21 | Acute sialoadenitis |
| K11.22 | Acute recurrent sialoadenitis |
| K11.23 | Chronic sialoadenitis |
| K11.3 | Abscess of salivary gland |
| K11.4 | Fistula of salivary gland |
| K11.5 | Sialolithiasis |
| K11.6 | Mucocele of salivary gland |
| K11.7 | Disturbances of salivary secretion |
| K12.0 | Recurrent oral aphthae |
| K12.2 | Cellulitis and abscess of mouth |
| K12.31 | Oral mucositis (ulcerative) due to antineoplastic therapy |
| K12.32 | Oral mucositis (ulcerative) due to other drugs |
| K12.33 | Oral mucositis (ulcerative) due to radiation |
| K13.21 | Leukoplakia of oral mucosa, including tongue |
| K13.22 | Minimal keratinized residual ridge mucosa |
| K13.23 | Excessive keratinized residual ridge mucosa |
| K13.24 | Leukokeratosis nicotina palati |
| K13.3 | Hairy leukoplakia |
| K13.4 | Granuloma and granuloma-like lesions of oral mucosa |
| K13.5 | Oral submucous fibrosis |
| K13.6 | Irritative hyperplasia of oral mucosa |
| K14.0 | Glossitis |
| K14.1 | Geographic tongue |
| K14.2 | Median rhomboid glossitis |
| K14.3 | Hypertrophy of tongue papillae |
| K14.4 | Atrophy of tongue papillae |
| K14.5 | Plicated tongue |
| K14.6 | Glossodynia |

## Relative Value Units/Medicare Edits

| Non-Facility RVU | Work | PE | MP | Total |
|---|---|---|---|---|
| **D0140** | 0.50 | 0.27 | 0.04 | 0.81 |
| **D0145** | 0.48 | 0.26 | 0.03 | 0.77 |
| **Facility RVU** | **Work** | **PE** | **MP** | **Total** |
| **D0140** | 0.50 | 0.27 | 0.04 | 0.81 |
| **D0145** | 0.48 | 0.26 | 0.03 | 0.77 |

| | FUD | Status | MUE | Modifiers | | | | IOM Reference |
|---|---|---|---|---|---|---|---|---|
| **D0140** | N/A | N | - | N/A | N/A | N/A | N/A | 100-03,260.6 |
| **D0145** | N/A | N | - | N/A | N/A | N/A | N/A | |

* with documentation

# D0150

**D0150** comprehensive oral evaluation - new or established patient

*Used by a general dentist and/or a specialist when evaluating a patient comprehensively. This applies to new patients; established patients who have had a significant change in health conditions or other unusual circumstances, by report, or established patients who have been absent from active treatment for three or more years. It is a thorough evaluation and recording of the extraoral and intraoral hard and soft tissues. It may require interpretation of information acquired through additional diagnostic procedures. Additional diagnostic procedures should be reported separately. This includes an evaluation for oral cancer, the evaluation and recording of the patient's dental and medical history and a general health assessment. It may include the evaluation and recording of dental caries, missing or unerupted teeth, restorations, existing prostheses, occlusal relationships, periodontal conditions (including periodontal screening and/or charting), hard and soft tissue anomalies, etc.*

## Explanation

A comprehensive oral evaluation is performed on a new or established patient who has had a significant change in health or has not been seen for active treatment in three or more years, including a thorough intra- and extra-oral examination of all hard and soft tissues with evaluation and recording of findings. A comprehensive oral evaluation includes the patient's dental and medical history, typically recording things such as anomalies, caries, missing or unerupted teeth, restorations, occlusal relationships, evaluation for oral cancer, and periodontal evaluation.

## Coding Tips

This service may require interpretation of information acquired by other diagnostic procedures that may be reported separately. To report a periodic evaluation, see code D0120. A detailed and extensive evaluation that is problem focused is reported using code D0160. When the provider performs a caries risk assessment using a standardized risk assessment tool, see D0601-D0603. When the patient is referred by another dentist for an opinion and/or advice regarding a particular condition, see code D9310. Any radiograph, prophylaxis, fluoride, restorative, or extraction service is reported separately. This procedure is a Medicare-covered service if its purpose is to identify a patient's existing infections prior to kidney transplantation.

## Documentation Tips

Documentation supporting an evaluation must indicate if the evaluation was complete, periodic, or limited. Any diagnostic studies performed elsewhere but reviewed should be recorded in the documentation. If the patient is established, the time interval between encounters should be recorded as well. Treatment plan documentation should reflect any treatment failure or change in diagnosis and/or a change in treatment plan. There should also be evidence of any initiation or reinstatement of a drug regime, which requires close and continuous skilled medical observation. Dentists should be certain that sufficient documentation is provided in the dental records to accurately verify and describe the services rendered. Additionally, records should be legible and signed with the appropriate name and title of the provider of the service. The following information can be documented on a tooth chart: treatment/location of caries, endodontic procedures, prosthetic services, preventive services, treatment of lesions and dental disease, or other special procedures.A tooth chart may also be used to identify structure and rationale of disease process and the type of service performed on intraoral structures other than teeth.

## Reimbursement Tips

Coverage of this procedure varies by payer and there may be frequency limitations.

## ICD-10-CM Diagnostic Codes

|  |  |
|---|---|
| K00.0 | Anodontia |
| K00.1 | Supernumerary teeth |
| K00.2 | Abnormalities of size and form of teeth |
| K00.3 | Mottled teeth |
| K00.4 | Disturbances in tooth formation |
| K00.5 | Hereditary disturbances in tooth structure, not elsewhere classified |
| K00.6 | Disturbances in tooth eruption |
| K00.7 | Teething syndrome |
| K01.0 | Embedded teeth |
| K01.1 | Impacted teeth |
| K02.3 | Arrested dental caries |
| K02.51 | Dental caries on pit and fissure surface limited to enamel |
| K02.52 | Dental caries on pit and fissure surface penetrating into dentin |
| K02.53 | Dental caries on pit and fissure surface penetrating into pulp |
| K02.61 | Dental caries on smooth surface limited to enamel |
| K02.62 | Dental caries on smooth surface penetrating into dentin |
| K02.63 | Dental caries on smooth surface penetrating into pulp |
| K02.7 | Dental root caries |
| K03.0 | Excessive attrition of teeth |
| K03.1 | Abrasion of teeth |
| K03.2 | Erosion of teeth |
| K03.3 | Pathological resorption of teeth |
| K03.4 | Hypercementosis |
| K03.5 | Ankylosis of teeth |
| K03.6 | Deposits [accretions] on teeth |
| K03.7 | Posteruptive color changes of dental hard tissues |
| K03.81 | Cracked tooth |
| K04.01 | Reversible pulpitis |
| K04.02 | Irreversible pulpitis |
| K04.1 | Necrosis of pulp |
| K04.2 | Pulp degeneration |
| K04.3 | Abnormal hard tissue formation in pulp |
| K04.4 | Acute apical periodontitis of pulpal origin |
| K04.5 | Chronic apical periodontitis |
| K04.6 | Periapical abscess with sinus |
| K04.7 | Periapical abscess without sinus |
| K04.8 | Radicular cyst |
| K05.00 | Acute gingivitis, plaque induced |
| K05.01 | Acute gingivitis, non-plaque induced |
| K05.10 | Chronic gingivitis, plaque induced |
| K05.11 | Chronic gingivitis, non-plaque induced |
| K05.211 | Aggressive periodontitis, localized, slight |
| K05.212 | Aggressive periodontitis, localized, moderate |
| K05.213 | Aggressive periodontitis, localized, severe |
| K05.221 | Aggressive periodontitis, generalized, slight |
| K05.222 | Aggressive periodontitis, generalized, moderate |
| K05.223 | Aggressive periodontitis, generalized, severe |
| K05.311 | Chronic periodontitis, localized, slight |
| K05.312 | Chronic periodontitis, localized, moderate |
| K05.313 | Chronic periodontitis, localized, severe |
| K05.321 | Chronic periodontitis, generalized, slight |

K05.322 Chronic periodontitis, generalized, moderate
K05.323 Chronic periodontitis, generalized, severe
K05.4 Periodontosis
K06.011 Localized gingival recession, minimal
K06.012 Localized gingival recession, moderate
K06.013 Localized gingival recession, severe
K06.021 Generalized gingival recession, minimal
K06.022 Generalized gingival recession, moderate
K06.023 Generalized gingival recession, severe
K06.1 Gingival enlargement
K06.2 Gingival and edentulous alveolar ridge lesions associated with trauma
K08.0 Exfoliation of teeth due to systemic causes
K08.111 Complete loss of teeth due to trauma, class I
K08.112 Complete loss of teeth due to trauma, class II
K08.113 Complete loss of teeth due to trauma, class III
K08.114 Complete loss of teeth due to trauma, class IV
K08.121 Complete loss of teeth due to periodontal diseases, class I
K08.122 Complete loss of teeth due to periodontal diseases, class II
K08.123 Complete loss of teeth due to periodontal diseases, class III
K08.124 Complete loss of teeth due to periodontal diseases, class IV
K08.131 Complete loss of teeth due to caries, class I
K08.132 Complete loss of teeth due to caries, class II
K08.133 Complete loss of teeth due to caries, class III
K08.134 Complete loss of teeth due to caries, class IV
K08.21 Minimal atrophy of the mandible
K08.22 Moderate atrophy of the mandible
K08.23 Severe atrophy of the mandible
K08.24 Minimal atrophy of maxilla
K08.25 Moderate atrophy of the maxilla
K08.26 Severe atrophy of the maxilla
K08.3 Retained dental root
K08.411 Partial loss of teeth due to trauma, class I
K08.412 Partial loss of teeth due to trauma, class II
K08.413 Partial loss of teeth due to trauma, class III
K08.414 Partial loss of teeth due to trauma, class IV
K08.421 Partial loss of teeth due to periodontal diseases, class I
K08.422 Partial loss of teeth due to periodontal diseases, class II
K08.423 Partial loss of teeth due to periodontal diseases, class III
K08.424 Partial loss of teeth due to periodontal diseases, class IV
K08.431 Partial loss of teeth due to caries, class I
K08.432 Partial loss of teeth due to caries, class II
K08.433 Partial loss of teeth due to caries, class III
K08.434 Partial loss of teeth due to caries, class IV
K08.491 Partial loss of teeth due to other specified cause, class I
K08.492 Partial loss of teeth due to other specified cause, class II
K08.493 Partial loss of teeth due to other specified cause, class III
K08.494 Partial loss of teeth due to other specified cause, class IV
K08.51 Open restoration margins of tooth
K08.52 Unrepairable overhanging of dental restorative materials
K08.530 Fractured dental restorative material without loss of material
K08.531 Fractured dental restorative material with loss of material
K08.54 Contour of existing restoration of tooth biologically incompatible with oral health
K08.55 Allergy to existing dental restorative material
K08.56 Poor aesthetic of existing restoration of tooth
K08.81 Primary occlusal trauma
K08.82 Secondary occlusal trauma
K09.0 Developmental odontogenic cysts
K09.1 Developmental (nonodontogenic) cysts of oral region
K11.0 Atrophy of salivary gland
K11.1 Hypertrophy of salivary gland
K11.21 Acute sialoadenitis
K11.22 Acute recurrent sialoadenitis
K11.23 Chronic sialoadenitis
K11.3 Abscess of salivary gland
K11.4 Fistula of salivary gland
K11.5 Sialolithiasis
K11.6 Mucocele of salivary gland
K11.7 Disturbances of salivary secretion
K12.0 Recurrent oral aphthae
K12.1 Other forms of stomatitis
K12.2 Cellulitis and abscess of mouth
K12.31 Oral mucositis (ulcerative) due to antineoplastic therapy
K12.32 Oral mucositis (ulcerative) due to other drugs
K12.33 Oral mucositis (ulcerative) due to radiation
K12.39 Other oral mucositis (ulcerative)
K13.0 Diseases of lips
K13.1 Cheek and lip biting
K13.21 Leukoplakia of oral mucosa, including tongue
K13.22 Minimal keratinized residual ridge mucosa
K13.23 Excessive keratinized residual ridge mucosa
K13.24 Leukokeratosis nicotina palati
K13.29 Other disturbances of oral epithelium, including tongue
K13.3 Hairy leukoplakia
K13.4 Granuloma and granuloma-like lesions of oral mucosa
K13.5 Oral submucous fibrosis
K13.6 Irritative hyperplasia of oral mucosa
K14.0 Glossitis
K14.1 Geographic tongue
K14.2 Median rhomboid glossitis
K14.3 Hypertrophy of tongue papillae
K14.4 Atrophy of tongue papillae
K14.5 Plicated tongue
K14.6 Glossodynia

## Relative Value Units/Medicare Edits

| Non-Facility RVU | Work | PE | MP | Total |
|---|---|---|---|---|
| **D0150** | 0.53 | 0.28 | 0.04 | 0.85 |
| **Facility RVU** | **Work** | **PE** | **MP** | **Total** |
| **D0150** | 0.53 | 0.28 | 0.04 | 0.85 |

| | FUD | Status | MUE | Modifiers | | | | IOM Reference |
|---|---|---|---|---|---|---|---|---|
| **D0150** | N/A | R | - | N/A | N/A | N/A | 80* | 100-02,1,70; 100-03,260.6; 100-04,4,20.5 |

* with documentation

# D0160

**D0160** detailed and extensive oral evaluation - problem focused, by report

*A detailed and extensive problem focused evaluation entails extensive diagnostic and cognitive modalities based on the findings of a comprehensive oral evaluation. Integration of more extensive diagnostic modalities to develop a treatment plan for a specific problem is required. The condition requiring this type of evaluation should be described and documented. Examples of conditions requiring this type of evaluation may include dentofacial anomalies, complicated perio-prosthetic conditions, complex temporomandibular dysfunction, facial pain of unknown origin, conditions requiring multi-disciplinary consultation, etc.*

## Explanation

The detailed, extensive oral evaluation focuses on a specific problem with extensive diagnostic and cognitive skills being used, based on the findings of a comprehensive oral exam. Developing a treatment plan through integrating more extensive diagnostic faculties for the specific problem is a requirement. Thorough documentation of the condition requiring this service should be made. Examples of such conditions may include acute peri-prosthetic complications, temporomandibular joint (TMJ) dysfunction, and pain of unknown origin.

## Coding Tips

When a comprehensive examination is performed and documented, see code D0150. When the patient is referred by another dentist for an opinion or advice regarding a particular condition, see code D9310. When a comprehensive periodontal evaluation is performed, report D0180. When the provider performs a caries risk assessment using a standardized risk assessment tool, see D0601-D0603. Any radiograph, prophylaxis, fluoride, restorative, or extraction service is reported separately. Pertinent documentation to evaluate medical appropriateness should be included when this code is reported.

## Documentation Tips

The following information can be documented on a tooth chart: treatment/location of caries, endodontic procedures, prosthetic services, preventive services, treatment of lesions and dental disease, or other special procedures. A tooth chart may also be used to identify structure and rationale of disease process and the type of service performed on intraoral structures other than teeth.

## Reimbursement Tips

Coverage of this procedure varies by payer and there may be frequency limitations.

## ICD-10-CM Diagnostic Codes

| | |
|---|---|
| K00.1 | Supernumerary teeth |
| K00.2 | Abnormalities of size and form of teeth |
| K00.3 | Mottled teeth |
| K00.4 | Disturbances in tooth formation |
| K00.5 | Hereditary disturbances in tooth structure, not elsewhere classified |
| K00.6 | Disturbances in tooth eruption |
| K00.7 | Teething syndrome |
| K01.0 | Embedded teeth |
| K01.1 | Impacted teeth |
| K02.3 | Arrested dental caries |
| K02.51 | Dental caries on pit and fissure surface limited to enamel |
| K02.52 | Dental caries on pit and fissure surface penetrating into dentin |
| K02.53 | Dental caries on pit and fissure surface penetrating into pulp |
| K02.61 | Dental caries on smooth surface limited to enamel |
| K02.62 | Dental caries on smooth surface penetrating into dentin |
| K02.63 | Dental caries on smooth surface penetrating into pulp |
| K02.7 | Dental root caries |
| K03.0 | Excessive attrition of teeth |
| K03.1 | Abrasion of teeth |
| K03.2 | Erosion of teeth |
| K03.3 | Pathological resorption of teeth |
| K03.4 | Hypercementosis |
| K03.5 | Ankylosis of teeth |
| K03.6 | Deposits [accretions] on teeth |
| K03.7 | Posteruptive color changes of dental hard tissues |
| K03.81 | Cracked tooth |
| K04.01 | Reversible pulpitis |
| K04.02 | Irreversible pulpitis |
| K04.1 | Necrosis of pulp |
| K04.2 | Pulp degeneration |
| K04.3 | Abnormal hard tissue formation in pulp |
| K04.4 | Acute apical periodontitis of pulpal origin |
| K04.5 | Chronic apical periodontitis |
| K04.6 | Periapical abscess with sinus |
| K04.7 | Periapical abscess without sinus |
| K04.8 | Radicular cyst |
| K05.00 | Acute gingivitis, plaque induced |
| K05.01 | Acute gingivitis, non-plaque induced |
| K05.10 | Chronic gingivitis, plaque induced |
| K05.11 | Chronic gingivitis, non-plaque induced |
| K05.211 | Aggressive periodontitis, localized, slight |
| K05.212 | Aggressive periodontitis, localized, moderate |
| K05.213 | Aggressive periodontitis, localized, severe |
| K05.221 | Aggressive periodontitis, generalized, slight |
| K05.222 | Aggressive periodontitis, generalized, moderate |
| K05.223 | Aggressive periodontitis, generalized, severe |
| K05.311 | Chronic periodontitis, localized, slight |
| K05.312 | Chronic periodontitis, localized, moderate |
| K05.313 | Chronic periodontitis, localized, severe |
| K05.321 | Chronic periodontitis, generalized, slight |
| K05.322 | Chronic periodontitis, generalized, moderate |
| K05.323 | Chronic periodontitis, generalized, severe |
| K05.4 | Periodontosis |
| K05.5 | Other periodontal diseases |
| K06.011 | Localized gingival recession, minimal |
| K06.012 | Localized gingival recession, moderate |
| K06.013 | Localized gingival recession, severe |
| K06.021 | Generalized gingival recession, minimal |
| K06.022 | Generalized gingival recession, moderate |
| K06.023 | Generalized gingival recession, severe |
| K06.1 | Gingival enlargement |
| K06.2 | Gingival and edentulous alveolar ridge lesions associated with trauma |
| K06.8 | Other specified disorders of gingiva and edentulous alveolar ridge |
| K08.0 | Exfoliation of teeth due to systemic causes |
| K08.111 | Complete loss of teeth due to trauma, class I |
| K08.112 | Complete loss of teeth due to trauma, class II |
| K08.113 | Complete loss of teeth due to trauma, class III |
| K08.114 | Complete loss of teeth due to trauma, class IV |

K08.121 Complete loss of teeth due to periodontal diseases, class I
K08.122 Complete loss of teeth due to periodontal diseases, class II
K08.123 Complete loss of teeth due to periodontal diseases, class III
K08.124 Complete loss of teeth due to periodontal diseases, class IV
K08.131 Complete loss of teeth due to caries, class I
K08.132 Complete loss of teeth due to caries, class II
K08.133 Complete loss of teeth due to caries, class III
K08.134 Complete loss of teeth due to caries, class IV
K08.191 Complete loss of teeth due to other specified cause, class I
K08.192 Complete loss of teeth due to other specified cause, class II
K08.193 Complete loss of teeth due to other specified cause, class III
K08.194 Complete loss of teeth due to other specified cause, class IV
K08.199 Complete loss of teeth due to other specified cause, unspecified class
K08.21 Minimal atrophy of the mandible
K08.22 Moderate atrophy of the mandible
K08.23 Severe atrophy of the mandible
K08.24 Minimal atrophy of maxilla
K08.25 Moderate atrophy of the maxilla
K08.26 Severe atrophy of the maxilla
K08.3 Retained dental root
K08.411 Partial loss of teeth due to trauma, class I
K08.412 Partial loss of teeth due to trauma, class II
K08.413 Partial loss of teeth due to trauma, class III
K08.414 Partial loss of teeth due to trauma, class IV
K08.421 Partial loss of teeth due to periodontal diseases, class I
K08.422 Partial loss of teeth due to periodontal diseases, class II
K08.423 Partial loss of teeth due to periodontal diseases, class III
K08.424 Partial loss of teeth due to periodontal diseases, class IV
K08.431 Partial loss of teeth due to caries, class I
K08.432 Partial loss of teeth due to caries, class II
K08.433 Partial loss of teeth due to caries, class III
K08.434 Partial loss of teeth due to caries, class IV
K08.491 Partial loss of teeth due to other specified cause, class I
K08.492 Partial loss of teeth due to other specified cause, class II
K08.493 Partial loss of teeth due to other specified cause, class III
K08.494 Partial loss of teeth due to other specified cause, class IV
K08.51 Open restoration margins of tooth
K08.52 Unrepairable overhanging of dental restorative materials
K08.530 Fractured dental restorative material without loss of material
K08.531 Fractured dental restorative material with loss of material
K08.54 Contour of existing restoration of tooth biologically incompatible with oral health
K08.55 Allergy to existing dental restorative material
K08.56 Poor aesthetic of existing restoration of tooth
K08.59 Other unsatisfactory restoration of tooth
K08.81 Primary occlusal trauma
K08.82 Secondary occlusal trauma
K08.89 Other specified disorders of teeth and supporting structures
K09.0 Developmental odontogenic cysts
K09.1 Developmental (nonodontogenic) cysts of oral region
K09.8 Other cysts of oral region, not elsewhere classified
K11.0 Atrophy of salivary gland
K11.1 Hypertrophy of salivary gland
K11.21 Acute sialoadenitis
K11.22 Acute recurrent sialoadenitis
K11.23 Chronic sialoadenitis
K11.3 Abscess of salivary gland
K11.4 Fistula of salivary gland
K11.5 Sialolithiasis
K11.6 Mucocele of salivary gland
K11.7 Disturbances of salivary secretion
K11.8 Other diseases of salivary glands
K12.0 Recurrent oral aphthae
K12.1 Other forms of stomatitis
K12.2 Cellulitis and abscess of mouth
K12.31 Oral mucositis (ulcerative) due to antineoplastic therapy
K12.32 Oral mucositis (ulcerative) due to other drugs
K12.33 Oral mucositis (ulcerative) due to radiation
K12.39 Other oral mucositis (ulcerative)
K13.0 Diseases of lips
K13.1 Cheek and lip biting
K13.21 Leukoplakia of oral mucosa, including tongue
K13.22 Minimal keratinized residual ridge mucosa
K13.23 Excessive keratinized residual ridge mucosa
K13.24 Leukokeratosis nicotina palati
K13.29 Other disturbances of oral epithelium, including tongue
K13.3 Hairy leukoplakia
K13.4 Granuloma and granuloma-like lesions of oral mucosa
K13.5 Oral submucous fibrosis
K13.6 Irritative hyperplasia of oral mucosa
K14.0 Glossitis
K14.1 Geographic tongue
K14.2 Median rhomboid glossitis
K14.3 Hypertrophy of tongue papillae
K14.4 Atrophy of tongue papillae
K14.5 Plicated tongue
K14.6 Glossodynia
K14.8 Other diseases of tongue

## Relative Value Units/Medicare Edits

| Non-Facility RVU | Work | PE | MP | Total |
|---|---|---|---|---|
| **D0160** | 1.03 | 0.55 | 0.07 | 1.65 |
| **Facility RVU** | **Work** | **PE** | **MP** | **Total** |
| **D0160** | 1.03 | 0.55 | 0.07 | 1.65 |

| | FUD | Status | MUE | Modifiers | | | | IOM Reference |
|---|---|---|---|---|---|---|---|---|
| **D0160** | N/A | N | - | N/A | N/A | N/A | N/A | 100-03,260.6 |

* with documentation

# D0170

**D0170** re-evaluation - limited, problem focused (established patient; not post-operative visit)

*Assessing the status of a previously existing condition. For example: - a traumatic injury where no treatment was rendered but patient needs follow-up monitoring; - evaluation for undiagnosed continuing pain; - soft tissue lesion requiring follow-up evaluation.*

## Explanation

Re-evaluation of an established patient, not being seen for a post-operative visit, is a limited, problem-focused assessment of the current status of a patient who has already presented with the existing condition, such as ongoing pain that continues undiagnosed, a non-healing soft tissue wound, or traumatic injury that did not receive surgical care.

## Coding Tips

Reevaluations performed postoperatively are reported with D0171. According to the ADA, code D0170 may be reported for a periodontal reevaluation when not monitoring postoperative tissue healing. When the examination is not problem focused, consider D0120 or D0150. To report an initial, limited, problem-focused oral examination, see codes D0140-D0145. When the provider performs a caries risk assessment using a standardized risk assessment tool, see D0601-D0603. Any radiograph, prophylaxis, fluoride, restorative, or extraction service is reported separately.

## Documentation Tips

Documentation supporting an evaluation must indicate if the evaluation was complete, periodic, or limited. Treatment plan documentation should reflect any treatment failure or change in diagnosis and/or a change in treatment plan. There should also be evidence of any initiation or reinstatement of a drug regime, which requires close and continuous skilled medical observation.

## Reimbursement Tips

Third-party payers may not reimburse separately for this service as it may be bundled into the payment for other services previously rendered. Check with the payer for specific guidelines.

## ICD-10-CM Diagnostic Codes

| | |
|---|---|
| K00.0 | Anodontia |
| K00.1 | Supernumerary teeth |
| K00.2 | Abnormalities of size and form of teeth |
| K00.3 | Mottled teeth |
| K00.4 | Disturbances in tooth formation |
| K00.5 | Hereditary disturbances in tooth structure, not elsewhere classified |
| K00.6 | Disturbances in tooth eruption |
| K01.0 | Embedded teeth |
| K01.1 | Impacted teeth |
| K02.51 | Dental caries on pit and fissure surface limited to enamel |
| K02.52 | Dental caries on pit and fissure surface penetrating into dentin |
| K02.53 | Dental caries on pit and fissure surface penetrating into pulp |
| K02.61 | Dental caries on smooth surface limited to enamel |
| K02.62 | Dental caries on smooth surface penetrating into dentin |
| K02.63 | Dental caries on smooth surface penetrating into pulp |
| K02.7 | Dental root caries |
| K03.0 | Excessive attrition of teeth |
| K03.1 | Abrasion of teeth |
| K03.2 | Erosion of teeth |
| K03.3 | Pathological resorption of teeth |
| K03.4 | Hypercementosis |
| K03.5 | Ankylosis of teeth |
| K03.6 | Deposits [accretions] on teeth |
| K03.7 | Posteruptive color changes of dental hard tissues |
| K03.81 | Cracked tooth |
| K04.1 | Necrosis of pulp |
| K04.2 | Pulp degeneration |
| K04.3 | Abnormal hard tissue formation in pulp |
| K04.4 | Acute apical periodontitis of pulpal origin |
| K04.5 | Chronic apical periodontitis |
| K04.6 | Periapical abscess with sinus |
| K04.7 | Periapical abscess without sinus |
| K04.8 | Radicular cyst |
| K05.00 | Acute gingivitis, plaque induced |
| K05.01 | Acute gingivitis, non-plaque induced |
| K05.10 | Chronic gingivitis, plaque induced |
| K05.11 | Chronic gingivitis, non-plaque induced |
| K05.4 | Periodontosis |
| K06.011 | Localized gingival recession, minimal |
| K06.012 | Localized gingival recession, moderate |
| K06.013 | Localized gingival recession, severe |
| K06.020 | Generalized gingival recession, unspecified |
| K06.021 | Generalized gingival recession, minimal |
| K06.022 | Generalized gingival recession, moderate |
| K06.023 | Generalized gingival recession, severe |
| K06.1 | Gingival enlargement |
| K06.2 | Gingival and edentulous alveolar ridge lesions associated with trauma |
| K08.0 | Exfoliation of teeth due to systemic causes |
| K08.111 | Complete loss of teeth due to trauma, class I |
| K08.112 | Complete loss of teeth due to trauma, class II |
| K08.113 | Complete loss of teeth due to trauma, class III |
| K08.114 | Complete loss of teeth due to trauma, class IV |
| K08.121 | Complete loss of teeth due to periodontal diseases, class I |
| K08.122 | Complete loss of teeth due to periodontal diseases, class II |
| K08.123 | Complete loss of teeth due to periodontal diseases, class III |
| K08.124 | Complete loss of teeth due to periodontal diseases, class IV |
| K08.131 | Complete loss of teeth due to caries, class I |
| K08.132 | Complete loss of teeth due to caries, class II |
| K08.133 | Complete loss of teeth due to caries, class III |
| K08.134 | Complete loss of teeth due to caries, class IV |
| K08.21 | Minimal atrophy of the mandible |
| K08.22 | Moderate atrophy of the mandible |
| K08.23 | Severe atrophy of the mandible |
| K08.24 | Minimal atrophy of maxilla |
| K08.25 | Moderate atrophy of the maxilla |
| K08.26 | Severe atrophy of the maxilla |
| K08.3 | Retained dental root |
| K08.411 | Partial loss of teeth due to trauma, class I |
| K08.412 | Partial loss of teeth due to trauma, class II |
| K08.413 | Partial loss of teeth due to trauma, class III |
| K08.414 | Partial loss of teeth due to trauma, class IV |
| K08.421 | Partial loss of teeth due to periodontal diseases, class I |
| K08.422 | Partial loss of teeth due to periodontal diseases, class II |
| K08.423 | Partial loss of teeth due to periodontal diseases, class III |
| K08.424 | Partial loss of teeth due to periodontal diseases, class IV |

| | |
|---|---|
| K08.431 | Partial loss of teeth due to caries, class I |
| K08.432 | Partial loss of teeth due to caries, class II |
| K08.433 | Partial loss of teeth due to caries, class III |
| K08.434 | Partial loss of teeth due to caries, class IV |
| K08.51 | Open restoration margins of tooth |
| K08.52 | Unrepairable overhanging of dental restorative materials |
| K08.530 | Fractured dental restorative material without loss of material |
| K08.531 | Fractured dental restorative material with loss of material |
| K08.54 | Contour of existing restoration of tooth biologically incompatible with oral health |
| K08.55 | Allergy to existing dental restorative material |
| K08.56 | Poor aesthetic of existing restoration of tooth |
| K09.0 | Developmental odontogenic cysts |
| K09.1 | Developmental (nonodontogenic) cysts of oral region |
| K09.8 | Other cysts of oral region, not elsewhere classified |
| K11.0 | Atrophy of salivary gland |
| K11.1 | Hypertrophy of salivary gland |
| K11.21 | Acute sialoadenitis |
| K11.22 | Acute recurrent sialoadenitis |
| K11.23 | Chronic sialoadenitis |
| K11.3 | Abscess of salivary gland |
| K11.4 | Fistula of salivary gland |
| K11.5 | Sialolithiasis |
| K11.6 | Mucocele of salivary gland |
| K11.7 | Disturbances of salivary secretion |
| K11.8 | Other diseases of salivary glands |
| K12.0 | Recurrent oral aphthae |
| K12.2 | Cellulitis and abscess of mouth |
| K12.31 | Oral mucositis (ulcerative) due to antineoplastic therapy |
| K12.32 | Oral mucositis (ulcerative) due to other drugs |
| K12.33 | Oral mucositis (ulcerative) due to radiation |
| K12.39 | Other oral mucositis (ulcerative) |
| K13.0 | Diseases of lips |
| K13.1 | Cheek and lip biting |
| K13.21 | Leukoplakia of oral mucosa, including tongue |
| K13.22 | Minimal keratinized residual ridge mucosa |
| K13.23 | Excessive keratinized residual ridge mucosa |
| K13.24 | Leukokeratosis nicotina palati |
| K13.3 | Hairy leukoplakia |

## Relative Value Units/Medicare Edits

| Non-Facility RVU | Work | PE | MP | Total |
|---|---|---|---|---|
| D0170 | 0.38 | 0.20 | 0.03 | 0.61 |
| **Facility RVU** | **Work** | **PE** | **MP** | **Total** |
| D0170 | 0.38 | 0.20 | 0.03 | 0.61 |

| | FUD | Status | MUE | Modifiers | | | | IOM Reference |
|---|---|---|---|---|---|---|---|---|
| D0170 | N/A | N | - | N/A | N/A | N/A | N/A | None |

* with documentation

# D0171

**D0171** re-evaluation - post-operative office visit

## Explanation

The provider reports this code to indicate a postoperative evaluation following a procedure. During the encounter, the provider examines the patient to determine healing and the lack of complications following the procedure.

## Coding Tips

Reevaluations other than postoperative are reported using D0170. To report routine oral evaluations, see D0120–D0180. Pre-diagnostic screening or assessments are reported using D0190–D0191. Additional services or procedures performed during the encounter should be reported separately.

## Reimbursement Tips

Third-party payers may not reimburse separately for this service but may bundle it into payment for the surgical service. Check with the payer for specific guidelines. When selecting the procedure or service that accurately identifies the service performed, dentists must use the most accurate code. If the CDT code more accurately identifies the service, this should be used rather than the CPT codes.

## Associated CPT Codes

| | |
|---|---|
| 99024 | Postoperative follow-up visit, normally included in the surgical package, to indicate that an evaluation and management service was performed during a postoperative period for a reason(s) related to the original procedure |
| 99211 | Office or other outpatient visit for the evaluation and management of an established patient that may not require the presence of a physician or other qualified health care professional |
| 99212 | Office or other outpatient visit for the evaluation and management of an established patient, which requires a medically appropriate history and/or examination and straightforward medical decision making. When using time for code selection, 10-19 minutes of total time is spent on the date of the encounter. |
| 99213 | Office or other outpatient visit for the evaluation and management of an established patient, which requires a medically appropriate history and/or examination and low level of medical decision making. When using time for code selection, 20-29 minutes of total time is spent on the date of the encounter. |
| 99214 | Office or other outpatient visit for the evaluation and management of an established patient, which requires a medically appropriate history and/or examination and moderate level of medical decision making. When using time for code selection, 30-39 minutes of total time is spent on the date of the encounter. |
| 99215 | Office or other outpatient visit for the evaluation and management of an established patient, which requires a medically appropriate history and/or examination and high level of medical decision making. When using time for code selection, 40-54 minutes of total time is spent on the date of the encounter. |

## ICD-10-CM Diagnostic Codes

| | |
|---|---|
| Z48.89 | Encounter for other specified surgical aftercare |

## Relative Value Units/Medicare Edits

| Non-Facility RVU | Work | PE | MP | Total |
|---|---|---|---|---|
| D0171 | 0.24 | 0.13 | 0.02 | 0.39 |
| **Facility RVU** | **Work** | **PE** | **MP** | **Total** |
| D0171 | 0.24 | 0.13 | 0.02 | 0.39 |

| | FUD | Status | MUE | Modifiers | | | | IOM Reference |
|---|---|---|---|---|---|---|---|---|
| D0171 | N/A | N | - | N/A | N/A | N/A | N/A | None |

* with documentation

## Terms To Know

**encounter.** Direct personal contact between a patient and a physician, or other person who is authorized by state licensure law and, if applicable, by hospital staff bylaws, to order or furnish hospital services for diagnosis or treatment of the patient.

**follow-up.** Visits or treatment following a procedure.

# D0180

Dental - Diagnostic

▲ **D0180** comprehensive periodontal evaluation - new or established patient

*This procedure is indicated for patients showing signs or symptoms of periodontal disease and for patients with risk factors such as smoking or diabetes. It includes evaluation of periodontal conditions, probing and charting, an evaluation for oral cancer, the evaluation and recording of the patient's dental and medical history, and general health assessment. It may include the evaluation and recording of dental caries, missing or unerupted teeth, restorations, and occlusal relationships.*

## Explanation

A comprehensive periodontal evaluation of a new or established patient is meant for patients showing signs and symptoms of periodontal disease, especially those with increased risk factors like tobacco use disorder or diabetes. The evaluation of the periodontal conditions is done with a general health and medical history assessment. Charting of the present condition of oral health may include things like caries, missing teeth, restorations, occlusal relationships, and oral cancer screening.

## Coding Tips

Any radiograph, prophylaxis, fluoride, restorative, or extraction service is reported separately. This code is not limited to use by periodontists. Dentists may report D0180. According to the ADA, code D0170 or D4999 may be used to report periodontal re-examinations. Check with third-party payers for their specific guidelines.

## Documentation Tips

The following information can be documented on a tooth chart: treatment/location of caries, endodontic procedures, prosthetic services, preventive services, treatment of lesions and dental disease, or other special procedures. A tooth chart may also be used to identify structure and rationale of disease process and the type of service performed on intraoral structures other than teeth.

## Reimbursement Tips

Coverage of this procedure varies by payer. Check with the payer for specific coverage guidelines.

## ICD-10-CM Diagnostic Codes

| | |
|---|---|
| K02.63 | Dental caries on smooth surface penetrating into pulp |
| K02.7 | Dental root caries |
| K03.89 | Other specified diseases of hard tissues of teeth |
| K04.01 | Reversible pulpitis |
| K04.02 | Irreversible pulpitis |
| K04.1 | Necrosis of pulp |
| K04.2 | Pulp degeneration |
| K04.3 | Abnormal hard tissue formation in pulp |
| K04.4 | Acute apical periodontitis of pulpal origin |
| K04.5 | Chronic apical periodontitis |
| K04.6 | Periapical abscess with sinus |
| K04.7 | Periapical abscess without sinus |
| K04.8 | Radicular cyst |
| K04.99 | Other diseases of pulp and periapical tissues |
| Z91.841 | Risk for dental caries, low |
| Z91.842 | Risk for dental caries, moderate |
| Z91.843 | Risk for dental caries, high |

## Relative Value Units/Medicare Edits

| Non-Facility RVU | Work | PE | MP | Total |
|---|---|---|---|---|
| D0180 | 0.56 | 0.30 | 0.04 | 0.90 |
| **Facility RVU** | **Work** | **PE** | **MP** | **Total** |
| D0180 | 0.56 | 0.30 | 0.04 | 0.90 |

| | FUD | Status | MUE | Modifiers | | | | IOM Reference |
|---|---|---|---|---|---|---|---|---|
| D0180 | N/A | N | - | N/A | N/A | N/A | N/A | None |

* with documentation

## Terms To Know

**periodontal.** Relating to the tissues that support and surround the teeth.

**periodontitis.** Inflammation of the tissue structures supporting the teeth leading to a loss of connective tissue attachments.

**pulp.** Living connective tissue within the tooth's root canal space that supplies blood vessels and nerves to the tooth.

# D0190-D0191

**D0190** screening of a patient

*A screening, including state or federally mandated screenings, to determine an individual's need to be seen by a dentist for diagnosis.*

**D0191** assessment of a patient

*A limited clinical inspection that is performed to identify possible signs of oral or systemic disease, malformation, or injury, and the potential need for referral for diagnosis and treatment.*

## Explanation

Code D0190 reports a screening, including state or federally mandated screenings to determine an individuals' need to be seen by a dentist of diagnosis. The provider performs a screening examination of the patient to determine if further examination is needed for diagnosis of the patient's dental health. Code D0191 reports a limited clinical inspection that is performed to identify possible signs of oral or systemic disease, malformation, or injury, and the potential need for referral for diagnosis and treatment. The provider performs a limited examination of a patient to determine the presence of oral or systemic dentoalveolar disease is present, or if there is malformation or injury. The objective of the examination is to determine if a referral to another provider is necessary.

## Coding Tips

Radiographs are reported separately. To report a problem-focused examination, see D0140-D0145. To report a detailed and extensive problem-focused oral evaluation, see D0160. A comprehensive examination is reported using D0150. Report D0180 when a comprehensive periodontal evaluation is performed. When the provider performs a caries risk assessment using a standardized risk assessment tool, see D0601-D0603. These codes do not distinguish between an established or new patient. When screening or assessment is performed by someone other than the dentist, for example, a licensed dental hygienist, some third-party payers may require that modifier DA Oral health assessment by a licensed health professional other than a dentist, be appended to these codes. Check with third-party payers for their specific requirements.

## Documentation Tips

The following information can be documented on a tooth chart: treatment/location of caries, endodontic procedures, prosthetic services, preventive services, treatment of lesions and dental disease, or other special procedures. A tooth chart may also be used to identify structure and rationale of disease process and the type of service performed on intraoral structures other than teeth.

## Reimbursement Tips

Coverage of this procedure varies by payer. Check with the payer for specific coverage guidelines.

## ICD-10-CM Diagnostic Codes

| | |
|---|---|
| Z01.20 | Encounter for dental examination and cleaning without abnormal findings |
| Z01.21 | Encounter for dental examination and cleaning with abnormal findings |

## Relative Value Units/Medicare Edits

| Non-Facility RVU | Work | PE | MP | Total |
|---|---|---|---|---|
| **D0190** | 0.24 | 0.13 | 0.02 | 0.39 |
| **D0191** | 0.17 | 0.09 | 0.01 | 0.27 |
| **Facility RVU** | **Work** | **PE** | **MP** | **Total** |
| **D0190** | 0.24 | 0.13 | 0.02 | 0.39 |
| **D0191** | 0.17 | 0.09 | 0.01 | 0.27 |

| | FUD | Status | MUE | Modifiers | | | | IOM Reference |
|---|---|---|---|---|---|---|---|---|
| **D0190** | N/A | N | - | N/A | N/A | N/A | N/A | None |
| **D0191** | N/A | N | - | N/A | N/A | N/A | N/A | |

* with documentation

## Terms To Know

**assessment.** Process of reviewing a patient's health status, including collecting and studying information and data such as test values, signs, and symptoms.

**examination.** Comprehensive visual and tactile screening and specific testing leading to diagnosis or, as appropriate, to a referral to another practitioner.

**screening test.** Exam or study used by a physician to identify abnormalities, regardless of whether the patient exhibits symptoms.

# D0210-D0240

**D0210** intraoral - complete series of radiographic images

*A radiographic survey of the whole mouth, usually consisting of 14-22 periapical and posterior bitewing images intended to display the crowns and roots of all teeth, periapical areas and alveolar bone.*

**D0220** intraoral - periapical first radiographic image

**D0230** intraoral - periapical each additional radiographic image

**D0240** intraoral - occlusal radiographic image



## Explanation

Intraoral x-rays are taken of the mouth to show teeth and/or surrounding bone. Code D0210 reports a complete series of 14–22 periapical and posterior bitewing radiographs that are intended to reveal the crown and root of all teeth, periapical areas as well as alveolar bone structures. Code D0220 is for a single film, periapical image that shows the whole tooth above and below the gum line. Report D0230 for each additional periapical film taken after the initial and D0240 for an occlusal film showing the chewing surfaces of the back teeth.

## Coding Tips

Appropriate code selection is dependent upon the type of film (periapical, occlusal, complete series) and the number of films taken. Report code D0230 for EACH additional periapical film taken. When periapical films are performed at the same time as a panoramic, most payers will bundle these services and reimburse as if a complete intraoral x-ray examination was performed. Code D0210 reports a full mouth series. For panoramic film, see D0330. For extraoral x-rays, see D0250; bitewing films, see D0270–D0277. When reporting digital subtraction of two or more images (of the same modality), report D0394 in addition to the appropriate code for obtaining the image. Any evaluation, prophylaxis, fluoride, restorative, or extraction service is reported separately.

## Reimbursement Tips

Most payers require that each periapical film be reported as a separate line item. For example, if three periapical films are taken, code D0220 would be reported on the first line and code D0230 would be reported on the second and third lines.

## Associated CPT Codes

| | |
|---|---|
| 70300 | Radiologic examination, teeth; single view |
| 70310 | Radiologic examination, teeth; partial examination, less than full mouth |
| 70320 | Radiologic examination, teeth; complete, full mouth |

## ICD-10-CM Diagnostic Codes

| | |
|---|---|
| K00.1 | Supernumerary teeth |
| K00.2 | Abnormalities of size and form of teeth |
| K00.3 | Mottled teeth |
| K00.4 | Disturbances in tooth formation |
| K00.5 | Hereditary disturbances in tooth structure, not elsewhere classified |
| K00.6 | Disturbances in tooth eruption |
| K00.7 | Teething syndrome |
| K00.8 | Other disorders of tooth development |
| K01.0 | Embedded teeth |
| K01.1 | Impacted teeth |
| K02.3 | Arrested dental caries |
| K02.51 | Dental caries on pit and fissure surface limited to enamel |
| K02.52 | Dental caries on pit and fissure surface penetrating into dentin |

Dental - Diagnostic

| | |
|---|---|
| K02.53 | Dental caries on pit and fissure surface penetrating into pulp |
| K02.61 | Dental caries on smooth surface limited to enamel |
| K02.62 | Dental caries on smooth surface penetrating into dentin |
| K02.63 | Dental caries on smooth surface penetrating into pulp |
| K02.7 | Dental root caries |
| K03.0 | Excessive attrition of teeth |
| K03.1 | Abrasion of teeth |
| K03.2 | Erosion of teeth |
| K03.3 | Pathological resorption of teeth |
| K03.4 | Hypercementosis |
| K03.5 | Ankylosis of teeth |
| K03.6 | Deposits [accretions] on teeth |
| K03.7 | Posteruptive color changes of dental hard tissues |
| K03.81 | Cracked tooth |
| K04.01 | Reversible pulpitis |
| K04.02 | Irreversible pulpitis |
| K04.1 | Necrosis of pulp |
| K04.2 | Pulp degeneration |
| K04.3 | Abnormal hard tissue formation in pulp |
| K04.4 | Acute apical periodontitis of pulpal origin |
| K04.5 | Chronic apical periodontitis |
| K04.6 | Periapical abscess with sinus |
| K04.7 | Periapical abscess without sinus |
| K04.8 | Radicular cyst |
| K04.99 | Other diseases of pulp and periapical tissues |
| K05.00 | Acute gingivitis, plaque induced |
| K05.01 | Acute gingivitis, non-plaque induced |
| K05.10 | Chronic gingivitis, plaque induced |
| K05.11 | Chronic gingivitis, non-plaque induced |
| K05.211 | Aggressive periodontitis, localized, slight |
| K05.212 | Aggressive periodontitis, localized, moderate |
| K05.213 | Aggressive periodontitis, localized, severe |
| K05.221 | Aggressive periodontitis, generalized, slight |
| K05.222 | Aggressive periodontitis, generalized, moderate |
| K05.223 | Aggressive periodontitis, generalized, severe |
| K05.311 | Chronic periodontitis, localized, slight |
| K05.312 | Chronic periodontitis, localized, moderate |
| K05.313 | Chronic periodontitis, localized, severe |
| K05.321 | Chronic periodontitis, generalized, slight |
| K05.322 | Chronic periodontitis, generalized, moderate |
| K05.323 | Chronic periodontitis, generalized, severe |
| K05.4 | Periodontosis |
| K05.5 | Other periodontal diseases |
| K06.011 | Localized gingival recession, minimal |
| K06.012 | Localized gingival recession, moderate |
| K06.013 | Localized gingival recession, severe |
| K06.021 | Generalized gingival recession, minimal |
| K06.022 | Generalized gingival recession, moderate |
| K06.023 | Generalized gingival recession, severe |
| K06.1 | Gingival enlargement |
| K06.2 | Gingival and edentulous alveolar ridge lesions associated with trauma |
| K06.8 | Other specified disorders of gingiva and edentulous alveolar ridge |
| K08.0 | Exfoliation of teeth due to systemic causes |
| K08.111 | Complete loss of teeth due to trauma, class I |
| K08.112 | Complete loss of teeth due to trauma, class II |
| K08.113 | Complete loss of teeth due to trauma, class III |
| K08.114 | Complete loss of teeth due to trauma, class IV |
| K08.121 | Complete loss of teeth due to periodontal diseases, class I |
| K08.122 | Complete loss of teeth due to periodontal diseases, class II |
| K08.123 | Complete loss of teeth due to periodontal diseases, class III |
| K08.124 | Complete loss of teeth due to periodontal diseases, class IV |
| K08.131 | Complete loss of teeth due to caries, class I |
| K08.132 | Complete loss of teeth due to caries, class II |
| K08.133 | Complete loss of teeth due to caries, class III |
| K08.134 | Complete loss of teeth due to caries, class IV |
| K08.191 | Complete loss of teeth due to other specified cause, class I |
| K08.192 | Complete loss of teeth due to other specified cause, class II |
| K08.193 | Complete loss of teeth due to other specified cause, class III |
| K08.194 | Complete loss of teeth due to other specified cause, class IV |
| K08.21 | Minimal atrophy of the mandible |
| K08.22 | Moderate atrophy of the mandible |
| K08.23 | Severe atrophy of the mandible |
| K08.24 | Minimal atrophy of maxilla |
| K08.25 | Moderate atrophy of the maxilla |
| K08.26 | Severe atrophy of the maxilla |
| K08.3 | Retained dental root |
| K08.411 | Partial loss of teeth due to trauma, class I |
| K08.412 | Partial loss of teeth due to trauma, class II |
| K08.413 | Partial loss of teeth due to trauma, class III |
| K08.414 | Partial loss of teeth due to trauma, class IV |
| K08.421 | Partial loss of teeth due to periodontal diseases, class I |
| K08.422 | Partial loss of teeth due to periodontal diseases, class II |
| K08.423 | Partial loss of teeth due to periodontal diseases, class III |
| K08.424 | Partial loss of teeth due to periodontal diseases, class IV |
| K08.431 | Partial loss of teeth due to caries, class I |
| K08.432 | Partial loss of teeth due to caries, class II |
| K08.433 | Partial loss of teeth due to caries, class III |
| K08.434 | Partial loss of teeth due to caries, class IV |
| K08.491 | Partial loss of teeth due to other specified cause, class I |
| K08.492 | Partial loss of teeth due to other specified cause, class II |
| K08.493 | Partial loss of teeth due to other specified cause, class III |
| K08.494 | Partial loss of teeth due to other specified cause, class IV |
| K08.51 | Open restoration margins of tooth |
| K08.52 | Unrepairable overhanging of dental restorative materials |
| K08.530 | Fractured dental restorative material without loss of material |
| K08.531 | Fractured dental restorative material with loss of material |
| K08.54 | Contour of existing restoration of tooth biologically incompatible with oral health |
| K08.55 | Allergy to existing dental restorative material |
| K08.56 | Poor aesthetic of existing restoration of tooth |
| K08.81 | Primary occlusal trauma |
| K08.82 | Secondary occlusal trauma |
| K08.89 | Other specified disorders of teeth and supporting structures |
| K09.0 | Developmental odontogenic cysts |
| K09.1 | Developmental (nonodontogenic) cysts of oral region |
| K09.8 | Other cysts of oral region, not elsewhere classified |
| K11.0 | Atrophy of salivary gland |
| K11.1 | Hypertrophy of salivary gland |
| K11.21 | Acute sialoadenitis |
| K11.22 | Acute recurrent sialoadenitis |
| K11.23 | Chronic sialoadenitis |
| K11.3 | Abscess of salivary gland |

| | |
|---|---|
| K11.4 | Fistula of salivary gland |
| K11.5 | Sialolithiasis |
| K11.6 | Mucocele of salivary gland |
| K11.7 | Disturbances of salivary secretion |
| K11.8 | Other diseases of salivary glands |
| K12.0 | Recurrent oral aphthae |
| K12.1 | Other forms of stomatitis |
| K12.2 | Cellulitis and abscess of mouth |
| K12.31 | Oral mucositis (ulcerative) due to antineoplastic therapy |
| K12.32 | Oral mucositis (ulcerative) due to other drugs |
| K12.33 | Oral mucositis (ulcerative) due to radiation |
| K12.39 | Other oral mucositis (ulcerative) |
| K13.0 | Diseases of lips |
| K13.1 | Cheek and lip biting |
| K13.21 | Leukoplakia of oral mucosa, including tongue |
| K13.22 | Minimal keratinized residual ridge mucosa |
| K13.23 | Excessive keratinized residual ridge mucosa |
| K13.24 | Leukokeratosis nicotina palati |
| K13.3 | Hairy leukoplakia |
| K13.4 | Granuloma and granuloma-like lesions of oral mucosa |
| K13.5 | Oral submucous fibrosis |
| K13.6 | Irritative hyperplasia of oral mucosa |
| K13.79 | Other lesions of oral mucosa |
| K14.0 | Glossitis |
| K14.1 | Geographic tongue |
| K14.2 | Median rhomboid glossitis |
| K14.3 | Hypertrophy of tongue papillae |
| K14.4 | Atrophy of tongue papillae |
| K14.5 | Plicated tongue |
| K14.6 | Glossodynia |
| K14.8 | Other diseases of tongue |

## Relative Value Units/Medicare Edits

| Non-Facility RVU | Work | PE | MP | Total |
|---|---|---|---|---|
| **D0210** | 0.30 | 1.15 | 0.02 | 1.47 |
| **D0220** | 0.06 | 0.24 | 0.00 | 0.30 |
| **D0230** | 0.05 | 0.19 | 0.00 | 0.24 |
| **D0240** | 0.09 | 0.35 | 0.01 | 0.45 |
| **Facility RVU** | **Work** | **PE** | **MP** | **Total** |
| **D0210** | 0.30 | 1.15 | 0.02 | 1.47 |
| **D0220** | 0.06 | 0.24 | 0.00 | 0.30 |
| **D0230** | 0.05 | 0.19 | 0.00 | 0.24 |
| **D0240** | 0.09 | 0.35 | 0.01 | 0.45 |

| | FUD | Status | MUE | Modifiers | | | | IOM Reference |
|---|---|---|---|---|---|---|---|---|
| **D0210** | N/A | I | - | N/A | N/A | N/A | N/A | 100-02,1,70; 100-04,4,20.5 |
| **D0220** | N/A | I | - | N/A | N/A | N/A | N/A | |
| **D0230** | N/A | I | - | N/A | N/A | N/A | N/A | |
| **D0240** | N/A | R | - | N/A | N/A | N/A | 80* | |

* with documentation

# D0250

**D0250** extra-oral - 2D projection radiographic image created using a stationary radiation source, and detector

*These images include, but are not limited to: Lateral Skull; Posterior-Anterior Skull; Submentovertex; Waters; Reverse Tomes; Oblique Mandibular Body; Lateral Ramus.*

## Explanation

Images are obtained from outside of the mouth and include but are not limited to the lateral skull, the posterior-anterior (PA) skull, submentovertex (SMV) (basal view), Waters (occipitomental view), reverse tomes, oblique mandibular body or the lateral ramus.

## Coding Tips

To report extra-oral imaging of the posterior teeth, see D0251. For intraoral x-ray images, see codes from range D0210–D0240; for bitewing x-ray images, see D0270–D0277. Panoramic images are reported using D0330. When reporting digital subtraction of two or more images (of the same modality), report D0394 in addition to the appropriate code for obtaining the image. Any evaluation, prophylaxis, fluoride, restorative, or extraction service is reported separately.

## Reimbursement Tips

Most payers require that each extraoral film be reported as a separate line item. For example, if three extraoral films are taken, code D0250 would be reported on the first line, and code D0260 would be reported on the second and third lines.

## Associated CPT Codes

| | |
|---|---|
| 70300 | Radiologic examination, teeth; single view |
| 70310 | Radiologic examination, teeth; partial examination, less than full mouth |
| 70320 | Radiologic examination, teeth; complete, full mouth |

## ICD-10-CM Diagnostic Codes

| | |
|---|---|
| K00.1 | Supernumerary teeth |
| K00.2 | Abnormalities of size and form of teeth |
| K00.3 | Mottled teeth |
| K00.4 | Disturbances in tooth formation |
| K00.5 | Hereditary disturbances in tooth structure, not elsewhere classified |
| K00.6 | Disturbances in tooth eruption |
| K00.7 | Teething syndrome |
| K00.8 | Other disorders of tooth development |
| K00.9 | Disorder of tooth development, unspecified |
| K01.0 | Embedded teeth |
| K01.1 | Impacted teeth |
| K02.3 | Arrested dental caries |
| K02.51 | Dental caries on pit and fissure surface limited to enamel |
| K02.52 | Dental caries on pit and fissure surface penetrating into dentin |
| K02.53 | Dental caries on pit and fissure surface penetrating into pulp |
| K02.61 | Dental caries on smooth surface limited to enamel |
| K02.62 | Dental caries on smooth surface penetrating into dentin |
| K02.63 | Dental caries on smooth surface penetrating into pulp |
| K02.7 | Dental root caries |
| K03.0 | Excessive attrition of teeth |
| K03.1 | Abrasion of teeth |
| K03.2 | Erosion of teeth |

| | |
|---|---|
| K03.3 | Pathological resorption of teeth |
| K03.4 | Hypercementosis |
| K03.5 | Ankylosis of teeth |
| K03.6 | Deposits [accretions] on teeth |
| K03.7 | Posteruptive color changes of dental hard tissues |
| K03.81 | Cracked tooth |
| K03.89 | Other specified diseases of hard tissues of teeth |
| K04.01 | Reversible pulpitis |
| K04.02 | Irreversible pulpitis |
| K04.1 | Necrosis of pulp |
| K04.2 | Pulp degeneration |
| K04.3 | Abnormal hard tissue formation in pulp |
| K04.4 | Acute apical periodontitis of pulpal origin |
| K04.5 | Chronic apical periodontitis |
| K04.6 | Periapical abscess with sinus |
| K04.7 | Periapical abscess without sinus |
| K04.8 | Radicular cyst |
| K04.99 | Other diseases of pulp and periapical tissues |
| K05.00 | Acute gingivitis, plaque induced |
| K05.01 | Acute gingivitis, non-plaque induced |
| K05.10 | Chronic gingivitis, plaque induced |
| K05.11 | Chronic gingivitis, non-plaque induced |
| K05.211 | Aggressive periodontitis, localized, slight |
| K05.212 | Aggressive periodontitis, localized, moderate |
| K05.213 | Aggressive periodontitis, localized, severe |
| K05.221 | Aggressive periodontitis, generalized, slight |
| K05.222 | Aggressive periodontitis, generalized, moderate |
| K05.223 | Aggressive periodontitis, generalized, severe |
| K05.311 | Chronic periodontitis, localized, slight |
| K05.312 | Chronic periodontitis, localized, moderate |
| K05.313 | Chronic periodontitis, localized, severe |
| K05.321 | Chronic periodontitis, generalized, slight |
| K05.322 | Chronic periodontitis, generalized, moderate |
| K05.323 | Chronic periodontitis, generalized, severe |
| K05.4 | Periodontosis |
| K05.5 | Other periodontal diseases |
| K06.011 | Localized gingival recession, minimal |
| K06.012 | Localized gingival recession, moderate |
| K06.013 | Localized gingival recession, severe |
| K06.021 | Generalized gingival recession, minimal |
| K06.022 | Generalized gingival recession, moderate |
| K06.023 | Generalized gingival recession, severe |
| K06.1 | Gingival enlargement |
| K06.2 | Gingival and edentulous alveolar ridge lesions associated with trauma |
| K06.8 | Other specified disorders of gingiva and edentulous alveolar ridge |
| K08.0 | Exfoliation of teeth due to systemic causes |
| K08.111 | Complete loss of teeth due to trauma, class I |
| K08.112 | Complete loss of teeth due to trauma, class II |
| K08.113 | Complete loss of teeth due to trauma, class III |
| K08.114 | Complete loss of teeth due to trauma, class IV |
| K08.121 | Complete loss of teeth due to periodontal diseases, class I |
| K08.122 | Complete loss of teeth due to periodontal diseases, class II |
| K08.123 | Complete loss of teeth due to periodontal diseases, class III |
| K08.124 | Complete loss of teeth due to periodontal diseases, class IV |
| K08.131 | Complete loss of teeth due to caries, class I |
| K08.132 | Complete loss of teeth due to caries, class II |
| K08.133 | Complete loss of teeth due to caries, class III |
| K08.134 | Complete loss of teeth due to caries, class IV |
| K08.191 | Complete loss of teeth due to other specified cause, class I |
| K08.192 | Complete loss of teeth due to other specified cause, class II |
| K08.193 | Complete loss of teeth due to other specified cause, class III |
| K08.194 | Complete loss of teeth due to other specified cause, class IV |
| K08.21 | Minimal atrophy of the mandible |
| K08.22 | Moderate atrophy of the mandible |
| K08.23 | Severe atrophy of the mandible |
| K08.24 | Minimal atrophy of maxilla |
| K08.25 | Moderate atrophy of the maxilla |
| K08.26 | Severe atrophy of the maxilla |
| K08.3 | Retained dental root |
| K08.411 | Partial loss of teeth due to trauma, class I |
| K08.412 | Partial loss of teeth due to trauma, class II |
| K08.413 | Partial loss of teeth due to trauma, class III |
| K08.414 | Partial loss of teeth due to trauma, class IV |
| K08.421 | Partial loss of teeth due to periodontal diseases, class I |
| K08.422 | Partial loss of teeth due to periodontal diseases, class II |
| K08.423 | Partial loss of teeth due to periodontal diseases, class III |
| K08.424 | Partial loss of teeth due to periodontal diseases, class IV |
| K08.431 | Partial loss of teeth due to caries, class I |
| K08.432 | Partial loss of teeth due to caries, class II |
| K08.433 | Partial loss of teeth due to caries, class III |
| K08.434 | Partial loss of teeth due to caries, class IV |
| K08.491 | Partial loss of teeth due to other specified cause, class I |
| K08.492 | Partial loss of teeth due to other specified cause, class II |
| K08.493 | Partial loss of teeth due to other specified cause, class III |
| K08.494 | Partial loss of teeth due to other specified cause, class IV |
| K08.51 | Open restoration margins of tooth |
| K08.52 | Unrepairable overhanging of dental restorative materials |
| K08.530 | Fractured dental restorative material without loss of material |
| K08.531 | Fractured dental restorative material with loss of material |
| K08.539 | Fractured dental restorative material, unspecified |
| K08.54 | Contour of existing restoration of tooth biologically incompatible with oral health |
| K08.55 | Allergy to existing dental restorative material |
| K08.56 | Poor aesthetic of existing restoration of tooth |
| K08.59 | Other unsatisfactory restoration of tooth |
| K08.81 | Primary occlusal trauma |
| K08.82 | Secondary occlusal trauma |
| K08.89 | Other specified disorders of teeth and supporting structures |
| K08.9 | Disorder of teeth and supporting structures, unspecified |
| K09.0 | Developmental odontogenic cysts |
| K09.1 | Developmental (nonodontogenic) cysts of oral region |
| K09.8 | Other cysts of oral region, not elsewhere classified |
| K09.9 | Cyst of oral region, unspecified |
| K11.0 | Atrophy of salivary gland |
| K11.1 | Hypertrophy of salivary gland |
| K11.21 | Acute sialoadenitis |
| K11.22 | Acute recurrent sialoadenitis |
| K11.23 | Chronic sialoadenitis |
| K11.3 | Abscess of salivary gland |
| K11.4 | Fistula of salivary gland |
| K11.5 | Sialolithiasis |
| K11.6 | Mucocele of salivary gland |

| | |
|---|---|
| K11.7 | Disturbances of salivary secretion |
| K11.8 | Other diseases of salivary glands |
| K13.3 | Hairy leukoplakia |
| K13.4 | Granuloma and granuloma-like lesions of oral mucosa |
| K13.5 | Oral submucous fibrosis |
| K13.6 | Irritative hyperplasia of oral mucosa |
| K13.79 | Other lesions of oral mucosa |

## Relative Value Units/Medicare Edits

| Non-Facility RVU | Work | PE | MP | Total |
|---|---|---|---|---|
| D0250 | 0.12 | 0.47 | 0.01 | 0.60 |
| **Facility RVU** | **Work** | **PE** | **MP** | **Total** |
| D0250 | 0.12 | 0.47 | 0.01 | 0.60 |

| | FUD | Status | MUE | Modifiers | | | | IOM Reference |
|---|---|---|---|---|---|---|---|---|
| D0250 | N/A | R | - | N/A | N/A | N/A | 80* | 100-02,1,70; 100-04,4,20.5 |

* with documentation

## Terms To Know

**bitewing x-ray.** Radiograph of the coronal portion of the tooth.

**extraoral.** Outside of the mouth or oral cavity.

**occlusal x-ray.** In dentistry, radiograph taken from inside the mouth with films that are held in place by the contacting teeth in a closed jaw.

**panoramic x-ray.** X-ray that contains views of both the maxilla and mandible on a single extraoral image.

**periapical x-ray.** X-ray of the terminal end of the root of a tooth.

**radiograph.** Image made by an x-ray.

# D0270-D0277

**D0270** bitewing - single radiographic image
**D0272** bitewings - two radiographic images
**D0273** bitewings - three radiographic images
**D0274** bitewings - four radiographic images
**D0277** vertical bitewings - 7 to 8 radiographic images

*This does not constitute a full mouth intraoral radiographic series.*

## Explanation

A bitewing is an x-ray that shows the upper and lower teeth's biting surfaces on the same film for the portion of teeth above the gum line. The vertical bitewing positioning allows an image of up to two molars to be taken, showing part of the periodontal ligaments. The horizontal bitewing positioning allows up to three molars to be viewed with one image. Report D0270 for a single film bitewing, D0272 for two bitewing films, D0273 for three bitewing films, D0274 for four bitewing films, and D0277 for vertical bitewings, seven to eight films.

## Coding Tips

Correct code selection is dependent on the number of films obtained. See D0240 for intraoral occlusal film. Code D0210 reports a full-mouth series. When reporting digital subtraction of two or more images (of the same modality), report D0394 in addition to the appropriate code for obtaining the image. Report D0277 when the service of seven or eight vertical bitewing films does not constitute a full-mouth intraoral radiographic series. Any evaluation, prophylaxis, fluoride, restorative, or extraction service is reported separately.

## Reimbursement Tips

When bitewings are performed at the same time as a panoramic, most payers will bundle these services and reimburse as if a complete intraoral x-ray examination was performed. When selecting the procedure or service that accurately identifies the service performed, dentists must use the most accurate code. If the CDT code more accurately identifies the service, this should be used rather than the CPT codes.

## Associated CPT Codes

| | |
|---|---|
| 70300 | Radiologic examination, teeth; single view |
| 70310 | Radiologic examination, teeth; partial examination, less than full mouth |

## ICD-10-CM Diagnostic Codes

| | |
|---|---|
| K00.0 | Anodontia |
| K00.1 | Supernumerary teeth |
| K00.2 | Abnormalities of size and form of teeth |
| K00.3 | Mottled teeth |
| K00.4 | Disturbances in tooth formation |
| K00.5 | Hereditary disturbances in tooth structure, not elsewhere classified |
| K00.6 | Disturbances in tooth eruption |
| K00.7 | Teething syndrome |
| K00.8 | Other disorders of tooth development |
| K01.0 | Embedded teeth |
| K01.1 | Impacted teeth |
| K02.3 | Arrested dental caries |
| K02.51 | Dental caries on pit and fissure surface limited to enamel |
| K02.52 | Dental caries on pit and fissure surface penetrating into dentin |
| K02.53 | Dental caries on pit and fissure surface penetrating into pulp |
| K02.61 | Dental caries on smooth surface limited to enamel |

| | |
|---|---|
| K02.62 | Dental caries on smooth surface penetrating into dentin |
| K02.63 | Dental caries on smooth surface penetrating into pulp |
| K02.7 | Dental root caries |
| K03.0 | Excessive attrition of teeth |
| K03.1 | Abrasion of teeth |
| K03.2 | Erosion of teeth |
| K03.3 | Pathological resorption of teeth |
| K03.4 | Hypercementosis |
| K03.5 | Ankylosis of teeth |
| K03.6 | Deposits [accretions] on teeth |
| K03.7 | Posteruptive color changes of dental hard tissues |
| K03.81 | Cracked tooth |
| K03.89 | Other specified diseases of hard tissues of teeth |
| K04.01 | Reversible pulpitis |
| K04.02 | Irreversible pulpitis |
| K04.1 | Necrosis of pulp |
| K04.2 | Pulp degeneration |
| K04.3 | Abnormal hard tissue formation in pulp |
| K04.4 | Acute apical periodontitis of pulpal origin |
| K04.5 | Chronic apical periodontitis |
| K04.6 | Periapical abscess with sinus |
| K04.7 | Periapical abscess without sinus |
| K04.8 | Radicular cyst |
| K04.99 | Other diseases of pulp and periapical tissues |
| K05.00 | Acute gingivitis, plaque induced |
| K05.01 | Acute gingivitis, non-plaque induced |
| K05.10 | Chronic gingivitis, plaque induced |
| K05.11 | Chronic gingivitis, non-plaque induced |
| K05.211 | Aggressive periodontitis, localized, slight |
| K05.212 | Aggressive periodontitis, localized, moderate |
| K05.213 | Aggressive periodontitis, localized, severe |
| K05.221 | Aggressive periodontitis, generalized, slight |
| K05.222 | Aggressive periodontitis, generalized, moderate |
| K05.223 | Aggressive periodontitis, generalized, severe |
| K05.311 | Chronic periodontitis, localized, slight |
| K05.312 | Chronic periodontitis, localized, moderate |
| K05.313 | Chronic periodontitis, localized, severe |
| K05.321 | Chronic periodontitis, generalized, slight |
| K05.322 | Chronic periodontitis, generalized, moderate |
| K05.323 | Chronic periodontitis, generalized, severe |
| K05.4 | Periodontosis |
| K05.5 | Other periodontal diseases |
| K06.011 | Localized gingival recession, minimal |
| K06.012 | Localized gingival recession, moderate |
| K06.013 | Localized gingival recession, severe |
| K06.021 | Generalized gingival recession, minimal |
| K06.022 | Generalized gingival recession, moderate |
| K06.023 | Generalized gingival recession, severe |
| K06.1 | Gingival enlargement |
| K06.2 | Gingival and edentulous alveolar ridge lesions associated with trauma |
| K06.8 | Other specified disorders of gingiva and edentulous alveolar ridge |
| K08.0 | Exfoliation of teeth due to systemic causes |
| K08.111 | Complete loss of teeth due to trauma, class I |
| K08.112 | Complete loss of teeth due to trauma, class II |
| K08.113 | Complete loss of teeth due to trauma, class III |
| K08.114 | Complete loss of teeth due to trauma, class IV |
| K08.121 | Complete loss of teeth due to periodontal diseases, class I |
| K08.122 | Complete loss of teeth due to periodontal diseases, class II |
| K08.123 | Complete loss of teeth due to periodontal diseases, class III |
| K08.124 | Complete loss of teeth due to periodontal diseases, class IV |
| K08.131 | Complete loss of teeth due to caries, class I |
| K08.132 | Complete loss of teeth due to caries, class II |
| K08.133 | Complete loss of teeth due to caries, class III |
| K08.134 | Complete loss of teeth due to caries, class IV |
| K08.191 | Complete loss of teeth due to other specified cause, class I |
| K08.192 | Complete loss of teeth due to other specified cause, class II |
| K08.193 | Complete loss of teeth due to other specified cause, class III |
| K08.194 | Complete loss of teeth due to other specified cause, class IV |
| K08.21 | Minimal atrophy of the mandible |
| K08.22 | Moderate atrophy of the mandible |
| K08.23 | Severe atrophy of the mandible |
| K08.24 | Minimal atrophy of maxilla |
| K08.25 | Moderate atrophy of the maxilla |
| K08.26 | Severe atrophy of the maxilla |
| K08.3 | Retained dental root |
| K08.411 | Partial loss of teeth due to trauma, class I |
| K08.412 | Partial loss of teeth due to trauma, class II |
| K08.413 | Partial loss of teeth due to trauma, class III |
| K08.414 | Partial loss of teeth due to trauma, class IV |
| K08.421 | Partial loss of teeth due to periodontal diseases, class I |
| K08.422 | Partial loss of teeth due to periodontal diseases, class II |
| K08.423 | Partial loss of teeth due to periodontal diseases, class III |
| K08.424 | Partial loss of teeth due to periodontal diseases, class IV |
| K08.431 | Partial loss of teeth due to caries, class I |
| K08.432 | Partial loss of teeth due to caries, class II |
| K08.433 | Partial loss of teeth due to caries, class III |
| K08.434 | Partial loss of teeth due to caries, class IV |
| K08.491 | Partial loss of teeth due to other specified cause, class I |
| K08.492 | Partial loss of teeth due to other specified cause, class II |
| K08.493 | Partial loss of teeth due to other specified cause, class III |
| K08.494 | Partial loss of teeth due to other specified cause, class IV |
| K08.51 | Open restoration margins of tooth |
| K08.52 | Unrepairable overhanging of dental restorative materials |
| K08.530 | Fractured dental restorative material without loss of material |
| K08.531 | Fractured dental restorative material with loss of material |
| K08.54 | Contour of existing restoration of tooth biologically incompatible with oral health |
| K08.55 | Allergy to existing dental restorative material |
| K08.56 | Poor aesthetic of existing restoration of tooth |
| K08.81 | Primary occlusal trauma |
| K08.82 | Secondary occlusal trauma |
| K08.89 | Other specified disorders of teeth and supporting structures |
| K09.0 | Developmental odontogenic cysts |
| K09.1 | Developmental (nonodontogenic) cysts of oral region |
| K09.8 | Other cysts of oral region, not elsewhere classified |
| K11.0 | Atrophy of salivary gland |
| K11.1 | Hypertrophy of salivary gland |
| K11.21 | Acute sialoadenitis |
| K11.22 | Acute recurrent sialoadenitis |
| K11.23 | Chronic sialoadenitis |
| K11.3 | Abscess of salivary gland |
| K11.4 | Fistula of salivary gland |

| | |
|---|---|
| K11.5 | Sialolithiasis |
| K11.6 | Mucocele of salivary gland |
| K11.7 | Disturbances of salivary secretion |
| K11.8 | Other diseases of salivary glands |
| K12.0 | Recurrent oral aphthae |
| K12.1 | Other forms of stomatitis |
| K12.2 | Cellulitis and abscess of mouth |
| K12.31 | Oral mucositis (ulcerative) due to antineoplastic therapy |
| K12.32 | Oral mucositis (ulcerative) due to other drugs |
| K12.33 | Oral mucositis (ulcerative) due to radiation |
| K13.0 | Diseases of lips |
| K13.1 | Cheek and lip biting |
| K13.21 | Leukoplakia of oral mucosa, including tongue |
| K13.22 | Minimal keratinized residual ridge mucosa |
| K13.23 | Excessive keratinized residual ridge mucosa |
| K13.24 | Leukokeratosis nicotina palati |
| K13.3 | Hairy leukoplakia |
| K13.4 | Granuloma and granuloma-like lesions of oral mucosa |
| K13.5 | Oral submucous fibrosis |
| K13.6 | Irritative hyperplasia of oral mucosa |
| K13.79 | Other lesions of oral mucosa |

## Relative Value Units/Medicare Edits

| Non-Facility RVU | Work | PE | MP | Total |
|---|---|---|---|---|
| **D0270** | 0.06 | 0.24 | 0.00 | 0.30 |
| **D0272** | 0.09 | 0.36 | 0.01 | 0.46 |
| **D0273** | 0.12 | 0.45 | 0.01 | 0.58 |
| **D0274** | 0.14 | 0.53 | 0.01 | 0.68 |
| **D0277** | 0.20 | 0.76 | 0.01 | 0.97 |
| **Facility RVU** | **Work** | **PE** | **MP** | **Total** |
| **D0270** | 0.06 | 0.24 | 0.00 | 0.30 |
| **D0272** | 0.09 | 0.36 | 0.01 | 0.46 |
| **D0273** | 0.12 | 0.45 | 0.01 | 0.58 |
| **D0274** | 0.14 | 0.53 | 0.01 | 0.68 |
| **D0277** | 0.20 | 0.76 | 0.01 | 0.97 |

| | FUD | Status | MUE | Modifiers | | | | IOM Reference |
|---|---|---|---|---|---|---|---|---|
| **D0270** | N/A | R | - | N/A | N/A | N/A | 80* | 100-02,1,70; 100-04,4,20.5 |
| **D0272** | N/A | R | - | N/A | N/A | N/A | 80* | |
| **D0273** | N/A | N | - | N/A | N/A | N/A | N/A | |
| **D0274** | N/A | R | - | N/A | N/A | N/A | 80* | |
| **D0277** | N/A | R | - | N/A | N/A | N/A | N/A | |

* with documentation

## Terms To Know

**bitewing x-ray.** Radiograph of the coronal portion of the tooth.

**occlusal x-ray.** In dentistry, radiograph taken from inside the mouth with films that are held in place by the contacting teeth in a closed jaw.

**panoramic x-ray.** X-ray that contains views of both the maxilla and mandible on a single extraoral image.

**periapical x-ray.** X-ray of the terminal end of the root of a tooth.

**radiograph.** Image made by an x-ray.

# D0310

**D0310** sialography

## Explanation

A radiographic contrast study is performed to visualize the salivary glands and ducts, typically to demonstrate possible lesions or tumors, salivary fistulae, or to localize calcium deposits within the gland. The radiologist injects the main salivary duct with radiopaque dye (contrast), after which it flows into the duct system and is examined with x-ray fluoroscopy. The projected image is amplified and displayed on a monitor.

## Coding Tips

Any evaluation, prophylaxis, fluoride, restorative, or extraction service is reported separately. To report sialolithotomy, see D7979–D7980.

## Reimbursement Tips

This service may not be covered by the patient's dental insurance. However, coverage may be available through the patient's medical insurance. Check with third-party payers for specific coverage information. Services submitted to the medical coverage will require that the service be reported with the appropriate CPT code on a CMS-1500 claim form.

## Associated CPT Codes

| | |
|---|---|
| 70390 | Sialography, radiological supervision and interpretation |

## Associated HCPCS Codes

| | |
|---|---|
| A4641 | Radiopharmaceutical, diagnostic, not otherwise classified |

## ICD-10-CM Diagnostic Codes

| | |
|---|---|
| C08.0 | Malignant neoplasm of submandibular gland |
| C08.1 | Malignant neoplasm of sublingual gland |
| C79.89 | Secondary malignant neoplasm of other specified sites |
| D00.06 | Carcinoma in situ of floor of mouth |
| D10.39 | Benign neoplasm of other parts of mouth |
| D11.0 | Benign neoplasm of parotid gland |
| D11.7 | Benign neoplasm of other major salivary glands |
| D37.030 | Neoplasm of uncertain behavior of the parotid salivary glands |
| D37.031 | Neoplasm of uncertain behavior of the sublingual salivary glands |
| D37.032 | Neoplasm of uncertain behavior of the submandibular salivary glands |
| K11.0 | Atrophy of salivary gland |
| K11.1 | Hypertrophy of salivary gland |
| K11.21 | Acute sialoadenitis |
| K11.22 | Acute recurrent sialoadenitis |
| K11.23 | Chronic sialoadenitis |
| K11.3 | Abscess of salivary gland |
| K11.4 | Fistula of salivary gland |
| K11.5 | Sialolithiasis |
| K11.6 | Mucocele of salivary gland |
| K11.7 | Disturbances of salivary secretion |
| K11.8 | Other diseases of salivary glands |
| R68.84 | Jaw pain |
| Z01.89 | Encounter for other specified special examinations |

## Relative Value Units/Medicare Edits

| Non-Facility RVU | Work | PE | MP | Total |
|---|---|---|---|---|
| D0310 | 0.82 | 3.21 | 0.06 | 4.09 |
| **Facility RVU** | **Work** | **PE** | **MP** | **Total** |
| D0310 | 0.82 | 3.21 | 0.06 | 4.09 |

| | FUD | Status | MUE | Modifiers | | | | IOM Reference |
|---|---|---|---|---|---|---|---|---|
| D0310 | N/A | I | - | N/A | N/A | N/A | N/A | None |

* with documentation

## Terms To Know

**fistula.** Abnormal tube-like passage between two body cavities or organs or from an organ to the outside surface.

**fluoroscopy.** Radiology technique that allows visual examination of part of the body or a function of an organ using a device that projects an x-ray image on a fluorescent screen.

**lesion.** Area of damaged tissue that has lost continuity or function, due to disease or trauma. Lesions may be located on internal structures such as the brain, nerves, or kidneys, or visible on the skin.

**radiopaque dye.** Medium injected into the body that is impenetrable by x-rays.

**sialography.** Radiographic examination of the ductal system of a salivary gland by instilling radiographic dye into a major duct and taking x-ray pictures.

**tumor.** Pathological swelling or enlargement; a neoplastic growth of uncontrolled, abnormal multiplication of cells.

# D0320-D0321

**D0320** temporomandibular joint arthrogram, including injection

**D0321** other temporomandibular joint radiographic images, by report

## Explanation

A radiographic contrast study, or arthrogram, is performed on the temporomandibular joint (TMJ) in D0320, which includes the injection of contrast material into the joint. A needle is first inserted through the skin and into the superior and/or inferior joint spaces to allow a small catheter to be threaded into the temporomandibular joint. Radiopaque dye is injected through the catheter and x-ray images are taken to study the soft tissue anatomy of the joint, such as the articular disc or ligaments. This allows the physician to see the position of the structures not normally seen on conventional x-ray. When conventional x-ray images are taken for imaging the temporomandibular joint, report D0321.

## Coding Tips

These codes include interpretation.

## Reimbursement Tips

This service may not be covered by the patient's dental insurance. However, coverage may be available through the patient's medical insurance. Check with third-party payers for specific coverage information. Services submitted to the medical coverage will require that the service be reported with the appropriate CPT code on a CMS-1500 claim form.

## Associated CPT Codes

| | |
|---|---|
| 21116 | Injection procedure for temporomandibular joint arthrography |
| 70328 | Radiologic examination, temporomandibular joint, open and closed mouth; unilateral |
| 70330 | Radiologic examination, temporomandibular joint, open and closed mouth; bilateral |
| 70332 | Temporomandibular joint arthrography, radiological supervision and interpretation |

## Associated HCPCS Codes

| | |
|---|---|
| A4641 | Radiopharmaceutical, diagnostic, not otherwise classified |

## ICD-10-CM Diagnostic Codes

| | |
|---|---|
| C41.1 | Malignant neoplasm of mandible |
| D16.4 | Benign neoplasm of bones of skull and face |
| D16.5 | Benign neoplasm of lower jaw bone |
| M26.601 | Right temporomandibular joint disorder, unspecified |
| M26.602 | Left temporomandibular joint disorder, unspecified |
| M26.603 | Bilateral temporomandibular joint disorder, unspecified |
| M26.609 | Unspecified temporomandibular joint disorder, unspecified side |
| M26.611 | Adhesions and ankylosis of right temporomandibular joint ☑ |
| M26.612 | Adhesions and ankylosis of left temporomandibular joint ☑ |
| M26.613 | Adhesions and ankylosis of bilateral temporomandibular joint ☑ |
| M26.619 | Adhesions and ankylosis of temporomandibular joint, unspecified side |
| M26.621 | Arthralgia of right temporomandibular joint ☑ |
| M26.622 | Arthralgia of left temporomandibular joint ☑ |
| M26.623 | Arthralgia of bilateral temporomandibular joint ☑ |
| M26.629 | Arthralgia of temporomandibular joint, unspecified side |
| M26.631 | Articular disc disorder of right temporomandibular joint ☑ |
| M26.632 | Articular disc disorder of left temporomandibular joint ☑ |
| M26.633 | Articular disc disorder of bilateral temporomandibular joint ☑ |

| | |
|---|---|
| M26.639 | Articular disc disorder of temporomandibular joint, unspecified side |
| M26.641 | Arthritis of right temporomandibular joint ☑ |
| M26.642 | Arthritis of left temporomandibular joint ☑ |
| M26.643 | Arthritis of bilateral temporomandibular joint ☑ |
| M26.651 | Arthropathy of right temporomandibular joint ☑ |
| M26.652 | Arthropathy of left temporomandibular joint ☑ |
| M26.653 | Arthropathy of bilateral temporomandibular joint ☑ |
| M26.69 | Other specified disorders of temporomandibular joint |
| M27.2 | Inflammatory conditions of jaws |
| R68.84 | Jaw pain |
| Z01.89 | Encounter for other specified special examinations |

## Relative Value Units/Medicare Edits

| Non-Facility RVU | Work | PE | MP | Total |
|---|---|---|---|---|
| **D0320** | 1.55 | 6.03 | 0.11 | 7.69 |
| **D0321** | 0.34 | 1.33 | 0.02 | 1.69 |
| **Facility RVU** | **Work** | **PE** | **MP** | **Total** |
| **D0320** | 1.55 | 6.03 | 0.11 | 7.69 |
| **D0321** | 0.34 | 1.33 | 0.02 | 1.69 |

| | FUD | Status | MUE | Modifiers | | | | IOM Reference |
|---|---|---|---|---|---|---|---|---|
| **D0320** | N/A | I | - | N/A | N/A | N/A | N/A | None |
| **D0321** | N/A | I | - | N/A | N/A | N/A | N/A | |

* with documentation

## Terms To Know

**arthrogram.** X-ray of a joint after the injection of contrast material.

**ligament.** Band or sheet of fibrous tissue that connects the articular surfaces of bones or supports visceral organs.

**radiopaque dye.** Medium injected into the body that is impenetrable by x-rays.

**temporomandibular joint.** Joint or hinge formed by the connection of the lower jaw to the temporal bone of the cranium, located in front of the ear on both sides of the face.

# D0322

**D0322** tomographic survey

## Explanation

Tomographic examination is performed, which provides a more accurate image of the quantity and quality of the osseous structures. The images allow the provider to accurately measure the amount of bone that is available typically for implants. The patient is asked to remove any jewelry from the head and neck, so that it does not interfere with the study. The patient is positioned face up on the CT scanner bed, and the head is placed on a padded cradle and immobilized with a Velcro strap. The scanner bed slides through the CT scanner and images are taken.

## Coding Tips

This code includes interpretation. When reporting digital subtraction of two or more images (of the same modality), report D0394 in addition to the appropriate code for obtaining the image.

## Reimbursement Tips

This service may not be covered by the patient's dental insurance. However, coverage may be available through the patient's medical insurance. Check with third-party payers for specific coverage information. Services submitted to the payer of medical coverage will require that the service be reported with the appropriate CPT code on the CMS-1500 claim form.

## Associated CPT Codes

| | |
|---|---|
| 70486 | Computed tomography, maxillofacial area; without contrast material |
| 70487 | Computed tomography, maxillofacial area; with contrast material(s) |
| 70488 | Computed tomography, maxillofacial area; without contrast material, followed by contrast material(s) and further sections |

## ICD-10-CM Diagnostic Codes

| | |
|---|---|
| C41.0 | Malignant neoplasm of bones of skull and face |
| C41.1 | Malignant neoplasm of mandible |
| C76.0 | Malignant neoplasm of head, face and neck |
| C79.51 | Secondary malignant neoplasm of bone |
| D10.39 | Benign neoplasm of other parts of mouth |
| D16.4 | Benign neoplasm of bones of skull and face |
| D16.5 | Benign neoplasm of lower jaw bone |
| D48.7 | Neoplasm of uncertain behavior of other specified sites |
| D49.2 | Neoplasm of unspecified behavior of bone, soft tissue, and skin |
| M26.601 | Right temporomandibular joint disorder, unspecified |
| M26.602 | Left temporomandibular joint disorder, unspecified |
| M26.603 | Bilateral temporomandibular joint disorder, unspecified |
| M26.609 | Unspecified temporomandibular joint disorder, unspecified side |
| M26.611 | Adhesions and ankylosis of right temporomandibular joint ☑ |
| M26.612 | Adhesions and ankylosis of left temporomandibular joint ☑ |
| M26.613 | Adhesions and ankylosis of bilateral temporomandibular joint ☑ |
| M26.619 | Adhesions and ankylosis of temporomandibular joint, unspecified side |
| M26.621 | Arthralgia of right temporomandibular joint ☑ |
| M26.622 | Arthralgia of left temporomandibular joint ☑ |
| M26.623 | Arthralgia of bilateral temporomandibular joint ☑ |
| M26.629 | Arthralgia of temporomandibular joint, unspecified side |
| M26.631 | Articular disc disorder of right temporomandibular joint ☑ |
| M26.632 | Articular disc disorder of left temporomandibular joint ☑ |

| | |
|---|---|
| M26.633 | Articular disc disorder of bilateral temporomandibular joint ☑ |
| M26.639 | Articular disc disorder of temporomandibular joint, unspecified side |
| M26.641 | Arthritis of right temporomandibular joint ☑ |
| M26.642 | Arthritis of left temporomandibular joint ☑ |
| M26.643 | Arthritis of bilateral temporomandibular joint ☑ |
| M26.651 | Arthropathy of right temporomandibular joint ☑ |
| M26.652 | Arthropathy of left temporomandibular joint ☑ |
| M26.653 | Arthropathy of bilateral temporomandibular joint ☑ |
| M27.0 | Developmental disorders of jaws |
| M27.2 | Inflammatory conditions of jaws |
| M27.49 | Other cysts of jaw |

## Relative Value Units/Medicare Edits

| Non-Facility RVU | Work | PE | MP | Total |
|---|---|---|---|---|
| D0322 | 1.17 | 4.53 | 0.08 | 5.78 |
| **Facility RVU** | **Work** | **PE** | **MP** | **Total** |
| D0322 | 1.17 | 4.53 | 0.08 | 5.78 |

| | FUD | Status | MUE | Modifiers | | | | IOM Reference |
|---|---|---|---|---|---|---|---|---|
| D0322 | N/A | I | - | N/A | N/A | N/A | N/A | None |

* with documentation

## Terms To Know

**contrast material.** Any internally administered substance that has a different opacity from soft tissue on radiography or computed tomograph; includes barium, used to opacify parts of the gastrointestinal tract; water-soluble iodinated compounds, used to opacify blood vessels or the genitourinary tract; may refer to air occurring naturally or introduced into the body; also, paramagnetic substances used in magnetic resonance imaging. Substances may also be documented as contrast agent or contrast medium.

**implant.** Material or device inserted or placed within the body for therapeutic, reconstructive, or diagnostic purposes.

**tomography.** Specialized type of imaging that provides slices through a body structure to obliterate overlying structures.

# D0330

**D0330** panoramic radiographic image

## Explanation

A panoramic image (x-ray) is taken that allows a comprehensive all-in-one view of the oral structures to be seen.

## Coding Tips

Any evaluation, prophylaxis, fluoride, restorative, or extraction service is reported separately. A panoramic image is an extraoral film. For full-mouth series, see D0120. When reporting digital subtraction of two or more images (of the same modality), report D0394 in addition to the appropriate code for obtaining the image.

## Reimbursement Tips

Many payer contracts allow EITHER a full-mouth series OR a panoramic film but not both during a specified time period. Check with individual payers for contract-specific guidelines. When selecting the procedure or service that accurately identifies the service performed, dentists must use the most accurate code. If the CDT code more accurately identifies the service, this should be used rather than the CPT codes.

## Associated CPT Codes

| | |
|---|---|
| 70320 | Radiologic examination, teeth; complete, full mouth |
| 70355 | Orthopantogram (eg, panoramic x-ray) |

## ICD-10-CM Diagnostic Codes

| | |
|---|---|
| K00.1 | Supernumerary teeth |
| K00.2 | Abnormalities of size and form of teeth |
| K00.3 | Mottled teeth |
| K00.4 | Disturbances in tooth formation |
| K00.5 | Hereditary disturbances in tooth structure, not elsewhere classified |
| K00.6 | Disturbances in tooth eruption |
| K00.7 | Teething syndrome |
| K00.8 | Other disorders of tooth development |
| K01.0 | Embedded teeth |
| K01.1 | Impacted teeth |
| K02.3 | Arrested dental caries |
| K02.51 | Dental caries on pit and fissure surface limited to enamel |
| K02.52 | Dental caries on pit and fissure surface penetrating into dentin |
| K02.53 | Dental caries on pit and fissure surface penetrating into pulp |
| K02.61 | Dental caries on smooth surface limited to enamel |
| K02.62 | Dental caries on smooth surface penetrating into dentin |
| K02.63 | Dental caries on smooth surface penetrating into pulp |
| K02.7 | Dental root caries |
| K03.0 | Excessive attrition of teeth |
| K03.1 | Abrasion of teeth |
| K03.2 | Erosion of teeth |
| K03.3 | Pathological resorption of teeth |
| K03.4 | Hypercementosis |
| K03.5 | Ankylosis of teeth |
| K03.6 | Deposits [accretions] on teeth |
| K03.7 | Posteruptive color changes of dental hard tissues |
| K03.81 | Cracked tooth |
| K04.01 | Reversible pulpitis |
| K04.02 | Irreversible pulpitis |

K04.2 Pulp degeneration
K04.3 Abnormal hard tissue formation in pulp
K04.4 Acute apical periodontitis of pulpal origin
K04.5 Chronic apical periodontitis
K04.6 Periapical abscess with sinus
K04.7 Periapical abscess without sinus
K04.8 Radicular cyst
K04.99 Other diseases of pulp and periapical tissues
K05.00 Acute gingivitis, plaque induced
K05.01 Acute gingivitis, non-plaque induced
K05.10 Chronic gingivitis, plaque induced
K05.11 Chronic gingivitis, non-plaque induced
K05.211 Aggressive periodontitis, localized, slight
K05.212 Aggressive periodontitis, localized, moderate
K05.213 Aggressive periodontitis, localized, severe
K05.221 Aggressive periodontitis, generalized, slight
K05.222 Aggressive periodontitis, generalized, moderate
K05.223 Aggressive periodontitis, generalized, severe
K05.311 Chronic periodontitis, localized, slight
K05.312 Chronic periodontitis, localized, moderate
K05.313 Chronic periodontitis, localized, severe
K05.321 Chronic periodontitis, generalized, slight
K05.322 Chronic periodontitis, generalized, moderate
K05.323 Chronic periodontitis, generalized, severe
K05.4 Periodontosis
K06.011 Localized gingival recession, minimal
K06.012 Localized gingival recession, moderate
K06.013 Localized gingival recession, severe
K06.021 Generalized gingival recession, minimal
K06.022 Generalized gingival recession, moderate
K06.023 Generalized gingival recession, severe
K06.1 Gingival enlargement
K06.2 Gingival and edentulous alveolar ridge lesions associated with trauma
K06.8 Other specified disorders of gingiva and edentulous alveolar ridge
K08.0 Exfoliation of teeth due to systemic causes
K08.111 Complete loss of teeth due to trauma, class I
K08.112 Complete loss of teeth due to trauma, class II
K08.113 Complete loss of teeth due to trauma, class III
K08.114 Complete loss of teeth due to trauma, class IV
K08.121 Complete loss of teeth due to periodontal diseases, class I
K08.122 Complete loss of teeth due to periodontal diseases, class II
K08.123 Complete loss of teeth due to periodontal diseases, class III
K08.124 Complete loss of teeth due to periodontal diseases, class IV
K08.131 Complete loss of teeth due to caries, class I
K08.132 Complete loss of teeth due to caries, class II
K08.133 Complete loss of teeth due to caries, class III
K08.134 Complete loss of teeth due to caries, class IV
K08.191 Complete loss of teeth due to other specified cause, class I
K08.192 Complete loss of teeth due to other specified cause, class II
K08.193 Complete loss of teeth due to other specified cause, class III
K08.194 Complete loss of teeth due to other specified cause, class IV
K08.21 Minimal atrophy of the mandible
K08.22 Moderate atrophy of the mandible
K08.23 Severe atrophy of the mandible
K08.24 Minimal atrophy of maxilla
K08.25 Moderate atrophy of the maxilla
K08.26 Severe atrophy of the maxilla
K08.3 Retained dental root
K08.411 Partial loss of teeth due to trauma, class I
K08.412 Partial loss of teeth due to trauma, class II
K08.413 Partial loss of teeth due to trauma, class III
K08.414 Partial loss of teeth due to trauma, class IV
K08.421 Partial loss of teeth due to periodontal diseases, class I
K08.422 Partial loss of teeth due to periodontal diseases, class II
K08.423 Partial loss of teeth due to periodontal diseases, class III
K08.424 Partial loss of teeth due to periodontal diseases, class IV
K08.431 Partial loss of teeth due to caries, class I
K08.432 Partial loss of teeth due to caries, class II
K08.433 Partial loss of teeth due to caries, class III
K08.434 Partial loss of teeth due to caries, class IV
K08.491 Partial loss of teeth due to other specified cause, class I
K08.492 Partial loss of teeth due to other specified cause, class II
K08.493 Partial loss of teeth due to other specified cause, class III
K08.494 Partial loss of teeth due to other specified cause, class IV
K08.51 Open restoration margins of tooth
K08.52 Unrepairable overhanging of dental restorative materials
K08.530 Fractured dental restorative material without loss of material
K08.531 Fractured dental restorative material with loss of material
K08.54 Contour of existing restoration of tooth biologically incompatible with oral health
K08.55 Allergy to existing dental restorative material
K08.56 Poor aesthetic of existing restoration of tooth
K08.81 Primary occlusal trauma
K08.82 Secondary occlusal trauma
K09.0 Developmental odontogenic cysts
K09.1 Developmental (nonodontogenic) cysts of oral region
K09.8 Other cysts of oral region, not elsewhere classified

## Relative Value Units/Medicare Edits

| Non-Facility RVU | Work | PE | MP | Total |
|---|---|---|---|---|
| **D0330** | 0.27 | 1.03 | 0.02 | 1.32 |
| **Facility RVU** | **Work** | **PE** | **MP** | **Total** |
| **D0330** | 0.27 | 1.03 | 0.02 | 1.32 |

| | FUD | Status | MUE | Modifiers | | | | IOM Reference |
|---|---|---|---|---|---|---|---|---|
| **D0330** | N/A | I | - | N/A | N/A | N/A | N/A | None |

* with documentation

## Terms To Know

**panoramic x-ray.** X-ray that contains views of both the maxilla and mandible on a single extraoral image.

# D0340

**D0340** 2D cephalometric radiographic image - acquisition, measurement and analysis

*Image of the head made using a cephalostat to standardize anatomic positioning, and with reproducible x-ray beam geometry.*

## Explanation

A lateral or frontal x-ray projection is taken to examine the entire skull, jaw, and related tooth positions in a cephalometric image. The machine holds the patient's head in the same position each time an image is taken so that a series of the individual cephalograms taken can be directly compared for growth and development over time.

## Coding Tips

Any evaluation, prophylaxis, fluoride, restorative, or extraction service is reported separately. When reporting digit subtraction of two or more images (of the same modality), report D0394 in addition to the appropriate code for obtaining the image.

## Reimbursement Tips

This procedure may be covered by the patient's medical insurance. When covered by medical insurance, the payer may require that the appropriate CPT code be reported on the CMS-1500 claim form.

## Associated CPT Codes

70350 Cephalogram, orthodontic

## ICD-10-CM Diagnostic Codes

K00.1 Supernumerary teeth
K00.2 Abnormalities of size and form of teeth
K00.3 Mottled teeth
K00.4 Disturbances in tooth formation
K00.5 Hereditary disturbances in tooth structure, not elsewhere classified
K00.6 Disturbances in tooth eruption
K01.0 Embedded teeth
K01.1 Impacted teeth
K03.0 Excessive attrition of teeth
K03.1 Abrasion of teeth
K03.2 Erosion of teeth
K03.3 Pathological resorption of teeth
K06.012 Localized gingival recession, moderate
K06.013 Localized gingival recession, severe
K06.022 Generalized gingival recession, moderate
K06.023 Generalized gingival recession, severe
K08.21 Minimal atrophy of the mandible
K08.22 Moderate atrophy of the mandible
K08.23 Severe atrophy of the mandible
K08.24 Minimal atrophy of maxilla
K08.25 Moderate atrophy of the maxilla
K08.26 Severe atrophy of the maxilla
K09.0 Developmental odontogenic cysts
K09.1 Developmental (nonodontogenic) cysts of oral region
M26.211 Malocclusion, Angle's class I
M26.212 Malocclusion, Angle's class II
M26.213 Malocclusion, Angle's class III
M26.220 Open anterior occlusal relationship
M26.221 Open posterior occlusal relationship
M26.23 Excessive horizontal overlap
M26.24 Reverse articulation
M26.31 Crowding of fully erupted teeth
M26.32 Excessive spacing of fully erupted teeth
M26.33 Horizontal displacement of fully erupted tooth or teeth
M26.34 Vertical displacement of fully erupted tooth or teeth
M26.35 Rotation of fully erupted tooth or teeth
M26.36 Insufficient interocclusal distance of fully erupted teeth (ridge)
M26.37 Excessive interocclusal distance of fully erupted teeth
M26.51 Abnormal jaw closure
M26.52 Limited mandibular range of motion
M26.53 Deviation in opening and closing of the mandible
M26.54 Insufficient anterior guidance
M26.55 Centric occlusion maximum intercuspation discrepancy
M26.56 Non-working side interference
M26.57 Lack of posterior occlusal support
M26.59 Other dentofacial functional abnormalities
M26.71 Alveolar maxillary hyperplasia
M26.72 Alveolar mandibular hyperplasia
M26.73 Alveolar maxillary hypoplasia
M26.74 Alveolar mandibular hypoplasia
M26.79 Other specified alveolar anomalies
M26.81 Anterior soft tissue impingement
M26.82 Posterior soft tissue impingement
S02.5XXA Fracture of tooth (traumatic), initial encounter for closed fracture
S02.5XXB Fracture of tooth (traumatic), initial encounter for open fracture
Z46.4 Encounter for fitting and adjustment of orthodontic device

## Relative Value Units/Medicare Edits

| Non-Facility RVU | Work | PE | MP | Total |
|---|---|---|---|---|
| **D0340** | 0.31 | 1.20 | 0.02 | 1.53 |
| **Facility RVU** | **Work** | **PE** | **MP** | **Total** |
| **D0340** | 0.31 | 1.20 | 0.02 | 1.53 |

| | FUD | Status | MUE | Modifiers | | | | IOM Reference |
|---|---|---|---|---|---|---|---|---|
| **D0340** | N/A | I | - | N/A | N/A | N/A | N/A | None |

* with documentation

## Terms To Know

**cephalad.** Toward the head.

**radiograph.** Image made by an x-ray.

# D0350

**D0350** 2D oral/facial photographic image obtained intra-orally or extra-orally

## Explanation

This code is used for reporting traditional two-dimensional photographic images taken of the face or the inside of the mouth with an intraoral or extraoral camera. This is not for conventional x-rays or any type of radiographic imaging.

## Coding Tips

To report three-dimensional photographic imaging for diagnostic purposes, see D0351. Any evaluation, prophylaxis, fluoride, restorative, or extraction service is reported separately. This code excludes conventional radiograph.

## Reimbursement Tips

Often, this service is covered only when performed in conjunction with covered orthodontic services. Check with payers to determine their specific requirements.

## ICD-10-CM Diagnostic Codes

| | |
|---|---|
| K08.21 | Minimal atrophy of the mandible |
| K08.22 | Moderate atrophy of the mandible |
| K08.23 | Severe atrophy of the mandible |
| K08.24 | Minimal atrophy of maxilla |
| K08.25 | Moderate atrophy of the maxilla |
| K08.26 | Severe atrophy of the maxilla |
| M26.211 | Malocclusion, Angle's class I |
| M26.212 | Malocclusion, Angle's class II |
| M26.213 | Malocclusion, Angle's class III |
| M26.220 | Open anterior occlusal relationship |
| M26.221 | Open posterior occlusal relationship |
| M26.23 | Excessive horizontal overlap |
| M26.24 | Reverse articulation |
| M26.51 | Abnormal jaw closure |
| M26.52 | Limited mandibular range of motion |
| M26.53 | Deviation in opening and closing of the mandible |
| M26.54 | Insufficient anterior guidance |
| M26.55 | Centric occlusion maximum intercuspation discrepancy |
| M26.56 | Non-working side interference |
| M26.57 | Lack of posterior occlusal support |
| M26.59 | Other dentofacial functional abnormalities |
| M26.71 | Alveolar maxillary hyperplasia |
| M26.72 | Alveolar mandibular hyperplasia |
| M26.73 | Alveolar maxillary hypoplasia |
| M26.74 | Alveolar mandibular hypoplasia |
| M26.79 | Other specified alveolar anomalies |
| M26.81 | Anterior soft tissue impingement |
| M26.82 | Posterior soft tissue impingement |

## Relative Value Units/Medicare Edits

| Non-Facility RVU | Work | PE | MP | Total |
|---|---|---|---|---|
| D0350 | 0.15 | 0.58 | 0.01 | 0.74 |
| **Facility RVU** | **Work** | **PE** | **MP** | **Total** |
| D0350 | 0.15 | 0.58 | 0.01 | 0.74 |

| | FUD | Status | MUE | Modifiers | | | | IOM Reference |
|---|---|---|---|---|---|---|---|---|
| D0350 | N/A | I | - | N/A | N/A | N/A | N/A | None |

* with documentation

## Terms To Know

**anomaly.** Irregularity in the structure or position of an organ or tissue.

**extraoral.** Outside of the mouth or oral cavity.

**imaging.** Radiologic means of producing pictures for clinical study of the internal structures and functions of the body, such as x-ray, ultrasound, magnetic resonance, or positron emission tomography.

**intraoral.** Within the mouth.

**malocclusion.** Condition in which the teeth are misaligned. Underlying causes may include accessory, impacted, or missing teeth; dentofacial abnormalities; thumb sucking; or sleeping positions.

**mandibular.** Having to do with the lower jaw.

**oral.** Pertaining to the mouth.

# D0351

**D0351** 3D photographic image

*This procedure is for dental or maxillofacial diagnostic purposes. Not applicable for a CAD-CAM procedure.*

## Explanation

A three-dimensional photographic image of the dental or maxillofacial structures is obtained for diagnostic purposes. Three-dimensional photography allows for hemispherical and full spherical output that assists in analyzing the aesthetic aspect of the smile, occlusal planes, wear patterns, and other details otherwise hard to detect during a regular patient examination.

## Coding Tips

For two-dimensional photographic imaging, see D0350. When computer-aided design/computer-aided manufacturing (CAD-CAM) device (therapeutic purposes) is performed, see D0393-D0395.

## Documentation Tips

Pertinent documentation to evaluate the medical appropriateness should be included with the claim when this code is reported.

## Reimbursement Tips

This procedure may be covered by the patient's medical insurance. When covered by medical insurance, the payer may require that the appropriate CPT code be reported on the CMS-1500 claim form.

## ICD-10-CM Diagnostic Codes

K08.21 Minimal atrophy of the mandible
K08.22 Moderate atrophy of the mandible
K08.23 Severe atrophy of the mandible
K08.24 Minimal atrophy of maxilla
K08.25 Moderate atrophy of the maxilla
K08.26 Severe atrophy of the maxilla
M26.01 Maxillary hyperplasia
M26.02 Maxillary hypoplasia
M26.03 Mandibular hyperplasia
M26.04 Mandibular hypoplasia
M26.05 Macrogenia
M26.06 Microgenia
M26.07 Excessive tuberosity of jaw
M26.09 Other specified anomalies of jaw size
M26.12 Other jaw asymmetry
M26.19 Other specified anomalies of jaw-cranial base relationship
M26.211 Malocclusion, Angle's class I
M26.212 Malocclusion, Angle's class II
M26.213 Malocclusion, Angle's class III
M26.220 Open anterior occlusal relationship
M26.221 Open posterior occlusal relationship
M26.23 Excessive horizontal overlap
M26.24 Reverse articulation
M26.25 Anomalies of interarch distance
M26.29 Other anomalies of dental arch relationship
M26.31 Crowding of fully erupted teeth
M26.32 Excessive spacing of fully erupted teeth
M26.33 Horizontal displacement of fully erupted tooth or teeth
M26.34 Vertical displacement of fully erupted tooth or teeth
M26.35 Rotation of fully erupted tooth or teeth
M26.36 Insufficient interocclusal distance of fully erupted teeth (ridge)
M26.37 Excessive interocclusal distance of fully erupted teeth
M26.39 Other anomalies of tooth position of fully erupted tooth or teeth
M26.51 Abnormal jaw closure
M26.52 Limited mandibular range of motion
M26.53 Deviation in opening and closing of the mandible
M26.54 Insufficient anterior guidance
M26.55 Centric occlusion maximum intercuspation discrepancy
M26.56 Non-working side interference
M26.57 Lack of posterior occlusal support
M26.59 Other dentofacial functional abnormalities

## Relative Value Units/Medicare Edits

| Non-Facility RVU | Work | PE | MP | Total |
|---|---|---|---|---|
| **D0351** | 0.14 | 0.56 | 0.01 | 0.71 |
| **Facility RVU** | **Work** | **PE** | **MP** | **Total** |
| **D0351** | 0.14 | 0.56 | 0.01 | 0.71 |

| | FUD | Status | MUE | Modifiers | | | | IOM Reference |
|---|---|---|---|---|---|---|---|---|
| **D0351** | N/A | I | - | N/A | N/A | N/A | N/A | None |

* with documentation

## Terms To Know

**maxillary.** Located between the eyes and the upper teeth.

**maxillofacial.** Referring to the face and jaws.

**photography.** Still image pictures that may be digital or film generated.

# D0364-D0368

**D0364** cone beam CT capture and interpretation with limited field of view - less than one whole jaw

**D0365** cone beam CT capture and interpretation with field of view of one full dental arch - mandible

**D0366** cone beam CT capture and interpretation with field of view of one full dental arch - maxilla, with or without cranium

**D0367** cone beam CT capture and interpretation with field of view of both jaws; with or without cranium

**D0368** cone beam CT capture and interpretation for TMJ series including two or more exposures

## Explanation

Cone-beam CT images are obtained and interpreted by the provider. Cone-beam CT is performed and a written interpretation is provided. Cone-beam CT capture emits an x-ray beam shaped like a cone as opposed to the conventional fan-shaped beam. The most common uses of cone-beam imaging in dentistry is for the evaluation of temporomandibular abnormalities and abnormalities of teeth /facial structures for orthodontic treatment planning. Cone-beam CT may is also useful used for evaluating the mandibular nerve proximity before extraction of the lower wisdom teeth. Cone-beam examination may also be used to identify signs of infection, cysts, or tumors. Report D0364 when less than one whole jaw is examined. When either the full mandible or maxilla are examined report D0365 or D0366, respectively. Report D0367 when both jaws are examined and D0368 when evaluation of the temporomandibular joint is performed.

## Coding Tips

When interpretation only is performed, see codes D0380–D0386. To report post processing of image or image sets, see D0393–D0395. When reporting digit subtraction of two or more images (of the same modality), report D0394 in addition to the appropriate code for obtaining the image.

## Reimbursement Tips

When selecting the procedure or service that accurately identifies the service performed, dentists must use the most accurate code. If the CDT code more accurately identifies the service, this should be used rather than the CPT codes. This procedure may be covered by the patient's medical insurance. When covered by medical insurance, the payer may require that the appropriate CPT code be reported on the CMS-1500 claim form.

## ICD-10-CM Diagnostic Codes

C08.0 Malignant neoplasm of submandibular gland
C08.1 Malignant neoplasm of sublingual gland
D10.2 Benign neoplasm of floor of mouth
D11.0 Benign neoplasm of parotid gland
D11.7 Benign neoplasm of other major salivary glands
K09.0 Developmental odontogenic cysts
K09.1 Developmental (nonodontogenic) cysts of oral region
K09.8 Other cysts of oral region, not elsewhere classified
K11.0 Atrophy of salivary gland
K11.1 Hypertrophy of salivary gland
K11.21 Acute sialoadenitis
K11.22 Acute recurrent sialoadenitis
K11.23 Chronic sialoadenitis
K11.3 Abscess of salivary gland
K11.4 Fistula of salivary gland
K11.5 Sialolithiasis
K11.6 Mucocele of salivary gland
K11.7 Disturbances of salivary secretion
K12.0 Recurrent oral aphthae
K12.1 Other forms of stomatitis
K12.2 Cellulitis and abscess of mouth
K12.31 Oral mucositis (ulcerative) due to antineoplastic therapy
K12.32 Oral mucositis (ulcerative) due to other drugs
K12.33 Oral mucositis (ulcerative) due to radiation
K13.0 Diseases of lips
K13.1 Cheek and lip biting
K13.21 Leukoplakia of oral mucosa, including tongue
K13.22 Minimal keratinized residual ridge mucosa
K13.23 Excessive keratinized residual ridge mucosa
K13.24 Leukokeratosis nicotina palati
K13.3 Hairy leukoplakia
K13.4 Granuloma and granuloma-like lesions of oral mucosa
K13.5 Oral submucous fibrosis
K13.6 Irritative hyperplasia of oral mucosa
K14.0 Glossitis
K14.1 Geographic tongue
K14.2 Median rhomboid glossitis
K14.3 Hypertrophy of tongue papillae
K14.4 Atrophy of tongue papillae
K14.5 Plicated tongue
K14.6 Glossodynia

## Relative Value Units/Medicare Edits

| Non-Facility RVU | Work | PE | MP | Total |
|---|---|---|---|---|
| **D0364** | 0.93 | 3.60 | 0.07 | 4.60 |
| **D0365** | 0.93 | 3.60 | 0.07 | 4.60 |
| **D0366** | 0.93 | 3.60 | 0.07 | 4.60 |
| **D0367** | 0.93 | 3.60 | 0.07 | 4.60 |
| **D0368** | 1.36 | 5.28 | 0.10 | 6.74 |
| **Facility RVU** | **Work** | **PE** | **MP** | **Total** |
| **D0364** | 0.93 | 3.60 | 0.07 | 4.60 |
| **D0365** | 0.93 | 3.60 | 0.07 | 4.60 |
| **D0366** | 0.93 | 3.60 | 0.07 | 4.60 |
| **D0367** | 0.93 | 3.60 | 0.07 | 4.60 |
| **D0368** | 1.36 | 5.28 | 0.10 | 6.74 |

| | FUD | Status | MUE | Modifiers | | | | IOM Reference |
|---|---|---|---|---|---|---|---|---|
| **D0364** | N/A | N | - | N/A | N/A | N/A | N/A | None |
| **D0365** | N/A | N | - | N/A | N/A | N/A | N/A | |
| **D0366** | N/A | N | - | N/A | N/A | N/A | N/A | |
| **D0367** | N/A | N | - | N/A | N/A | N/A | N/A | |
| **D0368** | N/A | N | - | N/A | N/A | N/A | N/A | |

* with documentation

# D0369

**D0369** maxillofacial MRI capture and interpretation

## Explanation

The provider obtains and interprets MRI images. MRI is a radiation-free, noninvasive technique to produce high-quality sectional images of the inside of the body in multiple planes. MRI uses the natural magnetic properties of the hydrogen atoms in our bodies that emit radiofrequency signals when exposed to radio waves within a strong electromagnetic field. These signals are processed and converted by the computer into high-resolution, three-dimensional, tomographic images. These images are captured and interpreted by the provider. The extension of a tumor or other lesion is clearer on MRI examination and MRI enhanced with Gd-DTPA is used in determining tumor extensions into bony structures.

## Coding Tips

When interpretation only is performed, see code D0385. When reporting digit subtraction of two or more images (of the same modality), report D0394 in addition to the appropriate code for obtaining the image.

## Reimbursement Tips

When selecting the procedure or service that accurately identifies the service performed, dentists must use the most accurate code. If the CDT code more accurately identifies the service, this should be used rather than the CPT codes. This procedure may be covered by the patient's medical insurance. When covered by medical insurance, the payer may require that the appropriate CPT code be reported on the CMS-1500 claim form.

## Associated CPT Codes

70540 Magnetic resonance (eg, proton) imaging, orbit, face, and/or neck; without contrast material(s)
70542 Magnetic resonance (eg, proton) imaging, orbit, face, and/or neck; with contrast material(s)
70543 Magnetic resonance (eg, proton) imaging, orbit, face, and/or neck; without contrast material(s), followed by contrast material(s) and further sequences

## ICD-10-CM Diagnostic Codes

C08.0 Malignant neoplasm of submandibular gland
C08.1 Malignant neoplasm of sublingual gland
D10.2 Benign neoplasm of floor of mouth
D11.0 Benign neoplasm of parotid gland
D11.7 Benign neoplasm of other major salivary glands
K09.0 Developmental odontogenic cysts
K09.1 Developmental (nonodontogenic) cysts of oral region
K09.8 Other cysts of oral region, not elsewhere classified
K11.0 Atrophy of salivary gland
K11.1 Hypertrophy of salivary gland
K11.21 Acute sialoadenitis
K11.22 Acute recurrent sialoadenitis
K11.23 Chronic sialoadenitis
K11.3 Abscess of salivary gland
K11.4 Fistula of salivary gland
K11.5 Sialolithiasis
K11.6 Mucocele of salivary gland
K11.7 Disturbances of salivary secretion
K11.8 Other diseases of salivary glands
K12.0 Recurrent oral aphthae
K12.1 Other forms of stomatitis
K12.2 Cellulitis and abscess of mouth
K12.31 Oral mucositis (ulcerative) due to antineoplastic therapy
K12.32 Oral mucositis (ulcerative) due to other drugs
K12.33 Oral mucositis (ulcerative) due to radiation
K12.39 Other oral mucositis (ulcerative)
K13.0 Diseases of lips
K13.1 Cheek and lip biting
K13.21 Leukoplakia of oral mucosa, including tongue
K13.22 Minimal keratinized residual ridge mucosa
K13.23 Excessive keratinized residual ridge mucosa
K13.24 Leukokeratosis nicotina palati
K13.29 Other disturbances of oral epithelium, including tongue
K13.3 Hairy leukoplakia
K13.4 Granuloma and granuloma-like lesions of oral mucosa
K13.5 Oral submucous fibrosis
K13.6 Irritative hyperplasia of oral mucosa
K13.79 Other lesions of oral mucosa
K14.0 Glossitis
K14.1 Geographic tongue
K14.2 Median rhomboid glossitis
K14.3 Hypertrophy of tongue papillae
K14.4 Atrophy of tongue papillae
K14.5 Plicated tongue
K14.6 Glossodynia
K14.8 Other diseases of tongue

## Relative Value Units/Medicare Edits

| Non-Facility RVU | Work | PE | MP | Total |
|---|---|---|---|---|
| D0369 | 2.43 | 9.43 | 0.17 | 12.03 |
| **Facility RVU** | **Work** | **PE** | **MP** | **Total** |
| D0369 | 2.43 | 9.43 | 0.17 | 12.03 |

| | FUD | Status | MUE | Modifiers | | | | IOM Reference |
|---|---|---|---|---|---|---|---|---|
| D0369 | N/A | N | - | N/A | N/A | N/A | N/A | None |

* with documentation

## Terms To Know

**MRI.** Magnetic resonance imaging. Radiation-free, noninvasive technique that produces high quality, multiple plane images of the inside of the body by using the natural magnetic properties of the hydrogen atoms within the body that emit radiofrequency signals when exposed to radio waves in a strong magnetic field.

# D0370

**D0370** maxillofacial ultrasound capture and interpretation

## Explanation

The provider obtains and interprets ultrasonic images of the maxillofacial structures. Ultrasound images are captured in real-time using a high-frequency linear probe that produces high-definition multi-linear images. These images capture the structure and movement of the body's internal organs, as well as blood flowing through blood vessels. These images are used in the examination of superficial structures.

## Coding Tips

When interpretation only is performed, see code D0385. When reporting digit subtraction of two or more images (of the same modality), report D0394 in addition to the appropriate code for obtaining the image.

## Reimbursement Tips

When selecting the procedure or service that accurately identifies the service performed, dentists must use the most accurate code. If the CDT code more accurately identifies the service, this should be used rather than the CPT codes. This procedure may be covered by medical insurance. When covered by medical insurance, the payer may require that the appropriate CPT code be reported on the CMS-1500 claim form.

## Associated CPT Codes

76536 Ultrasound, soft tissues of head and neck (eg, thyroid, parathyroid, parotid), real time with image documentation

## ICD-10-CM Diagnostic Codes

C08.0 Malignant neoplasm of submandibular gland
C08.1 Malignant neoplasm of sublingual gland
D10.2 Benign neoplasm of floor of mouth
D11.0 Benign neoplasm of parotid gland
D11.7 Benign neoplasm of other major salivary glands
K09.0 Developmental odontogenic cysts
K09.1 Developmental (nonodontogenic) cysts of oral region
K09.8 Other cysts of oral region, not elsewhere classified
K11.0 Atrophy of salivary gland
K11.1 Hypertrophy of salivary gland
K11.21 Acute sialoadenitis
K11.22 Acute recurrent sialoadenitis
K11.23 Chronic sialoadenitis
K11.3 Abscess of salivary gland
K11.4 Fistula of salivary gland
K11.5 Sialolithiasis
K11.6 Mucocele of salivary gland
K11.7 Disturbances of salivary secretion
K11.8 Other diseases of salivary glands
K12.0 Recurrent oral aphthae
K12.1 Other forms of stomatitis
K12.2 Cellulitis and abscess of mouth
K12.31 Oral mucositis (ulcerative) due to antineoplastic therapy
K12.32 Oral mucositis (ulcerative) due to other drugs
K12.33 Oral mucositis (ulcerative) due to radiation
K12.39 Other oral mucositis (ulcerative)
K13.0 Diseases of lips
K13.1 Cheek and lip biting
K13.21 Leukoplakia of oral mucosa, including tongue
K13.22 Minimal keratinized residual ridge mucosa
K13.23 Excessive keratinized residual ridge mucosa
K13.24 Leukokeratosis nicotina palati
K13.29 Other disturbances of oral epithelium, including tongue
K13.3 Hairy leukoplakia
K13.4 Granuloma and granuloma-like lesions of oral mucosa
K13.5 Oral submucous fibrosis
K13.6 Irritative hyperplasia of oral mucosa
K13.79 Other lesions of oral mucosa
K14.0 Glossitis
K14.1 Geographic tongue
K14.2 Median rhomboid glossitis
K14.3 Hypertrophy of tongue papillae
K14.4 Atrophy of tongue papillae
K14.5 Plicated tongue
K14.6 Glossodynia
K14.8 Other diseases of tongue

## Relative Value Units/Medicare Edits

| Non-Facility RVU | Work | PE | MP | Total |
|---|---|---|---|---|
| **D0370** | 0.82 | 3.17 | 0.06 | 4.05 |
| **Facility RVU** | **Work** | **PE** | **MP** | **Total** |
| **D0370** | 0.82 | 3.17 | 0.06 | 4.05 |

| | FUD | Status | MUE | Modifiers | | | | IOM Reference |
|---|---|---|---|---|---|---|---|---|
| **D0370** | N/A | N | - | N/A | N/A | N/A | N/A | None |

* with documentation

## Terms To Know

**maxillofacial.** Referring to the face and jaws.

**ultrasound.** Imaging using ultra-high sound frequency bounced off body structures.

# D0371

**D0371** sialoendoscopy capture and interpretation

## Explanation

The provider examines the salivary gland endoscopically. Local anesthetic is infiltrated at the papilla carefully avoiding the top of the papilla so that the orifice is not lost. Salivary dilators are inserted starting with the smallest and progressing to larger dilators until the papilla is dilated to the point that the endoscope can be inserted. The endoscope is advanced approximately 1 cm and the provider flushes the duct with a saline solution. Images are obtained via the endoscope.

## Coding Tips

When reporting digit subtraction of two or more images (of the same modality), report D0394 in addition to the appropriate code for obtaining the image.

## Reimbursement Tips

When covered by medical insurance, the payer may require that the appropriate CPT code be reported on the CMS-1500 claim form.

## ICD-10-CM Diagnostic Codes

| | |
|---|---|
| C08.0 | Malignant neoplasm of submandibular gland |
| C08.1 | Malignant neoplasm of sublingual gland |
| C79.89 | Secondary malignant neoplasm of other specified sites |
| D00.06 | Carcinoma in situ of floor of mouth |
| D10.39 | Benign neoplasm of other parts of mouth |
| D11.0 | Benign neoplasm of parotid gland |
| D11.7 | Benign neoplasm of other major salivary glands |
| K11.0 | Atrophy of salivary gland |
| K11.1 | Hypertrophy of salivary gland |
| K11.21 | Acute sialoadenitis |
| K11.22 | Acute recurrent sialoadenitis |
| K11.23 | Chronic sialoadenitis |
| K11.3 | Abscess of salivary gland |
| K11.4 | Fistula of salivary gland |
| K11.5 | Sialolithiasis |
| K11.6 | Mucocele of salivary gland |
| K11.7 | Disturbances of salivary secretion |
| K11.8 | Other diseases of salivary glands |

## Relative Value Units/Medicare Edits

| Non-Facility RVU | Work | PE | MP | Total |
|---|---|---|---|---|
| D0371 | 0.93 | 3.60 | 0.07 | 4.60 |
| **Facility RVU** | **Work** | **PE** | **MP** | **Total** |
| D0371 | 0.93 | 3.60 | 0.07 | 4.60 |

| | FUD | Status | MUE | Modifiers | | | | IOM Reference |
|---|---|---|---|---|---|---|---|---|
| D0371 | N/A | N | - | N/A | N/A | N/A | N/A | None |

* with documentation

## Terms To Know

**salivary gland.** One of several glands that secrete saliva into the oral cavity.

# D0380-D0384

**D0380** cone beam CT image capture with limited field of view - less than one whole jaw

**D0381** cone beam CT image capture with field of view of one full dental arch - mandible

**D0382** cone beam CT image capture with field of view of one full dental arch - maxilla, with or without cranium

**D0383** cone beam CT image capture with field of view of both jaws; with or without cranium

**D0384** cone beam CT image capture for TMJ series including two or more exposures

## Explanation

The provider interprets cone-beam CT images obtained elsewhere. Cone-beam CT capture emits an x-ray beam shaped like a cone as opposed to the conventional fan-shaped beam. The most common use of cone-beam imaging in dentistry is for the evaluation of temporomandibular abnormalities and teeth/facial structures for orthodontic treatment planning, as well as evaluating the mandibular nerve proximity before extraction of the lower wisdom teeth. Cone beam examination may also be used to identify signs of infections, cysts, or tumors. Report D0380 when films for less than one whole jaw are interpreted. Report D0380 for interpretation of mandibular films and D0382 for interpretation of films of the maxilla. Code D0383 reports the interpretation of the examination of both jaws and D0384 is reported when the interpretation is for two or more exposures of the temporomandibular joint.

## Coding Tips

When the radiologic procedure and interpretation are both performed by the same provider, see codes D0364–D0368. When reporting digit subtraction of two or more images (of the same modality), report D0394 in addition to the appropriate code for obtaining the image. When reporting digital subtraction of two or more images (of the same modality), report D0394 in addition to the appropriate code for obtaining the image.

## Reimbursement Tips

When selecting the procedure or service that accurately identifies the service performed, dentists must use the most accurate code. If the CDT code more accurately identifies the service, this should be used rather than the CPT codes. This procedure may be covered by the patient's medical insurance. When covered by medical insurance, the payer may require that the appropriate CPT code be reported on the CMS-1500 claim form. Note that when reporting with CPT codes, the appropriate CPT code (70486 or 76376) is reported with modifier 26 Professional component, appended.

## Associated CPT Codes

| | |
|---|---|
| 70486 | Computed tomography, maxillofacial area; without contrast material |
| 70487 | Computed tomography, maxillofacial area; with contrast material(s) |
| 70488 | Computed tomography, maxillofacial area; without contrast material, followed by contrast material(s) and further sections |

## ICD-10-CM Diagnostic Codes

| | |
|---|---|
| C08.0 | Malignant neoplasm of submandibular gland |
| C08.1 | Malignant neoplasm of sublingual gland |
| C08.9 | Malignant neoplasm of major salivary gland, unspecified |
| C79.89 | Secondary malignant neoplasm of other specified sites |
| D00.06 | Carcinoma in situ of floor of mouth |
| D10.39 | Benign neoplasm of other parts of mouth |

D11.0 Benign neoplasm of parotid gland
D11.7 Benign neoplasm of other major salivary glands
D37.030 Neoplasm of uncertain behavior of the parotid salivary glands
D37.031 Neoplasm of uncertain behavior of the sublingual salivary glands
D37.032 Neoplasm of uncertain behavior of the submandibular salivary glands
M26.01 Maxillary hyperplasia
M26.02 Maxillary hypoplasia
M26.03 Mandibular hyperplasia
M26.04 Mandibular hypoplasia
M26.05 Macrogenia
M26.06 Microgenia
M26.07 Excessive tuberosity of jaw
M26.09 Other specified anomalies of jaw size
M26.11 Maxillary asymmetry
M26.12 Other jaw asymmetry
M26.19 Other specified anomalies of jaw-cranial base relationship
M26.211 Malocclusion, Angle's class I
M26.212 Malocclusion, Angle's class II
M26.213 Malocclusion, Angle's class III
M26.220 Open anterior occlusal relationship
M26.221 Open posterior occlusal relationship
M26.23 Excessive horizontal overlap
M26.24 Reverse articulation
M26.25 Anomalies of interarch distance
M26.29 Other anomalies of dental arch relationship
M26.31 Crowding of fully erupted teeth
M26.32 Excessive spacing of fully erupted teeth
M26.33 Horizontal displacement of fully erupted tooth or teeth
M26.34 Vertical displacement of fully erupted tooth or teeth
M26.35 Rotation of fully erupted tooth or teeth
M26.36 Insufficient interocclusal distance of fully erupted teeth (ridge)
M26.37 Excessive interocclusal distance of fully erupted teeth
M26.39 Other anomalies of tooth position of fully erupted tooth or teeth
M26.51 Abnormal jaw closure
M26.52 Limited mandibular range of motion
M26.53 Deviation in opening and closing of the mandible
M26.54 Insufficient anterior guidance
M26.55 Centric occlusion maximum intercuspation discrepancy
M26.56 Non-working side interference
M26.57 Lack of posterior occlusal support
M26.59 Other dentofacial functional abnormalities
M26.611 Adhesions and ankylosis of right temporomandibular joint ☑
M26.612 Adhesions and ankylosis of left temporomandibular joint ☑
M26.613 Adhesions and ankylosis of bilateral temporomandibular joint ☑
M26.621 Arthralgia of right temporomandibular joint ☑
M26.622 Arthralgia of left temporomandibular joint ☑
M26.623 Arthralgia of bilateral temporomandibular joint ☑
M26.631 Articular disc disorder of right temporomandibular joint ☑
M26.632 Articular disc disorder of left temporomandibular joint ☑
M26.633 Articular disc disorder of bilateral temporomandibular joint ☑
M26.641 Arthritis of right temporomandibular joint ☑
M26.642 Arthritis of left temporomandibular joint ☑
M26.643 Arthritis of bilateral temporomandibular joint ☑
M26.651 Arthropathy of right temporomandibular joint ☑
M26.652 Arthropathy of left temporomandibular joint ☑
M26.653 Arthropathy of bilateral temporomandibular joint ☑
M26.69 Other specified disorders of temporomandibular joint
M26.71 Alveolar maxillary hyperplasia
M26.72 Alveolar mandibular hyperplasia
M26.73 Alveolar maxillary hypoplasia
M26.74 Alveolar mandibular hypoplasia
M26.81 Anterior soft tissue impingement
M26.82 Posterior soft tissue impingement
M27.0 Developmental disorders of jaws
M27.1 Giant cell granuloma, central
M27.2 Inflammatory conditions of jaws
M27.3 Alveolitis of jaws
M27.49 Other cysts of jaw
M27.51 Perforation of root canal space due to endodontic treatment
M27.52 Endodontic overfill
M27.53 Endodontic underfill
M27.59 Other periradicular pathology associated with previous endodontic treatment
M27.61 Osseointegration failure of dental implant
M27.62 Post-osseointegration biological failure of dental implant
M27.63 Post-osseointegration mechanical failure of dental implant
M27.69 Other endosseous dental implant failure
M27.8 Other specified diseases of jaws
M30.0 Polyarteritis nodosa
M30.1 Polyarteritis with lung involvement [Churg-Strauss]
M30.2 Juvenile polyarteritis

## Relative Value Units/Medicare Edits

| Non-Facility RVU | Work | PE | MP | Total |
|---|---|---|---|---|
| **D0380** | 0.74 | 2.88 | 0.05 | 3.67 |
| **D0381** | 0.74 | 2.88 | 0.05 | 3.67 |
| **D0382** | 0.74 | 2.88 | 0.05 | 3.67 |
| **D0383** | 0.74 | 2.88 | 0.05 | 3.67 |
| **D0384** | 1.08 | 4.20 | 0.08 | 5.36 |
| **Facility RVU** | **Work** | **PE** | **MP** | **Total** |
| **D0380** | 0.74 | 2.88 | 0.05 | 3.67 |
| **D0381** | 0.74 | 2.88 | 0.05 | 3.67 |
| **D0382** | 0.74 | 2.88 | 0.05 | 3.67 |
| **D0383** | 0.74 | 2.88 | 0.05 | 3.67 |
| **D0384** | 1.08 | 4.20 | 0.08 | 5.36 |

| | FUD | Status | MUE | Modifiers | | | | IOM Reference |
|---|---|---|---|---|---|---|---|---|
| **D0380** | N/A | N | - | N/A | N/A | N/A | N/A | None |
| **D0381** | N/A | N | - | N/A | N/A | N/A | N/A | |
| **D0382** | N/A | N | - | N/A | N/A | N/A | N/A | |
| **D0383** | N/A | N | - | N/A | N/A | N/A | N/A | |
| **D0384** | N/A | N | - | N/A | N/A | N/A | N/A | |

* with documentation

# D0385

**D0385** maxillofacial MRI image capture

## Explanation

A provider obtains maxillofacial MRI images but does not provide interpretation or report. MRI is a radiation-free, noninvasive technique to produce high-quality sectional images of the inside of the body in multiple planes. MRI uses the natural magnetic properties of the hydrogen atoms in our bodies that emit radiofrequency signals when exposed to radiowaves within a strong electromagnetic field. These signals are processed and converted by the computer into high-resolution, three-dimensional, tomographic images. These images are captured and interpreted by another entity. The extension of a tumor or other lesion is clearer on MRI examination and an MRI enhanced with Gd-DTPA can be used to determine tumor extensions into bony structures.

## Coding Tips

When the provider performs and interprets the MRI study, see D0369. When reporting digital subtraction of two or more images (of the same modality), report D0394 in addition to the appropriate code for obtaining the image.

## Reimbursement Tips

This procedure may be covered by the patient's medical insurance. When covered by medical insurance, the payer may require that the appropriate CPT code be reported on the CMS-1500 claim form. Note that when reporting with CPT codes, the appropriate CPT code (70544–70546) is reported with modifier 26 Professional component, appended.

## ICD-10-CM Diagnostic Codes

|  |  |
|---|---|
| C08.0 | Malignant neoplasm of submandibular gland |
| C08.1 | Malignant neoplasm of sublingual gland |
| C08.9 | Malignant neoplasm of major salivary gland, unspecified |
| C79.89 | Secondary malignant neoplasm of other specified sites |
| D00.00 | Carcinoma in situ of oral cavity, unspecified site |
| D00.06 | Carcinoma in situ of floor of mouth |
| D10.39 | Benign neoplasm of other parts of mouth |
| D11.0 | Benign neoplasm of parotid gland |
| D11.7 | Benign neoplasm of other major salivary glands |
| D11.9 | Benign neoplasm of major salivary gland, unspecified |
| D37.030 | Neoplasm of uncertain behavior of the parotid salivary glands |
| D37.031 | Neoplasm of uncertain behavior of the sublingual salivary glands |
| D37.032 | Neoplasm of uncertain behavior of the submandibular salivary glands |
| D37.039 | Neoplasm of uncertain behavior of the major salivary glands, unspecified |
| M26.00 | Unspecified anomaly of jaw size |
| M26.01 | Maxillary hyperplasia |
| M26.02 | Maxillary hypoplasia |
| M26.03 | Mandibular hyperplasia |
| M26.04 | Mandibular hypoplasia |
| M26.05 | Macrogenia |
| M26.06 | Microgenia |
| M26.07 | Excessive tuberosity of jaw |
| M26.09 | Other specified anomalies of jaw size |
| M26.10 | Unspecified anomaly of jaw-cranial base relationship |
| M26.11 | Maxillary asymmetry |
| M26.12 | Other jaw asymmetry |
| M26.19 | Other specified anomalies of jaw-cranial base relationship |
| M26.20 | Unspecified anomaly of dental arch relationship |
| M26.211 | Malocclusion, Angle's class I |
| M26.212 | Malocclusion, Angle's class II |
| M26.213 | Malocclusion, Angle's class III |
| M26.219 | Malocclusion, Angle's class, unspecified |
| M26.220 | Open anterior occlusal relationship |
| M26.221 | Open posterior occlusal relationship |
| M26.23 | Excessive horizontal overlap |
| M26.24 | Reverse articulation |
| M26.25 | Anomalies of interarch distance |
| M26.29 | Other anomalies of dental arch relationship |
| M26.30 | Unspecified anomaly of tooth position of fully erupted tooth or teeth |
| M26.31 | Crowding of fully erupted teeth |
| M26.32 | Excessive spacing of fully erupted teeth |
| M26.33 | Horizontal displacement of fully erupted tooth or teeth |
| M26.34 | Vertical displacement of fully erupted tooth or teeth |
| M26.35 | Rotation of fully erupted tooth or teeth |
| M26.36 | Insufficient interocclusal distance of fully erupted teeth (ridge) |
| M26.37 | Excessive interocclusal distance of fully erupted teeth |
| M26.39 | Other anomalies of tooth position of fully erupted tooth or teeth |
| M26.4 | Malocclusion, unspecified |
| M26.50 | Dentofacial functional abnormalities, unspecified |
| M26.51 | Abnormal jaw closure |
| M26.52 | Limited mandibular range of motion |
| M26.53 | Deviation in opening and closing of the mandible |
| M26.54 | Insufficient anterior guidance |
| M26.55 | Centric occlusion maximum intercuspation discrepancy |
| M26.56 | Non-working side interference |
| M26.57 | Lack of posterior occlusal support |
| M26.59 | Other dentofacial functional abnormalities |
| M26.601 | Right temporomandibular joint disorder, unspecified |
| M26.602 | Left temporomandibular joint disorder, unspecified |
| M26.603 | Bilateral temporomandibular joint disorder, unspecified |
| M26.609 | Unspecified temporomandibular joint disorder, unspecified side |
| M26.611 | Adhesions and ankylosis of right temporomandibular joint ☑ |
| M26.612 | Adhesions and ankylosis of left temporomandibular joint ☑ |
| M26.613 | Adhesions and ankylosis of bilateral temporomandibular joint ☑ |
| M26.619 | Adhesions and ankylosis of temporomandibular joint, unspecified side |
| M26.621 | Arthralgia of right temporomandibular joint ☑ |
| M26.622 | Arthralgia of left temporomandibular joint ☑ |
| M26.623 | Arthralgia of bilateral temporomandibular joint ☑ |
| M26.629 | Arthralgia of temporomandibular joint, unspecified side |
| M26.631 | Articular disc disorder of right temporomandibular joint ☑ |
| M26.632 | Articular disc disorder of left temporomandibular joint ☑ |
| M26.633 | Articular disc disorder of bilateral temporomandibular joint ☑ |
| M26.639 | Articular disc disorder of temporomandibular joint, unspecified side |
| M26.641 | Arthritis of right temporomandibular joint ☑ |
| M26.642 | Arthritis of left temporomandibular joint ☑ |
| M26.643 | Arthritis of bilateral temporomandibular joint ☑ |
| M26.651 | Arthropathy of right temporomandibular joint ☑ |
| M26.652 | Arthropathy of left temporomandibular joint ☑ |
| M26.653 | Arthropathy of bilateral temporomandibular joint ☑ |
| M26.69 | Other specified disorders of temporomandibular joint |
| M26.70 | Unspecified alveolar anomaly |

M26.71 Alveolar maxillary hyperplasia
M26.72 Alveolar mandibular hyperplasia
M26.73 Alveolar maxillary hypoplasia
M26.74 Alveolar mandibular hypoplasia
M26.81 Anterior soft tissue impingement
M26.82 Posterior soft tissue impingement
M26.9 Dentofacial anomaly, unspecified
M27.0 Developmental disorders of jaws
M27.1 Giant cell granuloma, central
M27.2 Inflammatory conditions of jaws
M27.3 Alveolitis of jaws
M27.40 Unspecified cyst of jaw
M27.49 Other cysts of jaw
M27.51 Perforation of root canal space due to endodontic treatment
M27.52 Endodontic overfill
M27.53 Endodontic underfill
M27.59 Other periradicular pathology associated with previous endodontic treatment
M27.61 Osseointegration failure of dental implant
M27.62 Post-osseointegration biological failure of dental implant
M27.63 Post-osseointegration mechanical failure of dental implant
M27.69 Other endosseous dental implant failure
M27.8 Other specified diseases of jaws
M27.9 Disease of jaws, unspecified
M30.0 Polyarteritis nodosa
M30.1 Polyarteritis with lung involvement [Churg-Strauss]
M30.2 Juvenile polyarteritis

## Relative Value Units/Medicare Edits

| Non-Facility RVU | Work | PE | MP | Total |
|---|---|---|---|---|
| D0385 | 1.76 | 6.86 | 0.13 | 8.75 |
| **Facility RVU** | **Work** | **PE** | **MP** | **Total** |
| D0385 | 1.76 | 6.86 | 0.13 | 8.75 |

| | FUD | Status | MUE | Modifiers | | | | IOM Reference |
|---|---|---|---|---|---|---|---|---|
| D0385 | N/A | N | - | N/A | N/A | N/A | N/A | None |

* with documentation

## Terms To Know

**MRI.** Magnetic resonance imaging. Radiation-free, noninvasive technique that produces high quality, multiple plane images of the inside of the body by using the natural magnetic properties of the hydrogen atoms within the body that emit radiofrequency signals when exposed to radio waves in a strong magnetic field.

**professional component.** Portion of a charge for health care services that represents the physician's (or other practitioner's) work in providing the service, including interpretation and report of the procedure. This component of the service usually is charged for and billed separately from the inpatient hospital charges.

# D0386

**D0386** maxillofacial ultrasound image capture

## Explanation

The provider obtains ultrasonic images of the maxillofacial structures but does not provide interpretation or report. Ultrasound images are captured in real-time using a high frequency linear probe that produces high-definition multilinear images. These images capture the structure and movement of the body's internal organs, as well as blood flowing through blood vessels. These images are also used in the examination of superficial structures.

## Coding Tips

When the provider obtains and interprets the ultrasound image, see code D0370. When reporting digital subtraction of two or more images (of the same modality), report D0394 in addition to the appropriate code for obtaining the image.

## Reimbursement Tips

When selecting the procedure or service that accurately identifies the service performed, dentists must use the most accurate code. If the CDT code more accurately identifies the service, this should be used rather than the CPT codes. This procedure may be covered by the patient's medical insurance. When covered by medical insurance, the payer may require that the appropriate CPT code be reported on the CMS-1500 claim form. Note that when reporting with CPT codes, the appropriate CPT code (76536) is reported with modifier 26 Professional component, appended.

## Associated CPT Codes

76536 Ultrasound, soft tissues of head and neck (eg, thyroid, parathyroid, parotid), real time with image documentation

## ICD-10-CM Diagnostic Codes

C08.0 Malignant neoplasm of submandibular gland
C08.1 Malignant neoplasm of sublingual gland
C08.9 Malignant neoplasm of major salivary gland, unspecified
C79.89 Secondary malignant neoplasm of other specified sites
D00.06 Carcinoma in situ of floor of mouth
D10.39 Benign neoplasm of other parts of mouth
D11.0 Benign neoplasm of parotid gland
D11.7 Benign neoplasm of other major salivary glands
D37.030 Neoplasm of uncertain behavior of the parotid salivary glands
D37.031 Neoplasm of uncertain behavior of the sublingual salivary glands
D37.032 Neoplasm of uncertain behavior of the submandibular salivary glands
M26.01 Maxillary hyperplasia
M26.02 Maxillary hypoplasia
M26.03 Mandibular hyperplasia
M26.04 Mandibular hypoplasia
M26.05 Macrogenia
M26.06 Microgenia
M26.07 Excessive tuberosity of jaw
M26.09 Other specified anomalies of jaw size
M26.11 Maxillary asymmetry
M26.12 Other jaw asymmetry
M26.19 Other specified anomalies of jaw-cranial base relationship
M26.211 Malocclusion, Angle's class I
M26.212 Malocclusion, Angle's class II
M26.213 Malocclusion, Angle's class III

M26.220 Open anterior occlusal relationship
M26.221 Open posterior occlusal relationship
M26.23 Excessive horizontal overlap
M26.24 Reverse articulation
M26.25 Anomalies of interarch distance
M26.29 Other anomalies of dental arch relationship
M26.31 Crowding of fully erupted teeth
M26.32 Excessive spacing of fully erupted teeth
M26.33 Horizontal displacement of fully erupted tooth or teeth
M26.34 Vertical displacement of fully erupted tooth or teeth
M26.35 Rotation of fully erupted tooth or teeth
M26.36 Insufficient interocclusal distance of fully erupted teeth (ridge)
M26.37 Excessive interocclusal distance of fully erupted teeth
M26.39 Other anomalies of tooth position of fully erupted tooth or teeth
M26.51 Abnormal jaw closure
M26.52 Limited mandibular range of motion
M26.53 Deviation in opening and closing of the mandible
M26.54 Insufficient anterior guidance
M26.55 Centric occlusion maximum intercuspation discrepancy
M26.56 Non-working side interference
M26.57 Lack of posterior occlusal support
M26.59 Other dentofacial functional abnormalities
M26.611 Adhesions and ankylosis of right temporomandibular joint ☑
M26.612 Adhesions and ankylosis of left temporomandibular joint ☑
M26.613 Adhesions and ankylosis of bilateral temporomandibular joint ☑
M26.621 Arthralgia of right temporomandibular joint ☑
M26.622 Arthralgia of left temporomandibular joint ☑
M26.623 Arthralgia of bilateral temporomandibular joint ☑
M26.631 Articular disc disorder of right temporomandibular joint ☑
M26.632 Articular disc disorder of left temporomandibular joint ☑
M26.633 Articular disc disorder of bilateral temporomandibular joint ☑
M26.641 Arthritis of right temporomandibular joint ☑
M26.642 Arthritis of left temporomandibular joint ☑
M26.643 Arthritis of bilateral temporomandibular joint ☑
M26.651 Arthropathy of right temporomandibular joint ☑
M26.652 Arthropathy of left temporomandibular joint ☑
M26.653 Arthropathy of bilateral temporomandibular joint ☑
M26.69 Other specified disorders of temporomandibular joint
M26.71 Alveolar maxillary hyperplasia
M26.72 Alveolar mandibular hyperplasia
M26.73 Alveolar maxillary hypoplasia
M26.74 Alveolar mandibular hypoplasia
M26.81 Anterior soft tissue impingement
M26.82 Posterior soft tissue impingement
M26.9 Dentofacial anomaly, unspecified
M27.0 Developmental disorders of jaws
M27.1 Giant cell granuloma, central
M27.2 Inflammatory conditions of jaws
M27.3 Alveolitis of jaws
M27.49 Other cysts of jaw
M27.51 Perforation of root canal space due to endodontic treatment
M27.52 Endodontic overfill
M27.53 Endodontic underfill
M27.59 Other periradicular pathology associated with previous endodontic treatment
M27.61 Osseointegration failure of dental implant
M27.62 Post-osseointegration biological failure of dental implant
M27.63 Post-osseointegration mechanical failure of dental implant
M27.69 Other endosseous dental implant failure
M27.8 Other specified diseases of jaws
M30.0 Polyarteritis nodosa
M30.1 Polyarteritis with lung involvement [Churg-Strauss]
M30.2 Juvenile polyarteritis

## Relative Value Units/Medicare Edits

| Non-Facility RVU | Work | PE | MP | Total |
|---|---|---|---|---|
| **D0386** | 0.44 | 1.72 | 0.03 | 2.19 |
| **Facility RVU** | **Work** | **PE** | **MP** | **Total** |
| **D0386** | 0.44 | 1.72 | 0.03 | 2.19 |

| | FUD | Status | MUE | Modifiers | | | | IOM Reference |
|---|---|---|---|---|---|---|---|---|
| **D0386** | N/A | N | - | N/A | N/A | N/A | N/A | None |

* with documentation

## Terms To Know

**professional component.** Portion of a charge for health care services that represents the physician's (or other practitioner's) work in providing the service, including interpretation and report of the procedure. This component of the service usually is charged for and billed separately from the inpatient hospital charges.

**ultrasound.** Imaging using ultra-high sound frequency bounced off body structures.

# D0391

**D0391** interpretation of diagnostic image by a practitioner not associated with capture of the image, including report

## Explanation

The provider interprets of radiological images that are obtained elsewhere and provides a written report of the findings.

## Coding Tips

This code should be used for the interpretation of studies other than cone-beam CT (D0380–D0384), MRI (D0385), or ultrasound (D0386). When the complete procedure is performed, see the appropriate code for the type of imaging study provided. Note, that when reporting with CPT codes, the appropriate CPT code is reported with modifier 26 Professional component, appended. When CT, MRI, or ultrasound image capture only is performed, report the appropriate code for the type of image from the D0380-D0386 range. When the complete procedure is performed (image capture AND interpretation and the reporting of the findings), report the appropriate code from the D0210-D0371 range. When reporting digital subtraction of two or more images (of the same modality), report D0394 in addition to the appropriate code for obtaining the image.

## Reimbursement Tips

When selecting the procedure or service that accurately identifies the service performed, dentists must use the most accurate code. If the CDT code more accurately identifies the service, this should be used rather than the CPT codes. This procedure may be covered by the patient's medical insurance. When covered by medical insurance, the payer may require that the appropriate CPT code be reported on the CMS-1500 claim form. Note that when reporting with CPT codes, the appropriate CPT code (76140) is reported with modifier 26 Professional component, appended.

## Associated CPT Codes

76140 Consultation on X-ray examination made elsewhere, written report

## ICD-10-CM Diagnostic Codes

The application of this code is too broad to adequately present ICD-10-CM diagnostic code links here. Refer to your ICD-10-CM book.

## Relative Value Units/Medicare Edits

| Non-Facility RVU | Work | PE | MP | Total |
|---|---|---|---|---|
| D0391 | 0.86 | 3.35 | 0.06 | 4.27 |
| **Facility RVU** | **Work** | **PE** | **MP** | **Total** |
| D0391 | 0.86 | 3.35 | 0.06 | 4.27 |

| | FUD | Status | MUE | Modifiers | | | | IOM Reference |
|---|---|---|---|---|---|---|---|---|
| D0391 | N/A | N | - | N/A | N/A | N/A | N/A | None |

* with documentation

## Terms To Know

**interpretation.** Professional health care provider's review of data with a written or verbal opinion.

# D0393

**D0393** treatment simulation using 3D image volume

*The use of 3D image volumes for simulation of treatment including, but not limited to, dental implant placement, orthognathic surgery and orthodontic tooth movement.*

## Explanation

A provider uses 3D cone imaging to evaluate relationships between bones, teeth, airways, nerves, and tissues to develop treatment plans. The patient is placed in the upright position and the 3D cone beam imager revolves in a 360 degree circle around the patient gathering the necessary imaging data.

## Coding Tips

To report three-dimensional photographic imaging for diagnostic purposes, see D0351.

## Reimbursement Tips

When selecting the procedure or service that accurately identifies the service performed, dentists must use the most accurate code. If the CDT code more accurately identifies the service, this should be used rather than the CPT codes. Coverage of this procedure varies by payer. Check with the payer for specific coverage guidelines.

## Associated CPT Codes

76376 3D rendering with interpretation and reporting of computed tomography, magnetic resonance imaging, ultrasound, or other tomographic modality with image postprocessing under concurrent supervision; not requiring image postprocessing on an independent workstation

76377 3D rendering with interpretation and reporting of computed tomography, magnetic resonance imaging, ultrasound, or other tomographic modality with image postprocessing under concurrent supervision; requiring image postprocessing on an independent workstation

## ICD-10-CM Diagnostic Codes

The application of this code is too broad to adequately present ICD-10-CM diagnostic code links here. Refer to your ICD-10-CM book.

## Relative Value Units/Medicare Edits

| Non-Facility RVU | Work | PE | MP | Total |
|---|---|---|---|---|
| D0393 | 1.10 | 4.29 | 0.08 | 5.47 |
| **Facility RVU** | **Work** | **PE** | **MP** | **Total** |
| D0393 | 1.10 | 4.29 | 0.08 | 5.47 |

| | FUD | Status | MUE | Modifiers | | | | IOM Reference |
|---|---|---|---|---|---|---|---|---|
| D0393 | N/A | N | - | N/A | N/A | N/A | N/A | None |

* with documentation

## Terms To Know

**imaging.** Radiologic means of producing pictures for clinical study of the internal structures and functions of the body, such as x-ray, ultrasound, magnetic resonance, or positron emission tomography.

**treatment.** Management of patient.

# D0394

**D0394** digital subtraction of two or more images or image volumes of the same modality

*To demonstrate changes that have occurred over time.*

## Explanation

Digital subtraction radiography (DSR) is employed to determine qualitative changes occurring over a period of time. A first baseline image is obtained. After a predetermined period of time, a second image is obtained and compared to the first by subtracting the pixel values from the first image from the pixel values of the second image. Anything that has been unchanged is removed by the process and thusly the changes that have transpired can be observed. DSR images may be used to detect continued disease processes or to demonstrate the effectiveness of the current treatment.

## Coding Tips

To report three-dimensional photographic images of the dental or maxillofacial structures for diagnostic purposes, see D0351.

## Reimbursement Tips

When selecting the procedure or service that accurately identifies the service performed, dentists must use the most accurate code. If the CDT code more accurately identifies the service, this should be used rather than the CPT codes. Coverage of this procedure varies by payer. Check with the payer for specific coverage guidelines.

## Associated CPT Codes

| | |
|---|---|
| 76376 | 3D rendering with interpretation and reporting of computed tomography, magnetic resonance imaging, ultrasound, or other tomographic modality with image postprocessing under concurrent supervision; not requiring image postprocessing on an independent workstation |
| 76377 | 3D rendering with interpretation and reporting of computed tomography, magnetic resonance imaging, ultrasound, or other tomographic modality with image postprocessing under concurrent supervision; requiring image postprocessing on an independent workstation |

## ICD-10-CM Diagnostic Codes

The application of this code is too broad to adequately present ICD-10-CM diagnostic code links here. Refer to your ICD-10-CM book.

## Relative Value Units/Medicare Edits

| Non-Facility RVU | Work | PE | MP | Total |
|---|---|---|---|---|
| D0394 | 0.13 | 0.52 | 0.01 | 0.66 |
| **Facility RVU** | **Work** | **PE** | **MP** | **Total** |
| D0394 | 0.13 | 0.52 | 0.01 | 0.66 |

| | FUD | Status | MUE | Modifiers | | | | IOM Reference |
|---|---|---|---|---|---|---|---|---|
| D0394 | N/A | N | - | N/A | N/A | N/A | N/A | None |

* with documentation

## Terms To Know

**baseline.** Starting point or place of reference from which to base progression or treatment of a condition.

# D0411

**D0411** HbA1c in-office point of service testing

## Explanation

This may also be known as glycosylated A1C. A blood specimen is collected. Glycosylated hemoglobin levels reflect the average level of glucose in the blood over a three-month period. Methods may include high-performance liquid chromatography and ion exchange chromatography or FDA approved home monitoring device.

## Coding Tips

Third-party payers may require that the CPT code (83036 or 83037) be used to report this service. When reported with a CPT code, note that these tests may be performed using a CLIA-waived test system. A national coverage determination (NCD) applies to code 83036. See the *Medicare National Coverage Determinations Manual*, IOM 100-03, section 190.21.

## Reimbursement Tips

When selecting the procedure or service that accurately identifies the service performed, dentists must use the most accurate code. If the CDT code more accurately identifies the service, this should be used rather than the CPT codes. Modifier QW would be appended to code 83036 or 83037 to report a Clinical Laboratory Improvement Amendments (CLIA) approved code when submitting a Medicare claim.

## Associated CPT Codes

| | |
|---|---|
| 83036 | Hemoglobin; glycosylated (A1C) |
| 83037 | Hemoglobin; glycosylated (A1C) by device cleared by FDA for home use |

## ICD-10-CM Diagnostic Codes

| | |
|---|---|
| E10.10 | Type 1 diabetes mellitus with ketoacidosis without coma |
| E10.21 | Type 1 diabetes mellitus with diabetic nephropathy |
| E10.22 | Type 1 diabetes mellitus with diabetic chronic kidney disease |
| E10.29 | Type 1 diabetes mellitus with other diabetic kidney complication |
| E10.3211 | Type 1 diabetes mellitus with mild nonproliferative diabetic retinopathy with macular edema, right eye ☑ |
| E10.3291 | Type 1 diabetes mellitus with mild nonproliferative diabetic retinopathy without macular edema, right eye ☑ |
| E10.3311 | Type 1 diabetes mellitus with moderate nonproliferative diabetic retinopathy with macular edema, right eye ☑ |
| E10.3391 | Type 1 diabetes mellitus with moderate nonproliferative diabetic retinopathy without macular edema, right eye ☑ |
| E10.3411 | Type 1 diabetes mellitus with severe nonproliferative diabetic retinopathy with macular edema, right eye ☑ |
| E10.3491 | Type 1 diabetes mellitus with severe nonproliferative diabetic retinopathy without macular edema, right eye ☑ |
| E10.3511 | Type 1 diabetes mellitus with proliferative diabetic retinopathy with macular edema, right eye ☑ |
| E10.3521 | Type 1 diabetes mellitus with proliferative diabetic retinopathy with traction retinal detachment involving the macula, right eye ☑ |
| E10.3531 | Type 1 diabetes mellitus with proliferative diabetic retinopathy with traction retinal detachment not involving the macula, right eye ☑ |
| E10.3541 | Type 1 diabetes mellitus with proliferative diabetic retinopathy with combined traction retinal detachment and rhegmatogenous retinal detachment, right eye ☑ |

E10.3551 Type 1 diabetes mellitus with stable proliferative diabetic retinopathy, right eye ☑
E10.3591 Type 1 diabetes mellitus with proliferative diabetic retinopathy without macular edema, right eye ☑
E10.36 Type 1 diabetes mellitus with diabetic cataract
E10.37X1 Type 1 diabetes mellitus with diabetic macular edema, resolved following treatment, right eye ☑
E10.39 Type 1 diabetes mellitus with other diabetic ophthalmic complication
E10.41 Type 1 diabetes mellitus with diabetic mononeuropathy
E10.42 Type 1 diabetes mellitus with diabetic polyneuropathy
E10.43 Type 1 diabetes mellitus with diabetic autonomic (poly)neuropathy
E10.44 Type 1 diabetes mellitus with diabetic amyotrophy
E10.49 Type 1 diabetes mellitus with other diabetic neurological complication
E10.51 Type 1 diabetes mellitus with diabetic peripheral angiopathy without gangrene
E10.52 Type 1 diabetes mellitus with diabetic peripheral angiopathy with gangrene
E10.59 Type 1 diabetes mellitus with other circulatory complications
E10.610 Type 1 diabetes mellitus with diabetic neuropathic arthropathy
E10.618 Type 1 diabetes mellitus with other diabetic arthropathy
E10.620 Type 1 diabetes mellitus with diabetic dermatitis
E10.621 Type 1 diabetes mellitus with foot ulcer
E10.622 Type 1 diabetes mellitus with other skin ulcer
E10.628 Type 1 diabetes mellitus with other skin complications
E10.630 Type 1 diabetes mellitus with periodontal disease
E10.638 Type 1 diabetes mellitus with other oral complications
E10.649 Type 1 diabetes mellitus with hypoglycemia without coma
E10.65 Type 1 diabetes mellitus with hyperglycemia
E10.69 Type 1 diabetes mellitus with other specified complication
E10.9 Type 1 diabetes mellitus without complications
E11.00 Type 2 diabetes mellitus with hyperosmolarity without nonketotic hyperglycemic-hyperosmolar coma (NKHHC)
E11.10 Type 2 diabetes mellitus with ketoacidosis without coma
E11.21 Type 2 diabetes mellitus with diabetic nephropathy
E11.22 Type 2 diabetes mellitus with diabetic chronic kidney disease
E11.29 Type 2 diabetes mellitus with other diabetic kidney complication
E11.3211 Type 2 diabetes mellitus with mild nonproliferative diabetic retinopathy with macular edema, right eye ☑
E11.3291 Type 2 diabetes mellitus with mild nonproliferative diabetic retinopathy without macular edema, right eye ☑
E11.3311 Type 2 diabetes mellitus with moderate nonproliferative diabetic retinopathy with macular edema, right eye ☑
E11.3391 Type 2 diabetes mellitus with moderate nonproliferative diabetic retinopathy without macular edema, right eye ☑
E11.3411 Type 2 diabetes mellitus with severe nonproliferative diabetic retinopathy with macular edema, right eye ☑
E11.3491 Type 2 diabetes mellitus with severe nonproliferative diabetic retinopathy without macular edema, right eye ☑
E11.3511 Type 2 diabetes mellitus with proliferative diabetic retinopathy with macular edema, right eye ☑
E11.3521 Type 2 diabetes mellitus with proliferative diabetic retinopathy with traction retinal detachment involving the macula, right eye ☑
E11.3531 Type 2 diabetes mellitus with proliferative diabetic retinopathy with traction retinal detachment not involving the macula, right eye ☑
E11.3541 Type 2 diabetes mellitus with proliferative diabetic retinopathy with combined traction retinal detachment and rhegmatogenous retinal detachment, right eye ☑
E11.3551 Type 2 diabetes mellitus with stable proliferative diabetic retinopathy, right eye ☑
E11.3591 Type 2 diabetes mellitus with proliferative diabetic retinopathy without macular edema, right eye ☑
E11.36 Type 2 diabetes mellitus with diabetic cataract
E11.37X1 Type 2 diabetes mellitus with diabetic macular edema, resolved following treatment, right eye ☑
E11.39 Type 2 diabetes mellitus with other diabetic ophthalmic complication
E11.41 Type 2 diabetes mellitus with diabetic mononeuropathy
E11.42 Type 2 diabetes mellitus with diabetic polyneuropathy
E11.43 Type 2 diabetes mellitus with diabetic autonomic (poly)neuropathy
E11.44 Type 2 diabetes mellitus with diabetic amyotrophy
E11.49 Type 2 diabetes mellitus with other diabetic neurological complication
E11.51 Type 2 diabetes mellitus with diabetic peripheral angiopathy without gangrene
E11.52 Type 2 diabetes mellitus with diabetic peripheral angiopathy with gangrene
E11.59 Type 2 diabetes mellitus with other circulatory complications
E11.610 Type 2 diabetes mellitus with diabetic neuropathic arthropathy
E11.618 Type 2 diabetes mellitus with other diabetic arthropathy
E11.620 Type 2 diabetes mellitus with diabetic dermatitis
E11.621 Type 2 diabetes mellitus with foot ulcer
E11.622 Type 2 diabetes mellitus with other skin ulcer
E11.628 Type 2 diabetes mellitus with other skin complications
E11.630 Type 2 diabetes mellitus with periodontal disease
E11.638 Type 2 diabetes mellitus with other oral complications
E11.649 Type 2 diabetes mellitus with hypoglycemia without coma
E11.65 Type 2 diabetes mellitus with hyperglycemia
E11.69 Type 2 diabetes mellitus with other specified complication
E11.9 Type 2 diabetes mellitus without complications
R73.03 Prediabetes
R73.09 Other abnormal glucose

## Relative Value Units/Medicare Edits

| Non-Facility RVU | Work | PE | MP | Total |
|---|---|---|---|---|
| **D0411** | 0.00 | 0.27 | 0.00 | 0.27 |
| **Facility RVU** | **Work** | **PE** | **MP** | **Total** |
| **D0411** | 0.00 | 0.27 | 0.00 | 0.27 |

| | FUD | Status | MUE | Modifiers | | | | IOM Reference |
|---|---|---|---|---|---|---|---|---|
| **D0411** | N/A | N | - | N/A | N/A | N/A | N/A | None |

* with documentation

# D0412

**D0412** blood glucose level test - in-office using a glucose meter

*This procedure provides an immediate finding of a patient's blood glucose level at the time of sample collection for the point-of-service analysis.*

## Explanation

Also referred to as blood sugar level. This test reports blood glucose monitoring by an FDA-approved device. While the HCPCS device code states that it is for home use, these devices may also be used in the dentist's office. Blood is obtained by finger stick. Method is enzymatic, electrochemical, or spectrophotometry by small portable device designed for home glucose testing.

## Coding Tips

To report the HbA1c, see D0411. Third-party payers may require that 82962 be used to report this service. When reported with a CPT code, note that these tests may be performed using a CLIA-waived test system. A national coverage determination (NCD) applies to 82962. See the *Medicare National Coverage Determinations Manual*, IOM 100-03, section 190.2.

## Reimbursement Tips

When selecting the procedure or service that accurately identifies the service performed, dentists must use the most accurate code. If the CDT code more accurately identifies the service, this should be used rather than the CPT codes. This procedure may be covered by the patient's medical insurance. When covered by medical insurance, the payer may require that CPT code 82962 be reported on the CMS-1500 claim form. Modifier QW may be required.

## Associated CPT Codes

82962 Glucose, blood by glucose monitoring device(s) cleared by the FDA specifically for home use

## ICD-10-CM Diagnostic Codes

E10.10 Type 1 diabetes mellitus with ketoacidosis without coma
E10.21 Type 1 diabetes mellitus with diabetic nephropathy
E10.22 Type 1 diabetes mellitus with diabetic chronic kidney disease
E10.29 Type 1 diabetes mellitus with other diabetic kidney complication
E10.3211 Type 1 diabetes mellitus with mild nonproliferative diabetic retinopathy with macular edema, right eye ☑
E10.3291 Type 1 diabetes mellitus with mild nonproliferative diabetic retinopathy without macular edema, right eye ☑
E10.3311 Type 1 diabetes mellitus with moderate nonproliferative diabetic retinopathy with macular edema, right eye ☑
E10.3391 Type 1 diabetes mellitus with moderate nonproliferative diabetic retinopathy without macular edema, right eye ☑
E10.3411 Type 1 diabetes mellitus with severe nonproliferative diabetic retinopathy with macular edema, right eye ☑
E10.3491 Type 1 diabetes mellitus with severe nonproliferative diabetic retinopathy without macular edema, right eye ☑
E10.3511 Type 1 diabetes mellitus with proliferative diabetic retinopathy with macular edema, right eye ☑
E10.3521 Type 1 diabetes mellitus with proliferative diabetic retinopathy with traction retinal detachment involving the macula, right eye ☑
E10.3531 Type 1 diabetes mellitus with proliferative diabetic retinopathy with traction retinal detachment not involving the macula, right eye ☑
E10.3541 Type 1 diabetes mellitus with proliferative diabetic retinopathy with combined traction retinal detachment and rhegmatogenous retinal detachment, right eye ☑
E10.3551 Type 1 diabetes mellitus with stable proliferative diabetic retinopathy, right eye ☑
E10.3591 Type 1 diabetes mellitus with proliferative diabetic retinopathy without macular edema, right eye ☑
E10.36 Type 1 diabetes mellitus with diabetic cataract
E10.37X1 Type 1 diabetes mellitus with diabetic macular edema, resolved following treatment, right eye ☑
E10.39 Type 1 diabetes mellitus with other diabetic ophthalmic complication
E10.41 Type 1 diabetes mellitus with diabetic mononeuropathy
E10.42 Type 1 diabetes mellitus with diabetic polyneuropathy
E10.43 Type 1 diabetes mellitus with diabetic autonomic (poly)neuropathy
E10.44 Type 1 diabetes mellitus with diabetic amyotrophy
E10.49 Type 1 diabetes mellitus with other diabetic neurological complication
E10.51 Type 1 diabetes mellitus with diabetic peripheral angiopathy without gangrene
E10.52 Type 1 diabetes mellitus with diabetic peripheral angiopathy with gangrene
E10.59 Type 1 diabetes mellitus with other circulatory complications
E10.610 Type 1 diabetes mellitus with diabetic neuropathic arthropathy
E10.618 Type 1 diabetes mellitus with other diabetic arthropathy
E10.620 Type 1 diabetes mellitus with diabetic dermatitis
E10.621 Type 1 diabetes mellitus with foot ulcer
E10.622 Type 1 diabetes mellitus with other skin ulcer
E10.628 Type 1 diabetes mellitus with other skin complications
E10.630 Type 1 diabetes mellitus with periodontal disease
E10.638 Type 1 diabetes mellitus with other oral complications
E10.649 Type 1 diabetes mellitus with hypoglycemia without coma
E10.65 Type 1 diabetes mellitus with hyperglycemia
E10.69 Type 1 diabetes mellitus with other specified complication
E10.9 Type 1 diabetes mellitus without complications
E11.00 Type 2 diabetes mellitus with hyperosmolarity without nonketotic hyperglycemic-hyperosmolar coma (NKHHC)
E11.10 Type 2 diabetes mellitus with ketoacidosis without coma
E11.21 Type 2 diabetes mellitus with diabetic nephropathy
E11.22 Type 2 diabetes mellitus with diabetic chronic kidney disease
E11.29 Type 2 diabetes mellitus with other diabetic kidney complication
E11.3211 Type 2 diabetes mellitus with mild nonproliferative diabetic retinopathy with macular edema, right eye ☑
E11.3291 Type 2 diabetes mellitus with mild nonproliferative diabetic retinopathy without macular edema, right eye ☑
E11.3311 Type 2 diabetes mellitus with moderate nonproliferative diabetic retinopathy with macular edema, right eye ☑
E11.3391 Type 2 diabetes mellitus with moderate nonproliferative diabetic retinopathy without macular edema, right eye ☑
E11.3411 Type 2 diabetes mellitus with severe nonproliferative diabetic retinopathy with macular edema, right eye ☑
E11.3491 Type 2 diabetes mellitus with severe nonproliferative diabetic retinopathy without macular edema, right eye ☑
E11.3511 Type 2 diabetes mellitus with proliferative diabetic retinopathy with macular edema, right eye ☑

| | |
|---|---|
| E11.3521 | Type 2 diabetes mellitus with proliferative diabetic retinopathy with traction retinal detachment involving the macula, right eye ☑ |
| E11.3531 | Type 2 diabetes mellitus with proliferative diabetic retinopathy with traction retinal detachment not involving the macula, right eye ☑ |
| E11.3541 | Type 2 diabetes mellitus with proliferative diabetic retinopathy with combined traction retinal detachment and rhegmatogenous retinal detachment, right eye ☑ |
| E11.3551 | Type 2 diabetes mellitus with stable proliferative diabetic retinopathy, right eye ☑ |
| E11.3591 | Type 2 diabetes mellitus with proliferative diabetic retinopathy without macular edema, right eye ☑ |
| E11.36 | Type 2 diabetes mellitus with diabetic cataract |
| E11.37X1 | Type 2 diabetes mellitus with diabetic macular edema, resolved following treatment, right eye ☑ |
| E11.39 | Type 2 diabetes mellitus with other diabetic ophthalmic complication |
| E11.41 | Type 2 diabetes mellitus with diabetic mononeuropathy |
| E11.42 | Type 2 diabetes mellitus with diabetic polyneuropathy |
| E11.43 | Type 2 diabetes mellitus with diabetic autonomic (poly)neuropathy |
| E11.44 | Type 2 diabetes mellitus with diabetic amyotrophy |
| E11.49 | Type 2 diabetes mellitus with other diabetic neurological complication |
| E11.51 | Type 2 diabetes mellitus with diabetic peripheral angiopathy without gangrene |
| E11.52 | Type 2 diabetes mellitus with diabetic peripheral angiopathy with gangrene |
| E11.59 | Type 2 diabetes mellitus with other circulatory complications |
| E11.610 | Type 2 diabetes mellitus with diabetic neuropathic arthropathy |
| E11.618 | Type 2 diabetes mellitus with other diabetic arthropathy |
| E11.620 | Type 2 diabetes mellitus with diabetic dermatitis |
| E11.621 | Type 2 diabetes mellitus with foot ulcer |
| E11.622 | Type 2 diabetes mellitus with other skin ulcer |
| E11.628 | Type 2 diabetes mellitus with other skin complications |
| E11.630 | Type 2 diabetes mellitus with periodontal disease |
| E11.638 | Type 2 diabetes mellitus with other oral complications |
| E11.649 | Type 2 diabetes mellitus with hypoglycemia without coma |
| E11.65 | Type 2 diabetes mellitus with hyperglycemia |
| E11.69 | Type 2 diabetes mellitus with other specified complication |
| E11.9 | Type 2 diabetes mellitus without complications |
| R73.03 | Prediabetes |
| R73.09 | Other abnormal glucose |

## Relative Value Units/Medicare Edits

| Non-Facility RVU | Work | PE | MP | Total |
|---|---|---|---|---|
| D0412 | 0.00 | 0.27 | 0.00 | 0.27 |
| **Facility RVU** | **Work** | **PE** | **MP** | **Total** |
| D0412 | 0.00 | 0.27 | 0.00 | 0.27 |

| | FUD | Status | MUE | Modifiers | | | | IOM Reference |
|---|---|---|---|---|---|---|---|---|
| D0412 | N/A | N | - | N/A | N/A | N/A | N/A | None |

* with documentation

# D0414-D0416

**D0414** laboratory processing of microbial specimen to include culture and sensitivity studies, preparation and transmission of written report

**D0415** collection of microorganisms for culture and sensitivity

**D0416** viral culture

*A diagnostic test to identify viral organisms, most often herpes virus.*

## Explanation

Samples are collected for diagnostic laboratory analysis to identify pathogens. In D4014, a microbial specimen is processed including culture and sensitivity and a written report must be performed. In D0415, a specimen is collected for bacteriologic examinations to identify a patient's existing infections and the causative organisms. In D0416, specimen is collected to determine if viral infection is present, most commonly herpes virus.

## Coding Tips

This service must include the preparation and transmission of a written report. Any evaluation, radiograph, prophylaxis, fluoride, restorative, or extraction service is reported separately.

## Reimbursement Tips

These procedures are Medicare-covered services if the purpose is to identify a patient's existing infections prior to kidney transplantation. When selecting the procedure or service that accurately identifies the service performed, dentists must use the most accurate code. If the CDT code more accurately identifies the service, this should be used rather than the CPT codes.

## Associated CPT Codes

| | |
|---|---|
| 87070 | Culture, bacterial; any other source except urine, blood or stool, aerobic, with isolation and presumptive identification of isolates |
| 87071 | Culture, bacterial; quantitative, aerobic with isolation and presumptive identification of isolates, any source except urine, blood or stool |
| 87081 | Culture, presumptive, pathogenic organisms, screening only; |
| 87181 | Susceptibility studies, antimicrobial agent; agar dilution method, per agent (eg, antibiotic gradient strip) |
| 87184 | Susceptibility studies, antimicrobial agent; disk method, per plate (12 or fewer agents) |
| 87207 | Smear, primary source with interpretation; special stain for inclusion bodies or parasites (eg, malaria, coccidia, microsporidia, trypanosomes, herpes viruses) |
| 87250 | Virus isolation; inoculation of embryonated eggs, or small animal, includes observation and dissection |
| 87252 | Virus isolation; tissue culture inoculation, observation, and presumptive identification by cytopathic effect |
| 87253 | Virus isolation; tissue culture, additional studies or definitive identification (eg, hemabsorption, neutralization, immunofluorescence stain), each isolate |
| 87254 | Virus isolation; centrifuge enhanced (shell vial) technique, includes identification with immunofluorescence stain, each virus |
| 87255 | Virus isolation; including identification by non-immunologic method, other than by cytopathic effect (eg, virus specific enzymatic activity) |

## ICD-10-CM Diagnostic Codes

The application of this code is too broad to adequately present ICD-10-CM diagnostic code links here. Refer to your ICD-10-CM book.

## Relative Value Units/Medicare Edits

| Non-Facility RVU | Work | PE | MP | Total |
|---|---|---|---|---|
| **D0414** | 0.00 | 0.82 | 0.00 | 0.82 |
| **D0415** | 0.00 | 0.76 | 0.00 | 0.76 |
| **D0416** | 0.00 | 0.87 | 0.00 | 0.87 |
| **Facility RVU** | **Work** | **PE** | **MP** | **Total** |
| **D0414** | 0.00 | 0.82 | 0.00 | 0.82 |
| **D0415** | 0.00 | 0.76 | 0.00 | 0.76 |
| **D0416** | 0.00 | 0.87 | 0.00 | 0.87 |

| | FUD | Status | MUE | Modifiers | | | | IOM Reference |
|---|---|---|---|---|---|---|---|---|
| **D0414** | N/A | N | - | N/A | N/A | N/A | N/A | None |
| **D0415** | N/A | N | - | N/A | N/A | N/A | N/A | |
| **D0416** | N/A | R | - | N/A | N/A | N/A | N/A | |

* with documentation

## Terms To Know

**culture.** Growth of microorganisms in a medium conducive to their development.

**infection.** Presence of microorganisms in body tissues that may result in cellular damage.

**salivary gland.** One of several glands that secrete saliva into the oral cavity.

**sarcoidosis.** Clustering of immune cells resulting in granuloma formation. Often affects the lungs and lymphatic system but can occur in other body sites.

# D0417-D0419

**D0417** collection and preparation of saliva sample for laboratory diagnostic testing

**D0418** analysis of saliva sample

*Chemical or biological analysis of saliva sample for diagnostic purposes.*

**D0419** assessment of salivary flow by measurement

*This procedure is for identification of low salivary flow in patients at risk for hyposalivation and xerostomia, as well as effectiveness of pharmacological agents used to stimulate saliva production.*

## Explanation

The provider performs a salivary flow by measurement to determine the presence of hypofunction. Hypofunction is used as a risk assessment for dental caries and periodontal diseases, diagnosis, and for monitoring high-risk behavior and disease progression. The procedure can be performed either in an unstimulated or stimulated whole saliva measurement. The patient is instructed to swallow at the beginning of the procedure. During a timed period (recommended for at least five minutes), the patient is told not to swallow and to drain any saliva into the funnel and test tube. The saliva is then measured. Stimulated testing should be performed prior to unstimulated saliva collection. The stimulated whole saliva is performed as above with the patient chewing gum base, sucking sugar-free lemon flavored candy, or both. Code D0417 describes the collection and preparation of saliva for testing. Code D0418 describes analysis of saliva to identify systemic disease. Code D0419 describes assessment of salivary flow measurement.

## Coding Tips

This service must include the preparation and transmission of a written report.

## Associated CPT Codes

| | |
|---|---|
| 87070 | Culture, bacterial; any other source except urine, blood or stool, aerobic, with isolation and presumptive identification of isolates |
| 87071 | Culture, bacterial; quantitative, aerobic with isolation and presumptive identification of isolates, any source except urine, blood or stool |
| 87081 | Culture, presumptive, pathogenic organisms, screening only; |
| 87181 | Susceptibility studies, antimicrobial agent; agar dilution method, per agent (eg, antibiotic gradient strip) |
| 87184 | Susceptibility studies, antimicrobial agent; disk method, per plate (12 or fewer agents) |
| 87207 | Smear, primary source with interpretation; special stain for inclusion bodies or parasites (eg, malaria, coccidia, microsporidia, trypanosomes, herpes viruses) |

## ICD-10-CM Diagnostic Codes

| | |
|---|---|
| D11.0 | Benign neoplasm of parotid gland |
| D11.7 | Benign neoplasm of other major salivary glands |
| D11.9 | Benign neoplasm of major salivary gland, unspecified |
| D37.030 | Neoplasm of uncertain behavior of the parotid salivary glands |
| D37.031 | Neoplasm of uncertain behavior of the sublingual salivary glands |
| D37.032 | Neoplasm of uncertain behavior of the submandibular salivary glands |
| D37.039 | Neoplasm of uncertain behavior of the major salivary glands, unspecified |
| D86.89 | Sarcoidosis of other sites |
| K11.20 | Sialoadenitis, unspecified |
| K11.21 | Acute sialoadenitis |
| K11.22 | Acute recurrent sialoadenitis |

K11.23 Chronic sialoadenitis
K11.5 Sialolithiasis
K11.7 Disturbances of salivary secretion
K11.8 Other diseases of salivary glands
K11.9 Disease of salivary gland, unspecified

### Relative Value Units/Medicare Edits

| Non-Facility RVU | Work | PE | MP | Total |
|---|---|---|---|---|
| **D0417** | 0.00 | 0.52 | 0.00 | 0.52 |
| **D0418** | 0.00 | 0.88 | 0.00 | 0.88 |
| **D0419** | 0.00 | 1.53 | 0.00 | 1.53 |
| **Facility RVU** | **Work** | **PE** | **MP** | **Total** |
| **D0417** | 0.00 | 0.52 | 0.00 | 0.52 |
| **D0418** | 0.00 | 0.88 | 0.00 | 0.88 |
| **D0419** | 0.00 | 1.53 | 0.00 | 1.53 |

| | FUD | Status | MUE | Modifiers | | | | IOM Reference |
|---|---|---|---|---|---|---|---|---|
| **D0417** | N/A | N | - | N/A | N/A | N/A | N/A | None |
| **D0418** | N/A | N | - | N/A | N/A | N/A | N/A | |
| **D0419** | N/A | N | - | N/A | N/A | N/A | N/A | |

* with documentation

### Terms To Know

**saliva.** Viscous fluid secreted from the salivary or mucous glands to keep the oral mucous membranes moist and aid in the digestive process.

**salivary gland.** One of several glands that secrete saliva into the oral cavity.

# D0422-D0423

**D0422** collection and preparation of genetic sample material for laboratory analysis and report

**D0423** genetic test for susceptibility to diseases - specimen analysis

*Certified laboratory analysis to detect specific genetic variations associated with increased susceptibility for diseases.*

### Explanation

In D0422, samples are collected for diagnostic laboratory analysis to detect specific genetic variations associated with increased susceptibility for certain oral diseases (i.e., severe periodontal disease). In D0423, testing is done to determine the patient's particular susceptibility to increased susceptibility for diseases.

### Coding Tips

Code D0422 is for the collection and necessary preparation of the material sent to the laboratory. Code D0423 is for the actual analysis of the materials. To report the collection of microorganisms for culture and sensitivity, see code D0415. To report the collection and preparation of saliva sample for diagnostic testing at the laboratory, see D0417.

### Reimbursement Tips

These procedures are Medicare-covered services when the purpose is to identify any existing infections in the patient prior to kidney transplantation.

### Associated CPT Codes

87999 Unlisted microbiology procedure
99000 Handling and/or conveyance of specimen for transfer from the office to a laboratory
99001 Handling and/or conveyance of specimen for transfer from the patient in other than an office to a laboratory (distance may be indicated)

### ICD-10-CM Diagnostic Codes

Z13.71 Encounter for nonprocreative screening for genetic disease carrier status

### Relative Value Units/Medicare Edits

| Non-Facility RVU | Work | PE | MP | Total |
|---|---|---|---|---|
| **D0422** | 0.00 | 0.27 | 0.00 | 0.27 |
| **D0423** | 0.00 | 0.00 | 0.00 | 0.00 |
| **Facility RVU** | **Work** | **PE** | **MP** | **Total** |
| **D0422** | 0.00 | 0.27 | 0.00 | 0.27 |
| **D0423** | 0.00 | 0.00 | 0.00 | 0.00 |

| | FUD | Status | MUE | Modifiers | | | | IOM Reference |
|---|---|---|---|---|---|---|---|---|
| **D0422** | N/A | N | - | N/A | N/A | N/A | N/A | None |
| **D0423** | N/A | N | - | N/A | N/A | N/A | N/A | |

* with documentation

### Terms To Know

**genetic test.** Test that is able to detect a gene mutation, either inherited or caused by the environment.

# D0431

**D0431** adjunctive pre-diagnostic test that aids in detection of mucosal abnormalities including premalignant and malignant lesions, not to include cytology or biopsy procedures

## Explanation

The dentist performs supplementary pre-diagnostic tests that aid in the detection of mucosal abnormalities. In addition to visual inspection of the oral mucosa with special instrumentation (i.e., a luminoscope) after the application of an acetic solution oral rinse may also be performed. Suspicious tissue appears white and can be identified for diagnostic biopsy or brushing. One of the systems also includes a special dye that can be used to highlight other specified types of suspicious tissue. Mucosal abnormalities include leukoplakia (white lesions) and erythroplakia (red lesions), which can be precursors to malignant lesions. Mucosal abnormalities tested also include possible premalignant and malignant lesions. This code reports any supplementary testing that does not have a more specific code. However, D0431 should not be used for cytology studies or biopsy procedures.

## Coding Tips

Report biopsy procedures and cytology separately. Report the appropriate evaluation code in addition to this procedure when supported by the medical record documentation, see codes D0120-D0180. If appropriate, a CPT code from the evaluation and management section may also be reported.

## Reimbursement Tips

When selecting the procedure or service that accurately identifies the service performed, dentists must use the most accurate code. If the CDT code more accurately identifies the service, this should be used rather than the CPT codes. Coverage of this procedure varies by payer. Check with the payer for specific coverage guidelines.

## Associated CPT Codes

| | |
|---|---|
| 82397 | Chemiluminescent assay |

## ICD-10-CM Diagnostic Codes

| | |
|---|---|
| C03.0 | Malignant neoplasm of upper gum |
| C03.1 | Malignant neoplasm of lower gum |
| C04.1 | Malignant neoplasm of lateral floor of mouth |
| C04.8 | Malignant neoplasm of overlapping sites of floor of mouth |
| C05.0 | Malignant neoplasm of hard palate |
| C05.1 | Malignant neoplasm of soft palate |
| C05.2 | Malignant neoplasm of uvula |
| C05.8 | Malignant neoplasm of overlapping sites of palate |
| C06.0 | Malignant neoplasm of cheek mucosa |
| C06.1 | Malignant neoplasm of vestibule of mouth |
| C06.2 | Malignant neoplasm of retromolar area |
| C07 | Malignant neoplasm of parotid gland |
| C08.0 | Malignant neoplasm of submandibular gland |
| C08.1 | Malignant neoplasm of sublingual gland |
| D10.0 | Benign neoplasm of lip |
| D10.1 | Benign neoplasm of tongue |
| D10.2 | Benign neoplasm of floor of mouth |
| D10.39 | Benign neoplasm of other parts of mouth |
| Z01.20 | Encounter for dental examination and cleaning without abnormal findings |
| Z01.21 | Encounter for dental examination and cleaning with abnormal findings |

## Relative Value Units/Medicare Edits

| Non-Facility RVU | Work | PE | MP | Total |
|---|---|---|---|---|
| D0431 | 0.00 | 0.64 | 0.00 | 0.64 |
| **Facility RVU** | **Work** | **PE** | **MP** | **Total** |
| D0431 | 0.00 | 0.64 | 0.00 | 0.64 |

| | FUD | Status | MUE | Modifiers | | | | IOM Reference |
|---|---|---|---|---|---|---|---|---|
| D0431 | N/A | R | - | N/A | N/A | N/A | N/A | None |

* with documentation

## Terms To Know

**cytology.** Examination of cells for pathology, physiology, and chemistry content.

**leukoplakia.** Thickened white patches or lesions appearing on a mucous membrane, such as oral mucosa or tongue.

**malignant.** Any condition tending to progress toward death, specifically an invasive tumor with a loss of cellular differentiation that has the ability to spread or metastasize to other body areas.

**mucosa.** Moist tissue lining the mouth (buccal mucosa), stomach (gastric mucosa), intestines, and respiratory tract.

**submandibular gland.** Salivary gland located beneath the floor of the mouth.

# D0460

**D0460** pulp vitality tests

*Includes multiple teeth and contra lateral comparison(s), as indicated.*

## Explanation

Pulp vitality testing is done to investigate the integrity of the nerve. The suspect tooth is tested with its neighbors and any contralateral comparisons, as needed. Cold may be applied to the tooth with ethyl chloride on a bit of cotton wool. Heat may also be used. An electric pulp tester may be used on a dry tooth with a conductive paste applied. When the canal is full of infected exudate or the nerve supply is damaged but the blood supply is intact, false results may be returned. Percussion may be done by tapping on the suspect tooth with the end of a hand instrument to identify apical abscess or exudate. The pain response may also be elicited by having the patient bite down on rubber.

## Coding Tips

This code includes multiple teeth and contralateral comparison(s) as indicated. This code is considered a stand-alone code by the ADA and may be reported in addition to other endodontic procedures. Any evaluation, radiograph, prophylaxis, fluoride, restorative, or extraction service is reported separately.

## Documentation Tips

The following information can be documented on a tooth chart: treatment/location of caries, endodontic procedures, prosthetic services, preventive services, treatment of lesions and dental disease, or other special procedures.

## Reimbursement Tips

This procedure is a Medicare-covered service if its purpose is to identify a patient's existing infections prior to kidney transplantation.

## ICD-10-CM Diagnostic Codes

| | |
|---|---|
| K02.53 | Dental caries on pit and fissure surface penetrating into pulp |
| K02.63 | Dental caries on smooth surface penetrating into pulp |
| K04.01 | Reversible pulpitis |
| K04.02 | Irreversible pulpitis |
| K04.1 | Necrosis of pulp |
| K04.2 | Pulp degeneration |
| K04.3 | Abnormal hard tissue formation in pulp |
| K04.4 | Acute apical periodontitis of pulpal origin |
| K04.5 | Chronic apical periodontitis |
| K04.6 | Periapical abscess with sinus |
| K04.7 | Periapical abscess without sinus |

## Relative Value Units/Medicare Edits

| Non-Facility RVU | Work | PE | MP | Total |
|---|---|---|---|---|
| D0460 | 0.00 | 0.59 | 0.00 | 0.59 |
| **Facility RVU** | **Work** | **PE** | **MP** | **Total** |
| D0460 | 0.00 | 0.59 | 0.00 | 0.59 |

| | FUD | Status | MUE | Modifiers | | | | IOM Reference |
|---|---|---|---|---|---|---|---|---|
| D0460 | N/A | R | - | N/A | N/A | N/A | 80* | 100-02,1,70; 100-04,4,20.5 |

* with documentation

# D0470

**D0470** diagnostic casts

*Also known as diagnostic models or study models.*

## Explanation

A plaster or stone model of teeth and adjoining tissues is created. Diagnostic casts are an essential tool that allows the dentist to analyze tooth size and shape; alignment and rotation of the teeth; the presence or absence of teeth; arch width, length, form, and symmetry; and the occlusal (bite) relationship. Diagnostic casts assist the dentist in determining the extent and type of orthodontia or other treatment required.

## Coding Tips

Diagnostic casts may also be referred to as diagnostic models or study models.

## Documentation Tips

The following information can be documented on a tooth chart: treatment/location of caries, endodontic procedures, prosthetic services, preventive services, treatment of lesions and dental disease, or other special procedures. A tooth chart may also be used to identify structure and rationale of disease process and the type of service performed on intraoral structures other than teeth.

## Reimbursement Tips

When performed for orthodontia, this service may be processed under orthodontial benefit plans. This service is not covered by Medicare. Some dental plans may apply a patient copayment to this procedure.

## ICD-10-CM Diagnostic Codes

| | |
|---|---|
| K00.1 | Supernumerary teeth |
| K00.2 | Abnormalities of size and form of teeth |
| K00.3 | Mottled teeth |
| K00.4 | Disturbances in tooth formation |
| K00.5 | Hereditary disturbances in tooth structure, not elsewhere classified |
| K00.6 | Disturbances in tooth eruption |
| K00.8 | Other disorders of tooth development |
| K01.0 | Embedded teeth |
| K01.1 | Impacted teeth |
| K03.0 | Excessive attrition of teeth |
| K03.1 | Abrasion of teeth |
| K03.2 | Erosion of teeth |
| K03.3 | Pathological resorption of teeth |
| K03.4 | Hypercementosis |
| K03.5 | Ankylosis of teeth |
| K03.6 | Deposits [accretions] on teeth |
| K03.7 | Posteruptive color changes of dental hard tissues |
| K03.81 | Cracked tooth |
| K03.89 | Other specified diseases of hard tissues of teeth |
| K08.21 | Minimal atrophy of the mandible |
| K08.22 | Moderate atrophy of the mandible |
| K08.23 | Severe atrophy of the mandible |
| K08.24 | Minimal atrophy of maxilla |
| K08.25 | Moderate atrophy of the maxilla |
| K08.26 | Severe atrophy of the maxilla |
| K08.3 | Retained dental root |
| K08.401 | Partial loss of teeth, unspecified cause, class I |

Dental - Diagnostic

| | |
|---|---|
| K08.402 | Partial loss of teeth, unspecified cause, class II |
| K08.403 | Partial loss of teeth, unspecified cause, class III |
| K08.404 | Partial loss of teeth, unspecified cause, class IV |
| K08.411 | Partial loss of teeth due to trauma, class I |
| K08.412 | Partial loss of teeth due to trauma, class II |
| K08.413 | Partial loss of teeth due to trauma, class III |
| K08.414 | Partial loss of teeth due to trauma, class IV |
| K08.421 | Partial loss of teeth due to periodontal diseases, class I |
| K08.422 | Partial loss of teeth due to periodontal diseases, class II |
| K08.423 | Partial loss of teeth due to periodontal diseases, class III |
| K08.424 | Partial loss of teeth due to periodontal diseases, class IV |
| K08.431 | Partial loss of teeth due to caries, class I |
| K08.432 | Partial loss of teeth due to caries, class II |
| K08.433 | Partial loss of teeth due to caries, class III |
| K08.434 | Partial loss of teeth due to caries, class IV |
| K08.491 | Partial loss of teeth due to other specified cause, class I |
| K08.492 | Partial loss of teeth due to other specified cause, class II |
| K08.493 | Partial loss of teeth due to other specified cause, class III |
| K08.494 | Partial loss of teeth due to other specified cause, class IV |
| K08.51 | Open restoration margins of tooth |
| K08.52 | Unrepairable overhanging of dental restorative materials |
| K08.530 | Fractured dental restorative material without loss of material |
| K08.531 | Fractured dental restorative material with loss of material |
| K08.54 | Contour of existing restoration of tooth biologically incompatible with oral health |
| K08.55 | Allergy to existing dental restorative material |
| K08.56 | Poor aesthetic of existing restoration of tooth |
| K08.59 | Other unsatisfactory restoration of tooth |

## Relative Value Units/Medicare Edits

| Non-Facility RVU | Work | PE | MP | Total |
|---|---|---|---|---|
| D0470 | 0.00 | 1.20 | 0.00 | 1.20 |
| **Facility RVU** | **Work** | **PE** | **MP** | **Total** |
| D0470 | 0.00 | 1.20 | 0.00 | 1.20 |

| | FUD | Status | MUE | Modifiers | | | | IOM Reference |
|---|---|---|---|---|---|---|---|---|
| D0470 | N/A | N | - | N/A | N/A | N/A | N/A | None |

* with documentation

## Terms To Know

**cast.** Rigid encasement or dressing molded to the body from a substance that hardens upon drying to hold a body part immobile during the healing period; a model or reproduction made from an impression or mold.

**occlusal.** Biting surfaces of premolar and molar teeth or the areas of contact between opposing teeth in the maxilla and mandible.

**tooth erosion.** Wearing away of a tooth's hard substance by abrasive, not bacterial, forces.

# D0472

**D0472** accession of tissue, gross examination, preparation and transmission of written report

*To be used in reporting architecturally intact tissue obtained by invasive means.*

## Explanation

This procedure may be called a gross pathology exam or gross exam of tissue. The tissue is harvested in the course of a surgery and sent for routine lab evaluation. A gross exam is done on any tissue that the pathologist feels can be accurately diagnosed without a microscopic exam. Tissue is submitted in a container labeled with the source, preoperative or tentative diagnosis, and patient identification information. This code includes preparation and transmission of a written report, but not the removal of the tissue sample itself from the patient.

## Coding Tips

Removal of tissue for examination is reported separately. For biopsy of hard oral tissues (tooth and bone), see D7285. For biopsy of soft oral tissues, see D7286.When microscopic examination is also performed, see D0473. When microscopic examination also includes the assessment of the surgical margin, see D0474. Code D0475 is used to report decalcification procedures although some payers may not allow this code to be reported separately.

## Associated CPT Codes

| | |
|---|---|
| 88300 | Level I - Surgical pathology, gross examination only |

## ICD-10-CM Diagnostic Codes

| | |
|---|---|
| C03.0 | Malignant neoplasm of upper gum |
| C03.1 | Malignant neoplasm of lower gum |
| C04.0 | Malignant neoplasm of anterior floor of mouth |
| C04.1 | Malignant neoplasm of lateral floor of mouth |
| C04.8 | Malignant neoplasm of overlapping sites of floor of mouth |
| C05.0 | Malignant neoplasm of hard palate |
| C05.1 | Malignant neoplasm of soft palate |
| C05.2 | Malignant neoplasm of uvula |
| C05.8 | Malignant neoplasm of overlapping sites of palate |
| C06.0 | Malignant neoplasm of cheek mucosa |
| C06.1 | Malignant neoplasm of vestibule of mouth |
| C06.2 | Malignant neoplasm of retromolar area |
| C07 | Malignant neoplasm of parotid gland |
| C08.0 | Malignant neoplasm of submandibular gland |
| C08.1 | Malignant neoplasm of sublingual gland |

## Relative Value Units/Medicare Edits

| Non-Facility RVU | Work | PE | MP | Total |
|---|---|---|---|---|
| D0472 | 0.00 | 0.88 | 0.00 | 0.88 |
| **Facility RVU** | **Work** | **PE** | **MP** | **Total** |
| D0472 | 0.00 | 0.88 | 0.00 | 0.88 |

| | FUD | Status | MUE | Modifiers | | | | IOM Reference |
|---|---|---|---|---|---|---|---|---|
| D0472 | N/A | R | - | N/A | N/A | N/A | N/A | None |

* with documentation

# D0473

**D0473** accession of tissue, gross and microscopic examination, preparation and transmission of written report

*To be used in reporting architecturally intact tissue obtained by invasive means.*

## Explanation

This examination is a gross and microscopic pathology exam or a gross and microscopic tissue exam. The tissue is harvested in the course of a surgery and sent for routine lab evaluation. Tissue is submitted in a container labeled with the tissue source, preoperative or tentative diagnosis, and patient identification information. Specimens from separate sites must be submitted in separate containers, each labeled with the tissue source. It includes both a gross and microscopic examination with the microscopic exam mainly to confirm the identification or the absence of disease. This code includes preparation and transmission of a written report, but not the removal of the tissue sample itself from the patient.

## Coding Tips

Removal of tissue for examination is reported separately. For biopsy of hard oral tissues (tooth and bone), see D7285. For biopsy of soft oral tissues, see D7286. For oral pathology procedures, see D0472, D0473, D0474, and D0475. When only gross examination is performed, see D0472. When microscopic examination also includes the assessment of the surgical margin see D0474. Code D0475 is used to report decalcification procedures although some payers may not allow this code to be reported separately.

## Documentation Tips

Third-party payers may require clinical documentation such as the pathology report and/or x-rays before making payment determination. Check with the specific payer to determine coverage.

## Associated CPT Codes

| | |
|---|---|
| 88302 | Level II - Surgical pathology, gross and microscopic examination |
| 88304 | Level III - Surgical pathology, gross and microscopic examination |
| 88305 | Level IV - Surgical pathology, gross and microscopic examination |
| 88307 | Level V - Surgical pathology, gross and microscopic examination |

## ICD-10-CM Diagnostic Codes

| | |
|---|---|
| C03.0 | Malignant neoplasm of upper gum |
| C03.1 | Malignant neoplasm of lower gum |
| C03.9 | Malignant neoplasm of gum, unspecified |
| C04.0 | Malignant neoplasm of anterior floor of mouth |
| C04.1 | Malignant neoplasm of lateral floor of mouth |
| C04.8 | Malignant neoplasm of overlapping sites of floor of mouth |
| C04.9 | Malignant neoplasm of floor of mouth, unspecified |
| C05.0 | Malignant neoplasm of hard palate |
| C05.1 | Malignant neoplasm of soft palate |
| C05.2 | Malignant neoplasm of uvula |
| C05.8 | Malignant neoplasm of overlapping sites of palate |
| C05.9 | Malignant neoplasm of palate, unspecified |
| C06.0 | Malignant neoplasm of cheek mucosa |
| C06.1 | Malignant neoplasm of vestibule of mouth |
| C06.2 | Malignant neoplasm of retromolar area |
| C06.9 | Malignant neoplasm of mouth, unspecified |
| C07 | Malignant neoplasm of parotid gland |
| C08.0 | Malignant neoplasm of submandibular gland |
| C08.1 | Malignant neoplasm of sublingual gland |
| C08.9 | Malignant neoplasm of major salivary gland, unspecified |

## Relative Value Units/Medicare Edits

| Non-Facility RVU | Work | PE | MP | Total |
|---|---|---|---|---|
| D0473 | 0.00 | 1.65 | 0.00 | 1.65 |
| **Facility RVU** | **Work** | **PE** | **MP** | **Total** |
| D0473 | 0.00 | 1.65 | 0.00 | 1.65 |

| | FUD | Status | MUE | Modifiers | | | | IOM Reference |
|---|---|---|---|---|---|---|---|---|
| D0473 | N/A | R | - | N/A | N/A | N/A | N/A | None |

* with documentation

## Terms To Know

**accession.** Process of identifying a specimen and entering a unique specimen identifier into laboratory records.

**gross.** Macroscopic, as in gross pathology; the study of tissue changes without magnification by microscope.

**tissue.** Group of similar cells with a similar function that form definite structures and organs. Tissue types include epithelial tissue, muscle tissue, connective tissue, and nervous tissue.

# D0474

**D0474** accession of tissue, gross and microscopic examination, including assessment of surgical margins for presence of disease, preparation and transmission of written report

*To be used in reporting architecturally intact tissue obtained by invasive means.*

## Explanation

This examination is a gross and microscopic pathology exam or a gross and microscopic tissue exam with the evaluation of surgical margins for the presence of disease. The tissue is harvested in the course of a surgery and sent for routine lab evaluation. Tissue is submitted in a container labeled with the tissue source, preoperative or tentative diagnosis, and patient identification information. Specimens from separate sites must be submitted in separate containers, each labeled with the tissue source. It includes both a gross and microscopic examination and an additional level of evaluation to determine whether the margins of the surgically excised tissue present with disease or have been removed clear of disease. This code includes preparation and transmission of a written report, but not the removal of the tissue sample itself from the patient.

## Coding Tips

Removal of tissue for examination is reported separately. For biopsy of hard oral tissues (tooth and bone), see D7285. For biopsy of soft oral tissues, see D7286. Third-party payers may require clinical documentation, such as a pathology report and/or x-rays before making payment determination. Check with payers to determine their specific requirements. Report code D0472 when only a gross examination is performed. When microscopic examination without margin assessment is performed, see D0473. Code D0475 is used to report decalcification procedures although some payers may not allow this code to be reported separately.

## Documentation Tips

Third-party payers may require clinical documentation such as the pathology report and/or x-rays before making payment determination. Check with the specific payer to determine coverage.

## Associated CPT Codes

88305 Level IV - Surgical pathology, gross and microscopic examination
88307 Level V - Surgical pathology, gross and microscopic examination
88309 Level VI - Surgical pathology, gross and microscopic examination

## ICD-10-CM Diagnostic Codes

C03.0 Malignant neoplasm of upper gum
C03.1 Malignant neoplasm of lower gum
C03.9 Malignant neoplasm of gum, unspecified
C04.0 Malignant neoplasm of anterior floor of mouth
C04.1 Malignant neoplasm of lateral floor of mouth
C04.8 Malignant neoplasm of overlapping sites of floor of mouth
C04.9 Malignant neoplasm of floor of mouth, unspecified
C05.0 Malignant neoplasm of hard palate
C05.1 Malignant neoplasm of soft palate
C05.2 Malignant neoplasm of uvula
C05.8 Malignant neoplasm of overlapping sites of palate
C05.9 Malignant neoplasm of palate, unspecified
C06.0 Malignant neoplasm of cheek mucosa
C06.1 Malignant neoplasm of vestibule of mouth
C06.2 Malignant neoplasm of retromolar area
C06.9 Malignant neoplasm of mouth, unspecified
C07 Malignant neoplasm of parotid gland
C08.0 Malignant neoplasm of submandibular gland
C08.1 Malignant neoplasm of sublingual gland
C08.9 Malignant neoplasm of major salivary gland, unspecified

## Relative Value Units/Medicare Edits

| Non-Facility RVU | Work | PE | MP | Total |
|---|---|---|---|---|
| D0474 | 0.00 | 1.88 | 0.00 | 1.88 |
| **Facility RVU** | **Work** | **PE** | **MP** | **Total** |
| D0474 | 0.00 | 1.88 | 0.00 | 1.88 |

| | FUD | Status | MUE | Modifiers | | | | IOM Reference |
|---|---|---|---|---|---|---|---|---|
| D0474 | N/A | R | - | N/A | N/A | N/A | N/A | None |

* with documentation

## Terms To Know

**accession.** Process of identifying a specimen and entering a unique specimen identifier into laboratory records.

**gross.** Macroscopic, as in gross pathology; the study of tissue changes without magnification by microscope.

**tissue.** Group of similar cells with a similar function that form definite structures and organs. Tissue types include epithelial tissue, muscle tissue, connective tissue, and nervous tissue.

# D0475

**D0475** decalcification procedure

*Procedure in which hard tissue is processed in order to allow sectioning and subsequent microscopic examination.*

## Explanation

Calcium or calcifications from a laboratory specimen are removed. It is generally performed in conjunction with the definitive laboratory test. The decalcification procedure may be considered integral to the laboratory service being performed and payers may not allow separate payment for decalcification procedures.

## Coding Tips

This code does not include the removal of tissue sample from the patient; see D7285 and D7286. Separate payment may not be allowed for this code, as it may be considered integral to the laboratory/pathology service being performed. When microscopic examination is also performed, see D0473. When microscopic examination also includes the assessment of the surgical margin, see D0474. To report enamel microabrasion, see D9970. The removal of calculus, plaque, and/or stains from tooth structures is reported using D1110-D1120.

## Reimbursement Tips

Some payers may require that the pathology report be attached to the claim. This service is not covered by Medicare. Some dental plans may apply a patient copayment to this procedure.

## Associated CPT Codes

88311 Decalcification procedure (List separately in addition to code for surgical pathology examination)

## ICD-10-CM Diagnostic Codes

Z01.20 Encounter for dental examination and cleaning without abnormal findings

Z98.811 Dental restoration status

Z98.818 Other dental procedure status

## Relative Value Units/Medicare Edits

| Non-Facility RVU | Work | PE | MP | Total |
|---|---|---|---|---|
| D0475 | 0.00 | 1.29 | 0.00 | 1.29 |
| **Facility RVU** | **Work** | **PE** | **MP** | **Total** |
| D0475 | 0.00 | 1.29 | 0.00 | 1.29 |

| | FUD | Status | MUE | Modifiers | | | | IOM Reference |
|---|---|---|---|---|---|---|---|---|
| D0475 | N/A | R | - | N/A | N/A | N/A | N/A | None |

* with documentation

## Terms To Know

**biopsy.** Tissue or fluid removed for diagnostic purposes through analysis of the cells in the biopsy material.

**calcification.** Normal process of calcium salts deposition in bone.

# D0476-D0477

**D0476** special stains for microorganisms

*Procedure in which additional stains are applied to biopsy or surgical specimen in order to identify microorganisms.*

**D0477** special stains, not for microorganisms

*Procedure in which additional stains are applied to a biopsy or surgical specimen in order to identify such things as melanin, mucin, iron, glycogen, etc.*

## Explanation

The provider stains tissue or other laboratory specimens to aid in the diagnosis of the patient's condition. Depending on the type of specimen and the reason for the laboratory or pathology examination, different stains may be required to highlight or outline the microorganism or cells for identification. Code D0476 reports the use of chemical dye stains that localize to microorganisms found in tissue or other laboratory specimens. Special stains for microorganisms are used to assist in the diagnosis of infectious diseases. Alcian yellow, Giemsa, GMS, PAS, and Brown & Brenn are examples of special stains for microorganisms. For code D0477, chemical dye stains that localize to specific cell types, such as cancer cells found in tissue samples or other laboratory specimens are used.

## Coding Tips

Code D0477 may be performed in order to identify substances such as glycogen, iron, melanin, mucin, etc. These codes do not include the removal of tissue sample from the patient; see D7285 and D7286. These codes do not include the removal of tissue sample from the patient; see D7285 and D7286. To report immunohistochemical stains, see D0478.

## Reimbursement Tips

Separate payment may not be allowed for these codes, as they may be considered integral to the laboratory/pathology service being performed. Some payers may require that the pathology report be attached to the claim.

## Associated CPT Codes

87207 Smear, primary source with interpretation; special stain for inclusion bodies or parasites (eg, malaria, coccidia, microsporidia, trypanosomes, herpes viruses)

87209 Smear, primary source with interpretation; complex special stain (eg, trichrome, iron hemotoxylin) for ova and parasites

88312 Special stain including interpretation and report; Group I for microorganisms (eg, acid fast, methenamine silver)

88313 Special stain including interpretation and report; Group II, all other (eg, iron, trichrome), except stain for microorganisms, stains for enzyme constituents, or immunocytochemistry and immunohistochemistry

## ICD-10-CM Diagnostic Codes

Z01.20 Encounter for dental examination and cleaning without abnormal findings

Z98.811 Dental restoration status

Z98.818 Other dental procedure status

## Relative Value Units/Medicare Edits

| Non-Facility RVU | Work | PE | MP | Total |
|---|---|---|---|---|
| D0476 | 0.00 | 1.61 | 0.00 | 1.61 |
| D0477 | 0.00 | 1.89 | 0.00 | 1.89 |
| **Facility RVU** | **Work** | **PE** | **MP** | **Total** |
| D0476 | 0.00 | 1.61 | 0.00 | 1.61 |
| D0477 | 0.00 | 1.89 | 0.00 | 1.89 |

| | FUD | Status | MUE | Modifiers | | | | IOM Reference |
|---|---|---|---|---|---|---|---|---|
| D0476 | N/A | R | - | N/A | N/A | N/A | N/A | None |
| D0477 | N/A | R | - | N/A | N/A | N/A | N/A | |

* with documentation

# D0478

**D0478** immunohistochemical stains

*A procedure in which specific antibody based reagents are applied to tissue samples in order to facilitate diagnosis.*

## Explanation

Immunohistochemical (IHC) stains are special stains used to identify antibody-antigen interactions and chemical components or activities in cells or tissues.

## Coding Tips

This code does not include the removal of tissue sample from the patient; see D7285 and D7286. To report special stains either for microorganisms or for other reasons, see D0476-D0477, respectively.

## Reimbursement Tips

Separate payment may not be allowed for this code, as it may be considered integral to the laboratory/pathology service being performed. Some payers may require that the pathology report be attached to the claim.

## Associated CPT Codes

88312 Special stain including interpretation and report; Group I for microorganisms (eg, acid fast, methenamine silver)

88313 Special stain including interpretation and report; Group II, all other (eg, iron, trichrome), except stain for microorganisms, stains for enzyme constituents, or immunocytochemistry and immunohistochemistry

88314 Special stain including interpretation and report; histochemical stain on frozen tissue block (List separately in addition to code for primary procedure)

## ICD-10-CM Diagnostic Codes

Z01.20 Encounter for dental examination and cleaning without abnormal findings

Z98.811 Dental restoration status

Z98.818 Other dental procedure status

## Relative Value Units/Medicare Edits

| Non-Facility RVU | Work | PE | MP | Total |
|---|---|---|---|---|
| D0478 | 0.00 | 1.34 | 0.00 | 1.34 |
| **Facility RVU** | **Work** | **PE** | **MP** | **Total** |
| D0478 | 0.00 | 1.34 | 0.00 | 1.34 |

| | FUD | Status | MUE | Modifiers | | | | IOM Reference |
|---|---|---|---|---|---|---|---|---|
| D0478 | N/A | R | - | N/A | N/A | N/A | N/A | None |

* with documentation

## Terms To Know

**antibody.** Immunoglobulin or protective protein encoded within its building block sequence to interact only with its specific antigen.

**antigen.** Substance inducing sensitivity or triggering an immune response and the production of antibodies.

# D0479

**D0479** tissue in-situ hybridization, including interpretation

*A procedure which allows for the identification of nucleic acids, DNA and RNA, in the tissue sample in order to aid in the diagnosis of microorganisms and tumors.*

## Explanation

This test is also known as DNA-to-DNA homology, or simply ISH. In situ hybridization involves isolating and detecting specific nucleotide (mRNA) sequences within morphologically preserved cells and tissues by hybridizing a complementary nucleic acid strand, called a probe, to the sequence of interest within the prepared cells. The cells of interest may be snap-frozen and fixed in paraformaldehyde, spun out of suspension onto glass slides and fixed with methanol, or fixed in formalin and embedded in paraffin. The probe is first labeled with an easily detectable substance, such as a radioactive isotope, before hybridization. Types of probes used are oligonucleotides, single-stranded DNA, double-stranded DNA, and RNA, or riboprobes. The labeled probe strand is added to the prepared cells. The pairing or bonding (hybridization) that occurs between the complementary sequences of nucleotide bases in the probe to the specific mRNA sequences allows the expression of the type of sequence being detected to be seen on the target gene. This code is reported once for each type of probe used.

## Coding Tips

Report this code once for each type of probe used. This code includes interpretation, but does not include the removal of tissue sample from the patient; see D7285 and D7286.

## Reimbursement Tips

Separate payment may not be allowed for this code, as it may be considered integral to the laboratory/pathology service being performed. Some payers may require that the pathology report be attached to the claim.

## ICD-10-CM Diagnostic Codes

Z01.89 Encounter for other specified special examinations

## Relative Value Units/Medicare Edits

| Non-Facility RVU | Work | PE | MP | Total |
|---|---|---|---|---|
| D0479 | 0.00 | 2.04 | 0.00 | 2.04 |
| **Facility RVU** | **Work** | **PE** | **MP** | **Total** |
| D0479 | 0.00 | 2.04 | 0.00 | 2.04 |

| | FUD | Status | MUE | Modifiers | | | | IOM Reference |
|---|---|---|---|---|---|---|---|---|
| D0479 | N/A | R | - | N/A | N/A | N/A | N/A | None |

* with documentation

## Terms To Know

**DNA.** Deoxyribonucleic acid.

**in situ.** Located in the natural position or contained within the origin site, not spread into neighboring tissue.

**tissue.** Group of similar cells with a similar function that form definite structures and organs. Tissue types include epithelial tissue, muscle tissue, connective tissue, and nervous tissue.

# D0480-D0483

**D0480** accession of exfoliative cytologic smears, microscopic examination, preparation and transmission of written report

*To be used in reporting disaggregated, non-transepithelial cell cytology sample via mild scraping of the oral mucosa.*

**D0481** electron microscopy

**D0482** direct immunofluorescence

*A technique used to identify immunoreactants which are localized to the patient's skin or mucous membranes.*

**D0483** indirect immunofluorescence

*A technique used to identify circulating immunoreactants.*

## Explanation

These codes report cytopathology analysis for oral tissue. The specimen is obtained by a separate procedure. The specimen is collected and processed in a spray or liquid fixative smear or direct smear. Screening, defined as the careful review of the specimen for abnormal cells, may then be accomplished by methods involving the use of automated systems. Code D0480 includes the processing and interpretation of the smears and the preparation and transmission of a written report. Code D0481 includes examination under extreme magnification enabling identification of cell components and microorganisms that are otherwise not identifiable under microscopy. Code D0482 identifies immunoreactants that are localized to skin or mucous membranes and D0483 identifies circulating immunoreactants.

## Coding Tips

Code D0480 is an out-of-sequence code and will not display in numeric order in the CDT manual. Removal of tissue for examination is reported separately. For collection of oral cytology sample by mild scraping of the oral mucosa, see D7287.

## Reimbursement Tips

Third-party payers may require clinical documentation, such as a pathology report and/or x-rays before making payment determination. Check with payers to determine their specific requirements.

## Associated CPT Codes

88104 Cytopathology, fluids, washings or brushings, except cervical or vaginal; smears with interpretation

88112 Cytopathology, selective cellular enhancement technique with interpretation (eg, liquid based slide preparation method), except cervical or vaginal

88346 Immunofluorescence, per specimen; initial single antibody stain procedure

88348 Electron microscopy, diagnostic

## ICD-10-CM Diagnostic Codes

C03.0 Malignant neoplasm of upper gum

C03.1 Malignant neoplasm of lower gum

C04.0 Malignant neoplasm of anterior floor of mouth

C04.1 Malignant neoplasm of lateral floor of mouth

C04.8 Malignant neoplasm of overlapping sites of floor of mouth

C05.0 Malignant neoplasm of hard palate

C05.1 Malignant neoplasm of soft palate

C05.2 Malignant neoplasm of uvula

C05.8 Malignant neoplasm of overlapping sites of palate

C06.0 Malignant neoplasm of cheek mucosa

| | |
|---|---|
| C06.1 | Malignant neoplasm of vestibule of mouth |
| C06.2 | Malignant neoplasm of retromolar area |
| C07 | Malignant neoplasm of parotid gland |
| C08.0 | Malignant neoplasm of submandibular gland |
| C08.1 | Malignant neoplasm of sublingual gland |

## Relative Value Units/Medicare Edits

| Non-Facility RVU | Work | PE | MP | Total |
|---|---|---|---|---|
| **D0480** | 0.00 | 1.31 | 0.00 | 1.31 |
| **D0481** | 0.00 | 3.76 | 0.00 | 3.76 |
| **D0482** | 0.00 | 1.33 | 0.00 | 1.33 |
| **D0483** | 0.00 | 1.40 | 0.00 | 1.40 |
| **Facility RVU** | **Work** | **PE** | **MP** | **Total** |
| **D0480** | 0.00 | 1.31 | 0.00 | 1.31 |
| **D0481** | 0.00 | 3.76 | 0.00 | 3.76 |
| **D0482** | 0.00 | 1.33 | 0.00 | 1.33 |
| **D0483** | 0.00 | 1.40 | 0.00 | 1.40 |

| | FUD | Status | MUE | Modifiers | | | | IOM Reference |
|---|---|---|---|---|---|---|---|---|
| **D0480** | N/A | R | - | N/A | N/A | N/A | N/A | None |
| **D0481** | N/A | R | - | N/A | N/A | N/A | N/A | |
| **D0482** | N/A | R | - | N/A | N/A | N/A | N/A | |
| **D0483** | N/A | R | - | N/A | N/A | N/A | N/A | |

* with documentation

### Terms To Know

**tissue.** Group of similar cells with a similar function that form definite structures and organs. Tissue types include epithelial tissue, muscle tissue, connective tissue, and nervous tissue.

# D0484-D0485

**D0484** consultation on slides prepared elsewhere

*A service provided in which microscopic slides of a biopsy specimen prepared at another laboratory are evaluated to aid in the diagnosis of a difficult case or to offer a consultative opinion at the patient's request. The findings are delivered by written report.*

**D0485** consultation, including preparation of slides from biopsy material supplied by referring source

*A service that requires the consulting pathologist to prepare the slides as well as render a written report. The slides are evaluated to aid in the diagnosis of a difficult case or to offer a consultative opinion at the patient's request.*

### Explanation

A pathology consultation involves an opinion or advice on the presence or absence of diseased or abnormal tissue provided at the request of another dentist. In D0484, the requesting dentist prepares the slides and the consulting dentist provides an interpretation with a written report. In D0485, the slides require routine preparation by the consulting dentist who also provides an interpretation with a written report.

### Coding Tips

Code D0484 pertains to biopsy specimen slides prepared at another laboratory. Code D0485 pertains to biopsy specimen slides that are prepared by the consulting pathologist. These codes do not include removal of tissue sample from the patient; see D7285 and D7286. To report a diagnostic consult by the dentist at the request of another dentist or physician, see D9310.

### Reimbursement Tips

This procedure may be covered by the patient's medical insurance. When covered by medical insurance, the payer may require that the appropriate CPT code be reported on the CMS-1500 claim form.

### Associated CPT Codes

| | |
|---|---|
| 88321 | Consultation and report on referred slides prepared elsewhere |
| 88323 | Consultation and report on referred material requiring preparation of slides |

### ICD-10-CM Diagnostic Codes

| | |
|---|---|
| C03.0 | Malignant neoplasm of upper gum |
| C03.1 | Malignant neoplasm of lower gum |
| C04.0 | Malignant neoplasm of anterior floor of mouth |
| C04.1 | Malignant neoplasm of lateral floor of mouth |
| C04.8 | Malignant neoplasm of overlapping sites of floor of mouth |
| C05.0 | Malignant neoplasm of hard palate |
| C05.1 | Malignant neoplasm of soft palate |
| C05.2 | Malignant neoplasm of uvula |
| C05.8 | Malignant neoplasm of overlapping sites of palate |
| C06.0 | Malignant neoplasm of cheek mucosa |
| C06.1 | Malignant neoplasm of vestibule of mouth |
| C06.2 | Malignant neoplasm of retromolar area |
| C07 | Malignant neoplasm of parotid gland |
| C08.0 | Malignant neoplasm of submandibular gland |
| C08.1 | Malignant neoplasm of sublingual gland |

## Relative Value Units/Medicare Edits

| Non-Facility RVU | Work | PE | MP | Total |
|---|---|---|---|---|
| **D0484** | 0.00 | 2.06 | 0.00 | 2.06 |
| **D0485** | 0.00 | 2.73 | 0.00 | 2.73 |
| **Facility RVU** | **Work** | **PE** | **MP** | **Total** |
| **D0484** | 0.00 | 2.06 | 0.00 | 2.06 |
| **D0485** | 0.00 | 2.73 | 0.00 | 2.73 |

| | FUD | Status | MUE | Modifiers | | | | IOM Reference |
|---|---|---|---|---|---|---|---|---|
| **D0484** | N/A | R | - | N/A | N/A | N/A | N/A | None |
| **D0485** | N/A | R | - | N/A | N/A | N/A | N/A | |

* with documentation

## Terms To Know

**consultation.** Advice or opinion regarding diagnosis and treatment or determination to accept transfer of care of a patient rendered by a medical professional at the request of the primary care provider.

**laboratory.** Facility for the virological, microbiological, serological, chemical, immunohematological, hematological, biophysical, cytological, pathological, or other examination of materials derived from the human body for the purpose of providing information for the diagnosis, prevention, or treatment of any disease or impairment of or the assessment of the health of human beings. These examinations also include procedures to determine, measure, or otherwise describe the presence or absence of various substances or organisms in the body. Facilities that only collect or prepare specimens (or both) or act only as a mailing service and do not perform tests are not considered laboratories.

# D0486

**D0486** laboratory accession of transepithelial cytologic sample, microscopic examination, preparation and transmission of written report

*Analysis, and written report of findings, of cytologic sample of disaggregated transepithelial cells.*



## Explanation

Pathological analysis of a cytologic sample for the presence or absence of diseased or abnormal tissue is performed. The sample is examined microscopically and a written report is provided.

## Coding Tips

This is an out-of-sequence code and will not display in numeric order in the CDT manual. This code does not include the removal of the tissue sample from the patient. To report the accession of exfoliative cytologic smears including microscopic examination and the preparation and transmission of a written report, see D0480.

## Reimbursement Tips

This procedure may be covered by the patient's medical insurance. When covered by medical insurance, the payer may require that the appropriate CPT code be reported on the CMS-1500 claim form. When reporting code D0486, some third-party payers may require clinical documentation, such as the pathology report and/or x-rays before making payment determination. Check with payers to determine their specific requirements.

## Associated CPT Codes

88160 Cytopathology, smears, any other source; screening and interpretation

88161 Cytopathology, smears, any other source; preparation, screening and interpretation

88162 Cytopathology, smears, any other source; extended study involving over 5 slides and/or multiple stains

## ICD-10-CM Diagnostic Codes

The application of this code is too broad to adequately present ICD-10-CM diagnostic code links here. Refer to your ICD-10-CM book.

## Relative Value Units/Medicare Edits

| Non-Facility RVU | Work | PE | MP | Total |
|---|---|---|---|---|
| **D0486** | 0.00 | 1.45 | 0.00 | 1.45 |
| **Facility RVU** | **Work** | **PE** | **MP** | **Total** |
| **D0486** | 0.00 | 1.45 | 0.00 | 1.45 |

| | FUD | Status | MUE | Modifiers | | | | IOM Reference |
|---|---|---|---|---|---|---|---|---|
| **D0486** | N/A | N | - | N/A | N/A | N/A | N/A | None |

* with documentation

## Terms To Know

**cytology.** Examination of cells for pathology, physiology, and chemistry content.

# D0502

**D0502** other oral pathology procedures, by report

## Explanation

This code is used to report oral pathology procedures that have not been assigned a more specific code. Unspecified procedure codes always require submission of a detailed report of the service or procedure provided by the dentist.

## Coding Tips

Report this code for pathology procedures performed on oral tissue samples for which there is no more specific code. Pertinent documentation to evaluate medical appropriateness should be included when this code is reported

## Reimbursement Tips

In some instances, a CPT code may be required to indicate the specific service provided, check third-party payer guidelines before assigning CPT codes. Medicare covers this procedure if its purpose is to identify a patient's existing infections prior to kidney transplantation. Some payers may require that the pathology report be attached to the claim.

## ICD-10-CM Diagnostic Codes

Z12.81 Encounter for screening for malignant neoplasm of oral cavity
Z13.810 Encounter for screening for upper gastrointestinal disorder

## Relative Value Units/Medicare Edits

| Non-Facility RVU | Work | PE | MP | Total |
|---|---|---|---|---|
| D0502 | 0.00 | 1.48 | 0.00 | 1.48 |
| Facility RVU | Work | PE | MP | Total |
| D0502 | 0.00 | 1.48 | 0.00 | 1.48 |

| | FUD | Status | MUE | Modifiers | | | | IOM Reference |
|---|---|---|---|---|---|---|---|---|
| D0502 | N/A | R | - | N/A | N/A | N/A | 80* | 100-03,260.6 |

* with documentation

## Terms To Know

**pathology.** Medical science, and specialty practice, regarding all aspects of disease, with special reference to the essential nature, causes, and development of abnormal conditions, as well as the structural and functional changes that result from the disease processes.

**specimen.** Tissue cells or sample of fluid taken for analysis, pathologic examination, and diagnosis.

**unlisted procedure.** Procedural descriptions used when the overall procedure and outcome of the procedure are not adequately described by an existing procedure code. Such codes are used as a last resort and only when there is not a more appropriate procedure code.

# D0600

**D0600** non-ionizing diagnostic procedure capable of quantifying, monitoring, and recording changes in structure of enamel, dentin, and cementum

## Explanation

The dentist, utilizing a portable caries detection device using transillumination technology, examines teeth for the identification of occlusal, interproximal, and recurrent carious lesions (caries) and/or cracks that cannot be diagnosed clinically or radiographically. There are a number of devices currently on the market with some using lasers that result in fluorescence of the mineral structure of the tooth. Other devices use transillumination to visualize through the enamel.

## Coding Tips

Report clinical oral evaluations using D0120–D0170. To report caries risk assessment, see D0601–D0603. To report diagnostic x-ray examination, see D0210–D0274.

## Documentation Tips

Medical record documentation must include all findings including changes in structure of enamel, dentin, and cementum.

## Reimbursement Tips

Third-party payers may consider this service as a limiting service and do not cover this service. Check with third-party payers prior to providing the service.

## ICD-10-CM Diagnostic Codes

K02.3 Arrested dental caries
K02.51 Dental caries on pit and fissure surface limited to enamel
K02.52 Dental caries on pit and fissure surface penetrating into dentin
K02.53 Dental caries on pit and fissure surface penetrating into pulp
K02.61 Dental caries on smooth surface limited to enamel
K02.62 Dental caries on smooth surface penetrating into dentin
K02.63 Dental caries on smooth surface penetrating into pulp
K02.7 Dental root caries

## Relative Value Units/Medicare Edits

| Non-Facility RVU | Work | PE | MP | Total |
|---|---|---|---|---|
| D0600 | 0.00 | 0.00 | 0.00 | 0.00 |
| Facility RVU | Work | PE | MP | Total |
| D0600 | 0.00 | 0.00 | 0.00 | 0.00 |

| | FUD | Status | MUE | Modifiers | | | | IOM Reference |
|---|---|---|---|---|---|---|---|---|
| D0600 | N/A | R | - | N/A | N/A | N/A | N/A | None |

* with documentation

## Terms To Know

**caries.** Localized section of tooth decay that begins on the tooth surface with destruction of the calcified enamel, allowing bacterial destruction to continue and form cavities and may extend to the dentin and pulp.

**cavity.** Tooth decay.

**noncovered procedure.** Health care treatment not reimbursable according to provisions of a given insurance policy, or in the case of Medicare, in accordance with Medicare laws and regulations.

# D0601-D0603

**D0601** caries risk assessment and documentation, with a finding of low risk

*Using recognized assessment tools.*

**D0602** caries risk assessment and documentation, with a finding of moderate risk

*Using recognized assessment tools.*

**D0603** caries risk assessment and documentation, with a finding of high risk

*Using recognized assessment tools.*

## Explanation

Using a standardized risk assessment tool, the provider evaluates the patient's level of risk for developing caries. Assessments and level of risk vary based on the age of the patient but include such factors as fluoride exposure, dietary risks, general health conditions, and dental clinical conditions including but not limited to visible plaque, xerostomia, dental/orthodontic appliances, and unusual tooth morphology. Report D0601 when the level of risk is low, D0602 when the level of risk is moderate, and D0603 when the level of risk is determined to be high.

## Coding Tips

These are out of sequence codes and will not display in numeric order in the CDT manual. After review of the assessment tool, the level of risk may be increased or decreased dependent upon clinical judgment and the review of other pertinent information. Documentation as to the reason for the revised level of risk should be recorded in the medical record. To report nutritional counseling, see D1310. To report oral hygiene counseling, see D1330. To report caries susceptibility testing, see D0425. Coverage of this procedure varies by payer. Check with payers for their specific coverage guidelines.

## Documentation Tips

After review of the assessment tool, the level of risk may be increased or decreased dependent upon clinical judgment and the review of other pertinent information. Documentation as to the reason for the revised level of risk should be recorded in the medical record.

## Reimbursement Tips

Coverage of this procedure varies by payer. Check with the payer for specific coverage guidelines.

## ICD-10-CM Diagnostic Codes

| | |
|---|---|
| Z01.20 | Encounter for dental examination and cleaning without abnormal findings |
| Z01.21 | Encounter for dental examination and cleaning with abnormal findings |
| Z71.3 | Dietary counseling and surveillance |
| Z91.841 | Risk for dental caries, low |
| Z91.842 | Risk for dental caries, moderate |
| Z91.843 | Risk for dental caries, high |

## Relative Value Units/Medicare Edits

| Non-Facility RVU | Work | PE | MP | Total |
|---|---|---|---|---|
| **D0601** | 0.00 | 0.16 | 0.00 | 0.16 |
| **D0602** | 0.00 | 0.16 | 0.00 | 0.16 |
| **D0603** | 0.00 | 0.16 | 0.00 | 0.16 |
| **Facility RVU** | **Work** | **PE** | **MP** | **Total** |
| **D0601** | 0.00 | 0.16 | 0.00 | 0.16 |
| **D0602** | 0.00 | 0.16 | 0.00 | 0.16 |
| **D0603** | 0.00 | 0.16 | 0.00 | 0.16 |

| | FUD | Status | MUE | Modifiers | | | | IOM Reference |
|---|---|---|---|---|---|---|---|---|
| **D0601** | N/A | R | - | N/A | N/A | N/A | N/A | None |
| **D0602** | N/A | R | - | N/A | N/A | N/A | N/A | |
| **D0603** | N/A | R | - | N/A | N/A | N/A | N/A | |

* with documentation

## Terms To Know

**caries.** Localized section of tooth decay that begins on the tooth surface with destruction of the calcified enamel, allowing bacterial destruction to continue and form cavities and may extend to the dentin and pulp.

**morphological.** Pertaining to structure and function.

**xerostomia.** Dry mouth due to lack of saliva.

# D0604-D0606

**D0604** antigen testing for a public health related pathogen, including coronavirus

**D0605** antibody testing for a public health related pathogen, including coronavirus

● **D0606** molecular testing for a public health related pathogen, including coronavirus

## Explanation

These codes are used to report the collection and testing of patients who may have been exposed to or have a public health related pathogen. Specimens may be obtained through a variety of sources, such as nasopharyngeal or oropharyngeal swab, nasopharyngeal wash or aspirate, nasal aspirate, or sputum. Report D0604 for antigen testing to determine if the patient currently has the condition and D0605 to determine if the patient has developed antigens to the condition by exposure or recovery from the condition. Report D0606 for molecular testing to the condition.

## Coding Tips

The current public health pathogen is a coronavirus identified as SARS-CoV-2 or COVID-19. Highly contagious patients with this condition are treated only for emergent conditions. The specimen may be obtained by the practitioner with actual testing performed by an outside laboratory.

## Reimbursement Tips

Testing for SARS-CoV-2 or COVID-19 may be covered by payers or governmental agencies without cost sharing by the patient.

## Associated CPT Codes

0224U Antibody, severe acute respiratory syndrome coronavirus 2 (SARS-CoV-2) (coronavirus disease [COVID-19]), includes titer(s), when performed

86328 Immunoassay for infectious agent antibody(ies), qualitative or semiquantitative, single step method (eg, reagent strip); severe acute respiratory syndrome coronavirus 2 (SARS-CoV-2) (Coronavirus disease [COVID-19])

86769 Antibody; severe acute respiratory syndrome coronavirus 2 (SARS-CoV-2) (Coronavirus disease [COVID-19])

87635 Infectious agent detection by nucleic acid (DNA or RNA); severe acute respiratory syndrome coronavirus 2 (SARS-CoV-2) (Coronavirus disease [COVID-19]), amplified probe technique

## ICD-10-CM Diagnostic Codes

R06.02 Shortness of breath

R50.9 Fever, unspecified

U07.1 COVID-19

Z03.818 Encounter for observation for suspected exposure to other biological agents ruled out

Z09 Encounter for follow-up examination after completed treatment for conditions other than malignant neoplasm

Z11.52 Encounter for screening for COVID-19

Z11.59 Encounter for screening for other viral diseases

Z20.822 Contact with and (suspected) exposure to COVID-19

Z20.828 Contact with and (suspected) exposure to other viral communicable diseases

## Relative Value Units/Medicare Edits

| Non-Facility RVU | Work | PE | MP | Total |
|---|---|---|---|---|
| D0604 | | | | |
| D0605 | | | | |
| D0606 | | | | |
| **Facility RVU** | **Work** | **PE** | **MP** | **Total** |
| D0604 | | | | |
| D0605 | | | | |
| D0606 | | | | |

| | FUD | Status | MUE | Modifiers | | | | IOM Reference |
|---|---|---|---|---|---|---|---|---|
| D0604 | N/A | | - | N/A | N/A | N/A | N/A | |
| D0605 | N/A | | - | N/A | N/A | N/A | N/A | |
| D0606 | N/A | | - | N/A | N/A | N/A | N/A | |

* with documentation

## Terms To Know

**COVID-19.** First diagnosed in December 2019 in China, coronavirus disease 2019 (COVID-19) is a respiratory infection caused by a newly identified (novel) virus not previously seen in humans, known as severe acute respiratory syndrome coronavirus 2 (SARS-CoV-2). Symptoms of this lower respiratory illness include fever, dry cough, loss of taste and/or smell, skin lesions of toes, gastrointestinal disturbances, and tiredness that may progress to include difficulty breathing and ventilator assistance. Older patients and those with high blood pressure, heart problems, diabetes, and obesity are more likely to develop serious symptoms of the illness, which may result in death of the patient.

**PHE.** Public health emergency.

# D0701

**D0701** panoramic radiographic image - image capture only

## Explanation

A panoramic image (x-ray) is taken that allows a comprehensive all-in-one view of the oral structures to be seen. Report D0701 for image capture only without interpretation and report.

## Coding Tips

Any evaluation, prophylaxis, fluoride, restorative, or extraction service is reported separately. A panoramic image is an extraoral film. When image capture with interpretation and report is performed, see D0330. For full-mouth series, see D0120.

## Reimbursement Tips

Many payer contracts allow EITHER a full-mouth series OR a panoramic film but not both during a specified time period. Check with individual payers for contract-specific guidelines. When selecting the procedure or service that accurately identifies the service performed, dentists must use the most accurate code. If the CDT code more accurately identifies the service, this should be used rather than the CPT codes.

## Associated CPT Codes

| | |
|---|---|
| 70320 | Radiologic examination, teeth; complete, full mouth |
| 70355 | Orthopantogram (eg, panoramic x-ray) |

## ICD-10-CM Diagnostic Codes

| | |
|---|---|
| K00.1 | Supernumerary teeth |
| K00.2 | Abnormalities of size and form of teeth |
| K00.3 | Mottled teeth |
| K00.4 | Disturbances in tooth formation |
| K00.5 | Hereditary disturbances in tooth structure, not elsewhere classified |
| K00.6 | Disturbances in tooth eruption |
| K00.7 | Teething syndrome |
| K00.8 | Other disorders of tooth development |
| K01.0 | Embedded teeth |
| K01.1 | Impacted teeth |
| K02.3 | Arrested dental caries |
| K02.51 | Dental caries on pit and fissure surface limited to enamel |
| K02.52 | Dental caries on pit and fissure surface penetrating into dentin |
| K02.53 | Dental caries on pit and fissure surface penetrating into pulp |
| K02.61 | Dental caries on smooth surface limited to enamel |
| K02.62 | Dental caries on smooth surface penetrating into dentin |
| K02.63 | Dental caries on smooth surface penetrating into pulp |
| K02.7 | Dental root caries |
| K03.0 | Excessive attrition of teeth |
| K03.1 | Abrasion of teeth |
| K03.2 | Erosion of teeth |
| K03.3 | Pathological resorption of teeth |
| K03.4 | Hypercementosis |
| K03.5 | Ankylosis of teeth |
| K03.6 | Deposits [accretions] on teeth |
| K03.7 | Posteruptive color changes of dental hard tissues |
| K03.81 | Cracked tooth |
| K04.01 | Reversible pulpitis |
| K04.02 | Irreversible pulpitis |
| K04.2 | Pulp degeneration |
| K04.3 | Abnormal hard tissue formation in pulp |
| K04.4 | Acute apical periodontitis of pulpal origin |
| K04.5 | Chronic apical periodontitis |
| K04.6 | Periapical abscess with sinus |
| K04.7 | Periapical abscess without sinus |
| K04.8 | Radicular cyst |
| K04.99 | Other diseases of pulp and periapical tissues |
| K05.00 | Acute gingivitis, plaque induced |
| K05.01 | Acute gingivitis, non-plaque induced |
| K05.10 | Chronic gingivitis, plaque induced |
| K05.11 | Chronic gingivitis, non-plaque induced |
| K05.211 | Aggressive periodontitis, localized, slight |
| K05.212 | Aggressive periodontitis, localized, moderate |
| K05.213 | Aggressive periodontitis, localized, severe |
| K05.221 | Aggressive periodontitis, generalized, slight |
| K05.222 | Aggressive periodontitis, generalized, moderate |
| K05.223 | Aggressive periodontitis, generalized, severe |
| K05.311 | Chronic periodontitis, localized, slight |
| K05.312 | Chronic periodontitis, localized, moderate |
| K05.313 | Chronic periodontitis, localized, severe |
| K05.321 | Chronic periodontitis, generalized, slight |
| K05.322 | Chronic periodontitis, generalized, moderate |
| K05.323 | Chronic periodontitis, generalized, severe |
| K05.4 | Periodontosis |
| K06.011 | Localized gingival recession, minimal |
| K06.012 | Localized gingival recession, moderate |
| K06.013 | Localized gingival recession, severe |
| K06.021 | Generalized gingival recession, minimal |
| K06.022 | Generalized gingival recession, moderate |
| K06.023 | Generalized gingival recession, severe |
| K06.1 | Gingival enlargement |
| K06.2 | Gingival and edentulous alveolar ridge lesions associated with trauma |
| K06.8 | Other specified disorders of gingiva and edentulous alveolar ridge |
| K08.0 | Exfoliation of teeth due to systemic causes |
| K08.111 | Complete loss of teeth due to trauma, class I |
| K08.112 | Complete loss of teeth due to trauma, class II |
| K08.113 | Complete loss of teeth due to trauma, class III |
| K08.114 | Complete loss of teeth due to trauma, class IV |
| K08.121 | Complete loss of teeth due to periodontal diseases, class I |
| K08.122 | Complete loss of teeth due to periodontal diseases, class II |
| K08.123 | Complete loss of teeth due to periodontal diseases, class III |
| K08.124 | Complete loss of teeth due to periodontal diseases, class IV |
| K08.131 | Complete loss of teeth due to caries, class I |
| K08.132 | Complete loss of teeth due to caries, class II |
| K08.133 | Complete loss of teeth due to caries, class III |
| K08.134 | Complete loss of teeth due to caries, class IV |
| K08.191 | Complete loss of teeth due to other specified cause, class I |
| K08.192 | Complete loss of teeth due to other specified cause, class II |
| K08.193 | Complete loss of teeth due to other specified cause, class III |
| K08.194 | Complete loss of teeth due to other specified cause, class IV |
| K08.21 | Minimal atrophy of the mandible |
| K08.22 | Moderate atrophy of the mandible |
| K08.23 | Severe atrophy of the mandible |
| K08.24 | Minimal atrophy of maxilla |

| | |
|---|---|
| K08.25 | Moderate atrophy of the maxilla |
| K08.26 | Severe atrophy of the maxilla |
| K08.3 | Retained dental root |
| K08.411 | Partial loss of teeth due to trauma, class I |
| K08.412 | Partial loss of teeth due to trauma, class II |
| K08.413 | Partial loss of teeth due to trauma, class III |
| K08.414 | Partial loss of teeth due to trauma, class IV |
| K08.421 | Partial loss of teeth due to periodontal diseases, class I |
| K08.422 | Partial loss of teeth due to periodontal diseases, class II |
| K08.423 | Partial loss of teeth due to periodontal diseases, class III |
| K08.424 | Partial loss of teeth due to periodontal diseases, class IV |
| K08.431 | Partial loss of teeth due to caries, class I |
| K08.432 | Partial loss of teeth due to caries, class II |
| K08.433 | Partial loss of teeth due to caries, class III |
| K08.434 | Partial loss of teeth due to caries, class IV |
| K08.491 | Partial loss of teeth due to other specified cause, class I |
| K08.492 | Partial loss of teeth due to other specified cause, class II |
| K08.493 | Partial loss of teeth due to other specified cause, class III |
| K08.494 | Partial loss of teeth due to other specified cause, class IV |
| K08.51 | Open restoration margins of tooth |
| K08.52 | Unrepairable overhanging of dental restorative materials |
| K08.530 | Fractured dental restorative material without loss of material |
| K08.531 | Fractured dental restorative material with loss of material |
| K08.54 | Contour of existing restoration of tooth biologically incompatible with oral health |
| K08.55 | Allergy to existing dental restorative material |
| K08.56 | Poor aesthetic of existing restoration of tooth |
| K08.81 | Primary occlusal trauma |
| K08.82 | Secondary occlusal trauma |
| K09.0 | Developmental odontogenic cysts |
| K09.1 | Developmental (nonodontogenic) cysts of oral region |
| K09.8 | Other cysts of oral region, not elsewhere classified |

## Relative Value Units/Medicare Edits

| Non-Facility RVU | Work | PE | MP | Total |
|---|---|---|---|---|
| D0701 | | | | |
| Facility RVU | Work | PE | MP | Total |
| D0701 | | | | |

| | FUD | Status | MUE | Modifiers | | | | IOM Reference |
|---|---|---|---|---|---|---|---|---|
| D0701 | N/A | | - | N/A | N/A | N/A | N/A | |

* with documentation

## Terms To Know

**panoramic x-ray.** X-ray that contains views of both the maxilla and mandible on a single extraoral image.

# D0702

**D0702** 2-D cephalometric radiographic image - image capture only

## Explanation

A lateral or frontal x-ray projection is taken to examine the entire skull, jaw, and related tooth positions in a cephalometric image. The machine holds the patient's head in the same position each time an image is taken so that a series of the individual cephalograms taken can be directly compared for growth and development over time. Report D0702 for image capture only without interpretation and report.

## Coding Tips

Any evaluation, prophylaxis, fluoride, restorative, or extraction service is reported separately. When image capture with interpretation and report is performed, see D0340.

## Reimbursement Tips

This procedure may be covered by the patient's medical insurance. When covered by medical insurance, the payer may require that the appropriate CPT code be reported on the CMS-1500 claim form.

## Associated CPT Codes

| | |
|---|---|
| 70350 | Cephalogram, orthodontic |

## ICD-10-CM Diagnostic Codes

| | |
|---|---|
| K00.1 | Supernumerary teeth |
| K00.2 | Abnormalities of size and form of teeth |
| K00.3 | Mottled teeth |
| K00.4 | Disturbances in tooth formation |
| K00.5 | Hereditary disturbances in tooth structure, not elsewhere classified |
| K00.6 | Disturbances in tooth eruption |
| K01.0 | Embedded teeth |
| K01.1 | Impacted teeth |
| K03.0 | Excessive attrition of teeth |
| K03.1 | Abrasion of teeth |
| K03.2 | Erosion of teeth |
| K03.3 | Pathological resorption of teeth |
| K06.012 | Localized gingival recession, moderate |
| K06.013 | Localized gingival recession, severe |
| K06.022 | Generalized gingival recession, moderate |
| K06.023 | Generalized gingival recession, severe |
| K08.21 | Minimal atrophy of the mandible |
| K08.22 | Moderate atrophy of the mandible |
| K08.23 | Severe atrophy of the mandible |
| K08.24 | Minimal atrophy of maxilla |
| K08.25 | Moderate atrophy of the maxilla |
| K08.26 | Severe atrophy of the maxilla |
| K09.0 | Developmental odontogenic cysts |
| K09.1 | Developmental (nonodontogenic) cysts of oral region |
| M26.211 | Malocclusion, Angle's class I |
| M26.212 | Malocclusion, Angle's class II |
| M26.213 | Malocclusion, Angle's class III |
| M26.220 | Open anterior occlusal relationship |
| M26.221 | Open posterior occlusal relationship |
| M26.23 | Excessive horizontal overlap |
| M26.24 | Reverse articulation |

| | |
|---|---|
| M26.31 | Crowding of fully erupted teeth |
| M26.32 | Excessive spacing of fully erupted teeth |
| M26.33 | Horizontal displacement of fully erupted tooth or teeth |
| M26.34 | Vertical displacement of fully erupted tooth or teeth |
| M26.35 | Rotation of fully erupted tooth or teeth |
| M26.36 | Insufficient interocclusal distance of fully erupted teeth (ridge) |
| M26.37 | Excessive interocclusal distance of fully erupted teeth |
| M26.51 | Abnormal jaw closure |
| M26.52 | Limited mandibular range of motion |
| M26.53 | Deviation in opening and closing of the mandible |
| M26.54 | Insufficient anterior guidance |
| M26.55 | Centric occlusion maximum intercuspation discrepancy |
| M26.56 | Non-working side interference |
| M26.57 | Lack of posterior occlusal support |
| M26.59 | Other dentofacial functional abnormalities |
| M26.71 | Alveolar maxillary hyperplasia |
| M26.72 | Alveolar mandibular hyperplasia |
| M26.73 | Alveolar maxillary hypoplasia |
| M26.74 | Alveolar mandibular hypoplasia |
| M26.79 | Other specified alveolar anomalies |
| M26.81 | Anterior soft tissue impingement |
| M26.82 | Posterior soft tissue impingement |
| S02.5XXA | Fracture of tooth (traumatic), initial encounter for closed fracture |
| S02.5XXB | Fracture of tooth (traumatic), initial encounter for open fracture |
| Z46.4 | Encounter for fitting and adjustment of orthodontic device |

## Relative Value Units/Medicare Edits

| Non-Facility RVU | Work | PE | MP | Total |
|---|---|---|---|---|
| D0702 | | | | |
| Facility RVU | Work | PE | MP | Total |
| D0702 | | | | |

| | FUD | Status | MUE | Modifiers | | | | IOM Reference |
|---|---|---|---|---|---|---|---|---|
| D0702 | N/A | | - | N/A | N/A | N/A | N/A | |

* with documentation

## Terms To Know

**radiograph.** Image made by an x-ray.

# D0703

**D0703** 2-D oral/facial photographic image obtained intra-orally or extra-orally - image capture only

## Explanation

This code is used for reporting traditional two-dimensional photographic images taken of the face or the inside of the mouth with an intraoral or extraoral camera. This is not for conventional x-rays or any type of radiographic imaging. Report D0703 for image capture only without interpretation and report.

## Coding Tips

To report three-dimensional photographic imaging for diagnostic purposes, see D0351. Any evaluation, prophylaxis, fluoride, restorative, or extraction service is reported separately. This code excludes conventional radiograph. When image capture with interpretation and report is performed, see D0350.

## Reimbursement Tips

This service is often only covered when performed in conjunction with covered orthodontic services. Check with payers to determine specific requirements.

## ICD-10-CM Diagnostic Codes

| | |
|---|---|
| K08.21 | Minimal atrophy of the mandible |
| K08.22 | Moderate atrophy of the mandible |
| K08.23 | Severe atrophy of the mandible |
| K08.24 | Minimal atrophy of maxilla |
| K08.25 | Moderate atrophy of the maxilla |
| K08.26 | Severe atrophy of the maxilla |
| M26.211 | Malocclusion, Angle's class I |
| M26.212 | Malocclusion, Angle's class II |
| M26.213 | Malocclusion, Angle's class III |
| M26.220 | Open anterior occlusal relationship |
| M26.221 | Open posterior occlusal relationship |
| M26.23 | Excessive horizontal overlap |
| M26.24 | Reverse articulation |
| M26.51 | Abnormal jaw closure |
| M26.52 | Limited mandibular range of motion |
| M26.53 | Deviation in opening and closing of the mandible |
| M26.54 | Insufficient anterior guidance |
| M26.55 | Centric occlusion maximum intercuspation discrepancy |
| M26.56 | Non-working side interference |
| M26.57 | Lack of posterior occlusal support |
| M26.59 | Other dentofacial functional abnormalities |
| M26.71 | Alveolar maxillary hyperplasia |
| M26.72 | Alveolar mandibular hyperplasia |
| M26.73 | Alveolar maxillary hypoplasia |
| M26.74 | Alveolar mandibular hypoplasia |
| M26.79 | Other specified alveolar anomalies |
| M26.81 | Anterior soft tissue impingement |
| M26.82 | Posterior soft tissue impingement |

## Relative Value Units/Medicare Edits

| Non-Facility RVU | Work | PE | MP | Total |
|---|---|---|---|---|
| D0703 | | | | |
| **Facility RVU** | **Work** | **PE** | **MP** | **Total** |
| D0703 | | | | |

| | FUD | Status | MUE | Modifiers | | | | IOM Reference |
|---|---|---|---|---|---|---|---|---|
| D0703 | N/A | | - | N/A | N/A | N/A | N/A | |

* with documentation

## Terms To Know

**atrophy.** Reduction in size or activity in an anatomic structure, due to wasting away from disease or other factors.

**extraoral.** Outside of the mouth or oral cavity.

**imaging.** Radiologic means of producing pictures for clinical study of the internal structures and functions of the body, such as x-ray, ultrasound, magnetic resonance, or positron emission tomography.

**intraoral.** Within the mouth.

**malocclusion.** Condition in which the teeth are misaligned. Underlying causes may include accessory, impacted, or missing teeth; dentofacial abnormalities; thumb sucking; or sleeping positions.

**oral.** Pertaining to the mouth.

**prophylaxis.** Intervention or protective therapy intended to prevent a disease.

# D0704

**D0704** 3-D photographic image - image capture only

## Explanation

A three-dimensional photographic image of the dental or maxillofacial structures is obtained for diagnostic purposes. Three-dimensional photography allows for hemispherical and full spherical output that assists in analyzing the aesthetic aspect of the smile, occlusal planes, wear patterns, and other details otherwise hard to detect during a regular patient examination. Report D0704 for image capture only without interpretation and report.

## Coding Tips

For two-dimensional photographic imaging, see D0350 or D0703. When computer-aided design/computer-aided manufacturing (CAD-CAM) device (therapeutic purposes) is performed, see D0393-D0395. When image capture with interpretation and report is performed, see D0351.

## Documentation Tips

Pertinent documentation to evaluate the medical appropriateness should be included with the claim when this code is reported.

## Reimbursement Tips

This procedure may be covered by the patient's medical insurance. When covered by medical insurance, the payer may require that the appropriate CPT code be reported on the CMS-1500 claim form.

## ICD-10-CM Diagnostic Codes

| | |
|---|---|
| K08.21 | Minimal atrophy of the mandible |
| K08.22 | Moderate atrophy of the mandible |
| K08.23 | Severe atrophy of the mandible |
| K08.24 | Minimal atrophy of maxilla |
| K08.25 | Moderate atrophy of the maxilla |
| K08.26 | Severe atrophy of the maxilla |
| M26.01 | Maxillary hyperplasia |
| M26.02 | Maxillary hypoplasia |
| M26.03 | Mandibular hyperplasia |
| M26.04 | Mandibular hypoplasia |
| M26.05 | Macrogenia |
| M26.06 | Microgenia |
| M26.07 | Excessive tuberosity of jaw |
| M26.09 | Other specified anomalies of jaw size |
| M26.12 | Other jaw asymmetry |
| M26.19 | Other specified anomalies of jaw-cranial base relationship |
| M26.211 | Malocclusion, Angle's class I |
| M26.212 | Malocclusion, Angle's class II |
| M26.213 | Malocclusion, Angle's class III |
| M26.220 | Open anterior occlusal relationship |
| M26.221 | Open posterior occlusal relationship |
| M26.23 | Excessive horizontal overlap |
| M26.24 | Reverse articulation |
| M26.25 | Anomalies of interarch distance |
| M26.29 | Other anomalies of dental arch relationship |
| M26.31 | Crowding of fully erupted teeth |
| M26.32 | Excessive spacing of fully erupted teeth |
| M26.33 | Horizontal displacement of fully erupted tooth or teeth |
| M26.34 | Vertical displacement of fully erupted tooth or teeth |
| M26.35 | Rotation of fully erupted tooth or teeth |

M26.36 Insufficient interocclusal distance of fully erupted teeth (ridge)
M26.37 Excessive interocclusal distance of fully erupted teeth
M26.39 Other anomalies of tooth position of fully erupted tooth or teeth
M26.51 Abnormal jaw closure
M26.52 Limited mandibular range of motion
M26.53 Deviation in opening and closing of the mandible
M26.54 Insufficient anterior guidance
M26.55 Centric occlusion maximum intercuspation discrepancy
M26.56 Non-working side interference
M26.57 Lack of posterior occlusal support
M26.59 Other dentofacial functional abnormalities

## Relative Value Units/Medicare Edits

| Non-Facility RVU | Work | PE | MP | Total |
|---|---|---|---|---|
| **D0704** | | | | |
| **Facility RVU** | **Work** | **PE** | **MP** | **Total** |
| **D0704** | | | | |

| | FUD | Status | MUE | Modifiers | | | | IOM Reference |
|---|---|---|---|---|---|---|---|---|
| **D0704** | N/A | | - | N/A | N/A | N/A | N/A | |

* with documentation

## Terms To Know

**photography.** Still image pictures that may be digital or film generated.

# D0705

**D0705** extra-oral posterior dental radiographic image - image capture only

*Image limited to exposure of complete posterior teeth in both dental arches. This is a unique image that is not derived from another image.*

## Explanation

Images are obtained of the complete posterior teeth in both dental arches from outside of the mouth. Report D0705 for image capture only without interpretation and report.

## Coding Tips

To report bitewing images, see D0270-D2074 and D0277. To report extraoral images of the skull or facial bones, see D0250. Intraoral images are reported using D0210-D0240. When image capture with interpretation and report is performed, see D0251.

## Reimbursement Tips

Most payers require that each type of image be reported as separate line items.

## Associated CPT Codes

70300 Radiologic examination, teeth; single view
70310 Radiologic examination, teeth; partial examination, less than full mouth
70320 Radiologic examination, teeth; complete, full mouth

## ICD-10-CM Diagnostic Codes

K08.21 Minimal atrophy of the mandible
K08.22 Moderate atrophy of the mandible
K08.23 Severe atrophy of the mandible
K08.24 Minimal atrophy of maxilla
K08.25 Moderate atrophy of the maxilla
K08.26 Severe atrophy of the maxilla
K09.0 Developmental odontogenic cysts
K09.1 Developmental (nonodontogenic) cysts of oral region
K09.8 Other cysts of oral region, not elsewhere classified
M26.211 Malocclusion, Angle's class I
M26.212 Malocclusion, Angle's class II
M26.213 Malocclusion, Angle's class III
M26.220 Open anterior occlusal relationship
M26.221 Open posterior occlusal relationship
M26.23 Excessive horizontal overlap
M26.24 Reverse articulation
M26.25 Anomalies of interarch distance
M26.29 Other anomalies of dental arch relationship
M26.31 Crowding of fully erupted teeth
M26.32 Excessive spacing of fully erupted teeth
M26.33 Horizontal displacement of fully erupted tooth or teeth
M26.34 Vertical displacement of fully erupted tooth or teeth
M26.35 Rotation of fully erupted tooth or teeth
M26.36 Insufficient interocclusal distance of fully erupted teeth (ridge)
M26.37 Excessive interocclusal distance of fully erupted teeth
M26.39 Other anomalies of tooth position of fully erupted tooth or teeth
M26.51 Abnormal jaw closure
M26.52 Limited mandibular range of motion
M26.53 Deviation in opening and closing of the mandible
M26.54 Insufficient anterior guidance
M26.55 Centric occlusion maximum intercuspation discrepancy

| | |
|---|---|
| M26.56 | Non-working side interference |
| M26.57 | Lack of posterior occlusal support |
| M26.59 | Other dentofacial functional abnormalities |
| M26.71 | Alveolar maxillary hyperplasia |
| M26.72 | Alveolar mandibular hyperplasia |
| M26.73 | Alveolar maxillary hypoplasia |
| M26.74 | Alveolar mandibular hypoplasia |
| M26.79 | Other specified alveolar anomalies |
| M26.81 | Anterior soft tissue impingement |
| M26.82 | Posterior soft tissue impingement |

## Relative Value Units/Medicare Edits

| Non-Facility RVU | Work | PE | MP | Total |
|---|---|---|---|---|
| D0705 | | | | |
| **Facility RVU** | **Work** | **PE** | **MP** | **Total** |
| D0705 | | | | |

| | FUD | Status | MUE | Modifiers | | | | IOM Reference |
|---|---|---|---|---|---|---|---|---|
| D0705 | N/A | | - | N/A | N/A | N/A | N/A | |

* with documentation

## Terms To Know

**extraoral.** Outside of the mouth or oral cavity.

**posterior.** Located in the back part or caudal end of the body.

**x-ray.** Images of the bones and internal organs obtained by sending small amounts of radiation through the body, leaving a shadow-like image of internal structures.

# D0706-D0709

**D0706** intraoral - occlusal radiographic image - image capture only
**D0707** intraoral - periapical radiographic image - image capture only
**D0708** intraoral - bitewing radiographic image - image capture only

*Image axis may be horizontal or vertical.*

**D0709** intraoral - complete series of radiographic images - image capture only

*A radiographic survey of the whole mouth, usually consisting of 14-22 images (periapical and posterior bitewing as indicated) intended to display the crowns and roots of all teeth, periapical areas and alveolar bone.*

## Explanation

Appropriate code selection is dependent upon the type (i.e., periapical, occlusal, complete series) and number of images taken. For image capture only of intraoral occlusal images, see D0706; for intraoral periapical images, see D0707; for bitewing images, see D0708; for complete series of intraoral images, see D0709.

## Coding Tips

Any evaluation, prophylaxis, fluoride, restorative, or extraction service is reported separately. For extraoral images, see D0250-D0251. When reporting digital subtraction of two or more images (of the same modality), report D0394 in addition to the appropriate code for obtaining the image. When image capture with interpretation and report is performed, see D0210, D0220, or D0270-D0274.

## Reimbursement Tips

When periapical images are performed at the same time as a panoramic, most payers will bundle these services and reimburse as if a complete intraoral x-ray examination was performed.

## ICD-10-CM Diagnostic Codes

| | |
|---|---|
| K00.1 | Supernumerary teeth |
| K00.2 | Abnormalities of size and form of teeth |
| K00.3 | Mottled teeth |
| K00.4 | Disturbances in tooth formation |
| K00.5 | Hereditary disturbances in tooth structure, not elsewhere classified |
| K00.6 | Disturbances in tooth eruption |
| K00.7 | Teething syndrome |
| K00.8 | Other disorders of tooth development |
| K01.0 | Embedded teeth |
| K01.1 | Impacted teeth |
| K02.3 | Arrested dental caries |
| K02.51 | Dental caries on pit and fissure surface limited to enamel |
| K02.52 | Dental caries on pit and fissure surface penetrating into dentin |
| K02.53 | Dental caries on pit and fissure surface penetrating into pulp |
| K02.61 | Dental caries on smooth surface limited to enamel |
| K02.62 | Dental caries on smooth surface penetrating into dentin |
| K02.63 | Dental caries on smooth surface penetrating into pulp |
| K02.7 | Dental root caries |
| K03.0 | Excessive attrition of teeth |
| K03.1 | Abrasion of teeth |
| K03.2 | Erosion of teeth |
| K03.3 | Pathological resorption of teeth |
| K03.4 | Hypercementosis |
| K03.5 | Ankylosis of teeth |

| | |
|---|---|
| K03.6 | Deposits [accretions] on teeth |
| K03.7 | Posteruptive color changes of dental hard tissues |
| K03.81 | Cracked tooth |
| K04.01 | Reversible pulpitis |
| K04.02 | Irreversible pulpitis |
| K04.1 | Necrosis of pulp |
| K04.2 | Pulp degeneration |
| K04.3 | Abnormal hard tissue formation in pulp |
| K04.4 | Acute apical periodontitis of pulpal origin |
| K04.5 | Chronic apical periodontitis |
| K04.6 | Periapical abscess with sinus |
| K04.7 | Periapical abscess without sinus |
| K04.8 | Radicular cyst |
| K04.99 | Other diseases of pulp and periapical tissues |
| K05.00 | Acute gingivitis, plaque induced |
| K05.01 | Acute gingivitis, non-plaque induced |
| K05.10 | Chronic gingivitis, plaque induced |
| K05.11 | Chronic gingivitis, non-plaque induced |
| K05.211 | Aggressive periodontitis, localized, slight |
| K05.212 | Aggressive periodontitis, localized, moderate |
| K05.213 | Aggressive periodontitis, localized, severe |
| K05.221 | Aggressive periodontitis, generalized, slight |
| K05.222 | Aggressive periodontitis, generalized, moderate |
| K05.223 | Aggressive periodontitis, generalized, severe |
| K05.311 | Chronic periodontitis, localized, slight |
| K05.312 | Chronic periodontitis, localized, moderate |
| K05.313 | Chronic periodontitis, localized, severe |
| K05.321 | Chronic periodontitis, generalized, slight |
| K05.322 | Chronic periodontitis, generalized, moderate |
| K05.323 | Chronic periodontitis, generalized, severe |
| K05.4 | Periodontosis |
| K05.5 | Other periodontal diseases |
| K06.011 | Localized gingival recession, minimal |
| K06.012 | Localized gingival recession, moderate |
| K06.013 | Localized gingival recession, severe |
| K06.021 | Generalized gingival recession, minimal |
| K06.022 | Generalized gingival recession, moderate |
| K06.023 | Generalized gingival recession, severe |
| K06.1 | Gingival enlargement |
| K06.2 | Gingival and edentulous alveolar ridge lesions associated with trauma |
| K06.8 | Other specified disorders of gingiva and edentulous alveolar ridge |
| K08.0 | Exfoliation of teeth due to systemic causes |
| K08.111 | Complete loss of teeth due to trauma, class I |
| K08.112 | Complete loss of teeth due to trauma, class II |
| K08.113 | Complete loss of teeth due to trauma, class III |
| K08.114 | Complete loss of teeth due to trauma, class IV |
| K08.121 | Complete loss of teeth due to periodontal diseases, class I |
| K08.122 | Complete loss of teeth due to periodontal diseases, class II |
| K08.123 | Complete loss of teeth due to periodontal diseases, class III |
| K08.124 | Complete loss of teeth due to periodontal diseases, class IV |
| K08.131 | Complete loss of teeth due to caries, class I |
| K08.132 | Complete loss of teeth due to caries, class II |
| K08.133 | Complete loss of teeth due to caries, class III |
| K08.134 | Complete loss of teeth due to caries, class IV |
| K08.191 | Complete loss of teeth due to other specified cause, class I |
| K08.192 | Complete loss of teeth due to other specified cause, class II |
| K08.193 | Complete loss of teeth due to other specified cause, class III |
| K08.194 | Complete loss of teeth due to other specified cause, class IV |
| K08.21 | Minimal atrophy of the mandible |
| K08.22 | Moderate atrophy of the mandible |
| K08.23 | Severe atrophy of the mandible |
| K08.24 | Minimal atrophy of maxilla |
| K08.25 | Moderate atrophy of the maxilla |
| K08.26 | Severe atrophy of the maxilla |
| K08.3 | Retained dental root |
| K08.411 | Partial loss of teeth due to trauma, class I |
| K08.412 | Partial loss of teeth due to trauma, class II |
| K08.413 | Partial loss of teeth due to trauma, class III |
| K08.414 | Partial loss of teeth due to trauma, class IV |
| K08.421 | Partial loss of teeth due to periodontal diseases, class I |
| K08.422 | Partial loss of teeth due to periodontal diseases, class II |
| K08.423 | Partial loss of teeth due to periodontal diseases, class III |
| K08.424 | Partial loss of teeth due to periodontal diseases, class IV |
| K08.431 | Partial loss of teeth due to caries, class I |
| K08.432 | Partial loss of teeth due to caries, class II |
| K08.433 | Partial loss of teeth due to caries, class III |
| K08.434 | Partial loss of teeth due to caries, class IV |
| K08.491 | Partial loss of teeth due to other specified cause, class I |
| K08.492 | Partial loss of teeth due to other specified cause, class II |
| K08.493 | Partial loss of teeth due to other specified cause, class III |
| K08.494 | Partial loss of teeth due to other specified cause, class IV |
| K08.51 | Open restoration margins of tooth |
| K08.52 | Unrepairable overhanging of dental restorative materials |
| K08.530 | Fractured dental restorative material without loss of material |
| K08.531 | Fractured dental restorative material with loss of material |
| K08.54 | Contour of existing restoration of tooth biologically incompatible with oral health |
| K08.55 | Allergy to existing dental restorative material |
| K08.56 | Poor aesthetic of existing restoration of tooth |
| K08.81 | Primary occlusal trauma |
| K08.82 | Secondary occlusal trauma |
| K08.89 | Other specified disorders of teeth and supporting structures |
| K09.0 | Developmental odontogenic cysts |
| K09.1 | Developmental (nonodontogenic) cysts of oral region |
| K09.8 | Other cysts of oral region, not elsewhere classified |
| K11.0 | Atrophy of salivary gland |
| K11.1 | Hypertrophy of salivary gland |
| K11.21 | Acute sialoadenitis |
| K11.22 | Acute recurrent sialoadenitis |
| K11.23 | Chronic sialoadenitis |
| K11.3 | Abscess of salivary gland |
| K11.4 | Fistula of salivary gland |
| K11.5 | Sialolithiasis |
| K11.6 | Mucocele of salivary gland |
| K11.7 | Disturbances of salivary secretion |
| K11.8 | Other diseases of salivary glands |
| K12.0 | Recurrent oral aphthae |
| K12.1 | Other forms of stomatitis |
| K12.2 | Cellulitis and abscess of mouth |
| K13.0 | Diseases of lips |
| K13.1 | Cheek and lip biting |
| K13.21 | Leukoplakia of oral mucosa, including tongue |

| | |
|---|---|
| K13.22 | Minimal keratinized residual ridge mucosa |
| K13.23 | Excessive keratinized residual ridge mucosa |
| K13.24 | Leukokeratosis nicotina palati |
| K13.3 | Hairy leukoplakia |
| K13.4 | Granuloma and granuloma-like lesions of oral mucosa |
| K13.5 | Oral submucous fibrosis |
| K13.6 | Irritative hyperplasia of oral mucosa |
| K13.79 | Other lesions of oral mucosa |

## Relative Value Units/Medicare Edits

| Non-Facility RVU | Work | PE | MP | Total |
|---|---|---|---|---|
| D0706 | | | | |
| D0707 | | | | |
| D0708 | | | | |
| D0709 | | | | |

| Facility RVU | Work | PE | MP | Total |
|---|---|---|---|---|
| D0706 | | | | |
| D0707 | | | | |
| D0708 | | | | |
| D0709 | | | | |

| | FUD | Status | MUE | Modifiers | | | | IOM Reference |
|---|---|---|---|---|---|---|---|---|
| D0706 | N/A | | - | N/A | N/A | N/A | N/A | |
| D0707 | N/A | | - | N/A | N/A | N/A | N/A | |
| D0708 | N/A | | - | N/A | N/A | N/A | N/A | |
| D0709 | N/A | | - | N/A | N/A | N/A | N/A | |

* with documentation

## Terms To Know

**imaging.** Radiologic means of producing pictures for clinical study of the internal structures and functions of the body, such as x-ray, ultrasound, magnetic resonance, or positron emission tomography.

**intraoral.** Within the mouth.

# D1110-D1120

**D1110** prophylaxis - adult

*Removal of plaque, calculus and stains from the tooth structures and implants in the permanent and transitional dentition. It is intended to control local irritational factors.*

**D1120** prophylaxis - child

*Removal of plaque, calculus and stains from the tooth structures and implants in the permanent and transitional dentition. It is intended to control local irritational factors.*

## Explanation

Dental prophylaxis includes the removal of coronal plaque, calculus buildup, or stains. Report D1110 for prophylaxis cleaning performed on dentition (tooth structures and implants) of adults and D1120 for a prophylaxis treatment on the primary or transitional teeth and implants of a child.

## Coding Tips

Appropriate code selection is determined by patient age. The ADA considers a patient to be an adult at age 12 for any service except orthodontics or sealants. However, plan guidelines vary and can range from 12 to 14 years of age. Check with payers for specific guidelines. Any evaluation, radiograph, prophylaxis, fluoride, restorative, or extraction service is reported separately. Codes D1110 and D1120 are used to report the removal of coronal plaque and calculus that may cause local irritations. When bone loss is present, however, more intense services reported with other codes may be more appropriate. According to the ADA, prophylaxis may be reported in addition to scaling and root planing, one to three teeth per quadrant (D4342). However, third-party payers may have restrictions prohibiting billing these procedures together. Check with payers for specific guidelines. The application of fluoride is not included and is reported using D1206 or D1208. These procedures are not covered by Medicare and by other payers as well; check for specific guidelines for payment.

## Documentation Tips

The following information can be documented on a tooth chart: treatment/location of caries, endodontic procedures, prosthetic services, preventive services, treatment of lesions and dental disease, or other special procedures. A tooth chart may also be used to identify structure and rationale of disease process and the type of service performed on intraoral structures other than teeth.

## Reimbursement Tips

When an oral health assessment is performed by someone other than the dentist (e.g., a licensed dental hygienist), some third-party payers may require that modifier DA Oral health assessment by a licensed health professional other than a dentist, be appended to the code. Check with third-party payers for specific requirements.

## ICD-10-CM Diagnostic Codes

K03.4 Hypercementosis
K03.6 Deposits [accretions] on teeth
K03.7 Posteruptive color changes of dental hard tissues
K05.00 Acute gingivitis, plaque induced
K05.10 Chronic gingivitis, plaque induced
K05.211 Aggressive periodontitis, localized, slight
K05.212 Aggressive periodontitis, localized, moderate
K05.213 Aggressive periodontitis, localized, severe
K05.221 Aggressive periodontitis, generalized, slight
K05.222 Aggressive periodontitis, generalized, moderate
K05.223 Aggressive periodontitis, generalized, severe
K05.311 Chronic periodontitis, localized, slight
K05.312 Chronic periodontitis, localized, moderate
K05.313 Chronic periodontitis, localized, severe
K05.321 Chronic periodontitis, generalized, slight
K05.322 Chronic periodontitis, generalized, moderate
K05.323 Chronic periodontitis, generalized, severe
K05.4 Periodontosis
K05.5 Other periodontal diseases
K06.011 Localized gingival recession, minimal
K06.012 Localized gingival recession, moderate
K06.013 Localized gingival recession, severe
K06.021 Generalized gingival recession, minimal
K06.022 Generalized gingival recession, moderate
K06.023 Generalized gingival recession, severe
K06.1 Gingival enlargement

## Relative Value Units/Medicare Edits

| Non-Facility RVU | Work | PE | MP | Total |
|---|---|---|---|---|
| **D1110** | 0.35 | 0.69 | 0.04 | 1.08 |
| **D1120** | 0.24 | 0.47 | 0.03 | 0.74 |
| **Facility RVU** | **Work** | **PE** | **MP** | **Total** |
| **D1110** | 0.35 | 0.69 | 0.04 | 1.08 |
| **D1120** | 0.24 | 0.47 | 0.03 | 0.74 |

| | FUD | Status | MUE | Modifiers | | | | IOM Reference |
|---|---|---|---|---|---|---|---|---|
| **D1110** | N/A | N | - | N/A | N/A | N/A | N/A | 100-01,5,70.2; 100-02,1,70 |
| **D1120** | N/A | N | - | N/A | N/A | N/A | N/A | |

* with documentation

## Terms To Know

**incident to.** Provision of a service concurrently with another service. For example, additional covered supplies and materials that are furnished after surgery typically are billed as "incident to" a physician's services and not as hospital services. This term is used specifically for revenue codes for pharmacy, supplies, and anesthesia furnished along with radiology and other diagnostic services.

**plaque.** Accumulation of a soft sticky substance on the teeth largely composed of bacteria and its byproducts.

**prophylaxis.** Intervention or protective therapy intended to prevent a disease.

**scaling.** Removal of plaque, calculus, and stains from teeth.

# D1206-D1208

**D1206** topical application of fluoride varnish
**D1208** topical application of fluoride - excluding varnish

## Explanation

Topically applied fluoride treatments are done in the office with a variety of solutions or gels and different application protocols, excluding rinsing or "swish." The fluoride may be applied with trays or specifically to a few, isolated teeth at a time to prevent a high systemic dose from occurring. Fluoride varnish is painted directly on certain areas to help prevent further decay. The fluoride treatment reported here must be applied separately from any prophylaxis paste. Report D1206 for therapeutic application of varnish or D1208 for topical application of fluoride other than varnish.

## Coding Tips

These services must be provided under direct supervision of the dental provider. Appropriate code selection is determined method used. Code D1206 should be used for the application of topical fluoride varnish only. Report D1208 for other topical applications. Any evaluation, radiograph, restorative, or extraction service is reported separately. Removal of coronal plaque is reported separately using D1110 or D1120. Report D9910 if the varnish is applied solely to desensitize the tooth. To report application of interim caries arresting medicament, see D1354.

## Documentation Tips

The following information can be documented on a tooth chart: treatment/location of caries, endodontic procedures, prosthetic services, preventive services, treatment of lesions and dental disease, or other special procedures. A tooth chart may also be used to identify structure and rationale of disease process and the type of service performed on intraoral structures other than teeth.

## Reimbursement Tips

When selecting the procedure or service that accurately identifies the service performed, dentists must use the most accurate code. If the CDT code more accurately identifies the service, this should be used rather than the CPT codes. When an oral health assessment is performed by someone other than the dentist, for example, a licensed dental hygienist, some third-party payers may require that modifier DA Oral health assessment by a licensed health professional other than a dentist, be appended to the code. Check with third-party payers for their specific requirements.

## Associated CPT Codes

99188 Application of topical fluoride varnish by a physician or other qualified health care professional

## ICD-10-CM Diagnostic Codes

Z01.20 Encounter for dental examination and cleaning without abnormal findings
Z01.21 Encounter for dental examination and cleaning with abnormal findings
Z41.8 Encounter for other procedures for purposes other than remedying health state
Z46.4 Encounter for fitting and adjustment of orthodontic device
Z91.120 Patient's intentional underdosing of medication regimen due to financial hardship
Z91.128 Patient's intentional underdosing of medication regimen for other reason
Z91.14 Patient's other noncompliance with medication regimen
Z91.841 Risk for dental caries, low
Z91.842 Risk for dental caries, moderate
Z91.843 Risk for dental caries, high
Z98.810 Dental sealant status
Z98.811 Dental restoration status
Z98.818 Other dental procedure status

## Relative Value Units/Medicare Edits

| Non-Facility RVU | Work | PE | MP | Total |
|---|---|---|---|---|
| **D1206** | 0.20 | 0.39 | 0.02 | 0.61 |
| **D1208** | 0.10 | 0.19 | 0.01 | 0.30 |
| **Facility RVU** | **Work** | **PE** | **MP** | **Total** |
| **D1206** | 0.20 | 0.39 | 0.02 | 0.61 |
| **D1208** | 0.10 | 0.19 | 0.01 | 0.30 |

| | FUD | Status | MUE | Modifiers | | | | IOM Reference |
|---|---|---|---|---|---|---|---|---|
| **D1206** | N/A | N | - | N/A | N/A | N/A | N/A | None |
| **D1208** | N/A | N | - | N/A | N/A | N/A | N/A | |

* with documentation

## Terms To Know

**fluoride.** Compound of the gaseous element fluorine that can be incorporated into bone and teeth and provides some protection in reducing dental decay.

**plaque.** Accumulation of a soft sticky substance on the teeth largely composed of bacteria and its byproducts.

**prophylaxis.** Intervention or protective therapy intended to prevent a disease.

**scaling.** Removal of plaque, calculus, and stains from teeth.

# D1310-D1321

**D1310** nutritional counseling for control of dental disease

*Counseling on food selection and dietary habits as a part of treatment and control of periodontal disease and caries.*

**D1320** tobacco counseling for the control and prevention of oral disease

*Tobacco prevention and cessation services reduce patient risks of developing tobacco-related oral diseases and conditions and improves prognosis for certain dental therapies.*

**D1321** counseling for the control and prevention of adverse oral, behavioral, and systemic health effects associated with high-risk substance use

*Counseling services may include patient education about adverse oral, behavioral, and systemic effects associated with high-risk substance use and administration routes. This includes ingesting, injecting, inhaling and vaping. Substances used in a high-risk manner may include but are not limited to alcohol, opioids, nicotine, cannabis, methamphetamine and other pharmaceuticals or chemicals.*

## Explanation

Diet, tobacco, and substance abuse can have a great effect on teeth and oral health. The goal is to reduce the overall risk for decay and disease due to the consumption of detrimental substances. The advice given during counseling needs to be customized to the patient and present pattern of nutrition, tobacco, vaping, or high-risk substance abuse identified. The counseling should include an explanation of the effects of certain habits, such as holding tobacco in the mouth, substance abuse, or eating sugary snacks between meals. Other choices are discussed and helpful hints for adjusting the present pattern of behavior are outlined. Dietary advice or nutritional counseling as regards the control and prevention of dental disease is given in D1310, tobacco counseling is given in D1320, and high-risk substance abuse is given in D1321.

## Coding Tips

Any evaluation, radiograph, restorative, or extraction service is reported separately. To report the evaluation, see D0120-D0180. These procedures may not be covered by the dental plan. Check with the third-party payer for coverage requirements. When the counseling is performed as the result of the findings of a caries risk assessment using a standardized risk assessment tool, report the risk assessment separately using the appropriate code from D0601-D0603.

## Documentation Tips

Treatment plan documentation should reflect any treatment failure or change in diagnosis and/or a change in treatment plan. There should also be evidence of any initiation or reinstatement of a drug regime, which requires close and continuous skilled medical observation.

## Reimbursement Tips

When selecting the procedure or service that accurately identifies the service performed, dentists must use the most accurate code. If the CDT code more accurately identifies the service, this should be used rather than the CPT codes. When an oral health assessment or counseling is performed by someone other than the dentist (e.g., a licensed dental hygienist), some third-party payers may require that modifier DA Oral health assessment by a licensed health professional other than a dentist, be appended to the code. Check with third-party payers for specific requirements.

## Associated CPT Codes

96156 Health behavior assessment, or re-assessment (ie, health-focused clinical interview, behavioral observations, clinical decision making)

96158 Health behavior intervention, individual, face-to-face; initial 30 minutes

96159 Health behavior intervention, individual, face-to-face; each additional 15 minutes (List separately in addition to code for primary service)

97802 Medical nutrition therapy; initial assessment and intervention, individual, face-to-face with the patient, each 15 minutes

97803 Medical nutrition therapy; re-assessment and intervention, individual, face-to-face with the patient, each 15 minutes

99406 Smoking and tobacco use cessation counseling visit; intermediate, greater than 3 minutes up to 10 minutes

99407 Smoking and tobacco use cessation counseling visit; intensive, greater than 10 minutes

## ICD-10-CM Diagnostic Codes

Z41.8 Encounter for other procedures for purposes other than remedying health state

Z86.39 Personal history of other endocrine, nutritional and metabolic disease

Z87.891 Personal history of nicotine dependence

Z91.120 Patient's intentional underdosing of medication regimen due to financial hardship

Z91.128 Patient's intentional underdosing of medication regimen for other reason

Z91.842 Risk for dental caries, moderate

Z91.843 Risk for dental caries, high

Z91.89 Other specified personal risk factors, not elsewhere classified

## Relative Value Units/Medicare Edits

| Non-Facility RVU | Work | PE | MP | Total |
|---|---|---|---|---|
| **D1310** | 0.20 | 0.40 | 0.02 | 0.62 |
| **D1320** | 0.20 | 0.40 | 0.02 | 0.62 |
| **D1321** | | | | |
| **Facility RVU** | **Work** | **PE** | **MP** | **Total** |
| **D1310** | 0.20 | 0.40 | 0.02 | 0.62 |
| **D1320** | 0.20 | 0.40 | 0.02 | 0.62 |
| **D1321** | | | | |

| | FUD | Status | MUE | Modifiers | | | | IOM Reference |
|---|---|---|---|---|---|---|---|---|
| **D1310** | N/A | N | - | N/A | N/A | N/A | N/A | None |
| **D1320** | N/A | N | - | N/A | N/A | N/A | N/A | |
| **D1321** | N/A | | - | N/A | N/A | N/A | N/A | |

* with documentation

## Terms To Know

**counseling.** Discussion with a patient and/or family concerning one or more of the following areas: diagnostic results, impressions, and/or recommended diagnostic studies; prognosis; risks and benefits of management (treatment) options; instructions for management (treatment) and/or follow-up; importance of compliance with chosen management (treatment) options; risk factor reduction; and patient and family education.

**tobacco use disorder.** Cases in which tobacco is used to the detriment of a person's health or social functioning or in which there is tobacco dependence.

# D1330

**D1330** oral hygiene instructions

*This may include instructions for home care. Examples include tooth brushing technique, flossing, use of special oral hygiene aids.*

## Explanation

Oral hygiene instructions are given to the individual to educate about maintaining good dental health and/or caring for a particular situation. The problem and its etiology must first be defined for the patient. The reason for a lack of proper oral hygiene and/or compliance is addressed with realistic objectives set, possible and desired outcomes discussed, specific instructions outlined, and relevant demonstrations provided for the patient.

## Coding Tips

Any evaluation, radiograph, restorative, or extraction service is reported separately. To report the evaluation, see codes D0120-D0180. When the oral hygiene instructions are provided as the result of the findings of a caries risk assessment using a standardized risk assessment tool, report the risk assessment separately using the appropriate code from D0601-D0603.This procedure may not be covered by the patient's dental plan. Check with the third-party payer for coverage requirements.

## Documentation Tips

Treatment plan documentation should reflect any treatment failure or change in diagnosis and/or a change in treatment plan. There should also be evidence of any initiation or reinstatement of a drug regime, which requires close and continuous skilled medical observation.

## Reimbursement Tips

When selecting the procedure or service that accurately identifies the service performed, dentists must use the most accurate code. If the CDT code more accurately identifies the service, this should be used rather than the CPT codes. When an oral health assessment is performed by someone other than the dentist, for example, a licensed dental hygienist, some third-party payers may require that modifier DA Oral health assessment by a licensed health professional other than a dentist, be appended to the code. Check with third-party payers for their specific requirements.

## Associated CPT Codes

| | |
|---|---|
| 96156 | Health behavior assessment, or re-assessment (ie, health-focused clinical interview, behavioral observations, clinical decision making) |
| 96158 | Health behavior intervention, individual, face-to-face; initial 30 minutes |
| 96159 | Health behavior intervention, individual, face-to-face; each additional 15 minutes (List separately in addition to code for primary service) |

## ICD-10-CM Diagnostic Codes

| | |
|---|---|
| Z01.20 | Encounter for dental examination and cleaning without abnormal findings |
| Z01.21 | Encounter for dental examination and cleaning with abnormal findings |
| Z41.8 | Encounter for other procedures for purposes other than remedying health state |
| Z46.4 | Encounter for fitting and adjustment of orthodontic device |
| Z91.120 | Patient's intentional underdosing of medication regimen due to financial hardship |
| Z91.128 | Patient's intentional underdosing of medication regimen for other reason |
| Z91.841 | Risk for dental caries, low |
| Z91.842 | Risk for dental caries, moderate |
| Z91.843 | Risk for dental caries, high |
| Z97.2 | Presence of dental prosthetic device (complete) (partial) |
| Z98.810 | Dental sealant status |
| Z98.811 | Dental restoration status |
| Z98.818 | Other dental procedure status |

## Relative Value Units/Medicare Edits

| Non-Facility RVU | Work | PE | MP | Total |
|---|---|---|---|---|
| D1330 | 0.22 | 0.43 | 0.03 | 0.68 |
| **Facility RVU** | **Work** | **PE** | **MP** | **Total** |
| D1330 | 0.22 | 0.43 | 0.03 | 0.68 |

| | FUD | Status | MUE | Modifiers | | | | IOM Reference |
|---|---|---|---|---|---|---|---|---|
| D1330 | N/A | N | - | N/A | N/A | N/A | N/A | None |

* with documentation

## Terms To Know

**assessment.** Process of reviewing a patient's health status, including collecting and studying information and data such as test values, signs, and symptoms.

**caries.** Localized section of tooth decay that begins on the tooth surface with destruction of the calcified enamel, allowing bacterial destruction to continue and form cavities and may extend to the dentin and pulp.

**oral.** Pertaining to the mouth.

# D1351

**D1351** sealant - per tooth

*Mechanically and/or chemically prepared enamel surface sealed to prevent decay.*

## Explanation

Sealant is applied to a particular tooth. First, the tooth is cleaned and polished, then an etching gel is placed onto the tooth, which creates a bonding surface so the sealant will bond to the tooth. When the tooth is etched, it is dried and the dentist can then paint the liquid sealant plastic. When the sealant is in place, a curing light is shined onto the tooth and causes the plastic sealant to set immediately. If necessary, the biting surface of the tooth is checked and buffed down.

## Coding Tips

This code is used to report the application of resin as a sealant in a pit or fissure. When resin is applied to a pit or fissure that has a cavitated lesion not extending into the dentin, see D1352. Any evaluation, radiograph, restorative, or extraction service is reported separately. Third-party payers often limit this benefit to permanent first and second molars with no caries or restorations on the occlusal surface and may include age limitations. Payers may also include replacement or repairs within a certain time frame in this code. Check with third-party payers for their specific policies. This code should be reported per tooth. To report the repair of sealant, see D1353.

## Documentation Tips

The following information can be documented on a tooth chart: treatment/location of caries, endodontic procedures, prosthetic services, preventive services, treatment of lesions and dental disease, or other special procedures.

## Reimbursement Tips

The tooth/root number should be indicated on the claim. The tooth number(s) reported should correspond to the number of teeth treated.

## ICD-10-CM Diagnostic Codes

| | |
|---|---|
| K02.51 | Dental caries on pit and fissure surface limited to enamel |
| K02.61 | Dental caries on smooth surface limited to enamel |
| M35.0C | Sjögren syndrome with dental involvement |
| Z91.841 | Risk for dental caries, low |
| Z91.842 | Risk for dental caries, moderate |
| Z91.843 | Risk for dental caries, high |

## Relative Value Units/Medicare Edits

| Non-Facility RVU | Work | PE | MP | Total |
|---|---|---|---|---|
| **D1351** | 0.19 | 0.38 | 0.02 | 0.59 |
| **Facility RVU** | **Work** | **PE** | **MP** | **Total** |
| **D1351** | 0.19 | 0.38 | 0.02 | 0.59 |

| | FUD | Status | MUE | Modifiers | | | | IOM Reference |
|---|---|---|---|---|---|---|---|---|
| **D1351** | N/A | N | - | N/A | N/A | N/A | N/A | None |

* with documentation

# D1352

**D1352** preventive resin restoration in a moderate to high caries risk patient - permanent tooth

*Conservative restoration of an active cavitated lesion in a pit or fissure that does not extend into dentin; includes placement of a sealant in any radiating non-carious fissures or pits.*

## Explanation

Preventive resin restoration is a minimally invasive procedure. The dentist removes carious pits and fissures using small burs. Tooth removal only includes carious enamel. The tooth surface is restored using an adhesive technique with a composite resin.

## Coding Tips

This code is used to report the application of resin into a pit or fissure that has a cavitated lesion that does not extend into the dentin. When no cavitated lesion is present, see D1351. When the cavitated lesion extends into the dentin, see D2391. When a caries risk assessment is performed during the same encounter (using standardized assessment tools), report the appropriate code from the D0600–D0603 series.

## Documentation Tips

The following information can be documented on a tooth chart: treatment/location of caries, endodontic procedures, prosthetic services, preventive services, treatment of lesions and dental disease, or other special procedures. A tooth chart may also be used to identify structure and rationale of disease process and the type of service performed on intraoral structures other than teeth.

## Reimbursement Tips

The tooth/root number should be indicated on the claim. Coverage of this procedure varies by payer. Check with payers for their specific coverage guidelines.

## ICD-10-CM Diagnostic Codes

| | |
|---|---|
| K00.3 | Mottled teeth |
| K00.4 | Disturbances in tooth formation |
| K02.3 | Arrested dental caries |
| K02.51 | Dental caries on pit and fissure surface limited to enamel |
| K02.52 | Dental caries on pit and fissure surface penetrating into dentin |
| K02.53 | Dental caries on pit and fissure surface penetrating into pulp |
| K02.61 | Dental caries on smooth surface limited to enamel |
| K02.62 | Dental caries on smooth surface penetrating into dentin |
| K02.63 | Dental caries on smooth surface penetrating into pulp |
| K02.7 | Dental root caries |
| K02.9 | Dental caries, unspecified |
| K03.0 | Excessive attrition of teeth |
| K03.1 | Abrasion of teeth |
| K03.2 | Erosion of teeth |
| K03.7 | Posteruptive color changes of dental hard tissues |
| K03.81 | Cracked tooth |
| K03.89 | Other specified diseases of hard tissues of teeth |
| K03.9 | Disease of hard tissues of teeth, unspecified |
| Z91.841 | Risk for dental caries, low |
| Z91.842 | Risk for dental caries, moderate |
| Z91.843 | Risk for dental caries, high |

## Relative Value Units/Medicare Edits

| Non-Facility RVU | Work | PE | MP | Total |
|---|---|---|---|---|
| D1352 | 0.24 | 0.47 | 0.03 | 0.74 |
| **Facility RVU** | **Work** | **PE** | **MP** | **Total** |
| D1352 | 0.24 | 0.47 | 0.03 | 0.74 |

| | FUD | Status | MUE | Modifiers | | | | IOM Reference |
|---|---|---|---|---|---|---|---|---|
| D1352 | N/A | I | - | N/A | N/A | N/A | N/A | None |

* with documentation

## Terms To Know

**caries.** Localized section of tooth decay that begins on the tooth surface with destruction of the calcified enamel, allowing bacterial destruction to continue and form cavities and may extend to the dentin and pulp.

**dentin.** Hard substance of the tooth found beneath the enamel on the crown and the cementum on the root that surrounds the living pulp tissue.

**fissure.** Deep furrow, groove, or cleft in tissue structures.

**permanent tooth.** One of 32 adult teeth that usually erupt between 6 years and adulthood with the third molar.

Dental - Preventive

# D1353

**D1353** sealant repair - per tooth

## Explanation

The dentist repairs the sealant previously placed on a particular tooth. Sealants are plastic-type coatings placed on the chewing surfaces to teeth to prevent tooth decay. The damaged tooth sealant is removed, the tooth is cleaned and polished, and then an etching gel is placed onto the tooth, which creates a bonding surface so the sealant will bond to the tooth. When the tooth is etched, it is dried and the dentist can then paint the liquid sealant plastic. When the sealant is in place, a curing light is shined onto the tooth and causes the plastic sealant to set immediately. If necessary, the biting surface of the tooth is checked and buffed down.

## Coding Tips

This code should be reported per tooth. To report the placement of a tooth sealant, see D1351. To report the preventive resin restoration of a permanent tooth that has a moderate to high caries risk, see D1352. To report interim caries arresting medicament, see D1354.

## Documentation Tips

The following information can be documented on a tooth chart: treatment/location of caries, endodontic procedures, prosthetic services, preventive services, treatment of lesions and dental disease, or other special procedures.

## Reimbursement Tips

The tooth number should be indicated on the claim. The tooth number(s) reported should correspond to the number of teeth treated.

## ICD-10-CM Diagnostic Codes

| | |
|---|---|
| K02.3 | Arrested dental caries |
| K02.51 | Dental caries on pit and fissure surface limited to enamel |
| K02.52 | Dental caries on pit and fissure surface penetrating into dentin |
| K02.53 | Dental caries on pit and fissure surface penetrating into pulp |
| K02.61 | Dental caries on smooth surface limited to enamel |
| K02.62 | Dental caries on smooth surface penetrating into dentin |
| K02.63 | Dental caries on smooth surface penetrating into pulp |
| K02.7 | Dental root caries |
| K02.9 | Dental caries, unspecified |
| Z41.8 | Encounter for other procedures for purposes other than remedying health state |
| Z91.841 | Risk for dental caries, low |
| Z91.842 | Risk for dental caries, moderate |
| Z91.843 | Risk for dental caries, high |

## Relative Value Units/Medicare Edits

| Non-Facility RVU | Work | PE | MP | Total |
|---|---|---|---|---|
| D1353 | 0.15 | 0.31 | 0.02 | 0.48 |
| **Facility RVU** | **Work** | **PE** | **MP** | **Total** |
| D1353 | 0.15 | 0.31 | 0.02 | 0.48 |

| | FUD | Status | MUE | Modifiers | | | | IOM Reference |
|---|---|---|---|---|---|---|---|---|
| D1353 | N/A | N | - | N/A | N/A | N/A | N/A | None |

* with documentation

# D1354

▲ **D1354** application of caries arresting medicament – per tooth

*Conservative treatment of an active, non-symptomatic carious lesion by topical application of a caries arresting or inhibiting medicament and without mechanical removal of sound tooth structure.*

## Explanation

The provider applies arresting caries treatment (ACT) by the topical application of a caries arresting or inhibiting medicament such as silver diamine fluoride (SDF) (with or without tannic acid) to prevent or arrest further decay. The provider isolates the area to be treated with cotton rolls and protects the gingival tissues with petroleum jelly. Alternatively, a rubber dam may be used. The medicament is transferred directly to the affected area using an applicator. Excessive medicament is removed, and the area is allowed to dry.

## Coding Tips

This service is reported once for each tooth treated. To report the topical application of fluoride varnish, see D1206. To report the topical application of fluoride other than fluoride varnish, see D1208.

## Documentation Tips

The following information can be documented on a tooth chart: treatment/location of caries, endodontic procedures, prosthetic services, preventive services, treatment of lesions and dental disease, or other special procedures. A tooth chart may also be used to identify structure and rationale of disease process and the type of service performed on intraoral structures other than teeth.

## ICD-10-CM Diagnostic Codes

| | |
|---|---|
| K02.3 | Arrested dental caries |
| K02.51 | Dental caries on pit and fissure surface limited to enamel |
| K02.52 | Dental caries on pit and fissure surface penetrating into dentin |
| Z91.841 | Risk for dental caries, low |
| Z91.842 | Risk for dental caries, moderate |
| Z91.843 | Risk for dental caries, high |

## Relative Value Units/Medicare Edits

| Non-Facility RVU | Work | PE | MP | Total |
|---|---|---|---|---|
| D1354 | 0.00 | 0.00 | 0.00 | 0.00 |
| **Facility RVU** | **Work** | **PE** | **MP** | **Total** |
| D1354 | 0.00 | 0.00 | 0.00 | 0.00 |

| | FUD | Status | MUE | Modifiers | | | | IOM Reference |
|---|---|---|---|---|---|---|---|---|
| D1354 | N/A | N | - | N/A | N/A | N/A | N/A | None |

* with documentation

## Terms To Know

**acid etching.** Process of using an acidic chemical substance to prepare a tooth surface for bonding.

# D1355

**D1355** caries preventive medicament application - per tooth

*For primary prevention or remineralization. Medicaments applied do not include topical fluorides.*

## Explanation

The provider uses topical application of a caries preventive medicament, such as antimicrobials or remineralization substance (calcium and phosphate), to prevent or arrest further decay. The provider isolates the area to be treated with cotton rolls and protects the gingival tissues with petroleum jelly. Alternatively, a rubber dam may be used. The medicament is transferred directly to the affected area using an applicator. Excessive medicament is removed and the area is allowed to dry.

## Coding Tips

This service is reported once for each tooth treated. To report the topical application of fluoride varnish, see D1206. To report the topical application of fluoride other than fluoride varnish, see D1208. For sealant application or repair, see D1351-D1353.

## Documentation Tips

The following information can be documented on a tooth chart: treatment/location of caries, endodontic procedures, prosthetic services, preventive services, treatment of lesions and dental disease, or other special procedures. A tooth chart may also be used to identify structure and rationale of disease process and the type of service performed on intraoral structures other than teeth.

## ICD-10-CM Diagnostic Codes

| | |
|---|---|
| K02.3 | Arrested dental caries |
| K02.51 | Dental caries on pit and fissure surface limited to enamel |
| K02.52 | Dental caries on pit and fissure surface penetrating into dentin |
| Z91.841 | Risk for dental caries, low |
| Z91.842 | Risk for dental caries, moderate |
| Z91.843 | Risk for dental caries, high |

## Relative Value Units/Medicare Edits

| Non-Facility RVU | Work | PE | MP | Total |
|---|---|---|---|---|
| D1355 | | | | |
| **Facility RVU** | **Work** | **PE** | **MP** | **Total** |
| D1355 | | | | |

| | FUD | Status | MUE | Modifiers | | | | IOM Reference |
|---|---|---|---|---|---|---|---|---|
| D1355 | N/A | | - | N/A | N/A | N/A | N/A | |

* with documentation

## Terms To Know

**caries.** Localized section of tooth decay that begins on the tooth surface with destruction of the calcified enamel, allowing bacterial destruction to continue and form cavities and may extend to the dentin and pulp.

**medicament.** Medical and therapeutic compound, drug, substance, or remedy.

Dental - Preventive

# D1510-D1517

**D1510** space maintainer - fixed, unilateral - per quadrant

*Excludes a distal shoe space maintainer.*

**D1516** space maintainer - fixed - bilateral, maxillary

**D1517** space maintainer - fixed - bilateral, mandibular

## Explanation

A space maintainer is an appliance made of plastic or metal that is custom fit to the patient's mouth to maintain the space intended for a permanent tooth. Normally children do not lose their primary teeth until a permanent tooth is ready to replace the baby tooth. However, when primary teeth are lost prematurely, due to severe dental disease (caries) or trauma, a space maintainer is used to keep the surrounding teeth from moving into the empty space left. There are a number of different types of space maintainers. Fixed devices include band-and-loop maintainers that consist of a stainless steel wire. The dentist must first create a mold of the patient's mouth. This is sent to a laboratory where the space maintainer is made. The space maintainer is then returned to the dentist and the dentist cements the metal band around the tooth behind the empty space. Next, a loop or brace is placed over the empty space. This loop or brace extends to and rests against the tooth in front of the empty space. Another method of attaching a band-and-loop maintainer is by use of a crown on one of the adjacent teeth. Code D1510 is reported when the fixed space maintainer is applied on one side of the mouth. Code D1516 is reported when the fixed space maintainer is applied on both sides of the upper jaw (maxilla). Code D1517 is reported when the fixed space maintainer is applied on both sides of the lower jaw (mandible). Report D1510 once per quadrant.

## Coding Tips

For removable space maintainers, see D1520 (unilateral) and D1526–D1527 (bilateral). Recementation (luting) or rebonding of space maintainer is reported with D1550; removal of fixed space maintainer is reported with D1555. Coverage may be dependent upon patient's age. Check with third-party payers regarding any age requirements. Payers frequently request identification of the space being maintained by identifying the quadrant/arch.

## Documentation Tips

The following information can be documented on a tooth chart: treatment/location of caries, endodontic procedures, prosthetic services, preventive services, treatment of lesions and dental disease, or other special procedures. A tooth chart may also be used to identify structure and rationale of disease process and the type of service performed on intraoral structures other than teeth.

## Reimbursement Tips

The tooth number should be indicated on the claim.

## ICD-10-CM Diagnostic Codes

| | |
|---|---|
| K00.6 | Disturbances in tooth eruption |
| K08.401 | Partial loss of teeth, unspecified cause, class I |
| K08.402 | Partial loss of teeth, unspecified cause, class II |
| K08.403 | Partial loss of teeth, unspecified cause, class III |
| K08.404 | Partial loss of teeth, unspecified cause, class IV |
| K08.411 | Partial loss of teeth due to trauma, class I |
| K08.412 | Partial loss of teeth due to trauma, class II |
| K08.413 | Partial loss of teeth due to trauma, class III |
| K08.414 | Partial loss of teeth due to trauma, class IV |
| K08.421 | Partial loss of teeth due to periodontal diseases, class I |
| K08.422 | Partial loss of teeth due to periodontal diseases, class II |
| K08.423 | Partial loss of teeth due to periodontal diseases, class III |
| K08.424 | Partial loss of teeth due to periodontal diseases, class IV |
| K08.431 | Partial loss of teeth due to caries, class I |
| K08.432 | Partial loss of teeth due to caries, class II |
| K08.433 | Partial loss of teeth due to caries, class III |
| K08.434 | Partial loss of teeth due to caries, class IV |
| K08.491 | Partial loss of teeth due to other specified cause, class I |
| K08.492 | Partial loss of teeth due to other specified cause, class II |
| K08.493 | Partial loss of teeth due to other specified cause, class III |
| K08.494 | Partial loss of teeth due to other specified cause, class IV |

## Relative Value Units/Medicare Edits

| Non-Facility RVU | Work | PE | MP | Total |
|---|---|---|---|---|
| **D1510** | 1.14 | 2.26 | 0.14 | 3.54 |
| **D1516** | 1.16 | 2.31 | 0.14 | 3.61 |
| **D1517** | 1.16 | 2.31 | 0.14 | 3.61 |
| **Facility RVU** | **Work** | **PE** | **MP** | **Total** |
| **D1510** | 1.14 | 2.26 | 0.14 | 3.54 |
| **D1516** | 1.16 | 2.31 | 0.14 | 3.61 |
| **D1517** | 1.16 | 2.31 | 0.14 | 3.61 |

| | FUD | Status | MUE | Modifiers | | | | IOM Reference |
|---|---|---|---|---|---|---|---|---|
| **D1510** | N/A | R | - | N/A | N/A | N/A | 80* | 100-02,1,70; 100-04,4,20.5; None |
| **D1516** | N/A | N | - | N/A | N/A | N/A | N/A | |
| **D1517** | N/A | N | - | N/A | N/A | N/A | N/A | |

* with documentation

## Terms To Know

**deciduous tooth.** Any of 20 teeth that usually erupt between the ages of 6 and 24 months and are later shed as the permanent, adult teeth displace them.

**space maintainer.** In dentistry, plastic or metal appliance that is custom fit to the patient's mouth to maintain the space intended for a permanent tooth.

# D1520-D1527

**D1520** space maintainer - removable, unilateral - per quadrant
**D1526** space maintainer - removable - bilateral, maxillary
**D1527** space maintainer - removable - bilateral, mandibular

## Explanation

A removable unilateral space maintainer is applied. A space maintainer is an appliance made of plastic or metal that is custom fit to the patient's mouth to maintain the space intended for a permanent tooth. Normally children do not lose their primary teeth until a permanent tooth is ready to replace the primary tooth. However, when primary teeth are lost prematurely, due to severe dental disease (caries) or trauma, a space maintainer is used to keep the surrounding teeth from moving into the empty space. There are a number of different types of space maintainers. Removable space maintainers consist of an artificial tooth. Removable space maintainers can only be used by older children. Report D1520 when the space maintainer is placed on one side of the mouth once per quadrant. Code D1526 is reported when the removable space maintainer is applied on both sides of the upper jaw (maxilla). Code D1527 is reported when the removable space maintainer is applied on both sides of the lower jaw (mandible).

## Coding Tips

For a fixed unilateral space maintainer, see D1510. For bilateral fixed space maintainer, see D1516–D1517. Recementation (luting) or rebonding of space maintainer is reported with D1550; removal of fixed space maintainer is reported with D1555. Coverage may be dependent upon patient's age. Check with third-party payers regarding any age requirements. Payers frequently request identification of the space being maintained by identifying the quadrant/arch.

## Documentation Tips

The following information can be documented on a tooth chart: treatment/location of caries, endodontic procedures, prosthetic services, preventive services, treatment of lesions and dental disease, or other special procedures. A tooth chart may also be used to identify structure and rationale of disease process and the type of service performed on intraoral structures other than teeth.

## Reimbursement Tips

The tooth number should be indicated on the claim.

## ICD-10-CM Diagnostic Codes

| | |
|---|---|
| K00.6 | Disturbances in tooth eruption |
| K08.401 | Partial loss of teeth, unspecified cause, class I |
| K08.402 | Partial loss of teeth, unspecified cause, class II |
| K08.403 | Partial loss of teeth, unspecified cause, class III |
| K08.404 | Partial loss of teeth, unspecified cause, class IV |
| K08.411 | Partial loss of teeth due to trauma, class I |
| K08.412 | Partial loss of teeth due to trauma, class II |
| K08.413 | Partial loss of teeth due to trauma, class III |
| K08.414 | Partial loss of teeth due to trauma, class IV |
| K08.421 | Partial loss of teeth due to periodontal diseases, class I |
| K08.422 | Partial loss of teeth due to periodontal diseases, class II |
| K08.423 | Partial loss of teeth due to periodontal diseases, class III |
| K08.424 | Partial loss of teeth due to periodontal diseases, class IV |
| K08.431 | Partial loss of teeth due to caries, class I |
| K08.432 | Partial loss of teeth due to caries, class II |
| K08.433 | Partial loss of teeth due to caries, class III |
| K08.434 | Partial loss of teeth due to caries, class IV |
| K08.491 | Partial loss of teeth due to other specified cause, class I |
| K08.492 | Partial loss of teeth due to other specified cause, class II |
| K08.493 | Partial loss of teeth due to other specified cause, class III |
| K08.494 | Partial loss of teeth due to other specified cause, class IV |

## Relative Value Units/Medicare Edits

| Non-Facility RVU | Work | PE | MP | Total |
|---|---|---|---|---|
| **D1520** | 1.29 | 2.56 | 0.16 | 4.01 |
| **D1526** | 1.36 | 2.70 | 0.16 | 4.22 |
| **D1527** | 1.36 | 2.70 | 0.16 | 4.22 |
| **Facility RVU** | **Work** | **PE** | **MP** | **Total** |
| **D1520** | 1.29 | 2.56 | 0.16 | 4.01 |
| **D1526** | 1.36 | 2.70 | 0.16 | 4.22 |
| **D1527** | 1.36 | 2.70 | 0.16 | 4.22 |

| | FUD | Status | MUE | Modifiers | | | | IOM Reference |
|---|---|---|---|---|---|---|---|---|
| **D1520** | N/A | R | - | N/A | N/A | N/A | 80* | None |
| **D1526** | N/A | N | - | N/A | N/A | N/A | N/A | |
| **D1527** | N/A | N | - | N/A | N/A | N/A | N/A | |

* with documentation

## Terms To Know

**deciduous tooth.** Any of 20 teeth that usually erupt between the ages of 6 and 24 months and are later shed as the permanent, adult teeth displace them.

**permanent tooth.** One of 32 adult teeth that usually erupt between 6 years and adulthood with the third molar.

**space maintainer.** In dentistry, plastic or metal appliance that is custom fit to the patient's mouth to maintain the space intended for a permanent tooth.

Dental - Preventive

# D1551-D1553

**D1551** re-cement or re-bond bilateral space maintainer - maxillary
**D1552** re-cement or re-bond bilateral space maintainer - mandibular
**D1553** re-cement or re-bond unilateral space maintainer - per quadrant

## Explanation

Recementation or rebonding of a fixed space maintainer is performed. A space maintainer is an appliance made of plastic or metal that is custom fit to the patient's mouth to maintain the space intended for a permanent tooth. Normally children do not lose their primary teeth until a permanent tooth is ready to replace the primary tooth. However, when primary teeth are lost prematurely due to disturbances in tooth eruption, severe dental disease (caries), or trauma, a space maintainer is used to keep the surrounding teeth from moving into the empty space. Fixed space maintainers must be cemented or bonded into place. Recementing or rebonding of the permanent space maintainer may be required if the space maintainer becomes loose or dislodged. When performed on a single tooth space on the upper jaw, report D1551; when performed on a single tooth space on the lower jaw report, D1552. When performed on a quadrant, report D1553.

## Coding Tips

Necessary clasps are included as part of the service. To report fixed space maintainer, see D1510 (unilateral) or D1516–D1517 (bilateral). For removable space maintainers, see D1520 (unilateral) and D1526–D1527 (bilateral). Coverage of space maintainers may be dependent upon patient's age. Check with third-party payers regarding any age requirements. Payers frequently request identification of the space being maintained by identifying the quadrant/arch.

## ICD-10-CM Diagnostic Codes

| | |
|---|---|
| Z46.4 | Encounter for fitting and adjustment of orthodontic device |
| Z98.811 | Dental restoration status |
| Z98.818 | Other dental procedure status |

## Relative Value Units/Medicare Edits

| Non-Facility RVU | Work | PE | MP | Total |
|---|---|---|---|---|
| D1551 | 0.23 | 0.46 | 0.03 | 0.72 |
| D1552 | 0.23 | 0.46 | 0.03 | 0.72 |
| D1553 | 0.23 | 0.46 | 0.03 | 0.72 |
| **Facility RVU** | **Work** | **PE** | **MP** | **Total** |
| D1551 | 0.23 | 0.46 | 0.03 | 0.72 |
| D1552 | 0.23 | 0.46 | 0.03 | 0.72 |
| D1553 | 0.23 | 0.46 | 0.03 | 0.72 |

| | FUD | Status | MUE | Modifiers | | | | IOM Reference |
|---|---|---|---|---|---|---|---|---|
| D1551 | N/A | R | - | N/A | N/A | N/A | 80* | None |
| D1552 | N/A | R | - | N/A | N/A | N/A | 80* | |
| D1553 | N/A | R | - | N/A | N/A | N/A | 80* | |

* with documentation

## Terms To Know

**deciduous tooth.** Any of 20 teeth that usually erupt between the ages of 6 and 24 months and are later shed as the permanent, adult teeth displace them.

**space maintainer.** In dentistry, plastic or metal appliance that is custom fit to the patient's mouth to maintain the space intended for a permanent tooth.

# D1556-D1558

**D1556** removal of fixed unilateral space maintainer - per quadrant
**D1557** removal of fixed bilateral space maintainer - maxillary
**D1558** removal of fixed bilateral space maintainer - mandibular

## Explanation

A fixed space maintainer that was placed is removed. A space maintainer is an appliance made of plastic or metal that is custom fit to the patient's mouth to maintain the space intended for a permanent tooth. Normally children do not lose their primary teeth until a permanent tooth is ready to replace the primary tooth. However, when primary teeth are lost prematurely, due to disturbances in tooth eruption, severe dental disease (caries), or trauma, a space maintainer is used to keep the surrounding teeth from moving into the empty space. Fixed space maintainers are cemented or bonded into place. The space maintainer may be removed once the permanent tooth is ready for eruption or if it becomes damaged. Removal techniques vary depending upon the type of fixation used. Report D1556 for removal of a unilateral fixed space maintainer, once per quadrant. Report D1557 for removal of a bilateral maxillary space maintainer. Report D1558 for a mandibular fixed bilateral space maintainer.

## Coding Tips

For re-cementation or re-bonding of the space maintainer, see D1551-D1553. For provision of a fixed space maintainer, see D1510-D1517. For provision of a removable space maintainer, see D1520-D1527.

## ICD-10-CM Diagnostic Codes

| | |
|---|---|
| Z98.811 | Dental restoration status |
| Z98.818 | Other dental procedure status |

## Relative Value Units/Medicare Edits

| Non-Facility RVU | Work | PE | MP | Total |
|---|---|---|---|---|
| D1556 | 0.21 | 0.42 | 0.03 | 0.66 |
| D1557 | 0.21 | 0.42 | 0.03 | 0.66 |
| D1558 | 0.21 | 0.42 | 0.03 | 0.66 |
| **Facility RVU** | **Work** | **PE** | **MP** | **Total** |
| D1556 | 0.21 | 0.42 | 0.03 | 0.66 |
| D1557 | 0.21 | 0.42 | 0.03 | 0.66 |
| D1558 | 0.21 | 0.42 | 0.03 | 0.66 |

| | FUD | Status | MUE | Modifiers | | | | IOM Reference |
|---|---|---|---|---|---|---|---|---|
| D1556 | N/A | N | - | N/A | N/A | N/A | N/A | None |
| D1557 | N/A | N | - | N/A | N/A | N/A | N/A | |
| D1558 | N/A | N | - | N/A | N/A | N/A | N/A | |

* with documentation

## Terms To Know

**space maintainer.** In dentistry, plastic or metal appliance that is custom fit to the patient's mouth to maintain the space intended for a permanent tooth.

**tooth bounded space.** Empty space in the mouth due to a missing tooth that is surrounded by a tooth on each side.

# D1701-D1704

**D1701** Pfizer-BioNTech Covid-19 vaccine administration - first dose

*SARSCOV2 COVID-19 VAC mRNA 30mcg/0.3mL IM DOSE 1*

**D1702** Pfizer-BioNTech Covid-19 vaccine administration - second dose

*SARSCOV2 COVID-19 VAC mRNA 30mcg/0.3mL IM DOSE 2*

**D1703** Moderna Covid-19 vaccine administration - first dose

*SARSCOV2 COVID-19 VAC mRNA 100mcg/0.5mL IM DOSE 1*

**D1704** Moderna Covid-19 vaccine administration - second dose

*SARSCOV2 COVID-19 VAC mRNA 100mcg/0.5mL IM DOSE 2*

## Explanation

A vaccine produces active immunization by inducing the immune system to build its own antibodies against specific microorganisms/viruses. The body retains memory of the antibody production pattern for long-term protection. These codes report the immunization administration only of a preservative-free spike protein vaccine against severe acute respiratory syndrome coronavirus 2, also known as SARS-CoV-2, coronavirus disease, or COVID-19. Based on messenger RNA (mRNA) that utilizes a lipid nanoparticle (LNP) as a delivery platform, these vaccines are intended for intramuscular use and have emergency use authorization (EUA) from the FDA. Report D1701 for administration of the first dose of the Pfizer-BioNTech 30 mcg/0.3mL dosage (diluent reconstituted) and D1702 for administration of the second dose. Report D1703 for administration of the first dose of the Moderna 100 mcg/0.5mL dosage and D1704 for administration of the second dose. These codes include vaccine risk/benefit counseling, when performed.

## Coding Tips

These codes are reported based upon the vaccine administered and first or second dose.

## Associated CPT Codes

0001A Immunization administration by intramuscular injection of severe acute respiratory syndrome coronavirus 2 (SARS-CoV-2) (coronavirus disease [COVID-19]) vaccine, mRNA-LNP, spike protein, preservative free, 30 mcg/0.3mL dosage, diluent reconstituted; first dose

0002A Immunization administration by intramuscular injection of severe acute respiratory syndrome coronavirus 2 (SARS-CoV-2) (coronavirus disease [COVID-19]) vaccine, mRNA-LNP, spike protein, preservative free, 30 mcg/0.3mL dosage, diluent reconstituted; second dose

0011A Immunization administration by intramuscular injection of severe acute respiratory syndrome coronavirus 2 (SARS-CoV-2) (coronavirus disease [COVID-19]) vaccine, mRNA-LNP, spike protein, preservative free, 100 mcg/0.5mL dosage; first dose

0012A Immunization administration by intramuscular injection of severe acute respiratory syndrome coronavirus 2 (SARS-CoV-2) (coronavirus disease [COVID-19]) vaccine, mRNA-LNP, spike protein, preservative free, 100 mcg/0.5mL dosage; second dose

## ICD-10-CM Diagnostic Codes

Z23 Encounter for immunization

Z29.8 Encounter for other specified prophylactic measures

## Relative Value Units/Medicare Edits

| Non-Facility RVU | Work | PE | MP | Total |
|---|---|---|---|---|
| D1701 | | | | |
| D1702 | | | | |
| D1703 | | | | |
| D1704 | | | | |

| Facility RVU | Work | PE | MP | Total |
|---|---|---|---|---|
| D1701 | | | | |
| D1702 | | | | |
| D1703 | | | | |
| D1704 | | | | |

| | FUD | Status | MUE | Modifiers | | | | IOM Reference |
|---|---|---|---|---|---|---|---|---|
| D1701 | N/A | | - | N/A | N/A | N/A | N/A | |
| D1702 | N/A | | - | N/A | N/A | N/A | N/A | |
| D1703 | N/A | | - | N/A | N/A | N/A | N/A | |
| D1704 | N/A | | - | N/A | N/A | N/A | N/A | |

* with documentation

## Terms To Know

**vaccine.** Preparation formed by microorganisms or viruses that have been altered to reduce their virulence but retain their ability to trigger the immune response.

# D1705-D1706

**D1705** AstraZeneca Covid-19 vaccine administration - first dose

*SARSCOV2 COVID-19 VAC rS-ChAdOx1 5x1010 VP/.5mL IM DOSE 1*

**D1706** AstraZeneca Covid-19 vaccine administration - second dose

*SARSCOV2 COVID-19 VAC rS-ChAdOx1 5x1010 VP/.5mL IM DOSE 2*

## Explanation

A vaccine produces active immunization by inducing the immune system to build its own antibodies against specific microorganisms/viruses. The body retains memory of the antibody production pattern for long-term protection. These codes report the immunization administration only of a preservative-free spike protein DNA vaccine against severe acute respiratory syndrome coronavirus 2, also known as SARS-CoV-2, coronavirus disease, or COVID-19. Using a genetically modified chimpanzee adenovirus vaccine vector as a delivery platform, these vaccines are intended for intramuscular use. Following vaccination, the immune system is groomed to attack the SARS-CoV-2 virus if it later infects the body. These codes are specific to the AstraZeneca vaccine, which is awaiting emergency use authorization (EUA) by the FDA. Report D1705 for administration of the first dose of the AstraZeneca $5x10^{10}$ viral particles/.5 mL and D1706 for administration of the second dose. Dosing interval is 28 days.

## Coding Tips

These codes are reported based upon the vaccine administered and first or second dose.

## Associated CPT Codes

0021A Immunization administration by intramuscular injection of severe acute respiratory syndrome coronavirus 2 (SARS-CoV-2) (coronavirus disease [COVID-19]) vaccine, DNA, spike protein, chimpanzee adenovirus Oxford 1 (ChAdOx1) vector, preservative free, $5x10^{10}$ viral particles/0.5mL dosage; first dose

0022A Immunization administration by intramuscular injection of severe acute respiratory syndrome coronavirus 2 (SARS-CoV-2) (coronavirus disease [COVID-19]) vaccine, DNA, spike protein, chimpanzee adenovirus Oxford 1 (ChAdOx1) vector, preservative free, 5x1010 viral particles/0.5mL dosage; second dose

## ICD-10-CM Diagnostic Codes

Z23 Encounter for immunization

Z29.8 Encounter for other specified prophylactic measures

## Relative Value Units/Medicare Edits

| Non-Facility RVU | Work | PE | MP | Total |
|---|---|---|---|---|
| D1705 | | | | |
| D1706 | | | | |
| **Facility RVU** | **Work** | **PE** | **MP** | **Total** |
| D1705 | | | | |
| D1706 | | | | |

| | FUD | Status | MUE | Modifiers | | | | IOM Reference |
|---|---|---|---|---|---|---|---|---|
| D1705 | N/A | | - | N/A | N/A | N/A | N/A | |
| D1706 | N/A | | - | N/A | N/A | N/A | N/A | |

* with documentation

# D1707

**D1707** Janssen Covid-19 vaccine administration

*SARSCOV2 COVID-19 VAC Ad26 5x1010 VP/.5mL IM SINGLE DOSE*

## Explanation

A vaccine produces active immunization by inducing the immune system to build its own antibodies against specific microorganisms/viruses. The body retains memory of the antibody production pattern for long-term protection. This code reports the immunization administration only of a preservative-free spike protein vaccine against severe acute respiratory syndrome coronavirus 2, also known as SARS-CoV-2, coronavirus disease, or COVID-19. A replication-incompetent adenovirus type 26 (Ad26)-vectored vaccine, it encodes a stabilized variant of the SARS-CoV-2 S protein and is specific to the Johnson & Johnson (Janssen) COVID-19 vaccine. Administered as a single-dose intramuscular injection, it is indicated for individuals 18 years of age and older and has been granted emergency use authorization (EUA) from the FDA.

## Coding Tips

This code is reported based upon the vaccine administered.

## Associated CPT Codes

0031A Immunization administration by intramuscular injection of severe acute respiratory syndrome coronavirus 2 (SARS-CoV-2) (coronavirus disease [COVID-19]) vaccine, DNA, spike protein, adenovirus type 26 (Ad26) vector, preservative free, $5x10^{10}$ viral particles/0.5mL dosage; single dose

## ICD-10-CM Diagnostic Codes

Z23 Encounter for immunization

Z29.8 Encounter for other specified prophylactic measures

## Relative Value Units/Medicare Edits

| Non-Facility RVU | Work | PE | MP | Total |
|---|---|---|---|---|
| D1707 | | | | |
| **Facility RVU** | **Work** | **PE** | **MP** | **Total** |
| D1707 | | | | |

| | FUD | Status | MUE | Modifiers | | | | IOM Reference |
|---|---|---|---|---|---|---|---|---|
| D1707 | N/A | | - | N/A | N/A | N/A | N/A | |

* with documentation

## Terms To Know

**COVID-19.** First diagnosed in December 2019 in China, coronavirus disease 2019 (COVID-19) is a respiratory infection caused by a newly identified (novel) virus not previously seen in humans, known as severe acute respiratory syndrome coronavirus 2 (SARS-CoV-2). Symptoms of this lower respiratory illness include fever, dry cough, loss of taste and/or smell, skin lesions of toes, gastrointestinal disturbances, and tiredness that may progress to include difficulty breathing and ventilator assistance. Older patients and those with high blood pressure, heart problems, diabetes, and obesity are more likely to develop serious symptoms of the illness, which may result in death of the patient.

**vaccine.** Preparation formed by microorganisms or viruses that have been altered to reduce their virulence but retain their ability to trigger the immune response.

# D2140-D2161

**D2140** amalgam - one surface, primary or permanent
**D2150** amalgam - two surfaces, primary or permanent
**D2160** amalgam - three surfaces, primary or permanent
**D2161** amalgam - four or more surfaces, primary or permanent

## Explanation

Amalgam is an alloy of (liquid) mercury mixed with other metals, such as silver, tin, copper, and zinc. The mercury is mixed with the pre-measured amalgam to be packed into the cavity. The tooth with decay is prepared to receive the filling by removing all the caries and even some healthy tooth substance to create undercuts to retain the filling in the tooth, since metal does not bond to the tooth. The dentist then packs the amalgam into the filling incrementally to ensure its fit. The filling is finally carved and polished to match the tooth and proper biting surface. Report D2140 for one surface amalgam, D2150 for two surfaces, D2160 for three surfaces, and D2161 for four or more surfaces. These codes are for primary or permanent teeth..

## Coding Tips

Report code D2140 when only one of the following surfaces is restored: mesial, distal, incisional, occlusal, lingual, buccal, or labial. Report code D2150 when two of the surfaces identified previously are restored without interruption for example, the mesial-lingual surfaces. Follow payer reporting guidelines for two-surface restorations on the same tooth. Report D2160 when three of the five surfaces are restored without interruption and report D2161 when four or more surfaces are restored without interruption. Preparation of the tooth surface, adhesives, bonding agents, liners, and bases are included in these services. An amalgam restoration placed the same day as a crown on the same tooth is often disallowed as part of the crown procedure. Local anesthesia is included in these services. Any evaluation or radiograph is reported separately. To report resin-based composite restorations, see D2330-D2394.

## Documentation Tips

Treatment plan documentation should reflect any treatment failure or change in diagnosis and/or a change in treatment plan. There should also be evidence of any initiation or reinstatement of a drug regime, which requires close and continuous skilled medical observation. The following information can be documented on a tooth chart: treatment/location of caries, endodontic procedures, prosthetic services, preventive services, treatment of lesions and dental disease, or other special procedures. A tooth chart may also be used to identify structure and rationale of disease process and the type of service performed on intraoral structures other than teeth.

## Reimbursement Tips

Tooth numbering may be required by some third-party payers.

## ICD-10-CM Diagnostic Codes

| | |
|---|---|
| K02.3 | Arrested dental caries |
| K02.51 | Dental caries on pit and fissure surface limited to enamel |
| K02.52 | Dental caries on pit and fissure surface penetrating into dentin |
| K02.53 | Dental caries on pit and fissure surface penetrating into pulp |
| K02.61 | Dental caries on smooth surface limited to enamel |
| K02.62 | Dental caries on smooth surface penetrating into dentin |
| K02.63 | Dental caries on smooth surface penetrating into pulp |
| K02.7 | Dental root caries |
| K03.81 | Cracked tooth |

## Relative Value Units/Medicare Edits

| Non-Facility RVU | Work | PE | MP | Total |
|---|---|---|---|---|
| **D2140** | 0.62 | 0.55 | 0.13 | 1.30 |
| **D2150** | 0.77 | 0.68 | 0.16 | 1.61 |
| **D2160** | 0.93 | 0.82 | 0.19 | 1.94 |
| **D2161** | 1.13 | 1.00 | 0.23 | 2.36 |
| **Facility RVU** | **Work** | **PE** | **MP** | **Total** |
| **D2140** | 0.62 | 0.55 | 0.13 | 1.30 |
| **D2150** | 0.77 | 0.68 | 0.16 | 1.61 |
| **D2160** | 0.93 | 0.82 | 0.19 | 1.94 |
| **D2161** | 1.13 | 1.00 | 0.23 | 2.36 |

| | FUD | Status | MUE | Modifiers | | | | IOM Reference |
|---|---|---|---|---|---|---|---|---|
| **D2140** | N/A | N | - | N/A | N/A | N/A | N/A | None |
| **D2150** | N/A | N | - | N/A | N/A | N/A | N/A | |
| **D2160** | N/A | N | - | N/A | N/A | N/A | N/A | |
| **D2161** | N/A | N | - | N/A | N/A | N/A | N/A | |

* with documentation

## Terms To Know

**amalgam.** Alloy that is used for dental restorations including fillings.

**attrition.** In dentistry, wearing away or erosion of tooth surface from abrasive food or grinding teeth.

**caries.** Localized section of tooth decay that begins on the tooth surface with destruction of the calcified enamel, allowing bacterial destruction to continue and form cavities and may extend to the dentin and pulp.

**cavity.** Tooth decay.

**erosion.** Eating away or gradual breaking down of the surface of a structure.

**permanent tooth.** One of 32 adult teeth that usually erupt between 6 years and adulthood with the third molar.

# D2330-D2335

**D2330** resin-based composite - one surface, anterior
**D2331** resin-based composite - two surfaces, anterior
**D2332** resin-based composite - three surfaces, anterior
**D2335** resin-based composite - four or more surfaces or involving incisal angle (anterior)

*Incisal angle to be defined as one of the angles formed by the junction of the incisal and the mesial or distal surface of an anterior tooth.*

## Explanation

Composite filling for tooth restoration is an alternative to silver amalgam. Also known as "white filling," it is made of composite quartz resin and is very strong. The tooth with decay is prepared to hold the filling by removing all the decay and preparing an etched surface for bonding. Composite, unlike metal, bonds to the tooth and requires less removal of the tooth structure to fill the cavity. A thin resin is applied, which bonds to the surface. The composite material is placed into the tooth and intense velvet blue light is directed at it for about 40 seconds, which hardens the composite material immediately. Report D2330 for one anterior surface resin-based composite filling, D2331 for two anterior surfaces, D2332 for three anterior surfaces, and D2335 for four or more surfaces or a resin-based composite restoration that involves an anterior incisal angle.

## Coding Tips

Anterior tooth surfaces are defined as the mesial, distal, incisal, lingual, or labial surfaces. When multiple surfaces are reported, those surfaces must be continuous. Follow payers reporting guidelines for two-surface restorations on the same tooth. Report D2332 when three of the five surfaces are restored without interruption and report D2335 when four or more surfaces are restored without interruption. Resin-based composite includes fiber or ceramic reinforced polymer compounds. Preparation of the tooth surface, acid etching, adhesives, bonding agents, liners, and bases and curing are included in these services. Local anesthesia is included in these services. Any evaluation or radiograph is reported separately. Report amalgam restorations using a code from the D2140–D2161 range. Codes from this range are used to report anterior restorations. To report posterior restorations, see D2391–D2394. Report D2390 if a full resin-based composite coverage of a tooth is performed. A resin restoration placed the same day as a crown on the same tooth is disallowed as part of the procedure.

## Documentation Tips

Treatment plan documentation should reflect any treatment failure or change in diagnosis and/or a change in treatment plan. There should also be evidence of any initiation or reinstatement of a drug regime, which requires close and continuous skilled medical observation. The following information can be documented on a tooth chart: treatment/location of caries, endodontic procedures, prosthetic services, preventive services, treatment of lesions and dental disease, or other special procedures. A tooth chart may also be used to identify structure and rationale of disease process and the type of service performed on intraoral structures other than teeth.

## Reimbursement Tips

Tooth numbering may be required by some third-party payers.

## ICD-10-CM Diagnostic Codes

| | |
|---|---|
| K02.3 | Arrested dental caries |
| K02.51 | Dental caries on pit and fissure surface limited to enamel |
| K02.52 | Dental caries on pit and fissure surface penetrating into dentin |
| K02.53 | Dental caries on pit and fissure surface penetrating into pulp |
| K02.61 | Dental caries on smooth surface limited to enamel |
| K02.62 | Dental caries on smooth surface penetrating into dentin |
| K02.63 | Dental caries on smooth surface penetrating into pulp |
| K02.7 | Dental root caries |
| K03.81 | Cracked tooth |

## Relative Value Units/Medicare Edits

| Non-Facility RVU | Work | PE | MP | Total |
|---|---|---|---|---|
| **D2330** | 0.72 | 0.64 | 0.15 | 1.51 |
| **D2331** | 0.96 | 0.85 | 0.20 | 2.01 |
| **D2332** | 1.16 | 1.03 | 0.24 | 2.43 |
| **D2335** | 1.36 | 1.20 | 0.28 | 2.84 |
| **Facility RVU** | **Work** | **PE** | **MP** | **Total** |
| **D2330** | 0.72 | 0.64 | 0.15 | 1.51 |
| **D2331** | 0.96 | 0.85 | 0.20 | 2.01 |
| **D2332** | 1.16 | 1.03 | 0.24 | 2.43 |
| **D2335** | 1.36 | 1.20 | 0.28 | 2.84 |

| | FUD | Status | MUE | Modifiers | | | | IOM Reference |
|---|---|---|---|---|---|---|---|---|
| **D2330** | N/A | N | - | N/A | N/A | N/A | N/A | None |
| **D2331** | N/A | N | - | N/A | N/A | N/A | N/A | |
| **D2332** | N/A | N | - | N/A | N/A | N/A | N/A | |
| **D2335** | N/A | N | - | N/A | N/A | N/A | N/A | |

* with documentation

## Terms To Know

**attrition.** In dentistry, wearing away or erosion of tooth surface from abrasive food or grinding teeth.

**caries.** Localized section of tooth decay that begins on the tooth surface with destruction of the calcified enamel, allowing bacterial destruction to continue and form cavities and may extend to the dentin and pulp.

**cavity.** Tooth decay.

**composite.** In dentistry, synthetic material such as acrylic resin and quartz particles used in tooth restoration.

**erosion.** Eating away or gradual breaking down of the surface of a structure.

**permanent tooth.** One of 32 adult teeth that usually erupt between 6 years and adulthood with the third molar.

# D2390

**D2390** resin-based composite crown, anterior

*Full resin-based composite coverage of tooth.*

## Explanation

A resin-based composite crown for the anterior teeth is applied. The dentist takes an upper and lower bite impression of the section of the mouth containing the tooth to be crowned and sends it to the lab. Plaster is poured into the impression mold with pins placed for later removal, connected to an articulator with more plaster, and then the poured model is removed. The prepped tooth is isolated. The margins are trimmed and marked. A spacer substance is painted on to represent the exact allowance needed for cementing the crown onto the tooth. A wax layer model, or coping, is made for the support layer of the crown and encased with a channel in high-density plaster. The wax is burned out. The coping model is filled with molten metal, spun on the arm of a centrifuge. If the crown is not made with a metal support, other pressing methods are used to cast the model. The metal support coping is tested on the tooth model, cleaned, and prepped for bonding so the resin layers of the crown may be completed over the metal coping support. The crown is contoured, shaped, checked for stain, color, and all contacts, and sent back to the dentist who tries the crown on the patient, checking all contact points, margins, and coloring. When the patient and dentist are satisfied with the results, the dentist cements the crown onto the tooth.

## Coding Tips

Resin-based composite includes fiber or ceramic reinforced polymer compounds. This code includes preparation of the tooth, acid etching, adhesives/bonding agents, liners, bases, and curing. Local anesthesia is generally considered to be part of restorative procedures. Pins should be reported separately, if used (see D2951). If less than full-tooth coverage is documented, see codes D2330–D2335 for anterior surface; D2391–D2394 for posterior surface. To report a provisional implant crown, see D6085.

## Documentation Tips

Treatment plan documentation should reflect any treatment failure or change in diagnosis and/or a change in treatment plan. There should also be evidence of any initiation or reinstatement of a drug regime, which requires close and continuous skilled medical observation. The following information can be documented on a tooth chart: treatment/location of caries, endodontic procedures, prosthetic services, preventive services, treatment of lesions and dental disease, or other special procedures. A tooth chart may also be used to identify structure and rationale of disease process and the type of service performed on intraoral structures other than teeth.

## Reimbursement Tips

Tooth numbering may be required by some third-party payers.

## ICD-10-CM Diagnostic Codes

| | |
|---|---|
| K02.3 | Arrested dental caries |
| K02.51 | Dental caries on pit and fissure surface limited to enamel |
| K02.52 | Dental caries on pit and fissure surface penetrating into dentin |
| K02.53 | Dental caries on pit and fissure surface penetrating into pulp |
| K02.61 | Dental caries on smooth surface limited to enamel |
| K02.62 | Dental caries on smooth surface penetrating into dentin |
| K02.63 | Dental caries on smooth surface penetrating into pulp |
| K02.7 | Dental root caries |
| K03.81 | Cracked tooth |

## Relative Value Units/Medicare Edits

| Non-Facility RVU | Work | PE | MP | Total |
|---|---|---|---|---|
| **D2390** | 1.70 | 1.50 | 0.35 | 3.55 |
| **Facility RVU** | **Work** | **PE** | **MP** | **Total** |
| **D2390** | 1.70 | 1.50 | 0.35 | 3.55 |

| | FUD | Status | MUE | Modifiers | | | | IOM Reference |
|---|---|---|---|---|---|---|---|---|
| **D2390** | N/A | N | - | N/A | N/A | N/A | N/A | None |

* with documentation

## Terms To Know

**bonding.** In dentistry, two or more components connected by chemical adhesion or mechanical means.

**coping.** Thin covering that is placed over a tooth before attaching a crown or overdenture.

**crown.** Dental restoration that completely caps or encircles a tooth or dental implant.

# D2391-D2394

**D2391** resin-based composite - one surface, posterior

*Used to restore a carious lesion into the dentin or a deeply eroded area into the dentin. Not a preventive procedure.*

**D2392** resin-based composite - two surfaces, posterior

**D2393** resin-based composite - three surfaces, posterior

**D2394** resin-based composite - four or more surfaces, posterior

## Explanation

Composite filling for tooth restoration is an alternative to silver amalgam. Also known as "white filling," it is made of composite quartz resin and is very strong. The tooth with decay is prepared to hold the filling by removing all the decay and preparing an etched surface for bonding. Composite, unlike metal, bonds to the tooth and requires less removal of the tooth structure to fill the cavity. A thin resin is applied which bonds to the surface. The composite material is placed into the tooth and intense velvet blue light is directed at it for about 40 seconds, which hardens the composite material immediately. Report D2391 for one posterior surface resin-based composite filling, D2392 for two posterior surfaces, and D2393 for three surfaces, and D2394 for four or more posterior surfaces.

## Coding Tips

Posterior tooth surfaces are defined as the mesial, distal, occlusal, lingual, or buccal surface. When assigning a code for multiple surfaces the surfaces must be continuous. Report D2391 for a single surface, D2392 when two of the surfaces identified previously are restored without interruption. Follow payer reporting guidelines for two-surface restorations on the same tooth. Report D2393 when three of the five surfaces are restored without interruption, and report D2394 when four or more surfaces are restored without interruption. Resin-based composite includes fiber or ceramic reinforced polymer compounds. Preparation of the tooth surface, acid etching, adhesives, bonding agents, liners, and bases and curing are included in these services. Local anesthesia is included in these services. Any evaluation or radiograph is reported separately. For anterior surface restorations, see D2330-D2335. For coverage of entire tooth surface (crown), see D2390. Report D2140-D2161 for amalgam restorations.

## Documentation Tips

Treatment plan documentation should reflect any treatment failure or change in diagnosis and/or a change in treatment plan. There should also be evidence of any initiation or reinstatement of a drug regime, which requires close and continuous skilled medical observation. The following information can be documented on a tooth chart: treatment/location of caries, endodontic procedures, prosthetic services, preventive services, treatment of lesions and dental disease, or other special procedures. A tooth chart may also be used to identify structure and rationale of disease process and the type of service performed on intraoral structures other than teeth.

## Reimbursement Tips

Tooth numbering may be required by some third-party payers.

## ICD-10-CM Diagnostic Codes

| | |
|---|---|
| K02.52 | Dental caries on pit and fissure surface penetrating into dentin |
| K02.53 | Dental caries on pit and fissure surface penetrating into pulp |
| K02.61 | Dental caries on smooth surface limited to enamel |
| K02.62 | Dental caries on smooth surface penetrating into dentin |
| K02.63 | Dental caries on smooth surface penetrating into pulp |
| K02.7 | Dental root caries |
| K03.0 | Excessive attrition of teeth |
| K03.1 | Abrasion of teeth |
| K03.2 | Erosion of teeth |

## Relative Value Units/Medicare Edits

| Non-Facility RVU | Work | PE | MP | Total |
|---|---|---|---|---|
| D2391 | 0.82 | 0.72 | 0.17 | 1.71 |
| D2392 | 1.19 | 1.05 | 0.24 | 2.48 |
| D2393 | 1.51 | 1.34 | 0.31 | 3.16 |
| D2394 | 1.77 | 1.56 | 0.36 | 3.69 |
| **Facility RVU** | **Work** | **PE** | **MP** | **Total** |
| D2391 | 0.82 | 0.72 | 0.17 | 1.71 |
| D2392 | 1.19 | 1.05 | 0.24 | 2.48 |
| D2393 | 1.51 | 1.34 | 0.31 | 3.16 |
| D2394 | 1.77 | 1.56 | 0.36 | 3.69 |

| | FUD | Status | MUE | Modifiers | | | | IOM Reference |
|---|---|---|---|---|---|---|---|---|
| D2391 | N/A | N | - | N/A | N/A | N/A | N/A | None |
| D2392 | N/A | N | - | N/A | N/A | N/A | N/A | |
| D2393 | N/A | N | - | N/A | N/A | N/A | N/A | |
| D2394 | N/A | N | - | N/A | N/A | N/A | N/A | |

* with documentation

## Terms To Know

**attrition.** In dentistry, wearing away or erosion of tooth surface from abrasive food or grinding teeth.

**caries.** Localized section of tooth decay that begins on the tooth surface with destruction of the calcified enamel, allowing bacterial destruction to continue and form cavities and may extend to the dentin and pulp.

**cavity.** Tooth decay.

**composite.** In dentistry, synthetic material such as acrylic resin and quartz particles used in tooth restoration.

**erosion.** Eating away or gradual breaking down of the surface of a structure.

**permanent tooth.** One of 32 adult teeth that usually erupt between 6 years and adulthood with the third molar.

# D2410-D2430

**D2410** gold foil - one surface
**D2420** gold foil - two surfaces
**D2430** gold foil - three surfaces

## Explanation

Gold foil restorations is an alternative to both composite and amalgam fillings. Although not commonly used today, it is the historical method of filling decayed areas of the tooth and dates back many centuries. Gold foil filling technique requires a high level of skill and attention to detail in placing these restorative fillings and is, of course, expensive. The gold is placed directly into the prepared tooth cavity and tapped into place with hand instruments, compacting it layer upon layer until the restoration is a solid filling and conformed to the tooth as needed. Report D2410 for one gold foil surface filling, D2420 for two surfaces, and D2430 for three surfaces.

## Coding Tips

When assigning a code for multiple surfaces the surfaces must be continuous. Local anesthesia is included in these services. Any evaluation or radiograph is reported separately.

## Documentation Tips

The following information can be documented on a tooth chart: treatment/location of caries, endodontic procedures, prosthetic services, preventive services, treatment of lesions and dental disease, or other special procedures.

## ICD-10-CM Diagnostic Codes

| | |
|---|---|
| K02.52 | Dental caries on pit and fissure surface penetrating into dentin |
| K02.53 | Dental caries on pit and fissure surface penetrating into pulp |
| K02.61 | Dental caries on smooth surface limited to enamel |
| K02.62 | Dental caries on smooth surface penetrating into dentin |
| K02.63 | Dental caries on smooth surface penetrating into pulp |
| K02.7 | Dental root caries |
| K03.0 | Excessive attrition of teeth |
| K03.1 | Abrasion of teeth |
| K03.2 | Erosion of teeth |

## Relative Value Units/Medicare Edits

| Non-Facility RVU | Work | PE | MP | Total |
|---|---|---|---|---|
| **D2410** | 1.86 | 1.64 | 0.38 | 3.88 |
| **D2420** | 2.78 | 2.46 | 0.57 | 5.81 |
| **D2430** | 4.43 | 3.91 | 0.91 | 9.25 |
| **Facility RVU** | **Work** | **PE** | **MP** | **Total** |
| **D2410** | 1.86 | 1.64 | 0.38 | 3.88 |
| **D2420** | 2.78 | 2.46 | 0.57 | 5.81 |
| **D2430** | 4.43 | 3.91 | 0.91 | 9.25 |

| | FUD | Status | MUE | Modifiers | | | | IOM Reference |
|---|---|---|---|---|---|---|---|---|
| **D2410** | N/A | N | - | N/A | N/A | N/A | N/A | None |
| **D2420** | N/A | N | - | N/A | N/A | N/A | N/A | |
| **D2430** | N/A | N | - | N/A | N/A | N/A | N/A | |

* with documentation

# D2510-D2530

**D2510** inlay - metallic - one surface
**D2520** inlay - metallic - two surfaces
**D2530** inlay - metallic - three or more surfaces

## Explanation

A metallic inlay is applied. An inlay, like a filling or a crown, is a type of dental restoration procedure. Inlays are constructed of metallic or non-metallic materials and are considered indirect restorations. An inlay fits like a puzzle piece into the tooth and is used to restore teeth that require more than a filling, but do not require a crown. The tooth is anesthetized and prepared for the inlay. If an old filling is present, it is removed, along with any decay. A mold is made of the tooth, the opposing tooth that the inlay bites against, and adjacent teeth. This mold is then sent to a laboratory where the inlay is constructed. While the inlay is being constructed, temporary inlay material is placed into the tooth. When the permanent inlay is returned from the laboratory, the patient returns to the dentist office and the inlay is cemented (luted) into the tooth. Report D2510 for a metallic inlay covering a single surface (top or side); D2520 for two surfaces (top and side or two sides); or D2530 for three or more surfaces.

## Coding Tips

Correct code assignment is dependent upon the number of surfaces involved. When assigning a code for multiple surfaces the surfaces must be continuous. See codes D2542-D2544 for metallic onlay procedures. See D2610-D2644 for porcelain/ceramic inlay/onlays. See D2650-D2664 for resin-based composite inlay/onlays.

## Documentation Tips

Treatment plan documentation should reflect any treatment failure or change in diagnosis and/or a change in treatment plan. There should also be evidence of any initiation or reinstatement of a drug regime, which requires close and continuous skilled medical observation. The following information can be documented on a tooth chart: treatment/location of caries, endodontic procedures, prosthetic services, preventive services, treatment of lesions and dental disease, or other special procedures. A tooth chart may also be used to identify structure and rationale of disease process and the type of service performed on intraoral structures other than teeth.

## Reimbursement Tips

Third-party payers often consider laboratory costs, tooth preparation, pulp caps, temporary restorations, porcelain margins, cement bases, impressions, and local anesthesia to be components of a complete restoration and, therefore, will not make separate payment for these services. Check with third-party payers for their specific guidelines.

## ICD-10-CM Diagnostic Codes

| | |
|---|---|
| K02.52 | Dental caries on pit and fissure surface penetrating into dentin |
| K02.53 | Dental caries on pit and fissure surface penetrating into pulp |
| K02.61 | Dental caries on smooth surface limited to enamel |
| K02.62 | Dental caries on smooth surface penetrating into dentin |
| K02.63 | Dental caries on smooth surface penetrating into pulp |
| K02.7 | Dental root caries |
| K03.0 | Excessive attrition of teeth |
| K03.1 | Abrasion of teeth |
| K03.2 | Erosion of teeth |

## Relative Value Units/Medicare Edits

| Non-Facility RVU | Work | PE | MP | Total |
|---|---|---|---|---|
| **D2510** | 4.10 | 3.62 | 0.85 | 8.57 |
| **D2520** | 4.65 | 4.11 | 0.96 | 9.72 |
| **D2530** | 5.20 | 4.59 | 1.07 | 10.86 |
| **Facility RVU** | **Work** | **PE** | **MP** | **Total** |
| **D2510** | 4.10 | 3.62 | 0.85 | 8.57 |
| **D2520** | 4.65 | 4.11 | 0.96 | 9.72 |
| **D2530** | 5.20 | 4.59 | 1.07 | 10.86 |

| | FUD | Status | MUE | Modifiers | | | | IOM Reference |
|---|---|---|---|---|---|---|---|---|
| **D2510** | N/A | N | - | N/A | N/A | N/A | N/A | None |
| **D2520** | N/A | N | - | N/A | N/A | N/A | N/A | |
| **D2530** | N/A | N | - | N/A | N/A | N/A | N/A | |

* with documentation

## Terms To Know

**inlay.** Restoration made outside of the mouth to fit a prepared cavity and placed on the tooth.

**permanent tooth.** One of 32 adult teeth that usually erupt between 6 years and adulthood with the third molar.

**primary tooth.** Any of 20 deciduous teeth that usually erupt between the ages of 6 and 24 months.

# D2542-D2544

**D2542** onlay - metallic - two surfaces
**D2543** onlay - metallic - three surfaces
**D2544** onlay - metallic - four or more surfaces

## Explanation

A metallic onlay is applied. An onlay, like a filling or a crown, is a type of dental restoration procedure. Onlays are constructed of metallic or non-metallic materials and are considered indirect restorations. An onlay fits like a puzzle piece onto the tooth, covering the cusp or pointed portion of the tooth. An onlay is used to restore teeth that require more than a filling, but do not require a crown. The tooth is anesthetized and prepared for the onlay. If an old filling is present, it is removed, along with any decay. A mold is made of the tooth, the opposing tooth that the inlay bites against, and adjacent teeth. This mold is then sent to a laboratory where the onlay is constructed. While the onlay is being constructed, temporary onlay material is placed onto the tooth cusp. When the permanent onlay is returned from the laboratory, the patient returns to the dentist office and the onlay is cemented (luted) onto the tooth cusp. Report D2542 when the metallic onlay covers two surfaces (top of the tooth and one side, or two sides); D2543 when it covers three surfaces; or D2544 when four or more surfaces are covered.

## Coding Tips

Correct code assignment is dependent upon the number of surfaces involved. When assigning a code for multiple surfaces the surfaces must be continuous. To report metallic inlay procedures, see D2510–D2530. To report porcelain/ceramic inlay/onlay procedures, see D2610–D2644; for resin-based composite inlay/onlay services, see D2650–D2664.

## Documentation Tips

Treatment plan documentation should reflect any treatment failure or change in diagnosis and/or a change in treatment plan. There should also be evidence of any initiation or reinstatement of a drug regime, which requires close and continuous skilled medical observation. The following information can be documented on a tooth chart: treatment/location of caries, endodontic procedures, prosthetic services, preventive services, treatment of lesions and dental disease, or other special procedures. A tooth chart may also be used to identify structure and rationale of disease process and the type of service performed on intraoral structures other than teeth.

## Reimbursement Tips

Third-party payers often consider laboratory costs, tooth preparation, pulp caps, temporary restorations, porcelain margins, cement bases, impressions, and local anesthesia to be components of a complete restoration and, therefore, will not make separate payment for these services. Payers may require documentation including the tooth number, surface(s), and preoperative periapical x-ray.

## ICD-10-CM Diagnostic Codes

K02.52 Dental caries on pit and fissure surface penetrating into dentin
K02.53 Dental caries on pit and fissure surface penetrating into pulp
K02.61 Dental caries on smooth surface limited to enamel
K02.62 Dental caries on smooth surface penetrating into dentin
K02.63 Dental caries on smooth surface penetrating into pulp
K02.7 Dental root caries
K03.0 Excessive attrition of teeth
K03.1 Abrasion of teeth
K03.2 Erosion of teeth

## Relative Value Units/Medicare Edits

| Non-Facility RVU | Work | PE | MP | Total |
|---|---|---|---|---|
| **D2542** | 5.28 | 4.66 | 1.09 | 11.03 |
| **D2543** | 5.52 | 4.87 | 1.14 | 11.53 |
| **D2544** | 5.82 | 5.13 | 1.20 | 12.15 |
| **Facility RVU** | **Work** | **PE** | **MP** | **Total** |
| **D2542** | 5.28 | 4.66 | 1.09 | 11.03 |
| **D2543** | 5.52 | 4.87 | 1.14 | 11.53 |
| **D2544** | 5.82 | 5.13 | 1.20 | 12.15 |

| | FUD | Status | MUE | Modifiers | | | | IOM Reference |
|---|---|---|---|---|---|---|---|---|
| **D2542** | N/A | N | - | N/A | N/A | N/A | N/A | None |
| **D2543** | N/A | N | - | N/A | N/A | N/A | N/A | |
| **D2544** | N/A | N | - | N/A | N/A | N/A | N/A | |

* with documentation

## Terms To Know

**cusp.** In dentistry, the rounded or pointed portion of the surface of the tooth used for mastication.

**indirect restoration.** In dentistry, restoration produced outside of the mouth.

**onlay.** In dentistry, restoration made outside of the mouth that is cemented over a cusp or cusps of the tooth.

# D2610-D2630

**D2610** inlay - porcelain/ceramic - one surface
**D2620** inlay - porcelain/ceramic - two surfaces
**D2630** inlay - porcelain/ceramic - three or more surfaces

## Explanation

A porcelain or ceramic inlay is applied. An inlay, like a filling or a crown, is a type of dental restoration procedure. Inlays are constructed of metallic or non-metallic materials and are considered indirect restorations. An inlay fits like a puzzle piece into the tooth and is used to restore teeth that require more than a filling, but do not require a crown. The tooth is anesthetized and prepared for the inlay. If an old filling is present, it is removed, along with any decay. A mold is made of the tooth, the opposing tooth that the inlay bites against, and adjacent teeth. When a ceramic or porcelain inlay is used, the dentist also uses a color chart to match the color of the inlay to the color of the tooth. The mold and the tooth color information are sent to a laboratory where the inlay is constructed. While the inlay is being constructed, temporary inlay material is placed into the tooth. When the permanent inlay is returned from the laboratory, the patient returns to the dentist office and the inlay is cemented (luted) into the tooth. The inlay covers a single surface (top or side) of the tooth in D2610; two surfaces (top and side or two sides) in D2620; and three or more surfaces in D2630.

## Coding Tips

Porcelain/ceramic refers to pressed, fired, polished, or milled substances, which predominantly contain inorganic refractory compounds such as porcelains, glasses, ceramics, and glass-ceramics. Correct code assignment is dependent upon the number of surfaces involved. When assigning a code for multiple surfaces, the surfaces must be continuous. Ceramic/porcelain onlay procedures are reported with D2642–D2644. For metallic inlay/onlay procedures, see D2510–D2544. For resin-based composite inlay/onlay procedures, see D2650–D2664.

## Documentation Tips

Treatment plan documentation should reflect any treatment failure or change in diagnosis and/or a change in treatment plan. There should also be evidence of any initiation or reinstatement of a drug regime, which requires close and continuous skilled medical observation. The following information can be documented on a tooth chart: treatment/location of caries, endodontic procedures, prosthetic services, preventive services, treatment of lesions and dental disease, or other special procedures. A tooth chart may also be used to identify structure and rationale of disease process and the type of service performed on intraoral structures other than teeth.

## Reimbursement Tips

Third-party payers often consider laboratory costs, tooth preparation, pulp caps, temporary restorations, porcelain margins, cement bases, impressions, and local anesthesia to be components of a complete restoration and, therefore, will not make separate payment for these services.

## ICD-10-CM Diagnostic Codes

| | |
|---|---|
| K02.52 | Dental caries on pit and fissure surface penetrating into dentin |
| K02.53 | Dental caries on pit and fissure surface penetrating into pulp |
| K02.61 | Dental caries on smooth surface limited to enamel |
| K02.62 | Dental caries on smooth surface penetrating into dentin |
| K02.63 | Dental caries on smooth surface penetrating into pulp |
| K02.7 | Dental root caries |
| K02.9 | Dental caries, unspecified |
| K03.0 | Excessive attrition of teeth |

K03.1 Abrasion of teeth
K03.2 Erosion of teeth

## Relative Value Units/Medicare Edits

| Non-Facility RVU | Work | PE | MP | Total |
|---|---|---|---|---|
| **D2610** | 4.75 | 4.19 | 0.98 | 9.92 |
| **D2620** | 5.00 | 4.41 | 1.03 | 10.44 |
| **D2630** | 5.59 | 4.93 | 1.15 | 11.67 |
| **Facility RVU** | **Work** | **PE** | **MP** | **Total** |
| **D2610** | 4.75 | 4.19 | 0.98 | 9.92 |
| **D2620** | 5.00 | 4.41 | 1.03 | 10.44 |
| **D2630** | 5.59 | 4.93 | 1.15 | 11.67 |

| | FUD | Status | MUE | Modifiers | | | | IOM Reference |
|---|---|---|---|---|---|---|---|---|
| **D2610** | N/A | N | - | N/A | N/A | N/A | N/A | None |
| **D2620** | N/A | N | - | N/A | N/A | N/A | N/A | |
| **D2630** | N/A | N | - | N/A | N/A | N/A | N/A | |

* with documentation

## Terms To Know

**inlay.** Restoration made outside of the mouth to fit a prepared cavity and placed on the tooth.

**onlay.** In dentistry, restoration made outside of the mouth that is cemented over a cusp or cusps of the tooth.

Dental - Restoration

# D2642-D2644

**D2642** onlay - porcelain/ceramic - two surfaces
**D2643** onlay - porcelain/ceramic - three surfaces
**D2644** onlay - porcelain/ceramic - four or more surfaces

## Explanation

A porcelain or ceramic onlay applied. An onlay, like a filling or a crown, is a type of dental restoration procedure. Onlays are constructed of metallic or non-metallic materials and are considered indirect restorations. An onlay fits like a puzzle piece onto the tooth, covering the cusp or pointed portion of the tooth. An onlay is used to restore teeth that require more than a filling, but do not require a crown. The tooth is anesthetized and prepared for the onlay. If an old filling is present, it is removed, along with any decay. A mold is made of the tooth, the opposing tooth that the inlay bites against, and adjacent teeth. When a ceramic or porcelain onlay is used, the dentist uses a color chart to match the color of the onlay to the color of the tooth. The mold and the tooth color information are then sent to a laboratory where the onlay is constructed. While the onlay is being constructed, temporary onlay material is placed onto the tooth cusp. When the permanent onlay is returned from the laboratory, the patient returns to the dentist office and the onlay is cemented (luted) onto the tooth cusp. Report D2642 if onlay is applied to two surfaces; D2643 for three surfaces; or D2644 for four or more surfaces.

## Coding Tips

Porcelain/ceramic refers to pressed, fired, polished, or milled substances, which predominantly contain inorganic refractory compounds such as porcelains, glasses, ceramics, and glass-ceramics. Correct code assignment is dependent upon the number of surfaces involved. When assigning a code for multiple surfaces, the surfaces must be continuous. Ceramic/porcelain inlay procedures are reported with D2610–D2630. For metallic inlay/onlay procedures, see D2510–D2544. For resin-based composite inlay/onlay procedures, see D2650–D2664.

## Documentation Tips

Treatment plan documentation should reflect any treatment failure or change in diagnosis and/or a change in treatment plan. There should also be evidence of any initiation or reinstatement of a drug regime, which requires close and continuous skilled medical observation. The following information can be documented on a tooth chart: treatment/location of caries, endodontic procedures, prosthetic services, preventive services, treatment of lesions and dental disease, or other special procedures. A tooth chart may also be used to identify structure and rationale of disease process and the type of service performed on intraoral structures other than teeth.

## Reimbursement Tips

Third-party payers often consider laboratory costs, tooth preparation, pulp caps, temporary restorations, porcelain margins, cement bases, impressions, and local anesthesia to be components of a complete restoration and, therefore, will not make separate payment for these services. Payers may require documentation including the tooth number, surface(s), and preoperative periapical x-ray.

## ICD-10-CM Diagnostic Codes

K02.52 Dental caries on pit and fissure surface penetrating into dentin
K02.53 Dental caries on pit and fissure surface penetrating into pulp
K02.61 Dental caries on smooth surface limited to enamel
K02.62 Dental caries on smooth surface penetrating into dentin
K02.63 Dental caries on smooth surface penetrating into pulp
K02.7 Dental root caries

K03.0 Excessive attrition of teeth
K03.1 Abrasion of teeth
K03.2 Erosion of teeth

## Relative Value Units/Medicare Edits

| Non-Facility RVU | Work | PE | MP | Total |
|---|---|---|---|---|
| D2642 | 5.22 | 4.61 | 1.07 | 10.90 |
| D2643 | 5.71 | 5.04 | 1.18 | 11.93 |
| D2644 | 6.18 | 5.46 | 1.27 | 12.91 |
| **Facility RVU** | **Work** | **PE** | **MP** | **Total** |
| D2642 | 5.22 | 4.61 | 1.07 | 10.90 |
| D2643 | 5.71 | 5.04 | 1.18 | 11.93 |
| D2644 | 6.18 | 5.46 | 1.27 | 12.91 |

| | FUD | Status | MUE | Modifiers | | | | IOM Reference |
|---|---|---|---|---|---|---|---|---|
| D2642 | N/A | N | - | N/A | N/A | N/A | N/A | None |
| D2643 | N/A | N | - | N/A | N/A | N/A | N/A | |
| D2644 | N/A | N | - | N/A | N/A | N/A | N/A | |

* with documentation

## Terms To Know

**cusp.** In dentistry, the rounded or pointed portion of the surface of the tooth used for mastication.

**indirect restoration.** In dentistry, restoration produced outside of the mouth.

**onlay.** In dentistry, restoration made outside of the mouth that is cemented over a cusp or cusps of the tooth.

# D2650-D2652

**D2650** inlay - resin-based composite - one surface
**D2651** inlay - resin-based composite - two surfaces
**D2652** inlay - resin-based composite - three or more surfaces

## Explanation

A resin-based composite or composite/resin inlay is applied. An inlay, like a filling or a crown, is a type of dental restoration procedure. Inlays are constructed of metallic or nonmetallic materials and are considered indirect restorations. An inlay fits like a puzzle piece into the tooth and is used to restore teeth that require more than a filling, but do not require a crown. The tooth is anesthetized and prepared for the inlay. If an old filling is present, it is removed, along with any decay. A mold is made of the tooth, the opposing tooth that the inlay bites against, and adjacent teeth. When a resin-based composite or composite/resin inlay is used, the dentist uses a color chart to match the color of the inlay to the color of the tooth. The mold and the tooth color information are then sent to a laboratory where the inlay is constructed. Inlays made with resin-based composite include all reinforced heat or pressure-cured polymer materials. While the inlay is being constructed, temporary inlay material is placed into the tooth. When the permanent inlay is returned from the laboratory, the patient returns to the dentist office and the inlay is cemented (luted) into the tooth. The inlay covers a single tooth surface (top or side) in D2650; two surfaces in D2651; or three or more surfaces in D2652.

## Coding Tips

Resin-based composite includes fiber or ceramic reinforced polymer compounds. Correct code assignment is dependent upon the number of surfaces involved. When assigning a code for multiple surfaces, the surfaces must be continuous. For resin-based composite onlay services, see D2662–D2664. Ceramic/porcelain inlay/onlay procedures are reported with D2610–D2644. For metallic inlay/onlay procedures, see D2510–D2544.

## Documentation Tips

Treatment plan documentation should reflect any treatment failure or change in diagnosis and/or a change in treatment plan. There should also be evidence of any initiation or reinstatement of a drug regime, which requires close and continuous skilled medical observation. The following information can be documented on a tooth chart: treatment/location of caries, endodontic procedures, prosthetic services, preventive services, treatment of lesions and dental disease, or other special procedures. A tooth chart may also be used to identify structure and rationale of disease process and the type of service performed on intraoral structures other than teeth.

## Reimbursement Tips

Third-party payers often consider laboratory costs, tooth preparation, pulp caps, temporary restorations, porcelain margins, cement bases, impressions, and local anesthesia to be components of a complete restoration and, therefore, will not make separate payment for these services.

## ICD-10-CM Diagnostic Codes

K02.52 Dental caries on pit and fissure surface penetrating into dentin
K02.53 Dental caries on pit and fissure surface penetrating into pulp
K02.61 Dental caries on smooth surface limited to enamel
K02.62 Dental caries on smooth surface penetrating into dentin
K02.63 Dental caries on smooth surface penetrating into pulp
K02.7 Dental root caries
K03.0 Excessive attrition of teeth
K03.1 Abrasion of teeth

K03.2 Erosion of teeth

## Relative Value Units/Medicare Edits

| Non-Facility RVU | Work | PE | MP | Total |
|---|---|---|---|---|
| **D2650** | 3.39 | 3.00 | 0.70 | 7.09 |
| **D2651** | 3.99 | 3.52 | 0.82 | 8.33 |
| **D2652** | 4.47 | 3.95 | 0.92 | 9.34 |
| **Facility RVU** | **Work** | **PE** | **MP** | **Total** |
| **D2650** | 3.39 | 3.00 | 0.70 | 7.09 |
| **D2651** | 3.99 | 3.52 | 0.82 | 8.33 |
| **D2652** | 4.47 | 3.95 | 0.92 | 9.34 |

| | FUD | Status | MUE | Modifiers | | | | IOM Reference |
|---|---|---|---|---|---|---|---|---|
| **D2650** | N/A | N | - | N/A | N/A | N/A | N/A | None |
| **D2651** | N/A | N | - | N/A | N/A | N/A | N/A | |
| **D2652** | N/A | N | - | N/A | N/A | N/A | N/A | |

* with documentation

## Terms To Know

**composite.** In dentistry, synthetic material such as acrylic resin and quartz particles used in tooth restoration.

**facial surface.** In dentistry, tooth surface that is facing the cheeks or lips.

**indirect restoration.** In dentistry, restoration produced outside of the mouth.

**inlay.** Restoration made outside of the mouth to fit a prepared cavity and placed on the tooth.

# D2662-D2664

**D2662** onlay - resin-based composite - two surfaces
**D2663** onlay - resin-based composite - three surfaces
**D2664** onlay - resin-based composite - four or more surfaces

## Explanation

A resin-based composite or composite/resin onlay covering two surfaces (top of the tooth and one side of the tooth) is applied. An onlay, like a filling or a crown, is a type of dental restoration procedure. Onlays are constructed of metallic or non-metallic materials and are considered indirect restorations. An onlay fits like a puzzle piece onto the tooth, covering the cusp or pointed portion of the tooth. An onlay is used to restore teeth that require more than a filling, but do not require a crown. The tooth is anesthetized and prepared for the onlay. If an old filling is present, it is removed, along with any decay. A mold is made of the tooth, the opposing tooth that the inlay bites against, and adjacent teeth. When a resin-based composite or composite/resin onlay is used, the dentist uses a color chart to match the color of the onlay to the color of the tooth. The mold and the tooth color information are then sent to a laboratory where the onlay is constructed. Onlays made with resin-based composite include all reinforced heat or pressure-cured polymer materials. While the onlay is being constructed, temporary onlay material is placed onto the tooth cusp. When the permanent onlay is returned from the laboratory, the patient returns to the dentist office and the onlay is cemented (luted) onto the tooth cusp. The onlay covers two surfaces (top and one side) of the tooth in D2662; three surfaces in D2663; or four or more surfaces in D2664.

## Coding Tips

Resin-based composite includes fiber or ceramic reinforced polymer compounds. Correct code assignment is dependent upon the number of surfaces involved. When assigning a code for multiple surfaces, the surfaces must be continuous. For resin-based inlay procedures, see D2650–D2652. Ceramic/porcelain inlay/onlay procedures are reported with D2610–D2644. For metallic inlay/onlay procedures, see D2510–D2544.

## Documentation Tips

Treatment plan documentation should reflect any treatment failure or change in diagnosis and/or a change in treatment plan. There should also be evidence of any initiation or reinstatement of a drug regime, which requires close and continuous skilled medical observation. The following information can be documented on a tooth chart: treatment/location of caries, endodontic procedures, prosthetic services, preventive services, treatment of lesions and dental disease, or other special procedures. A tooth chart may also be used to identify structure and rationale of disease process and the type of service performed on intraoral structures other than teeth.

## Reimbursement Tips

Third-party payers often consider laboratory costs, tooth preparation, pulp caps, temporary restorations, porcelain margins, cement bases, impressions, and local anesthesia to be components of a complete restoration and, therefore, will not make separate payment for these services.

## ICD-10-CM Diagnostic Codes

K02.52 Dental caries on pit and fissure surface penetrating into dentin
K02.53 Dental caries on pit and fissure surface penetrating into pulp
K02.61 Dental caries on smooth surface limited to enamel
K02.62 Dental caries on smooth surface penetrating into dentin
K02.63 Dental caries on smooth surface penetrating into pulp
K02.7 Dental root caries
K03.0 Excessive attrition of teeth

K03.1 Abrasion of teeth
K03.2 Erosion of teeth

## Relative Value Units/Medicare Edits

| Non-Facility RVU | Work | PE | MP | Total |
|---|---|---|---|---|
| D2662 | 3.73 | 3.30 | 0.77 | 7.80 |
| D2663 | 4.45 | 3.93 | 0.92 | 9.30 |
| D2664 | 4.76 | 4.20 | 0.98 | 9.94 |
| **Facility RVU** | **Work** | **PE** | **MP** | **Total** |
| D2662 | 3.73 | 3.30 | 0.77 | 7.80 |
| D2663 | 4.45 | 3.93 | 0.92 | 9.30 |
| D2664 | 4.76 | 4.20 | 0.98 | 9.94 |

| | FUD | Status | MUE | Modifiers | | | | IOM Reference |
|---|---|---|---|---|---|---|---|---|
| D2662 | N/A | N | - | N/A | N/A | N/A | N/A | None |
| D2663 | N/A | N | - | N/A | N/A | N/A | N/A | |
| D2664 | N/A | N | - | N/A | N/A | N/A | N/A | |

* with documentation

## Terms To Know

**composite.** In dentistry, synthetic material such as acrylic resin and quartz particles used in tooth restoration.

**cusp.** In dentistry, the rounded or pointed portion of the surface of the tooth used for mastication.

**indirect restoration.** In dentistry, restoration produced outside of the mouth.

**onlay.** In dentistry, restoration made outside of the mouth that is cemented over a cusp or cusps of the tooth.

# D2710-D2722

**D2710** crown - resin-based composite (indirect)
**D2712** crown - 3/4 resin-based composite (indirect)

*This procedure does not include facial veneers.*

**D2720** crown - resin with high noble metal
**D2721** crown - resin with predominantly base metal
**D2722** crown - resin with noble metal

## Explanation

A crown is a restorative "cap" for a tooth made in exact reproduction to the tooth's anatomy. Crowns made with resin-based composite include all reinforced heat or pressure-cured polymer materials. The dentist takes an upper and lower bite impression of the section of the mouth containing the tooth to be crowned and sends it to the lab. Plaster is poured into the impression mould with pins placed for later removal, connected to an articulator with more plaster, and then the poured model is removed. The prepped tooth is isolated. The margins are trimmed and marked. A spacer substance is painted on to represent the exact allowance needed for cementing the crown onto the tooth. A wax layer model, or coping, is made for the support layer of the crown and encased with a channel in high-density plaster. The wax is burned out. The coping model is filled with molten metal, spun on the arm of a centrifuge. If the crown is not made with a metal support, other pressing methods are used to cast the model. The metal support coping is tested on the tooth model, cleaned, and prepped for bonding so the resin layers of the crown may be completed over the metal coping support. The crown is contoured, shaped, checked for stain, color, and all contacts and sent back to the dentist who tries the crown on the patient, checking all contact points, margins, and coloring, and then cements the crown onto the tooth when the patient is satisfied. Report D2710 for an all resin crown, D2712 for resin-based composite, D2720 for resin bonded to high noble metal, D2721 for resin with predominantly base metal, and D2722 for resin with noble metal.

## Coding Tips

Local anesthesia is included in these services. Any evaluation or radiograph, root canal, core buildup, or post or preparation service is reported separately. Porcelain/ceramic crowns are reported with the appropriate code from D2740–D2752. To report 3/4 cast metal crowns, see D2780–D2782. Full cast metal crowns are reported with a code from D2790–D2792. High noble metals include gold, palladium, and platinum. The content must be ≤ 60 percent gold plus platinum and ≤ 40 percent gold. Noble metals include 25 percent or less gold plus platinum group. Predominantly base alloys contain a noble metal content of < 25 percent gold plus platinum group. The metals of the platinum group include platinum, palladium, rhodium, iridium, osmium, and ruthenium. Resin-based composite includes fiber or ceramic-reinforced polymer compounds. Porcelain/ceramic refers to pressed, fired, polished, or milled substances that predominantly contain inorganic refractory compounds such as porcelains, glasses, ceramics, and glass-ceramics. Resin-based crowns used as a temporary restoration are usually considered part of the final restoration and should not be billed separately. Restoration using a prefabricated resin crown is reported with code D2932; a stainless steel crown with resin window is reported with D2933. To report a provisional implant crown, see D6085.

## Documentation Tips

Payers may require documentation including the tooth number, surface(s), and preoperative periapical x-ray.

## Reimbursement Tips

Third-party payers often consider laboratory costs, tooth preparation, pulp caps, temporary restorations, porcelain margins, cement bases, impressions, and local anesthesia to be components of a complete restoration and, therefore, will not make separate payment for these services. Third-party payers may consider the buildup under a crown as included in the fee for a crown. A payer may allow an exception where extensive buildup is needed to gain retention and make additional payment in these instances. When this occurs, a written report and x-rays should be submitted with the claim. However, most payers will not reimburse separately for a buildup when placed to remove undercuts or to add bulk to the preparation.

## ICD-10-CM Diagnostic Codes

| | |
|---|---|
| K02.52 | Dental caries on pit and fissure surface penetrating into dentin |
| K02.53 | Dental caries on pit and fissure surface penetrating into pulp |
| K02.61 | Dental caries on smooth surface limited to enamel |
| K02.62 | Dental caries on smooth surface penetrating into dentin |
| K02.63 | Dental caries on smooth surface penetrating into pulp |
| K02.7 | Dental root caries |
| K03.0 | Excessive attrition of teeth |
| K03.1 | Abrasion of teeth |
| K03.2 | Erosion of teeth |

## Relative Value Units/Medicare Edits

| Non-Facility RVU | Work | PE | MP | Total |
|---|---|---|---|---|
| D2710 | 2.71 | 2.40 | 0.56 | 5.67 |
| D2712 | 3.09 | 2.73 | 0.64 | 6.46 |
| D2720 | 6.31 | 5.57 | 1.30 | 13.18 |
| D2721 | 5.60 | 4.94 | 1.15 | 11.69 |
| D2722 | 5.86 | 5.17 | 1.21 | 12.24 |
| **Facility RVU** | **Work** | **PE** | **MP** | **Total** |
| D2710 | 2.71 | 2.40 | 0.56 | 5.67 |
| D2712 | 3.09 | 2.73 | 0.64 | 6.46 |
| D2720 | 6.31 | 5.57 | 1.30 | 13.18 |
| D2721 | 5.60 | 4.94 | 1.15 | 11.69 |
| D2722 | 5.86 | 5.17 | 1.21 | 12.24 |

| | FUD | Status | MUE | Modifiers | | | | IOM Reference |
|---|---|---|---|---|---|---|---|---|
| D2710 | N/A | N | - | N/A | N/A | N/A | N/A | None |
| D2712 | N/A | N | - | N/A | N/A | N/A | N/A | |
| D2720 | N/A | N | - | N/A | N/A | N/A | N/A | |
| D2721 | N/A | N | - | N/A | N/A | N/A | N/A | |
| D2722 | N/A | N | - | N/A | N/A | N/A | N/A | |

* with documentation

## Terms To Know

**artificial crown.** In dentistry, a ceramic or metal restoration made to cover or replace a major part of the top of a tooth.

**bonding.** In dentistry, two or more components connected by chemical adhesion or mechanical means.

# D2740-D2753

**D2740** crown - porcelain/ceramic
**D2750** crown - porcelain fused to high noble metal
**D2751** crown - porcelain fused to predominantly base metal
**D2752** crown - porcelain fused to noble metal
**D2753** crown - porcelain fused to titanium and titanium alloys

## Explanation

A crown is a restorative "cap" for a tooth made in exact reproduction to the tooth's anatomy. Eighty percent of crowns are porcelain fused to metal, whether noble, high noble, or a base metal. The dentist takes an upper and lower bite impression of the section of the mouth containing the tooth to be crowned and sends it to the lab. Plaster is poured into the impression mould with pins placed for later removal, connected to an articulator with more plaster, and then the poured model is removed. The prepped tooth is isolated. The margins are trimmed and marked. A spacer substance is painted on to the exact allowance needed for cementing the crown onto the tooth. A wax layer model, or coping, is made for the support layer of the crown and encased with a channel in high-density plaster. The wax is burned out. The coping model is filled with molten metal, spun on the arm of a centrifuge. If the crown is not made with a metal support, other pressing methods under controlled firing temperatures are used to cast the model. The metal support coping is tested on the tooth model, cleaned, and prepped for bonding. The porcelain layers of the crown are completed, the crown is contoured, shaped, checked for stain, color, and all contacts and sent back to the dentist who tries the crown on the patient, checking all contact points, margins, and coloring, and then cements the crown onto the tooth when the patient is satisfied. Report D2740 for an all porcelain/ceramic substrate crown, D2750 for porcelain fused to high noble metal, D2751 for porcelain fused to predominantly base metal, D2752 for porcelain fused to noble metal, and D2753 for porcelain fused to titanium and titanium alloys.

## Coding Tips

Local anesthesia is included in these services. Any evaluation, radiograph, root canal, core buildup, or post or preparation service is reported separately. To report 3/4 cast metal crowns, see D2780-D2782. Resin crowns are reported with the appropriate code from D2710-D2722. To report full cast metal crowns, see D2790-D2794. High noble metals include gold, palladium, and platinum. The content must be ≥ 60 percent gold plus platinum and ≥ 40 percent gold. Noble metals include 25 percent or less gold plus platinum group. Predominantly base alloys contain a noble metal content of < 25 percent gold plus platinum group. The metals of the platinum group include platinum, palladium, rhodium, iridium, osmium, and ruthenium. Resin-based composite includes fiber or ceramic reinforced polymer compounds. Porcelain/ceramic refers to pressed, fired, polished, or milled substances, which predominantly contain inorganic refractory compounds such as porcelains, glasses, ceramics, and glass-ceramics. To report a provisional implant crown, see D6085.

## Documentation Tips

Treatment plan documentation should reflect any treatment failure or change in diagnosis and/or a change in treatment plan. There should also be evidence of any initiation or reinstatement of a drug regime, which requires close and continuous skilled medical observation. The following information can be documented on a tooth chart: treatment/location of caries, endodontic procedures, prosthetic services, preventive services, treatment of lesions and dental disease, or other special procedures. A tooth chart may also be used to identify structure and rationale of disease process and the type of service performed on intraoral structures other than teeth.

## Reimbursement Tips

Third-party payers often consider laboratory costs, tooth preparation, pulp caps, temporary restorations, porcelain margins, cement bases, impressions, and local anesthesia to be components of a complete restoration and, therefore, will not make separate payment for these services. Third-party payers may consider the buildup under a crown as included in the fee for a crown. A payer may allow an exception where extensive buildup is needed to gain retention and make additional payment in these instances. When this occurs, a written report and x-rays should be submitted with the claim. However, most payers will not reimburse separately for a buildup when placed to remove undercuts or to add bulk to the preparation. Payers may require documentation including the tooth number, surface(s), and preoperative periapical x-ray.

## ICD-10-CM Diagnostic Codes

| | |
|---|---|
| K02.52 | Dental caries on pit and fissure surface penetrating into dentin |
| K02.53 | Dental caries on pit and fissure surface penetrating into pulp |
| K02.61 | Dental caries on smooth surface limited to enamel |
| K02.62 | Dental caries on smooth surface penetrating into dentin |
| K02.63 | Dental caries on smooth surface penetrating into pulp |
| K02.7 | Dental root caries |
| K03.0 | Excessive attrition of teeth |
| K03.1 | Abrasion of teeth |
| K03.2 | Erosion of teeth |

## Relative Value Units/Medicare Edits

| Non-Facility RVU | Work | PE | MP | Total |
|---|---|---|---|---|
| **D2740** | 6.43 | 5.67 | 1.32 | 13.42 |
| **D2750** | 6.53 | 5.76 | 1.34 | 13.63 |
| **D2751** | 5.71 | 5.04 | 1.18 | 11.93 |
| **D2752** | 5.98 | 5.28 | 1.23 | 12.49 |
| **D2753** | 4.35 | 3.84 | 0.90 | 9.09 |
| **Facility RVU** | **Work** | **PE** | **MP** | **Total** |
| **D2740** | 6.43 | 5.67 | 1.32 | 13.42 |
| **D2750** | 6.53 | 5.76 | 1.34 | 13.63 |
| **D2751** | 5.71 | 5.04 | 1.18 | 11.93 |
| **D2752** | 5.98 | 5.28 | 1.23 | 12.49 |
| **D2753** | 4.35 | 3.84 | 0.90 | 9.09 |

| | FUD | Status | MUE | Modifiers | | | | IOM Reference |
|---|---|---|---|---|---|---|---|---|
| **D2740** | N/A | N | - | N/A | N/A | N/A | N/A | None |
| **D2750** | N/A | N | - | N/A | N/A | N/A | N/A | |
| **D2751** | N/A | N | - | N/A | N/A | N/A | N/A | |
| **D2752** | N/A | N | - | N/A | N/A | N/A | N/A | |
| **D2753** | N/A | N | - | N/A | N/A | N/A | N/A | |

* with documentation

## Terms To Know

**artificial crown.** In dentistry, a ceramic or metal restoration made to cover or replace a major part of the top of a tooth.

**bonding.** In dentistry, two or more components connected by chemical adhesion or mechanical means.

# D2780-D2783

**D2780** crown - 3/4 cast high noble metal
**D2781** crown - 3/4 cast predominantly base metal
**D2782** crown - 3/4 cast noble metal
**D2783** crown - 3/4 porcelain/ceramic

*This procedure does not include facial veneers.*

## Explanation

A cast metal crown or porcelain crown is one made to cap of the tooth's anatomy (i.e., one cusp of a molar is left outside the crown). These are not commonly done as the entire tooth is almost always capped when a crown is made (see other codes for crown procedures). The metal classification is based on the content of noble metal to other alloys. High noble metal has the highest content of precious noble metal, at least 60 percent of gold, palladium, or platinum; noble metal has less gold content, and predominantly base metal is less than 25 percent precious noble metal. Report D2780 for a cast high noble metal crown, D2781 for a cast predominately base metal, D2782 for a cast noble metal, and D2783 for a porcelain or ceramic substrate 3/4 crown.

## Coding Tips

Local anesthesia is included in these services. Any evaluation, radiograph, root canal, core buildup, or post or preparation service is reported separately. Fascial veneers are not included in code D2783 and may be billed separately; see codes D2960–D2962. To report full cast crowns, see codes D2790–D2792. Resin-based or porcelain/ceramic crowns are reported with the appropriate code from the D2710–D2722 range. When metallic inlays and onlays are provided, report D2510–D2544 as appropriate. High noble metals include gold, palladium, and platinum. The content must be ≥ 60 percent gold plus platinum and ≥ 40 percent gold. Noble metals include 25 percent or less gold plus platinum group. Predominantly base alloys contain a noble metal content of < 25 percent gold plus platinum group. The metals of the platinum group include platinum, palladium, rhodium, iridium, osmium, and ruthenium. Porcelain/ceramic refers to pressed, fired, polished, or milled substances, which predominantly contain inorganic refractory compounds such as porcelains, glasses, ceramics, and glass-ceramics. To report a provisional implant crown, see D6085.

## Documentation Tips

Treatment plan documentation should reflect any treatment failure or change in diagnosis and/or a change in treatment plan. There should also be evidence of any initiation or reinstatement of a drug regime, which requires close and continuous skilled medical observation. The following information can be documented on a tooth chart: treatment/location of caries, endodontic procedures, prosthetic services, preventive services, treatment of lesions and dental disease, or other special procedures. A tooth chart may also be used to identify structure and rationale of disease process and the type of service performed on intraoral structures other than teeth.

## Reimbursement Tips

Third-party payers often consider laboratory costs, tooth preparation, pulp caps, temporary restorations, porcelain margins, cement bases, impressions, and local anesthesia to be components of a complete restoration and, therefore, will not make separate payment for these services. Third-party payers may consider the buildup under a crown as included in the fee for a crown. A payer may allow an exception where extensive buildup is needed to gain retention and make additional payment in these instances. When this occurs, a written report and x-rays should be submitted with the claim. However, most payers will not reimburse separately for a buildup when placed to remove undercuts or to add bulk to the preparation. Payers may require documentation including the tooth number, surface(s), and preoperative periapical x-ray.

## ICD-10-CM Diagnostic Codes

| | |
|---|---|
| K02.52 | Dental caries on pit and fissure surface penetrating into dentin |
| K02.53 | Dental caries on pit and fissure surface penetrating into pulp |
| K02.61 | Dental caries on smooth surface limited to enamel |
| K02.62 | Dental caries on smooth surface penetrating into dentin |
| K02.63 | Dental caries on smooth surface penetrating into pulp |
| K02.7 | Dental root caries |
| K03.0 | Excessive attrition of teeth |
| K03.1 | Abrasion of teeth |
| K03.2 | Erosion of teeth |

## Relative Value Units/Medicare Edits

| Non-Facility RVU | Work | PE | MP | Total |
|---|---|---|---|---|
| **D2780** | 6.00 | 5.30 | 1.24 | 12.54 |
| **D2781** | 5.32 | 4.70 | 1.10 | 11.12 |
| **D2782** | 5.63 | 4.97 | 1.16 | 11.76 |
| **D2783** | 6.21 | 5.49 | 1.28 | 12.98 |
| **Facility RVU** | **Work** | **PE** | **MP** | **Total** |
| **D2780** | 6.00 | 5.30 | 1.24 | 12.54 |
| **D2781** | 5.32 | 4.70 | 1.10 | 11.12 |
| **D2782** | 5.63 | 4.97 | 1.16 | 11.76 |
| **D2783** | 6.21 | 5.49 | 1.28 | 12.98 |

| | FUD | Status | MUE | Modifiers | | | | IOM Reference |
|---|---|---|---|---|---|---|---|---|
| **D2780** | N/A | N | - | N/A | N/A | N/A | N/A | None |
| **D2781** | N/A | N | - | N/A | N/A | N/A | N/A | |
| **D2782** | N/A | N | - | N/A | N/A | N/A | N/A | |
| **D2783** | N/A | N | - | N/A | N/A | N/A | N/A | |

* with documentation

## Terms To Know

**artificial crown.** In dentistry, a ceramic or metal restoration made to cover or replace a major part of the top of a tooth.

**bonding.** In dentistry, two or more components connected by chemical adhesion or mechanical means.

**root canal.** Inner soft tissue, or pulp, of the tooth containing the lymph vessels, veins, arteries, and nerves of the tooth within small channels (up to five) running from the top of the tooth down to the tip of the root. When the tooth is cracked or decayed, bacteria enter the pulp and infect it, causing damage or death to the pulpal tissue and possibly an abscess that can infect bone. Root canal therapy repairs the root canal by removing the damaged pulp and cleaning out bacteria to prevent further damage and save the tooth.

# D2790-D2792

**D2790** crown - full cast high noble metal
**D2791** crown - full cast predominantly base metal
**D2792** crown - full cast noble metal

## Explanation

A crown is a restorative "cap" for a tooth made in exact reproduction to the tooth's anatomy. The dentist takes an upper and lower bite impression of the section of the mouth containing the tooth to be crowned and sends it to the lab. Plaster is poured into the impression mold with pins placed for later removal, connected to an articulator with more plaster, and then the poured model is removed. The prepped tooth is isolated. The margins are trimmed and marked. A spacer substance is painted on to the exact allowance needed for cementing the crown onto the tooth. A wax model is made of the full crown over the die model of the tooth, removed, and encased with a channel in high-density plaster. The wax is burned out. The model is filled with molten metal, spun on the arm of a centrifuge. The cast metal crown is tested on the tooth model, shaped, polished, and sent back to the dentist who tries the crown on the patient, checks all contact points and margins, then cements the crown onto the tooth. Report D2790 for a full cast high noble metal crown, D2791 for a full cast predominantly base metal crown, and D2792 for a full cast noble metal crown.

## Coding Tips

Local anesthesia is included in these services. Any evaluation, radiograph, root canal, core buildup, or post or preparation service is reported separately. Tooth numbering and preoperative periapical x-rays may be required by some third-party payers. To report 3/4 cast metal crowns see, D2780–D2782. Crowns made with a resin are reported using codes D2710–D2722. Porcelain crowns are reported with D2740–D2752. High noble metals include gold, palladium, and platinum. The content must be ≥ 60 percent gold plus platinum and ≥ 40 percent gold. Noble metals include 25 percent or less gold plus platinum group. Predominantly base alloys contain a noble metal content of < 25 percent gold plus platinum group. The metals of the platinum group include platinum, palladium, rhodium, iridium, osmium, and ruthenium. Resin-based composite includes fiber or ceramic reinforced polymer compounds. Porcelain/ceramic refers to pressed, fired, polished, or milled substances, which predominantly contain inorganic refractory compounds such as porcelains, glasses, ceramics, and glass-ceramics. Report prefabricated stainless steel crown restorations using D2930–D2931, D2933, or D2934. To report a provisional implant crown, see D6085.

## Documentation Tips

Treatment plan documentation should reflect any treatment failure or change in diagnosis and/or a change in treatment plan. There should also be evidence of any initiation or reinstatement of a drug regime, which requires close and continuous skilled medical observation. The following information can be documented on a tooth chart: treatment/location of caries, endodontic procedures, prosthetic services, preventive services, treatment of lesions and dental disease, or other special procedures. A tooth chart may also be used to identify structure and rationale of disease process and the type of service performed on intraoral structures other than teeth.

## Reimbursement Tips

Third-party payers often consider laboratory costs, tooth preparation, pulp caps, temporary restorations, porcelain margins, cement bases, impressions, and local anesthesia to be components of a complete restoration and, therefore, will not make separate payment for these services. Third-party payers may consider the buildup under a crown as included in the fee for a crown. A payer may allow an exception where extensive buildup is needed to gain retention and make additional payment in these instances. When this occurs, a written report and x-rays should be submitted with the claim. However, most payers will not reimburse separately for a buildup when placed to remove undercuts or to add bulk to the preparation. Payers may require documentation including the tooth number, surface(s), and preoperative periapical x-ray.

## ICD-10-CM Diagnostic Codes

| | |
|---|---|
| K02.52 | Dental caries on pit and fissure surface penetrating into dentin |
| K02.53 | Dental caries on pit and fissure surface penetrating into pulp |
| K02.61 | Dental caries on smooth surface limited to enamel |
| K02.62 | Dental caries on smooth surface penetrating into dentin |
| K02.63 | Dental caries on smooth surface penetrating into pulp |
| K02.7 | Dental root caries |
| K03.0 | Excessive attrition of teeth |
| K03.1 | Abrasion of teeth |
| K03.2 | Erosion of teeth |

## Relative Value Units/Medicare Edits

| Non-Facility RVU | Work | PE | MP | Total |
|---|---|---|---|---|
| **D2790** | 6.11 | 5.40 | 1.26 | 12.77 |
| **D2791** | 5.46 | 4.82 | 1.12 | 11.40 |
| **D2792** | 5.71 | 5.04 | 1.18 | 11.93 |
| **Facility RVU** | **Work** | **PE** | **MP** | **Total** |
| **D2790** | 6.11 | 5.40 | 1.26 | 12.77 |
| **D2791** | 5.46 | 4.82 | 1.12 | 11.40 |
| **D2792** | 5.71 | 5.04 | 1.18 | 11.93 |

| | FUD | Status | MUE | Modifiers | | | | IOM Reference |
|---|---|---|---|---|---|---|---|---|
| **D2790** | N/A | N | - | N/A | N/A | N/A | N/A | None |
| **D2791** | N/A | N | - | N/A | N/A | N/A | N/A | |
| **D2792** | N/A | N | - | N/A | N/A | N/A | N/A | |

* with documentation

## Terms To Know

**artificial crown.** In dentistry, a ceramic or metal restoration made to cover or replace a major part of the top of a tooth.

**bonding.** In dentistry, two or more components connected by chemical adhesion or mechanical means.

**coping.** Thin covering that is placed over a tooth before attaching a crown or overdenture.

**moulage.** Model of an anatomical structure formed via a negative impression in wax or plaster.

**root canal.** Inner soft tissue, or pulp, of the tooth containing the lymph vessels, veins, arteries, and nerves of the tooth within small channels (up to five) running from the top of the tooth down to the tip of the root. When the tooth is cracked or decayed, bacteria enter the pulp and infect it, causing damage or death to the pulpal tissue and possibly an abscess that can infect bone. Root canal therapy repairs the root canal by removing the damaged pulp and cleaning out bacteria to prevent further damage and save the tooth.

# D2794

**D2794** crown - titanium and titanium alloys

## Explanation

A titanium or titanium alloy crown is applied. A crown is a restorative "cap" for a tooth made in exact reproduction to the tooth's anatomy. A titanium dental crown is an extremely strong metal that is used when maximum strength is desired, appearance is not a factor, and a gold alloy is not considered biocompatible. The tooth is anesthetized and prepared for the crown. If an old filling is present, it is removed, along with any decay. The dentist takes an upper and lower bite impression of the section of the mouth containing the tooth to be crowned and sends it to the laboratory. This mold is then used to construct the crown. While the crown is being constructed, a temporary crown is placed on the tooth. When the permanent crown is returned from the laboratory, the patient returns to the dentist office. The temporary crown is removed from the tooth. The new crown is placed over the tooth and checked for fit, including fit between teeth and seal against the tooth, shape and appearance, and bite. If everything is correct, the permanent crown is cemented into place with long-term cement.

## Coding Tips

Local anesthesia is included. To report a provisional implant crown, see D6085. To report 3/4 cast metal crowns, see D2780–D2782. Full metal crowns other than titanium are reported using the appropriate code from the D2790–D2792 range.

## Documentation Tips

Treatment plan documentation should reflect any treatment failure or change in diagnosis and/or a change in treatment plan. There should also be evidence of any initiation or reinstatement of a drug regime, which requires close and continuous skilled medical observation. The following information can be documented on a tooth chart: treatment/location of caries, endodontic procedures, prosthetic services, preventive services, treatment of lesions and dental disease, or other special procedures. A tooth chart may also be used to identify structure and rationale of disease process and the type of service performed on intraoral structures other than teeth.

## Reimbursement Tips

Any evaluation, radiograph, root canal, core buildup, or post or preparation service is reported separately. Third-party payers often consider laboratory costs, tooth preparation, pulp caps, temporary restorations, porcelain margins, cement bases, impressions, and local anesthesia to be components of a complete restoration and, therefore, will not make separate payment for these services. Third-party payers may consider the buildup under a crown as included in the fee for a crown. A payer may allow an exception where extensive buildup is needed to gain retention and make additional payment in these instances. When this occurs, a written report and x-rays should be submitted with the claim. Payers may require documentation including the tooth number, surface(s), and preoperative periapical x-ray.

## ICD-10-CM Diagnostic Codes

| | |
|---|---|
| K02.52 | Dental caries on pit and fissure surface penetrating into dentin |
| K02.53 | Dental caries on pit and fissure surface penetrating into pulp |
| K02.61 | Dental caries on smooth surface limited to enamel |
| K02.62 | Dental caries on smooth surface penetrating into dentin |
| K02.63 | Dental caries on smooth surface penetrating into pulp |
| K02.7 | Dental root caries |
| K03.0 | Excessive attrition of teeth |
| K03.1 | Abrasion of teeth |

K03.2 Erosion of teeth

## Relative Value Units/Medicare Edits

| Non-Facility RVU | Work | PE | MP | Total |
|---|---|---|---|---|
| D2794 | 5.94 | 5.24 | 1.22 | 12.40 |
| **Facility RVU** | **Work** | **PE** | **MP** | **Total** |
| D2794 | 5.94 | 5.24 | 1.22 | 12.40 |

| | FUD | Status | MUE | Modifiers | | | | IOM Reference |
|---|---|---|---|---|---|---|---|---|
| D2794 | N/A | N | - | N/A | N/A | N/A | N/A | None |

* with documentation

## Terms To Know

**artificial crown.** In dentistry, a ceramic or metal restoration made to cover or replace a major part of the top of a tooth.

**bonding.** In dentistry, two or more components connected by chemical adhesion or mechanical means.

**dental cement.** Any substance used in the mouth that sets from a viscous to a hard form and functions as a restorative material, a bonding force for fabricated restorations and orthodontics, or protective filling for insulation.

Dental - Restoration

# D2799

▲ **D2799** interim crown – further treatment or completion of diagnosis necessary prior to final impression

*Not to be used as a temporary crown for a routine prosthetic restoration.*

## Explanation

A provisional crown is made and cemented onto the tooth for an interim restoration period of at least six months when healing time is required before permanent restoration or when longer restorative procedures must also be undertaken, such as completing periodontal therapy or treatment for cracked-tooth syndrome. This is not a temporary crown for routine prosthetic restoration.

## Coding Tips

Local anesthesia is included in this service. Any evaluation, radiograph, root canal, core buildup, or post or preparation service is reported separately.To report a crown that is used temporarily for a routine prosthetic restoration, see D2790. To report a provisional implant crown see D6085.

## Documentation Tips

Treatment plan documentation should reflect any treatment failure or change in diagnosis and/or a change in treatment plan. There should also be evidence of any initiation or reinstatement of a drug regime, which requires close and continuous skilled medical observation. The following information can be documented on a tooth chart: treatment/location of caries, endodontic procedures, prosthetic services, preventive services, treatment of lesions and dental disease, or other special procedures. A tooth chart may also be used to identify structure and rationale of disease process and the type of service performed on intraoral structures other than teeth.

## Reimbursement Tips

Many third-party payers consider provisional or temporary crowns to be part of the permanent restoration and will not make a separate payment for this service. However, when final restoration will not be performed for longer than six months or in other more unusual circumstances, payers may provide reimbursement after individual consideration. Check with payers to determine their specific guidelines and the type and extent of additional information required to process the claim. Payers may require documentation including the tooth number, surface(s), and preoperative periapical x-ray.

## ICD-10-CM Diagnostic Codes

K02.52 Dental caries on pit and fissure surface penetrating into dentin
K02.53 Dental caries on pit and fissure surface penetrating into pulp
K02.61 Dental caries on smooth surface limited to enamel
K02.62 Dental caries on smooth surface penetrating into dentin
K02.63 Dental caries on smooth surface penetrating into pulp
K02.7 Dental root caries
K03.0 Excessive attrition of teeth
K03.1 Abrasion of teeth
K03.2 Erosion of teeth

## Relative Value Units/Medicare Edits

| Non-Facility RVU | Work | PE | MP | Total |
|---|---|---|---|---|
| **D2799** | 2.37 | 2.09 | 0.49 | 4.95 |
| **Facility RVU** | **Work** | **PE** | **MP** | **Total** |
| **D2799** | 2.37 | 2.09 | 0.49 | 4.95 |

| | FUD | Status | MUE | Modifiers | | | | IOM Reference |
|---|---|---|---|---|---|---|---|---|
| **D2799** | N/A | N | - | N/A | N/A | N/A | N/A | None |

* with documentation

## Terms To Know

**artificial crown.** In dentistry, a ceramic or metal restoration made to cover or replace a major part of the top of a tooth.

**bonding.** In dentistry, two or more components connected by chemical adhesion or mechanical means.

**coping.** Thin covering that is placed over a tooth before attaching a crown or overdenture.

**moulage.** Model of an anatomical structure formed via a negative impression in wax or plaster.

**root canal.** Inner soft tissue, or pulp, of the tooth containing the lymph vessels, veins, arteries, and nerves of the tooth within small channels (up to five) running from the top of the tooth down to the tip of the root. When the tooth is cracked or decayed, bacteria enter the pulp and infect it, causing damage or death to the pulpal tissue and possibly an abscess that can infect bone. Root canal therapy repairs the root canal by removing the damaged pulp and cleaning out bacteria to prevent further damage and save the tooth.

# D2910

**D2910** re-cement or re-bond inlay, onlay, veneer or partial coverage restoration

## Explanation

An inlay, onlay, or partial coverage restoration is recemented if it becomes loose or dislodged. The inlay, onlay, or partial coverage restoration is removed from the tooth. It is cleaned and prepared for recementing. The tooth is also cleaned and prepared for recementing or rebonding. The inlay, onlay, or partial coverage restoration is recemented into place.

## Coding Tips

Local anesthesia is generally considered to be part of restorative procedures. For recementation or rebonding of cast or prefabricated post and core, see D2915; for crown, see D2920.

## Documentation Tips

Treatment plan documentation should reflect any treatment failure or change in diagnosis and/or a change in treatment plan. There should also be evidence of any initiation or reinstatement of a drug regime, which requires close and continuous skilled medical observation.

## Reimbursement Tips

Most payers require that the tooth number be indicated on the claim.

## ICD-10-CM Diagnostic Codes

| | |
|---|---|
| K08.51 | Open restoration margins of tooth |
| K08.52 | Unrepairable overhanging of dental restorative materials |
| K08.530 | Fractured dental restorative material without loss of material |
| K08.531 | Fractured dental restorative material with loss of material |
| K08.54 | Contour of existing restoration of tooth biologically incompatible with oral health |
| K08.55 | Allergy to existing dental restorative material |
| K08.56 | Poor aesthetic of existing restoration of tooth |
| K08.59 | Other unsatisfactory restoration of tooth |

## Relative Value Units/Medicare Edits

| Non-Facility RVU | Work | PE | MP | Total |
|---|---|---|---|---|
| **D2910** | 0.51 | 0.45 | 0.10 | 1.06 |
| **Facility RVU** | **Work** | **PE** | **MP** | **Total** |
| **D2910** | 0.51 | 0.45 | 0.10 | 1.06 |

| | FUD | Status | MUE | Modifiers | | | | IOM Reference |
|---|---|---|---|---|---|---|---|---|
| **D2910** | N/A | N | - | N/A | N/A | N/A | N/A | None |

* with documentation

## Terms To Know

**dental cement.** Any substance used in the mouth that sets from a viscous to a hard form and functions as a restorative material, a bonding force for fabricated restorations and orthodontics, or protective filling for insulation.

**inlay.** Restoration made outside of the mouth to fit a prepared cavity and placed on the tooth.

**onlay.** In dentistry, restoration made outside of the mouth that is cemented over a cusp or cusps of the tooth.

# D2915

**D2915** re-cement or re-bond indirectly fabricated or prefabricated post and core

## Explanation

A prefabricated or cast post and core that becomes loose or dislodged is recemented or rebonded after first cleaning and preparing the canal. This procedure code applies to a prefabricated or an individually fitted and specially cast post (including a core and coping) that was placed into the endodontically treated canal. A prefabricated post and core is any commercial product such as a screw post, endo post, Kurer anchor, or crown saver, or any preformed post of any material or shape.

## Coding Tips

For recementation or rebonding of a crown, see D2920. Code D2915 is considered an integral part of crown recementation or rebonding by most third-party payers and should not be reported in addition to D2920. Local anesthesia is generally considered to be part of restorative procedures. For recementation or rebonding of an inlay, onlay, or partial coverage restoration, see D2910.

## Documentation Tips

Treatment plan documentation should reflect any treatment failure or change in diagnosis and/or a change in treatment plan. There should also be evidence of any initiation or reinstatement of a drug regime, which requires close and continuous skilled medical observation. The following information can be documented on a tooth chart: treatment/location of caries, endodontic procedures, prosthetic services, preventive services, treatment of lesions and dental disease, or other special procedures. A tooth chart may also be used to identify structure and rationale of disease process and the type of service performed on intraoral structures other than teeth.

## ICD-10-CM Diagnostic Codes

K08.51 Open restoration margins of tooth
K08.52 Unrepairable overhanging of dental restorative materials
K08.530 Fractured dental restorative material without loss of material
K08.531 Fractured dental restorative material with loss of material
K08.54 Contour of existing restoration of tooth biologically incompatible with oral health
K08.55 Allergy to existing dental restorative material
K08.56 Poor aesthetic of existing restoration of tooth
K08.59 Other unsatisfactory restoration of tooth

## Relative Value Units/Medicare Edits

| Non-Facility RVU | Work | PE | MP | Total |
|---|---|---|---|---|
| D2915 | 0.52 | 0.46 | 0.11 | 1.09 |
| **Facility RVU** | **Work** | **PE** | **MP** | **Total** |
| D2915 | 0.52 | 0.46 | 0.11 | 1.09 |

| | FUD | Status | MUE | Modifiers | | | | IOM Reference |
|---|---|---|---|---|---|---|---|---|
| D2915 | N/A | N | - | N/A | N/A | N/A | N/A | None |

* with documentation

# D2920

**D2920** re-cement or re-bond crown

## Explanation

A crown is recemented or rebonded after becoming loose or dislodged. The crown is removed from the tooth. It is cleaned, residual cement removed, and prepared for recementing or rebonding. The tooth is also cleaned of any residual cement or foreign matter and prepared for recementing or rebonding. The crown is recemented or rebonded into place.

## Coding Tips

Local anesthesia is generally considered to be part of restorative procedures. Code D2915 is considered an integral part of crown recementation or rebonding by most third-party payers and should not be reported in addition to D2920. To report recementation or rebonding of inlay, onlay, or partial coverage restorations, see D2910.

## Documentation Tips

Treatment plan documentation should reflect any treatment failure or change in diagnosis and/or a change in treatment plan. There should also be evidence of any initiation or reinstatement of a drug regime, which requires close and continuous skilled medical observation.

## Reimbursement Tips

Most third-party payers require that the tooth number be indicated on the claim.

## ICD-10-CM Diagnostic Codes

K08.51 Open restoration margins of tooth
K08.52 Unrepairable overhanging of dental restorative materials
K08.530 Fractured dental restorative material without loss of material
K08.531 Fractured dental restorative material with loss of material
K08.539 Fractured dental restorative material, unspecified
K08.54 Contour of existing restoration of tooth biologically incompatible with oral health
K08.55 Allergy to existing dental restorative material
K08.56 Poor aesthetic of existing restoration of tooth
K08.59 Other unsatisfactory restoration of tooth

## Relative Value Units/Medicare Edits

| Non-Facility RVU | Work | PE | MP | Total |
|---|---|---|---|---|
| D2920 | 0.51 | 0.45 | 0.11 | 1.07 |
| **Facility RVU** | **Work** | **PE** | **MP** | **Total** |
| D2920 | 0.51 | 0.45 | 0.11 | 1.07 |

| | FUD | Status | MUE | Modifiers | | | | IOM Reference |
|---|---|---|---|---|---|---|---|---|
| D2920 | N/A | N | - | N/A | N/A | N/A | N/A | None |

* with documentation

## Terms To Know

**artificial crown.** In dentistry, a ceramic or metal restoration made to cover or replace a major part of the top of a tooth.

**dental cement.** Any substance used in the mouth that sets from a viscous to a hard form and functions as a restorative material, a bonding force for fabricated restorations and orthodontics, or protective filling for insulation.

# D2921

**D2921** reattachment of tooth fragment, incisal edge or cusp

## Explanation

The provider reattaches a tooth fragment to the incisal edge or cusp of the residual tooth. By using the incisal edge reattachment technique the provider is able to re-establish the contour, the architecture, and the original brightness of the tooth. When the fractured portion is intact and has adequate and correctly preserved margins, it is reattached using adhesive to the residual tooth. This technique is also used when there is a dental fracture but the detached fragment does not completely align with the remaining tooth structure. However, in this scenario the provider must also determine the best technique required to fill the gap between the tooth and the fragment, thus improving the adhesion.

## Coding Tips

Any evaluation or radiograph is reported separately. To report the reimplantation and/or stabilization of a tooth occurring accidentally, see D7270.

## Documentation Tips

Treatment plan documentation should reflect any treatment failure or change in diagnosis and/or a change in treatment plan. There should also be evidence of any initiation or reinstatement of a drug regime, which requires close and continuous skilled medical observation.

## Reimbursement Tips

Most third-party payers require that the tooth number be indicated on the claim.

## ICD-10-CM Diagnostic Codes

| | |
|---|---|
| K03.81 | Cracked tooth |
| S02.5XXA | Fracture of tooth (traumatic), initial encounter for closed fracture |
| S02.5XXB | Fracture of tooth (traumatic), initial encounter for open fracture |
| S03.2XXA | Dislocation of tooth, initial encounter |

## Relative Value Units/Medicare Edits

| Non-Facility RVU | Work | PE | MP | Total |
|---|---|---|---|---|
| D2921 | 0.48 | 0.43 | 0.10 | 1.01 |
| **Facility RVU** | **Work** | **PE** | **MP** | **Total** |
| D2921 | 0.48 | 0.43 | 0.10 | 1.01 |

| | FUD | Status | MUE | Modifiers | | | | IOM Reference |
|---|---|---|---|---|---|---|---|---|
| D2921 | N/A | N | - | N/A | N/A | N/A | N/A | None |

* with documentation

## Terms To Know

**cusp.** In dentistry, the rounded or pointed portion of the surface of the tooth used for mastication.

**fragment.** Small piece broken off a larger whole; to divide into pieces.

**incisal.** Biting edge of an incisor or a cuspid tooth.

# D2928-D2931

**D2928** prefabricated porcelain/ceramic crown - permanent tooth
**D2929** prefabricated porcelain/ceramic crown - primary tooth
**D2930** prefabricated stainless steel crown - primary tooth
**D2931** prefabricated stainless steel crown - permanent tooth

## Explanation

Prefabricated porcelain or ceramic crowns are most often used to cover fractured or decayed anterior (front) teeth while stainless steel crowns are most often used to restore back teeth and are a reasonable temporary alternative restoration to custom-made crowns. Some last long enough to be considered as a long-term temporary restoration. Prefabricated crowns are purchased by the dentist and made in a variety of graduated sizes and shapes to fit the type of tooth they are intended to restore. They are basically thin, tooth-shaped shells. Most are applied to primary teeth because of poor marginal fit, but they may also be used on adult teeth as well. Prefabricated stainless steel crowns are bulky by comparison and generally do not fit the tooth very well. The dentist makes some alterations to the prefabricated crown for fitting it to the specified tooth at the time of insertion. The extra space inside the stainless steel crown, the space between it and the actual tooth structure, is filled in by a heavy mixture of temporary filling material. Code D2928 is for a prefabricated porcelain or ceramic crown applied to a permanent tooth and D2929 is used for a primary tooth. Code D2930 is for a prefabricated stainless steel crown applied to a primary tooth. Report D2931 for a prefabricated stainless steel crown applied to a permanent tooth.

## Coding Tips

When documentation indicates that the prefabricated stainless crown also has a resin window, report D2933; for crown with exterior esthetic coating, see D2934. To report custom-fabricated porcelain or ceramic crowns, see D2740–D2752. To report custom-fabricated metal crowns, see codes D2780–D2794.

## Documentation Tips

Treatment plan documentation should reflect any treatment failure or change in diagnosis and/or a change in treatment plan. There should also be evidence of any initiation or reinstatement of a drug regime, which requires close and continuous skilled medical observation. The following information can be documented on a tooth chart: treatment/location of caries, endodontic procedures, prosthetic services, preventive services, treatment of lesions and dental disease, or other special procedures. A tooth chart may also be used to identify structure and rationale of disease process and the type of service performed on intraoral structures other than teeth.

## Reimbursement Tips

Third-party payers often consider laboratory costs, tooth preparation, pulp caps, temporary restorations, porcelain margins, cement bases, impressions, and local anesthesia to be components of a complete restoration and, therefore, will not make separate payment for these services. Third-party payers may consider the buildup under a crown as included in the fee for a crown. A payer may allow an exception where extensive buildup is needed to gain retention and make additional payment in these instances. When this occurs, a written report and x-rays should be submitted with the claim. However, most payers will not reimburse separately for a buildup when placed to remove undercuts or to add bulk to the preparation.

## ICD-10-CM Diagnostic Codes

| | |
|---|---|
| K03.81 | Cracked tooth |
| K08.51 | Open restoration margins of tooth |
| K08.52 | Unrepairable overhanging of dental restorative materials |

| | |
|---|---|
| K08.530 | Fractured dental restorative material without loss of material |
| K08.531 | Fractured dental restorative material with loss of material |
| K08.54 | Contour of existing restoration of tooth biologically incompatible with oral health |
| K08.55 | Allergy to existing dental restorative material |
| K08.56 | Poor aesthetic of existing restoration of tooth |
| K08.59 | Other unsatisfactory restoration of tooth |

## Relative Value Units/Medicare Edits

| Non-Facility RVU | Work | PE | MP | Total |
|---|---|---|---|---|
| **D2928** | | | | |
| **D2929** | 1.45 | 1.28 | 0.30 | 3.03 |
| **D2930** | 1.39 | 1.23 | 0.29 | 2.91 |
| **D2931** | 1.69 | 1.50 | 0.35 | 3.54 |
| **Facility RVU** | **Work** | **PE** | **MP** | **Total** |
| **D2928** | | | | |
| **D2929** | 1.45 | 1.28 | 0.30 | 3.03 |
| **D2930** | 1.39 | 1.23 | 0.29 | 2.91 |
| **D2931** | 1.69 | 1.50 | 0.35 | 3.54 |

| | FUD | Status | MUE | Modifiers | | | | IOM Reference |
|---|---|---|---|---|---|---|---|---|
| **D2928** | N/A | | - | N/A | N/A | N/A | N/A | None |
| **D2929** | N/A | N | - | N/A | N/A | N/A | N/A | |
| **D2930** | N/A | N | - | N/A | N/A | N/A | N/A | |
| **D2931** | N/A | N | - | N/A | N/A | N/A | N/A | |

* with documentation

## Terms To Know

**artificial crown.** In dentistry, a ceramic or metal restoration made to cover or replace a major part of the top of a tooth.

**bonding.** In dentistry, two or more components connected by chemical adhesion or mechanical means.

**coping.** Thin covering that is placed over a tooth before attaching a crown or overdenture.

**moulage.** Model of an anatomical structure formed via a negative impression in wax or plaster.

**root canal.** Inner soft tissue, or pulp, of the tooth containing the lymph vessels, veins, arteries, and nerves of the tooth within small channels (up to five) running from the top of the tooth down to the tip of the root. When the tooth is cracked or decayed, bacteria enter the pulp and infect it, causing damage or death to the pulpal tissue and possibly an abscess that can infect bone. Root canal therapy repairs the root canal by removing the damaged pulp and cleaning out bacteria to prevent further damage and save the tooth.

# D2932

**D2932** prefabricated resin crown

## Explanation

A prefabricated resin crown is applied. Prefabricated crowns are available in a variety of materials that are used for both short-and long-term coverage. Prefabricated resin crowns are composed of polycarbonate resin with microglass fibers and are used primarily on the incisors, cuspids, and bicuspids. The tooth is anesthetized. The dentist prepares the tooth for the prefabricated crown by removing the old filling, if present, along with any decay. A prefabricated crown is selected in a size and configuration that will best match the tooth being replaced. The prefabricated crown is placed over the tooth and checked for fit. It is then reconfigured and adjusted as needed. When a good fit is achieved, it is cemented into place.

## Coding Tips

Resin-based composite includes fiber or ceramic reinforced polymer compounds. Resin-based composite includes fiber or ceramic reinforced polymer compounds. For custom fabricated resin-based composite crown, see D2710–D2722.

## Documentation Tips

Treatment plan documentation should reflect any treatment failure or change in diagnosis and/or a change in treatment plan. There should also be evidence of any initiation or reinstatement of a drug regime, which requires close and continuous skilled medical observation. The following information can be documented on a tooth chart: treatment/location of caries, endodontic procedures, prosthetic services, preventive services, treatment of lesions and dental disease, or other special procedures. A tooth chart may also be used to identify structure and rationale of disease process and the type of service performed on intraoral structures other than teeth.

## Reimbursement Tips

Third-party payers often consider laboratory costs, tooth preparation, pulp caps, temporary restorations, porcelain margins, cement bases, impressions, and local anesthesia to be components of a complete restoration and, therefore, will not make separate payment for these services. Third-party payers may consider the buildup under a crown as included in the fee for a crown. A payer may allow an exception where extensive buildup is needed to gain retention and make additional payment in these instances. When this occurs, a written report and x-rays should be submitted with the claim. However, most payers will not reimburse separately for a buildup when placed to remove undercuts or to add bulk to the preparation.

## ICD-10-CM Diagnostic Codes

| | |
|---|---|
| K08.50 | Unsatisfactory restoration of tooth, unspecified |
| K08.51 | Open restoration margins of tooth |
| K08.52 | Unrepairable overhanging of dental restorative materials |
| K08.530 | Fractured dental restorative material without loss of material |
| K08.531 | Fractured dental restorative material with loss of material |
| K08.539 | Fractured dental restorative material, unspecified |
| K08.54 | Contour of existing restoration of tooth biologically incompatible with oral health |
| K08.55 | Allergy to existing dental restorative material |
| K08.56 | Poor aesthetic of existing restoration of tooth |
| K08.59 | Other unsatisfactory restoration of tooth |

## Relative Value Units/Medicare Edits

| Non-Facility RVU | Work | PE | MP | Total |
|---|---|---|---|---|
| D2932 | 1.67 | 1.47 | 0.34 | 3.48 |
| Facility RVU | Work | PE | MP | Total |
| D2932 | 1.67 | 1.47 | 0.34 | 3.48 |

| | FUD | Status | MUE | Modifiers | | | | IOM Reference |
|---|---|---|---|---|---|---|---|---|
| D2932 | N/A | N | - | N/A | N/A | N/A | N/A | None |

* with documentation

## Terms To Know

**artificial crown.** In dentistry, a ceramic or metal restoration made to cover or replace a major part of the top of a tooth.

**dental cement.** Any substance used in the mouth that sets from a viscous to a hard form and functions as a restorative material, a bonding force for fabricated restorations and orthodontics, or protective filling for insulation.

# D2933

**D2933** prefabricated stainless steel crown with resin window

*Open-face stainless steel crown with aesthetic resin facing or veneer.*

## Explanation

A prefabricated stainless steal crown with a resin window is applied. Prefabricated crowns are available in a variety of materials that are used for both short-and long-term coverage. The tooth is anesthetized. The dentist prepares the tooth for the prefabricated crown by removing the old filling, if present, along with any decay. A prefabricated crown is selected in a size and configuration that will best match the tooth being replaced. The prefabricated crown is placed over the tooth and checked for fit. It is then reconfigured and adjusted as needed. When a good fit is achieved, it is cemented into place.

## Coding Tips

To report prefabricated stainless steel crown without resin window, see D2930-D2931; prefabricated stainless steel crown with esthetic coating see D2934. To report custom fabricated metal crowns, see D2780-D2794.

## Reimbursement Tips

Third-party payers often consider laboratory costs, tooth preparation, pulp caps, temporary restorations, porcelain margins, cement bases, impressions, and local anesthesia to be components of a complete restoration and, therefore, will not make separate payment for these services. Third-party payers may consider the buildup under a crown as included in the fee for a crown. A payer may allow an exception where extensive buildup is needed to gain retention and make additional payment in these instances. When this occurs, a written report and x-rays should be submitted with the claim. However, most payers will not reimburse separately for a buildup when placed to remove undercuts or to add bulk to the preparation.

## ICD-10-CM Diagnostic Codes

| | |
|---|---|
| K08.51 | Open restoration margins of tooth |
| K08.52 | Unrepairable overhanging of dental restorative materials |
| K08.530 | Fractured dental restorative material without loss of material |
| K08.531 | Fractured dental restorative material with loss of material |
| K08.54 | Contour of existing restoration of tooth biologically incompatible with oral health |
| K08.55 | Allergy to existing dental restorative material |
| K08.56 | Poor aesthetic of existing restoration of tooth |
| K08.59 | Other unsatisfactory restoration of tooth |

## Relative Value Units/Medicare Edits

| Non-Facility RVU | Work | PE | MP | Total |
|---|---|---|---|---|
| D2933 | 1.83 | 1.62 | 0.38 | 3.83 |
| Facility RVU | Work | PE | MP | Total |
| D2933 | 1.83 | 1.62 | 0.38 | 3.83 |

| | FUD | Status | MUE | Modifiers | | | | IOM Reference |
|---|---|---|---|---|---|---|---|---|
| D2933 | N/A | N | - | N/A | N/A | N/A | N/A | None |

* with documentation

Dental - Restoration

# D2934

**D2934** prefabricated esthetic coated stainless steel crown - primary tooth

*Stainless steel primary crown with exterior esthetic coating.*

## Explanation

An esthetic coated stainless steel crown for use on a primary (primary) tooth is applied. Prefabricated crowns are available in a variety of materials that are used for both short-and long-term coverage. The tooth is anesthetized. The dentist prepares the tooth for the prefabricated crown by removing the old filling, if present, along with any decay. A prefabricated crown is selected in a size and configuration that will best match the tooth being replaced. The prefabricated crown is placed over the tooth and checked for fit. It is then reconfigured and adjusted as needed. When a good fit is achieved, it is cemented into place.

## Coding Tips

For prefabricated stainless crown without esthetic coating, see D2930-D2931; with resin window report D2934. For custom fabricated metal crowns, see D2780-D2794.

## Reimbursement Tips

Third-party payers often consider laboratory costs, tooth preparation, pulp caps, temporary restorations, porcelain margins, cement bases, impressions, and local anesthesia to be components of a complete restoration and, therefore, will not make separate payment for these services. Third-party payers may consider the buildup under a crown as included in the fee for a crown. A payer may allow an exception where extensive buildup is needed to gain retention and make additional payment in these instances. When this occurs, a written report and x-rays should be submitted with the claim. However, most payers will not reimburse separately for a buildup when placed to remove undercuts or to add bulk to the preparation.

## ICD-10-CM Diagnostic Codes

| | |
|---|---|
| K08.51 | Open restoration margins of tooth |
| K08.52 | Unrepairable overhanging of dental restorative materials |
| K08.530 | Fractured dental restorative material without loss of material |
| K08.531 | Fractured dental restorative material with loss of material |
| K08.54 | Contour of existing restoration of tooth biologically incompatible with oral health |
| K08.55 | Allergy to existing dental restorative material |
| K08.56 | Poor aesthetic of existing restoration of tooth |
| K08.59 | Other unsatisfactory restoration of tooth |

## Relative Value Units/Medicare Edits

| Non-Facility RVU | Work | PE | MP | Total |
|---|---|---|---|---|
| D2934 | 1.91 | 1.68 | 0.39 | 3.98 |
| **Facility RVU** | **Work** | **PE** | **MP** | **Total** |
| D2934 | 1.91 | 1.68 | 0.39 | 3.98 |

| | FUD | Status | MUE | Modifiers | | | | IOM Reference |
|---|---|---|---|---|---|---|---|---|
| D2934 | N/A | N | - | N/A | N/A | N/A | N/A | None |

* with documentation

# D2940

**D2940** protective restoration

*Direct placement of a restorative material to protect tooth and/or tissue form. This procedure may be used to relieve pain, promote healing, or prevent further deterioration. Not to be used for endodontic access closure, or as a base or liner under a restoration.*

## Explanation

A protective restoration is a temporary restorative procedure typically performed on an emergency basis to relieve pain, such as sedative fillings or to protect tooth ingegrity until a final restorative treatment can be performed.

## Coding Tips

This code is appropriate to use for all porcelain crowns and, in some instances, intermediate restorative materials. Check with third-party payers for their specific guidelines when reporting this code for one of these procedures.

## Documentation Tips

Treatment plan documentation should reflect any treatment failure or change in diagnosis and/or a change in treatment plan. There should also be evidence of any initiation or reinstatement of a drug regime, which requires close and continuous skilled medical observation. The following information can be documented on a tooth chart: treatment/location of caries, endodontic procedures, prosthetic services, preventive services, treatment of lesions and dental disease, or other special procedures. A tooth chart may also be used to identify structure and rationale of disease process and the type of service performed on intraoral structures other than teeth.

## Reimbursement Tips

Third-party payers often consider laboratory costs, tooth preparation, pulp caps, temporary restorations, porcelain margins, cement bases, impressions, and local anesthesia to be components of a complete restoration and, therefore, will not make separate payment for these services. Third-party payers may consider the buildup under a crown as included in the fee for a crown. A payer may allow an exception where extensive buildup is needed to gain retention and make additional payment in these instances. When this occurs, a written report and x-rays should be submitted with the claim. However, most payers will not reimburse separately for a buildup when placed to remove undercuts or to add bulk to the preparation.

## ICD-10-CM Diagnostic Codes

| | |
|---|---|
| K02.3 | Arrested dental caries |
| K02.51 | Dental caries on pit and fissure surface limited to enamel |
| K02.52 | Dental caries on pit and fissure surface penetrating into dentin |
| K02.53 | Dental caries on pit and fissure surface penetrating into pulp |
| K02.61 | Dental caries on smooth surface limited to enamel |
| K02.62 | Dental caries on smooth surface penetrating into dentin |
| K02.63 | Dental caries on smooth surface penetrating into pulp |
| K02.7 | Dental root caries |
| K03.0 | Excessive attrition of teeth |
| K03.1 | Abrasion of teeth |
| K03.2 | Erosion of teeth |
| K03.3 | Pathological resorption of teeth |
| K03.4 | Hypercementosis |
| K03.5 | Ankylosis of teeth |
| S02.5XXA | Fracture of tooth (traumatic), initial encounter for closed fracture |
| S02.5XXB | Fracture of tooth (traumatic), initial encounter for open fracture |
| S03.2XXA | Dislocation of tooth, initial encounter |

## Relative Value Units/Medicare Edits

| Non-Facility RVU | Work | PE | MP | Total |
|---|---|---|---|---|
| **D2940** | 0.53 | 0.46 | 0.11 | 1.10 |
| **Facility RVU** | **Work** | **PE** | **MP** | **Total** |
| **D2940** | 0.53 | 0.46 | 0.11 | 1.10 |

| | FUD | Status | MUE | Modifiers | | | | IOM Reference |
|---|---|---|---|---|---|---|---|---|
| **D2940** | N/A | N | - | N/A | N/A | N/A | N/A | None |

* with documentation

## Terms To Know

**base.** In dentistry, material utilized beneath a filling to take the place of lost tooth structure.

**dentin.** Hard substance of the tooth found beneath the enamel on the crown and the cementum on the root that surrounds the living pulp tissue.

**direct restoration.** In dentistry, restoration produced inside of the mouth.

**filling.** In dentistry, restoration of lost tooth structure by utilizing substances such as metal, alloy, plastic, or porcelain.

**fissure.** Deep furrow, groove, or cleft in tissue structures.

**pulp.** Living connective tissue within the tooth's root canal space that supplies blood vessels and nerves to the tooth.

# D2941

**D2941** interim therapeutic restoration - primary dentition

*Placement of an adhesive restorative material following caries debridement by hand or other method for the management of early childhood caries. Not considered a definitive restoration.*

## Explanation

The provider places adhesive restorative material after removing the carious lesion from the tooth. The removal of the caries is achieved by using hand or slow speed rotary instruments with careful attention so as the pulp is not exposed. Following preparation (dependent upon the type of restorative material to be used), the tooth is restored with an adhesive restorative material such as self-setting or resin-modified glass ionomer cement. This type of restoration is recognized by the American Academy of Pediatric Dentistry (AAPD) as a provisional technique for the restoration and prevention of dental caries in young patients or in patients who are uncooperative or who have special needs. The AAPD also recognizes this treatment for the control of caries in young children with multiple carious lesions prior to definitive restoration of the teeth.

## Coding Tips

To report protective restoration, see D2940. For permanent restorations, see the appropriate code for the type of restoration performed.

## Documentation Tips

Treatment plan documentation should reflect any treatment failure or change in diagnosis and/or a change in treatment plan. There should also be evidence of any initiation or reinstatement of a drug regime, which requires close and continuous skilled medical observation. The following information can be documented on a tooth chart: treatment/location of caries, endodontic procedures, prosthetic services, preventive services, treatment of lesions and dental disease, or other special procedures. A tooth chart may also be used to identify structure and rationale of disease process and the type of service performed on intraoral structures other than teeth.

## Reimbursement Tips

The third-party payer may require an x-ray or x-ray report before processing the claim.

## ICD-10-CM Diagnostic Codes

| | |
|---|---|
| K02.3 | Arrested dental caries |
| K02.51 | Dental caries on pit and fissure surface limited to enamel |
| K02.52 | Dental caries on pit and fissure surface penetrating into dentin |
| K02.53 | Dental caries on pit and fissure surface penetrating into pulp |
| K02.61 | Dental caries on smooth surface limited to enamel |
| K02.62 | Dental caries on smooth surface penetrating into dentin |
| K02.63 | Dental caries on smooth surface penetrating into pulp |
| K02.7 | Dental root caries |
| K03.0 | Excessive attrition of teeth |
| K03.1 | Abrasion of teeth |
| K03.2 | Erosion of teeth |
| K03.3 | Pathological resorption of teeth |
| K03.4 | Hypercementosis |
| K03.5 | Ankylosis of teeth |
| S02.5XXA | Fracture of tooth (traumatic), initial encounter for closed fracture |
| S02.5XXB | Fracture of tooth (traumatic), initial encounter for open fracture |
| S03.2XXA | Dislocation of tooth, initial encounter |

Dental - Restoration

## Relative Value Units/Medicare Edits

| Non-Facility RVU | Work | PE | MP | Total |
|---|---|---|---|---|
| D2941 | 0.51 | 0.45 | 0.10 | 1.06 |
| **Facility RVU** | **Work** | **PE** | **MP** | **Total** |
| D2941 | 0.51 | 0.45 | 0.10 | 1.06 |

| | FUD | Status | MUE | Modifiers | | | | IOM Reference |
|---|---|---|---|---|---|---|---|---|
| D2941 | N/A | N | - | N/A | N/A | N/A | N/A | None |

* with documentation

## Terms To Know

**caries.** Localized section of tooth decay that begins on the tooth surface with destruction of the calcified enamel, allowing bacterial destruction to continue and form cavities and may extend to the dentin and pulp.

**debridement.** Removal of dead or contaminated tissue and foreign matter from a wound.

**dentin.** Hard substance of the tooth found beneath the enamel on the crown and the cementum on the root that surrounds the living pulp tissue.

**direct restoration.** In dentistry, restoration produced inside of the mouth.

**fissure.** Deep furrow, groove, or cleft in tissue structures.

**pulp.** Living connective tissue within the tooth's root canal space that supplies blood vessels and nerves to the tooth.

# D2950

**D2950** core buildup, including any pins when required

*Refers to building up of coronal structure when there is insufficient retention for a separate extracoronal restorative procedure. A core buildup is not a filler to eliminate any undercut, box form, or concave irregularity in a preparation.*

## Explanation

Core build-up is done as part of a tooth's preparation for restorative measures when there is insufficient strength or not enough of the tooth anatomy remaining to securely fix the restorative crown to the tooth, as in cases of bad decay. The dentist must build up enough of the tooth anatomy, such as recreating a cusp of a molar, in order to make the tooth into the ideal prep for the crown. Sometimes the dentist must first place a pin down into the tooth structure and then proceed to build-up the tooth anatomy around the pin to hold it in place. When the tooth is sufficiently prepared for restoration, impressions may be taken for other restorative services.

## Coding Tips

Payers may require that x-rays be reported with the claim. An amalgam post/core is considered to be a crown buildup and, therefore, is not separately reportable in addition to a crown unless the above noted exceptions are documented.

## Documentation Tips

Treatment plan documentation should reflect any treatment failure or change in diagnosis and/or a change in treatment plan. There should also be evidence of any initiation or reinstatement of a drug regime, which requires close and continuous skilled medical observation. The following information can be documented on a tooth chart: treatment/location of caries, endodontic procedures, prosthetic services, preventive services, treatment of lesions and dental disease, or other special procedures. A tooth chart may also be used to identify structure and rationale of disease process and the type of service performed on intraoral structures other than teeth.

## Reimbursement Tips

Third-party payers usually consider the buildup under a crown as included in the fee for a crown. A payer may allow an exception where extensive buildup is needed to gain retention and make additional payment in these instances. When this occurs, a written report and x-rays should be submitted with the claim. However, most payers will not reimburse separately for a buildup when placed to remove undercuts or to add bulk to the preparation.

## ICD-10-CM Diagnostic Codes

| | |
|---|---|
| K02.51 | Dental caries on pit and fissure surface limited to enamel |
| K02.52 | Dental caries on pit and fissure surface penetrating into dentin |
| K02.53 | Dental caries on pit and fissure surface penetrating into pulp |
| K02.61 | Dental caries on smooth surface limited to enamel |
| K02.62 | Dental caries on smooth surface penetrating into dentin |
| K02.63 | Dental caries on smooth surface penetrating into pulp |
| K02.7 | Dental root caries |
| K03.0 | Excessive attrition of teeth |
| K03.1 | Abrasion of teeth |
| K03.2 | Erosion of teeth |
| K03.3 | Pathological resorption of teeth |
| K03.4 | Hypercementosis |
| K03.5 | Ankylosis of teeth |
| K03.6 | Deposits [accretions] on teeth |
| K03.7 | Posteruptive color changes of dental hard tissues |

K03.81 Cracked tooth
K03.89 Other specified diseases of hard tissues of teeth
K03.9 Disease of hard tissues of teeth, unspecified
K04.01 Reversible pulpitis
K04.02 Irreversible pulpitis
K04.1 Necrosis of pulp
K04.2 Pulp degeneration
K04.3 Abnormal hard tissue formation in pulp
K04.4 Acute apical periodontitis of pulpal origin
K04.5 Chronic apical periodontitis
K04.6 Periapical abscess with sinus
K04.7 Periapical abscess without sinus
K04.8 Radicular cyst
K04.90 Unspecified diseases of pulp and periapical tissues
K04.99 Other diseases of pulp and periapical tissues
K05.00 Acute gingivitis, plaque induced
K05.01 Acute gingivitis, non-plaque induced
K05.10 Chronic gingivitis, plaque induced
K05.11 Chronic gingivitis, non-plaque induced

## Relative Value Units/Medicare Edits

| Non-Facility RVU | Work | PE | MP | Total |
|---|---|---|---|---|
| D2950 | 1.34 | 1.18 | 0.28 | 2.80 |
| Facility RVU | Work | PE | MP | Total |
| D2950 | 1.34 | 1.18 | 0.28 | 2.80 |

| | FUD | Status | MUE | Modifiers | | | | IOM Reference |
|---|---|---|---|---|---|---|---|---|
| D2950 | N/A | N | - | N/A | N/A | N/A | N/A | None |

* with documentation

## Terms To Know

**artificial crown.** In dentistry, a ceramic or metal restoration made to cover or replace a major part of the top of a tooth.

**bonding.** In dentistry, two or more components connected by chemical adhesion or mechanical means.

**coping.** Thin covering that is placed over a tooth before attaching a crown or overdenture.

**moulage.** Model of an anatomical structure formed via a negative impression in wax or plaster.

**root canal.** Inner soft tissue, or pulp, of the tooth containing the lymph vessels, veins, arteries, and nerves of the tooth within small channels (up to five) running from the top of the tooth down to the tip of the root. When the tooth is cracked or decayed, bacteria enter the pulp and infect it, causing damage or death to the pulpal tissue and possibly an abscess that can infect bone. Root canal therapy repairs the root canal by removing the damaged pulp and cleaning out bacteria to prevent further damage and save the tooth.

# D2951

**D2951** pin retention - per tooth, in addition to restoration

## Explanation

Pins are sometimes required along with core build-up materials to replace missing coronal tooth structure. Placement of pins is reported separately, once per tooth, in addition to the restorative procedures.

## Coding Tips

Local anesthesia is generally considered to be part of restorative procedures. Core and coping is considered an integral part of these procedures and is not reported separately. Report this code once per tooth. Report restorations separately.

## Documentation Tips

Treatment plan documentation should reflect any treatment failure or change in diagnosis and/or a change in treatment plan. There should also be evidence of any initiation or reinstatement of a drug regime, which requires close and continuous skilled medical observation. The following information can be documented on a tooth chart: treatment/location of caries, endodontic procedures, prosthetic services, preventive services, treatment of lesions and dental disease, or other special procedures. A tooth chart may also be used to identify structure and rationale of disease process and the type of service performed on intraoral structures other than teeth.

## Reimbursement Tips

The third-party payer may require an x-ray or x-ray report before processing the claim.

## ICD-10-CM Diagnostic Codes

K02.51 Dental caries on pit and fissure surface limited to enamel
K02.52 Dental caries on pit and fissure surface penetrating into dentin
K02.53 Dental caries on pit and fissure surface penetrating into pulp
K02.61 Dental caries on smooth surface limited to enamel
K02.62 Dental caries on smooth surface penetrating into dentin
K02.63 Dental caries on smooth surface penetrating into pulp
K02.7 Dental root caries
K03.0 Excessive attrition of teeth
K03.1 Abrasion of teeth
K03.2 Erosion of teeth
K03.3 Pathological resorption of teeth
K03.4 Hypercementosis
K03.5 Ankylosis of teeth
K03.6 Deposits [accretions] on teeth
K03.7 Posteruptive color changes of dental hard tissues
K03.81 Cracked tooth
K03.89 Other specified diseases of hard tissues of teeth
K03.9 Disease of hard tissues of teeth, unspecified
K04.01 Reversible pulpitis
K04.02 Irreversible pulpitis
K04.1 Necrosis of pulp
K04.2 Pulp degeneration
K04.3 Abnormal hard tissue formation in pulp
K04.4 Acute apical periodontitis of pulpal origin
K04.5 Chronic apical periodontitis
K04.6 Periapical abscess with sinus
K04.7 Periapical abscess without sinus

| | |
|---|---|
| K04.8 | Radicular cyst |
| K04.90 | Unspecified diseases of pulp and periapical tissues |
| K04.99 | Other diseases of pulp and periapical tissues |
| K05.00 | Acute gingivitis, plaque induced |
| K05.01 | Acute gingivitis, non-plaque induced |
| K05.10 | Chronic gingivitis, plaque induced |
| K05.11 | Chronic gingivitis, non-plaque induced |

### Relative Value Units/Medicare Edits

| Non-Facility RVU | Work | PE | MP | Total |
|---|---|---|---|---|
| D2951 | 0.31 | 0.27 | 0.06 | 0.64 |
| **Facility RVU** | **Work** | **PE** | **MP** | **Total** |
| D2951 | 0.31 | 0.27 | 0.06 | 0.64 |

| | FUD | Status | MUE | Modifiers | | | | IOM Reference |
|---|---|---|---|---|---|---|---|---|
| D2951 | N/A | N | - | N/A | N/A | N/A | N/A | None |

* with documentation

### Terms To Know

**core buildup.** Replacement of all or a portion of the tooth's crown in order to provide a base for the retention of a crown that has been indirectly fabricated.

**coronal.** Relating to the top of a tooth or the crown of the head.

**PIN.** In dentistry, a restoration retention aid consisting of a metal rod that has been cemented or driven into the dentin.

Dental - Restoration

# D2952-D2954, D2957

**D2952** post and core in addition to crown, indirectly fabricated

*Post and core are custom fabricated as a single unit.*

**D2953** each additional indirectly fabricated post - same tooth

*To be used with D2952.*

**D2954** prefabricated post and core in addition to crown

*Core is built around a prefabricated post. This procedure includes the core material.*

**D2957** each additional prefabricated post - same tooth

*To be used with D2954.*

### Explanation

When a root canal must be done prior to restoration, the tooth is left with open channels that must be filled for the completion of tooth preparation before crowning. The dentist takes an impression of the open tooth to be filled and sends it to the lab. The impression is filled with wax, shaped, and built up to have a central core "build-up" extending above the post "filling" part to function as the necessary preparatory buildup for the crown restoration. This wax model of post and core is cast as one piece. It is first invested in high density plaster and the wax burned out. The three-dimensional mold inside the plaster is filled with molten metal and, when ready, serves as a custom-made post filling with core build-up for the root-therapy treated tooth. This cast post and core is fitted into the die model of the tooth and the crown is then made over that model (see crown procedure descriptions). The crown should not be connected to the cast post and core piece. The dentist fits in the cast post and core filling and cements the crown on or bonds the crown to the tooth over it. When the tooth has more than one "open channel" from the root therapy to be filled in by the cast post and core piece, the model must be made to accommodate more than one post fitting down into the tooth. Report D2953 for each additional cast post per tooth. If a prefabricated post and core is used and fitted into the tooth with the crown made over that instead of casting the post and core piece as custom-made, report D2954 and D2957 for each additional prefabricated post used in the same tooth.

### Coding Tips

In code D2952 the cost and core are fabricated as a single custom unit. Code D2954 should be used when the post is cast as part of a crown. Codes D2952 and D2953 indicate indirect fabrication of components. Use D2953 for each additional cast post, same tooth, when reporting D2952. Post and any core build up is included in these codes and should not be billed separately. When reporting D2954, see D2957 for each additional prefabricated post on the same tooth. Local anesthesia is included in these services. Any evaluation, radiograph, root canal, or crown service is reported separately.

### Documentation Tips

Treatment plan documentation should reflect any treatment failure or change in diagnosis and/or a change in treatment plan. There should also be evidence of any initiation or reinstatement of a drug regime, which requires close and continuous skilled medical observation. The following information can be documented on a tooth chart: treatment/location of caries, endodontic procedures, prosthetic services, preventive services, treatment of lesions and dental disease, or other special procedures. A tooth chart may also be used to identify structure and rationale of disease process and the type of service performed on intraoral structures other than teeth.

### Reimbursement Tips

Payers may require documentation including the tooth number and postoperative endo periapical x-ray.

## ICD-10-CM Diagnostic Codes

| | |
|---|---|
| K02.51 | Dental caries on pit and fissure surface limited to enamel |
| K02.52 | Dental caries on pit and fissure surface penetrating into dentin |
| K02.53 | Dental caries on pit and fissure surface penetrating into pulp |
| K02.61 | Dental caries on smooth surface limited to enamel |
| K02.62 | Dental caries on smooth surface penetrating into dentin |
| K02.63 | Dental caries on smooth surface penetrating into pulp |
| K02.7 | Dental root caries |
| K03.0 | Excessive attrition of teeth |
| K03.1 | Abrasion of teeth |
| K03.2 | Erosion of teeth |
| K03.3 | Pathological resorption of teeth |
| K03.4 | Hypercementosis |
| K03.5 | Ankylosis of teeth |
| K03.6 | Deposits [accretions] on teeth |
| K03.7 | Posteruptive color changes of dental hard tissues |
| K03.81 | Cracked tooth |
| K03.89 | Other specified diseases of hard tissues of teeth |
| K03.9 | Disease of hard tissues of teeth, unspecified |
| K04.1 | Necrosis of pulp |
| K04.2 | Pulp degeneration |
| K04.3 | Abnormal hard tissue formation in pulp |
| K04.4 | Acute apical periodontitis of pulpal origin |
| K04.5 | Chronic apical periodontitis |
| K04.6 | Periapical abscess with sinus |
| K04.7 | Periapical abscess without sinus |
| K04.8 | Radicular cyst |
| K04.99 | Other diseases of pulp and periapical tissues |
| K05.00 | Acute gingivitis, plaque induced |
| K05.01 | Acute gingivitis, non-plaque induced |
| K05.10 | Chronic gingivitis, plaque induced |
| K05.11 | Chronic gingivitis, non-plaque induced |

## Relative Value Units/Medicare Edits

| Non-Facility RVU | Work | PE | MP | Total |
|---|---|---|---|---|
| D2952 | 2.26 | 1.99 | 0.46 | 4.71 |
| D2953 | 1.34 | 1.18 | 0.28 | 2.80 |
| D2954 | 1.69 | 1.49 | 0.35 | 3.53 |
| D2957 | 0.93 | 0.82 | 0.19 | 1.94 |
| **Facility RVU** | **Work** | **PE** | **MP** | **Total** |
| D2952 | 2.26 | 1.99 | 0.46 | 4.71 |
| D2953 | 1.34 | 1.18 | 0.28 | 2.80 |
| D2954 | 1.69 | 1.49 | 0.35 | 3.53 |
| D2957 | 0.93 | 0.82 | 0.19 | 1.94 |

| | FUD | Status | MUE | Modifiers | | | | IOM Reference |
|---|---|---|---|---|---|---|---|---|
| D2952 | N/A | N | - | N/A | N/A | N/A | N/A | None |
| D2953 | N/A | N | - | N/A | N/A | N/A | N/A | |
| D2954 | N/A | N | - | N/A | N/A | N/A | N/A | |
| D2957 | N/A | N | - | N/A | N/A | N/A | N/A | |

* with documentation

# D2955

**D2955** post removal

## Explanation

When a root canal must be done prior to restoration, the tooth is left with open channels that must be filled for the completion of tooth preparation before crowning. The dentist takes an impression of the open tooth to be filled and sends it to the lab. The impression is filled with wax, shaped, and built up to have a central core "build-up" extending above the post "filling" part to function as the necessary preparatory buildup for the crown restoration. Report D2955 for the removal of a post that has already been fitted in and placed into the tooth, such as a fractured post but not for retreatment of previous root canal therapy.

## Coding Tips

Local anesthesia is included in this service. Any evaluation, radiograph, root canal, or crown service is reported separately.

## Reimbursement Tips

Payers may require documentation including the tooth number and postoperative endoperiapical x-ray.

## ICD-10-CM Diagnostic Codes

| | |
|---|---|
| K02.3 | Arrested dental caries |
| K02.51 | Dental caries on pit and fissure surface limited to enamel |
| K02.52 | Dental caries on pit and fissure surface penetrating into dentin |
| K02.53 | Dental caries on pit and fissure surface penetrating into pulp |
| K02.61 | Dental caries on smooth surface limited to enamel |
| K02.62 | Dental caries on smooth surface penetrating into dentin |
| K02.63 | Dental caries on smooth surface penetrating into pulp |
| K02.7 | Dental root caries |
| K02.9 | Dental caries, unspecified |
| K03.81 | Cracked tooth |
| K08.51 | Open restoration margins of tooth |
| K08.52 | Unrepairable overhanging of dental restorative materials |
| K08.530 | Fractured dental restorative material without loss of material |
| K08.531 | Fractured dental restorative material with loss of material |
| K08.539 | Fractured dental restorative material, unspecified |
| Z98.811 | Dental restoration status |
| Z98.818 | Other dental procedure status |

## Relative Value Units/Medicare Edits

| Non-Facility RVU | Work | PE | MP | Total |
|---|---|---|---|---|
| D2955 | 1.31 | 1.16 | 0.27 | 2.74 |
| **Facility RVU** | **Work** | **PE** | **MP** | **Total** |
| D2955 | 1.31 | 1.16 | 0.27 | 2.74 |

| | FUD | Status | MUE | Modifiers | | | | IOM Reference |
|---|---|---|---|---|---|---|---|---|
| D2955 | N/A | N | - | N/A | N/A | N/A | N/A | None |

* with documentation

## Terms To Know

**artificial crown.** In dentistry, a ceramic or metal restoration made to cover or replace a major part of the top of a tooth.

Dental - Restoration

Dental - Restoration

# D2960-D2961

**D2960** labial veneer (resin laminate) - direct

*Refers to labial/facial direct resin bonded veneers.*

**D2961** labial veneer (resin laminate) - indirect

*Refers to labial/facial indirect resin bonded veneers.*

## Explanation

A labial resin veneer, also referred to as a partial crown, is a restorative procedure performed on the anterior teeth (incisors, cuspids) in which a layer of tooth-colored material is luted (cemented) to the surface of the tooth. The procedure may be performed as a direct restorative service, which involves applying the veneer in the office (chair side). Veneers cover the surface of the tooth and are used to treat conditions such as amelogenesis imperfecta, dentinogenesis imperfecta, congenitally missing anterior teeth, maxillary midline diastema, pegged lateral incisors, severe fluorosis, and severe tetracycline staining. However, labial veneers may also be performed as purely cosmetic procedures to improve the appearance of the anterior teeth. Report D2960 for a direct labial veneer fabricated chairside and D2961 for an indirect veneer fabricated at a laboratory.

## Coding Tips

Local anesthesia is generally considered to be part of restorative procedures. These procedures are usually performed on permanent teeth. To report facial veneers that extend interproximally and/or cover the incisal edge, see D2962.

## Reimbursement Tips

Some payers may require that x-rays or x-ray reports be submitted with the claim. When performed for cosmetic reasons, these services are not covered by most third-party payers.

## ICD-10-CM Diagnostic Codes

| | |
|---|---|
| K02.51 | Dental caries on pit and fissure surface limited to enamel |
| K02.52 | Dental caries on pit and fissure surface penetrating into dentin |
| K02.53 | Dental caries on pit and fissure surface penetrating into pulp |
| K02.61 | Dental caries on smooth surface limited to enamel |
| K02.62 | Dental caries on smooth surface penetrating into dentin |
| K02.63 | Dental caries on smooth surface penetrating into pulp |
| K02.7 | Dental root caries |
| K02.9 | Dental caries, unspecified |
| K03.81 | Cracked tooth |

## Relative Value Units/Medicare Edits

| Non-Facility RVU | Work | PE | MP | Total |
|---|---|---|---|---|
| D2960 | 3.57 | 3.15 | 0.74 | 7.46 |
| D2961 | 4.32 | 3.81 | 0.89 | 9.02 |
| **Facility RVU** | **Work** | **PE** | **MP** | **Total** |
| D2960 | 3.57 | 3.15 | 0.74 | 7.46 |
| D2961 | 4.32 | 3.81 | 0.89 | 9.02 |

| | FUD | Status | MUE | Modifiers | | | | IOM Reference |
|---|---|---|---|---|---|---|---|---|
| D2960 | N/A | N | - | N/A | N/A | N/A | N/A | None |
| D2961 | N/A | N | - | N/A | N/A | N/A | N/A | |

* with documentation

# D2962

**D2962** labial veneer (porcelain laminate) - indirect

*Refers also to facial veneers that extend interproximally and/or cover the incisal edge. Porcelain/ceramic veneers presently include all ceramic and porcelain veneers.*

## Explanation

A porcelain laminate labial veneer that is fabricated in a laboratory is applied. A labial veneer, also referred to as a partial crown, is a restorative procedure performed on the anterior teeth (incisors, cuspids) in which a layer of tooth-colored material is luted (cemented) to the surface of the tooth. The procedure may be performed as indirect (laboratory). Veneers cover the surface of the tooth and are used to treat conditions such as amelogenesis imperfecta, dentinogenesis imperfecta, congenitally missing anterior teeth, maxillary midline diastema, pegged lateral incisors, severe fluorosis, and severe tetracycline staining. However, labial veneers may also be performed as purely cosmetic procedures to improve the appearance of the anterior teeth.

## Coding Tips

Local anesthesia is generally considered to be part of restorative procedures. This code is appropriate when reporting facial veneers that extend interproximally and/or cover the incisal edge.

## Documentation Tips

Treatment plan documentation should reflect any treatment failure or change in diagnosis and/or a change in treatment plan. There should also be evidence of any initiation or reinstatement of a drug regime, which requires close and continuous skilled medical observation. The following information can be documented on a tooth chart: treatment/location of caries, endodontic procedures, prosthetic services, preventive services, treatment of lesions and dental disease, or other special procedures. A tooth chart may also be used to identify structure and rationale of disease process and the type of service performed on intraoral structures other than teeth.

## Reimbursement Tips

Payers may require documentation including the tooth number and preoperative periapical x-ray. This procedure is usually performed on permanent teeth. When performed for cosmetic reasons, the service is not covered by most third-party payers. However, some payers may provide coverage when performed for the conditions described above. Check with payers for their specific coverage guidelines.

## ICD-10-CM Diagnostic Codes

| | |
|---|---|
| K00.0 | Anodontia |
| K00.1 | Supernumerary teeth |
| K00.2 | Abnormalities of size and form of teeth |
| K00.3 | Mottled teeth |
| K00.4 | Disturbances in tooth formation |
| K00.5 | Hereditary disturbances in tooth structure, not elsewhere classified |
| K00.6 | Disturbances in tooth eruption |
| K00.8 | Other disorders of tooth development |
| K02.51 | Dental caries on pit and fissure surface limited to enamel |
| K02.52 | Dental caries on pit and fissure surface penetrating into dentin |
| K02.53 | Dental caries on pit and fissure surface penetrating into pulp |
| K02.61 | Dental caries on smooth surface limited to enamel |
| K02.62 | Dental caries on smooth surface penetrating into dentin |
| K02.63 | Dental caries on smooth surface penetrating into pulp |
| K02.7 | Dental root caries |

| | |
|---|---|
| K03.0 | Excessive attrition of teeth |
| K03.1 | Abrasion of teeth |
| K03.2 | Erosion of teeth |
| K03.3 | Pathological resorption of teeth |
| K03.4 | Hypercementosis |
| K03.5 | Ankylosis of teeth |
| K03.6 | Deposits [accretions] on teeth |
| K03.7 | Posteruptive color changes of dental hard tissues |
| K03.81 | Cracked tooth |
| K03.89 | Other specified diseases of hard tissues of teeth |

## Relative Value Units/Medicare Edits

| Non-Facility RVU | Work | PE | MP | Total |
|---|---|---|---|---|
| D2962 | 4.99 | 4.40 | 1.03 | 10.42 |
| **Facility RVU** | **Work** | **PE** | **MP** | **Total** |
| D2962 | 4.99 | 4.40 | 1.03 | 10.42 |

| | FUD | Status | MUE | Modifiers | | | | IOM Reference |
|---|---|---|---|---|---|---|---|---|
| D2962 | N/A | N | - | N/A | N/A | N/A | N/A | None |

* with documentation

## Terms To Know

**veneer.** In dentistry, restoration that is cemented to the front (facial) surface of a tooth. Also refers to a layer of tooth-colored material made of composite, porcelain, ceramic, or acrylic resin, used to construct crowns or pontics and attached by direct fusion, cementation, or mechanical retention.

# D2971

▲ **D2971** additional procedures to customize a crown to fit under an existing partial denture framework

*This procedure is in addition to the separate crown procedure documented with its own code.*

## Explanation

A new crown is retrofitted to an existing removable partial denture framework. The crown is attached using existing clasp assembly. The type of procedure determines whether the patient will go without the partial during the fabrication process. In the traditional process, the dentist makes an impression that is sent to the lab, along with the partial, for the crown prep. The lab seats the partial onto a stone cast, fabricates the crown, and returns the partial and fitted crown to the dentist for placement. New techniques let the patient keep the partial during crown fabrication since the dentist seats the partial on the soft tissue in the mouth and makes the impression by squirting the material into the clasp area and over the prep. After the material sets, the partial is removed from the patient's mouth and a second impression of the mouth is taken. The set material is slid off the partial and sent to the lab for fabricating the crown. The patient wears the partial, and the crown is placed in the clasp assembly once completed in the lab.

## Coding Tips

Local anesthesia is generally considered part of a restorative procedure. Additional procedures, such as impressions and fittings, required to construct a new crown under existing partial denture framework, are reported with D2971. This code should be reported in addition to the appropriate code for the crown.

## Documentation Tips

Treatment plan documentation should reflect any treatment failure or change in diagnosis and/or a change in treatment plan. There should also be evidence of any initiation or reinstatement of a drug regime, which requires close and continuous skilled medical observation. The following information can be documented on a tooth chart: treatment/location of caries, endodontic procedures, prosthetic services, preventive services, treatment of lesions and dental disease, or other special procedures. A tooth chart may also be used to identify structure and rationale of disease process and the type of service performed on intraoral structures other than teeth.

## ICD-10-CM Diagnostic Codes

| | |
|---|---|
| K02.3 | Arrested dental caries |
| K02.51 | Dental caries on pit and fissure surface limited to enamel |
| K02.52 | Dental caries on pit and fissure surface penetrating into dentin |
| K02.53 | Dental caries on pit and fissure surface penetrating into pulp |
| K02.61 | Dental caries on smooth surface limited to enamel |
| K02.62 | Dental caries on smooth surface penetrating into dentin |
| K02.63 | Dental caries on smooth surface penetrating into pulp |
| K02.7 | Dental root caries |
| K03.0 | Excessive attrition of teeth |
| K03.1 | Abrasion of teeth |
| K03.2 | Erosion of teeth |
| K03.3 | Pathological resorption of teeth |
| K03.4 | Hypercementosis |
| K03.5 | Ankylosis of teeth |
| K03.6 | Deposits [accretions] on teeth |
| K03.7 | Posteruptive color changes of dental hard tissues |
| K03.81 | Cracked tooth |

| | |
|---|---|
| K03.89 | Other specified diseases of hard tissues of teeth |
| K04.01 | Reversible pulpitis |
| K04.02 | Irreversible pulpitis |
| K04.1 | Necrosis of pulp |
| K04.2 | Pulp degeneration |
| K04.3 | Abnormal hard tissue formation in pulp |
| K04.4 | Acute apical periodontitis of pulpal origin |
| K04.5 | Chronic apical periodontitis |
| K04.6 | Periapical abscess with sinus |
| K04.7 | Periapical abscess without sinus |
| K04.8 | Radicular cyst |

## Relative Value Units/Medicare Edits

| Non-Facility RVU | Work | PE | MP | Total |
|---|---|---|---|---|
| D2971 | 0.81 | 0.72 | 0.17 | 1.70 |
| **Facility RVU** | **Work** | **PE** | **MP** | **Total** |
| D2971 | 0.81 | 0.72 | 0.17 | 1.70 |

| | FUD | Status | MUE | Modifiers | | | | IOM Reference |
|---|---|---|---|---|---|---|---|---|
| D2971 | N/A | N | - | N/A | N/A | N/A | N/A | None |

* with documentation

## Terms To Know

**cast.** In dentistry, model or reproduction made from an impression or mold.

**coping.** Thin covering that is placed over a tooth before attaching a crown or overdenture.

**core buildup.** Replacement of all or a portion of the tooth's crown in order to provide a base for the retention of a crown that has been indirectly fabricated.

**post.** In dentistry, elongated supportive device that is fitted and cemented into the root canal of the tooth, which functions to reinforce and retain crown restorations or other restorative material.

# D2975

**D2975** coping

*A thin covering of the coronal portion of a tooth, usually devoid of anatomic contour, that can be used as a definitive restoration.*

## Explanation

The dentist provides a thin covering over a tooth as a method of restoring the tooth. This code reports custom fabrication of the coping component of a crown. Crowns can be manufactured of a combination of resin or porcelain exteriors with a metal interior coping.

## Coding Tips

Local anesthesia is generally considered to be part of restorative procedures. This code reports a definitive restoration.

## Documentation Tips

The following information can be documented on a tooth chart: treatment/location of caries, endodontic procedures, prosthetic services, preventive services, treatment of lesions and dental disease, or other special procedures. A tooth chart may also be used to identify structure and rationale of disease process and the type of service performed on intraoral structures other than teeth.

## Reimbursement Tips

Generally, the coping component is not reported separately, as it is considered integral to the construction of the crown. Consult individual payers to determine when this should be reported separately.

## ICD-10-CM Diagnostic Codes

| | |
|---|---|
| K00.2 | Abnormalities of size and form of teeth |
| K00.3 | Mottled teeth |
| K00.4 | Disturbances in tooth formation |
| K00.5 | Hereditary disturbances in tooth structure, not elsewhere classified |
| K02.3 | Arrested dental caries |
| K02.51 | Dental caries on pit and fissure surface limited to enamel |
| K02.52 | Dental caries on pit and fissure surface penetrating into dentin |
| K02.53 | Dental caries on pit and fissure surface penetrating into pulp |
| K02.61 | Dental caries on smooth surface limited to enamel |
| K02.62 | Dental caries on smooth surface penetrating into dentin |
| K02.63 | Dental caries on smooth surface penetrating into pulp |
| K02.7 | Dental root caries |
| K02.9 | Dental caries, unspecified |
| K03.0 | Excessive attrition of teeth |
| K03.1 | Abrasion of teeth |
| K03.2 | Erosion of teeth |
| K03.3 | Pathological resorption of teeth |
| K03.4 | Hypercementosis |
| K03.5 | Ankylosis of teeth |
| K03.6 | Deposits [accretions] on teeth |
| K03.7 | Posteruptive color changes of dental hard tissues |
| K03.81 | Cracked tooth |
| K03.89 | Other specified diseases of hard tissues of teeth |
| K03.9 | Disease of hard tissues of teeth, unspecified |
| K04.90 | Unspecified diseases of pulp and periapical tissues |

## Relative Value Units/Medicare Edits

| Non-Facility RVU | Work | PE | MP | Total |
|---|---|---|---|---|
| D2975 | 2.56 | 2.26 | 0.53 | 5.35 |
| **Facility RVU** | **Work** | **PE** | **MP** | **Total** |
| D2975 | 2.56 | 2.26 | 0.53 | 5.35 |

| | FUD | Status | MUE | Modifiers | | | | IOM Reference |
|---|---|---|---|---|---|---|---|---|
| D2975 | N/A | N | - | N/A | N/A | N/A | N/A | None |

* with documentation

### Terms To Know

**coping.** Thin covering that is placed over a tooth before attaching a crown or overdenture.

**crown.** Dental restoration that completely caps or encircles a tooth or dental implant.

**dentin.** Hard substance of the tooth found beneath the enamel on the crown and the cementum on the root that surrounds the living pulp tissue.

**direct restoration.** In dentistry, restoration produced inside of the mouth.

**fissure.** Deep furrow, groove, or cleft in tissue structures.

**pulp.** Living connective tissue within the tooth's root canal space that supplies blood vessels and nerves to the tooth.

# D2980

**D2980** crown repair necessitated by restorative material failure

### Explanation

Work required to repair a damaged crown may vary considerably. A detailed report of the specific procedures and services performed is required for this by report procedure.

### Coding Tips

Report this code when the repair is performed because of restorative material failure. Local anesthesia is generally considered to be part of restorative procedures. Providers should submit a detailed description of services and procedures when reporting this code. Third-party payers may require clinical documentation and/or x-rays before making payment determination. Check with payers to determine their specific requirements. This code includes removal of the crown, if necessary.

### Documentation Tips

A tooth chart may also be used to identify structure and rationale of disease process and the type of service performed on intraoral structures other than teeth. Providers should submit a detailed description of services and procedures when reporting this code. Third-party payers may require clinical documentation and/or x-rays before making payment determination. Check with payers to determine their specific requirements.

### ICD-10-CM Diagnostic Codes

| | |
|---|---|
| K08.530 | Fractured dental restorative material without loss of material |
| K08.531 | Fractured dental restorative material with loss of material |
| K08.539 | Fractured dental restorative material, unspecified |
| K08.54 | Contour of existing restoration of tooth biologically incompatible with oral health |
| K08.55 | Allergy to existing dental restorative material |
| K08.56 | Poor aesthetic of existing restoration of tooth |
| K08.59 | Other unsatisfactory restoration of tooth |

### Relative Value Units/Medicare Edits

| Non-Facility RVU | Work | PE | MP | Total |
|---|---|---|---|---|
| D2980 | 0.99 | 0.87 | 0.20 | 2.06 |
| **Facility RVU** | **Work** | **PE** | **MP** | **Total** |
| D2980 | 0.99 | 0.87 | 0.20 | 2.06 |

| | FUD | Status | MUE | Modifiers | | | | IOM Reference |
|---|---|---|---|---|---|---|---|---|
| D2980 | N/A | N | - | N/A | N/A | N/A | N/A | None |

* with documentation

### Terms To Know

**artificial crown.** In dentistry, a ceramic or metal restoration made to cover or replace a major part of the top of a tooth.

**tooth bounded space.** Empty space in the mouth due to a missing tooth that is surrounded by a tooth on each side.

# D2981-D2983

**D2981** inlay repair necessitated by restorative material failure
**D2982** onlay repair necessitated by restorative material failure
**D2983** veneer repair necessitated by restorative material failure

## Explanation

The provider repairs a previous restoration due to marginal defects. The repair of limited defects allows the previous restoration to be left undisturbed for several years or more. In D2981 the provider creates a fixed restoration outside of the mouth, which is then luted onto the tooth with the failed restorative material. In D2982 the repair restores one or more cusps and adjoining occlusal surfaces and is then retained by adhesive means. In D2983 a thin covering is placed over the damaged restorative material.

## Coding Tips

When the failed restoration is replaced, see the appropriate code for the type of procedure performed.

## Reimbursement Tips

The tooth/root number should be indicated on the claim.

## ICD-10-CM Diagnostic Codes

| | |
|---|---|
| K08.530 | Fractured dental restorative material without loss of material |
| K08.531 | Fractured dental restorative material with loss of material |
| K08.539 | Fractured dental restorative material, unspecified |
| K08.54 | Contour of existing restoration of tooth biologically incompatible with oral health |
| K08.55 | Allergy to existing dental restorative material |
| K08.56 | Poor aesthetic of existing restoration of tooth |
| K08.59 | Other unsatisfactory restoration of tooth |

## Relative Value Units/Medicare Edits

| Non-Facility RVU | Work | PE | MP | Total |
|---|---|---|---|---|
| D2981 | 0.00 | 0.00 | 0.00 | 0.00 |
| D2982 | 0.00 | 0.00 | 0.00 | 0.00 |
| D2983 | 0.00 | 0.00 | 0.00 | 0.00 |
| **Facility RVU** | **Work** | **PE** | **MP** | **Total** |
| D2981 | 0.00 | 0.00 | 0.00 | 0.00 |
| D2982 | 0.00 | 0.00 | 0.00 | 0.00 |
| D2983 | 0.00 | 0.00 | 0.00 | 0.00 |

| | FUD | Status | MUE | Modifiers | | | | IOM Reference |
|---|---|---|---|---|---|---|---|---|
| D2981 | N/A | N | - | N/A | N/A | N/A | N/A | None |
| D2982 | N/A | N | - | N/A | N/A | N/A | N/A | |
| D2983 | N/A | N | - | N/A | N/A | N/A | N/A | |

* with documentation

## Terms To Know

**inlay.** Restoration made outside of the mouth to fit a prepared cavity and placed on the tooth.

**onlay.** In dentistry, restoration made outside of the mouth that is cemented over a cusp or cusps of the tooth.

# D2990

**D2990** resin infiltration of incipient smooth surface lesions

*Placement of an infiltrating resin restoration for strengthening, stabilizing and/or limiting the progression of the lesion.*

## Explanation

The provider applies a resin infiltrant to a caries lesion to stop lesion progression. Low viscosity resins are drawn deep into the pore system of the lesion replacing lost tooth structure and stopping caries progression by blocking nutrients from entering into the pore system while stabilizing the anatomical shape and color of the tooth. A rubber dam is placed to protect the gingiva. The tooth surface is etched with a hydrochloric acid solution. The resin infiltrant is applied. Excessive materials are removed and the area is light cured. Application of the infiltrant may be repeated to ensure coverage.

## Coding Tips

This is an out of sequence code and will not display in numeric order in the CDT manual. When done at the same time a topical application of fluoride varnish, code D1206 may also be reported.

## Reimbursement Tips

Coverage of this procedure varies by payer. Check with payers for their specific coverage guidelines.

## ICD-10-CM Diagnostic Codes

| | |
|---|---|
| K02.3 | Arrested dental caries |
| K02.51 | Dental caries on pit and fissure surface limited to enamel |
| K02.52 | Dental caries on pit and fissure surface penetrating into dentin |
| K02.53 | Dental caries on pit and fissure surface penetrating into pulp |
| K02.61 | Dental caries on smooth surface limited to enamel |
| K02.62 | Dental caries on smooth surface penetrating into dentin |
| K02.63 | Dental caries on smooth surface penetrating into pulp |
| K02.7 | Dental root caries |
| K08.530 | Fractured dental restorative material without loss of material |
| K08.531 | Fractured dental restorative material with loss of material |
| K08.54 | Contour of existing restoration of tooth biologically incompatible with oral health |
| K08.55 | Allergy to existing dental restorative material |
| K08.56 | Poor aesthetic of existing restoration of tooth |

## Relative Value Units/Medicare Edits

| Non-Facility RVU | Work | PE | MP | Total |
|---|---|---|---|---|
| D2990 | 0.24 | 0.21 | 0.05 | 0.50 |
| **Facility RVU** | **Work** | **PE** | **MP** | **Total** |
| D2990 | 0.24 | 0.21 | 0.05 | 0.50 |

| | FUD | Status | MUE | Modifiers | | | | IOM Reference |
|---|---|---|---|---|---|---|---|---|
| D2990 | N/A | N | - | N/A | N/A | N/A | N/A | None |

* with documentation

## Terms To Know

**lesion.** Area of damaged tissue that has lost continuity or function, due to disease or trauma.

# D3110

**D3110** pulp cap - direct (excluding final restoration)

*Procedure in which the exposed pulp is covered with a dressing or cement that protects the pulp and promotes healing and repair.*

## Explanation

When direct exposure to the pulp occurs with a small, traumatic exposure that has not become contaminated, a direct pulp cap is performed. Local anesthesia is given and calcium hydroxide is applied. Calcium hydroxide in contact with pulp will form an area of necrosis, which then remineralizes with calcium ions. Calcium hydroxide is also bacteriostatic. Restoration may be done at this point, but is not included in this code. Root canal therapy may be required later when continued vitality of the pulp is questionable. Direct pulp capping may also be done when pulp extirpation needs to be delayed.

## Coding Tips

Local anesthesia is included in this service. Any evaluation, radiograph, or restoration service is reported separately. This code should not be used to report bases at the time of a restorative procedure.

## Reimbursement Tips

The third-party payer may require an x-ray or x-ray report before processing the claim.

## ICD-10-CM Diagnostic Codes

| | |
|---|---|
| K02.53 | Dental caries on pit and fissure surface penetrating into pulp |
| K02.63 | Dental caries on smooth surface penetrating into pulp |
| K04.01 | Reversible pulpitis |
| K04.02 | Irreversible pulpitis |
| K04.1 | Necrosis of pulp |
| K04.2 | Pulp degeneration |
| K04.3 | Abnormal hard tissue formation in pulp |
| K04.4 | Acute apical periodontitis of pulpal origin |
| K04.5 | Chronic apical periodontitis |

## Relative Value Units/Medicare Edits

| Non-Facility RVU | Work | PE | MP | Total |
|---|---|---|---|---|
| D3110 | 0.44 | 0.39 | 0.09 | 0.92 |
| **Facility RVU** | **Work** | **PE** | **MP** | **Total** |
| D3110 | 0.44 | 0.39 | 0.09 | 0.92 |

| | FUD | Status | MUE | Modifiers | | | | IOM Reference |
|---|---|---|---|---|---|---|---|---|
| D3110 | N/A | N | - | N/A | N/A | N/A | N/A | None |

* with documentation

## Terms To Know

**dental cement.** Any substance used in the mouth that sets from a viscous to a hard form and functions as a restorative material, a bonding force for fabricated restorations and orthodontics, or protective filling for insulation.

**indirect pulp cap.** In dentistry, insertion of a protective dressing to cover nearly exposed pulp.

**necrosis.** Death of cells or tissue within a living organ or structure.

# D3120

**D3120** pulp cap - indirect (excluding final restoration)

*Procedure in which the nearly exposed pulp is covered with a protective dressing to protect the pulp from additional injury and to promote healing and repair via formation of secondary dentin. This code is not to be used for bases and liners when all caries has been removed.*

## Explanation

When cavity preparation in a vital tooth would risk pulp exposure with the removal of all caries, an indirect pulp cap is done. This leaves a small amount of softened dentine at the base of the cavity and arrests bacterial spread while maintaining the viability of the pulp. Local anesthesia is given and a rubber dam is applied to contain bacterial spread. The cavity outline is prepared and caries removed. Softened dentine is carefully removed, but not to the point where exposure is likely to occur. Non-setting calcium hydroxide is applied to the floor and covered with glass ionomer cement. The margins are adjusted and restoration may be done at this point, but is not included in this code.

## Coding Tips

Local anesthesia is included in this service. Any evaluation, radiograph, or restoration service is reported separately. This code should not be used to report bases at the time of restorative procedures.

## Reimbursement Tips

Coverage of this procedure may vary by payer and patient contract. Check with the payer for specific coverage guidelines.

## ICD-10-CM Diagnostic Codes

| | |
|---|---|
| K02.53 | Dental caries on pit and fissure surface penetrating into pulp |
| K02.63 | Dental caries on smooth surface penetrating into pulp |
| K04.01 | Reversible pulpitis |
| K04.02 | Irreversible pulpitis |
| K04.1 | Necrosis of pulp |
| K04.2 | Pulp degeneration |
| K04.3 | Abnormal hard tissue formation in pulp |
| K04.4 | Acute apical periodontitis of pulpal origin |
| K04.5 | Chronic apical periodontitis |
| K04.99 | Other diseases of pulp and periapical tissues |

## Relative Value Units/Medicare Edits

| Non-Facility RVU | Work | PE | MP | Total |
|---|---|---|---|---|
| D3120 | 0.35 | 0.31 | 0.07 | 0.73 |
| **Facility RVU** | **Work** | **PE** | **MP** | **Total** |
| D3120 | 0.35 | 0.31 | 0.07 | 0.73 |

| | FUD | Status | MUE | Modifiers | | | | IOM Reference |
|---|---|---|---|---|---|---|---|---|
| D3120 | N/A | N | - | N/A | N/A | N/A | N/A | None |

* with documentation

## Terms To Know

**indirect pulp cap.** In dentistry, insertion of a protective dressing to cover nearly exposed pulp.

**pulp.** Living connective tissue within the tooth's root canal space that supplies blood vessels and nerves to the tooth.

# D3220

**D3220** therapeutic pulpotomy (excluding final restoration) - removal of pulp coronal to the dentinocemental junction and application of medicament

*Pulpotomy is the surgical removal of a portion of the pulp with the aim of maintaining the vitality of the remaining portion by means of an adequate dressing.*

## Explanation

Therapeutic pulpotomy is done to eliminate damaged, contaminated pulp tissue when trying to retain pulp vitality is not prudent, such as in a child's molar where pulpal involvement is very likely and difficult to determine or when the apices of the teeth are not fully mature. In pulpotomy, the dentist removes the coronal part of the pulp near the dentinocemental junction and leaves the radicular pulp tissue, treated with medicaments such as formalin/creosol preparations or devitalizing paste. The remaining viable apical pulp allows the root formation to continue maturing.

## Coding Tips

Do not use this code to report the first stage of root canal therapy, see codes D3310–D3330. Do not use this code to report apexogenesis. To report apexogenesis (partial pulpotomy), see D3222. Local anesthesia is included in this service. Any evaluation, radiograph, or restoration service is reported separately. For pulpal debridement, see D3221.

## Reimbursement Tips

Payers may bundle this procedure into more complex endodontic procedures. Check with third-party payers for their specific guidelines.

## ICD-10-CM Diagnostic Codes

| | |
|---|---|
| K04.01 | Reversible pulpitis |
| K04.02 | Irreversible pulpitis |
| K04.1 | Necrosis of pulp |
| K04.2 | Pulp degeneration |
| K04.3 | Abnormal hard tissue formation in pulp |
| K04.4 | Acute apical periodontitis of pulpal origin |
| K04.5 | Chronic apical periodontitis |
| K04.6 | Periapical abscess with sinus |
| K04.7 | Periapical abscess without sinus |
| K04.99 | Other diseases of pulp and periapical tissues |

## Relative Value Units/Medicare Edits

| Non-Facility RVU | Work | PE | MP | Total |
|---|---|---|---|---|
| D3220 | 0.95 | 0.84 | 0.20 | 1.99 |
| **Facility RVU** | **Work** | **PE** | **MP** | **Total** |
| D3220 | 0.95 | 0.84 | 0.20 | 1.99 |

| | FUD | Status | MUE | Modifiers | | | | IOM Reference |
|---|---|---|---|---|---|---|---|---|
| D3220 | N/A | N | - | N/A | N/A | N/A | N/A | None |

* with documentation

## Terms To Know

**pulpotomy.** In dentistry, partial excision or amputation of pulp from a root canal, with some vital tissue remaining in the rest of the pulp.

# D3221

**D3221** pulpal debridement, primary and permanent teeth

*Pulpal debridement for the relief of acute pain prior to conventional root canal therapy. This procedure is not to be used when endodontic treatment is completed on the same day.*

## Explanation

Pulpal debridement is performed on primary or permanent teeth. The pulp is the soft tissue inside the root canal. If it becomes inflamed or infected, debridement may be required. Inflammation or infection can occur from a variety of causes including deep decay, repeated dental procedures on the tooth, a crack or chip in the tooth, or an injury to the tooth with or without visible damage to the exterior tooth. If pulp inflammation or infection is left untreated, it can cause pain or lead to an abscess. Pulpal debridement involves removing the inflamed or infected pulpal tissue and cleaning the inside of the root canal. Following debridement, the canal is filled and sealed. The patient returns later for restorative care such as placement of a filling, crown, or bridgework.

## Coding Tips

Do not use this code to report the first stage of root canal therapy, see codes D3310–D3330. Local anesthesia is generally considered to be part of endodontic procedures. Report this code when pulpal debridement is performed to relieve acute pain prior to conventional root canal therapy. Do not report this code when endodontic treatment is completed on the same day.

## Documentation Tips

The following information can be documented on a tooth chart: treatment/location of caries, endodontic procedures, prosthetic services, preventive services, treatment of lesions and dental disease, or other special procedures. A tooth chart may also be used to identify structure and rationale of disease process and the type of service performed on intraoral structures other than teeth.

## ICD-10-CM Diagnostic Codes

| | |
|---|---|
| K04.01 | Reversible pulpitis |
| K04.02 | Irreversible pulpitis |
| K04.2 | Pulp degeneration |
| K04.3 | Abnormal hard tissue formation in pulp |
| K04.4 | Acute apical periodontitis of pulpal origin |
| K04.5 | Chronic apical periodontitis |
| K04.6 | Periapical abscess with sinus |
| K04.7 | Periapical abscess without sinus |
| K04.99 | Other diseases of pulp and periapical tissues |

## Relative Value Units/Medicare Edits

| Non-Facility RVU | Work | PE | MP | Total |
|---|---|---|---|---|
| D3221 | 1.12 | 0.98 | 0.23 | 2.33 |
| **Facility RVU** | **Work** | **PE** | **MP** | **Total** |
| D3221 | 1.12 | 0.98 | 0.23 | 2.33 |

| | FUD | Status | MUE | Modifiers | | | | IOM Reference |
|---|---|---|---|---|---|---|---|---|
| D3221 | N/A | N | - | N/A | N/A | N/A | N/A | None |

* with documentation

Dental - Endodontics

# D3222

**D3222** partial pulpotomy for apexogenesis - permanent tooth with incomplete root development

*Removal of a portion of the pulp and application of a medicament with the aim of maintaining the vitality of the remaining portion to encourage continued physiological development and formation of the root. This procedure is not to be construed as the first stage of root canal therapy.*

## Explanation

Apexogenesis is performed to promote development and formation of the root end. The dental provider removes of a portion of the pulp and then applies medicament for the purpose of maintaining the vitality of the remaining portion of the pulp and encourage growth.

## Coding Tips

This code should be used to report apexogenesis. For therapeutic pulpotomy, see code D3220. Pulpal debridement is reported using code D3221. Do not use this code to report the first stage of root canal therapy, see codes D3310–D3330. For pulpal therapy performed on molars, see D3240.

## Reimbursement Tips

Third-party payers may require clinical documentation and/or x-rays before making payment determination. Check with payers to determine their specific requirements.

## ICD-10-CM Diagnostic Codes

K04.01 Reversible pulpitis
K04.02 Irreversible pulpitis
K04.1 Necrosis of pulp
K04.2 Pulp degeneration
K04.3 Abnormal hard tissue formation in pulp
K04.4 Acute apical periodontitis of pulpal origin
K04.5 Chronic apical periodontitis
K04.6 Periapical abscess with sinus
K04.7 Periapical abscess without sinus
K04.99 Other diseases of pulp and periapical tissues

## Relative Value Units/Medicare Edits

| Non-Facility RVU | Work | PE | MP | Total |
|---|---|---|---|---|
| D3222 | 0.98 | 0.87 | 0.20 | 2.05 |
| **Facility RVU** | **Work** | **PE** | **MP** | **Total** |
| D3222 | 0.98 | 0.87 | 0.20 | 2.05 |

| | FUD | Status | MUE | Modifiers | | | | IOM Reference |
|---|---|---|---|---|---|---|---|---|
| D3222 | N/A | N | - | N/A | N/A | N/A | N/A | None |

* with documentation

## Terms To Know

**apexogenesis.** Procedure performed to remove a portion of the pulp of a tooth; medication is then applied to encourage root growth and vitality.

**root.** Part of the tooth located in the socket, covered by cementum, and attached by the periodontal structures.

# D3230

**D3230** pulpal therapy (resorbable filling) - anterior, primary tooth (excluding final restoration)

*Primary incisors and cuspids.*

## Explanation

Pulpal therapy is performed on the anterior primary teeth, which include the primary incisors and cuspids. The procedure includes only the resorbable filling placement. Final restoration services are reported separately.

## Coding Tips

Local anesthesia is generally considered to be part of endodontic procedures. Pulpectomy is considered an integral part of the procedure and should not be reported separately. Report final restoration services separately. When performed on a posterior tooth, see D3240.

## Reimbursement Tips

Coverage of this procedure may vary by payer and patient contract. Check with the payer for specific coverage guidelines.

## ICD-10-CM Diagnostic Codes

K04.01 Reversible pulpitis
K04.02 Irreversible pulpitis
K04.1 Necrosis of pulp
K04.2 Pulp degeneration
K04.3 Abnormal hard tissue formation in pulp
K04.4 Acute apical periodontitis of pulpal origin
K04.5 Chronic apical periodontitis
K04.6 Periapical abscess with sinus
K04.7 Periapical abscess without sinus
K04.99 Other diseases of pulp and periapical tissues

## Relative Value Units/Medicare Edits

| Non-Facility RVU | Work | PE | MP | Total |
|---|---|---|---|---|
| D3230 | 1.02 | 0.90 | 0.21 | 2.13 |
| **Facility RVU** | **Work** | **PE** | **MP** | **Total** |
| D3230 | 1.02 | 0.90 | 0.21 | 2.13 |

| | FUD | Status | MUE | Modifiers | | | | IOM Reference |
|---|---|---|---|---|---|---|---|---|
| D3230 | N/A | N | - | N/A | N/A | N/A | N/A | None |

* with documentation

## Terms To Know

**anterior teeth.** Six upper and six lower front teeth; the upper and lower incisors and cuspids.

**primary tooth.** Any of 20 deciduous teeth that usually erupt between the ages of 6 and 24 months.

**pulp.** Living connective tissue within the tooth's root canal space that supplies blood vessels and nerves to the tooth.

**retrograde filling.** Filling of a root canal by sealing it from the root apex.

# D3240

**D3240** pulpal therapy (resorbable filling) - posterior, primary tooth (excluding final restoration)

*Primary first and second molars.*

## Explanation

Pulpal therapy is performed on the posterior primary teeth, which include the primary first and second molars. The procedure includes only the resorbable filling placement. Final restoration services are reported separately.

## Coding Tips

Local anesthesia is generally considered to be part of endodontic procedures. Report final restoration services separately. When performed on an anterior tooth (incisor or cuspid), report D3230.

## Reimbursement Tips

Pulpectomy is considered an integral part of the procedure and should not be reported separately.

## ICD-10-CM Diagnostic Codes

K04.01 Reversible pulpitis
K04.02 Irreversible pulpitis
K04.1 Necrosis of pulp
K04.2 Pulp degeneration
K04.3 Abnormal hard tissue formation in pulp
K04.4 Acute apical periodontitis of pulpal origin
K04.5 Chronic apical periodontitis
K04.6 Periapical abscess with sinus
K04.7 Periapical abscess without sinus
K04.99 Other diseases of pulp and periapical tissues

## Relative Value Units/Medicare Edits

| Non-Facility RVU | Work | PE | MP | Total |
|---|---|---|---|---|
| D3240 | 1.22 | 1.07 | 0.25 | 2.54 |
| **Facility RVU** | **Work** | **PE** | **MP** | **Total** |
| D3240 | 1.22 | 1.07 | 0.25 | 2.54 |

| | FUD | Status | MUE | Modifiers | | | | IOM Reference |
|---|---|---|---|---|---|---|---|---|
| D3240 | N/A | N | - | N/A | N/A | N/A | N/A | None |

* with documentation

## Terms To Know

**molars.** Posterior teeth used for grinding.

**necrosis.** Death of cells or tissue within a living organ or structure.

**posterior teeth.** Teeth that are located toward the back of the mouth, distal to the canines; includes maxillary and mandibular premolars and molars.

**primary tooth.** Any of 20 deciduous teeth that usually erupt between the ages of 6 and 24 months.

**pulp.** Living connective tissue within the tooth's root canal space that supplies blood vessels and nerves to the tooth.

# D3310

**D3310** endodontic therapy, anterior tooth (excluding final restoration)

## Explanation

Root canal therapy is performed on the primary or permanent anterior teeth, which include the upper and lower incisors and cuspids. Underneath each tooth is a soft tissue area, called the pulp, that contains nerves, veins, arteries, and lymph vessels. The pulp with its network of nerves, veins, arteries, and lymph vessels extends from the top of the tooth down to its root by way of a root canal. Each tooth has at least one root and one root canal, but some teeth have as many as four or five root and root canals. Root canal therapy is performed when the pulp becomes inflamed or infected due to deep decay, repeated dental procedures on the tooth, a crack or chip in the tooth, or an injury to the tooth with or without visible damage to the exterior tooth. After discussing treatment options with the patient, a plan for the root canal therapy is developed. The tooth is anesthetized. An opening is made in the tooth and the diseased pulp is removed. The root canal is thoroughly cleaned and enlarged. Temporary antibacterial filler is placed into the canal to prevent bacteria from reentering the canal. Once the infection has healed, the canal is permanently sealed and separately reportable restoration work such as a filling, crown, or bridgework is performed. Root canal therapy may be performed during a single visit or multiple visits. This code should be reported only once regardless of the number of visits required.

## Coding Tips

Local anesthesia is generally considered to be part of endodontic procedures. This code reports complete root canal therapy, including pulpectomy, intraoperative radiographs, and all appointments necessary to complete treatment. This code does not include final restoration. When performed on a bicuspid tooth, see D3320. When performed on a molar, see D3330. To report pulpotomy, see D3220–D3222.

## ICD-10-CM Diagnostic Codes

K02.53 Dental caries on pit and fissure surface penetrating into pulp
K02.61 Dental caries on smooth surface limited to enamel
K02.62 Dental caries on smooth surface penetrating into dentin
K02.63 Dental caries on smooth surface penetrating into pulp
K02.7 Dental root caries
K03.0 Excessive attrition of teeth
K03.1 Abrasion of teeth
K03.2 Erosion of teeth
K03.81 Cracked tooth
K03.89 Other specified diseases of hard tissues of teeth
K04.01 Reversible pulpitis
K04.02 Irreversible pulpitis
K04.1 Necrosis of pulp
K04.2 Pulp degeneration
K04.3 Abnormal hard tissue formation in pulp
K04.4 Acute apical periodontitis of pulpal origin
K04.5 Chronic apical periodontitis
K04.6 Periapical abscess with sinus
K04.7 Periapical abscess without sinus
K04.8 Radicular cyst
K04.99 Other diseases of pulp and periapical tissues
K05.00 Acute gingivitis, plaque induced
K05.01 Acute gingivitis, non-plaque induced
K05.10 Chronic gingivitis, plaque induced
K05.11 Chronic gingivitis, non-plaque induced

| | |
|---|---|
| K05.20 | Aggressive periodontitis, unspecified |
| K05.211 | Aggressive periodontitis, localized, slight |
| K05.212 | Aggressive periodontitis, localized, moderate |
| K05.213 | Aggressive periodontitis, localized, severe |
| K05.222 | Aggressive periodontitis, generalized, moderate |
| K05.223 | Aggressive periodontitis, generalized, severe |
| K05.311 | Chronic periodontitis, localized, slight |
| K05.312 | Chronic periodontitis, localized, moderate |
| K05.313 | Chronic periodontitis, localized, severe |
| K05.321 | Chronic periodontitis, generalized, slight |
| K05.322 | Chronic periodontitis, generalized, moderate |
| K05.323 | Chronic periodontitis, generalized, severe |
| K05.4 | Periodontosis |
| K05.5 | Other periodontal diseases |
| K05.6 | Periodontal disease, unspecified |
| K06.011 | Localized gingival recession, minimal |
| K06.012 | Localized gingival recession, moderate |
| K06.013 | Localized gingival recession, severe |
| K06.021 | Generalized gingival recession, minimal |
| K06.022 | Generalized gingival recession, moderate |
| K06.023 | Generalized gingival recession, severe |
| K06.1 | Gingival enlargement |
| K06.2 | Gingival and edentulous alveolar ridge lesions associated with trauma |
| K06.8 | Other specified disorders of gingiva and edentulous alveolar ridge |
| K08.0 | Exfoliation of teeth due to systemic causes |
| K08.51 | Open restoration margins of tooth |
| K08.52 | Unrepairable overhanging of dental restorative materials |
| K08.530 | Fractured dental restorative material without loss of material |
| K08.531 | Fractured dental restorative material with loss of material |
| K08.539 | Fractured dental restorative material, unspecified |
| K08.54 | Contour of existing restoration of tooth biologically incompatible with oral health |
| K08.55 | Allergy to existing dental restorative material |
| K08.56 | Poor aesthetic of existing restoration of tooth |
| K08.59 | Other unsatisfactory restoration of tooth |
| K08.81 | Primary occlusal trauma |
| K08.82 | Secondary occlusal trauma |

## Relative Value Units/Medicare Edits

| Non-Facility RVU | Work | PE | MP | Total |
|---|---|---|---|---|
| **D3310** | 3.72 | 3.28 | 0.77 | 7.77 |
| **Facility RVU** | **Work** | **PE** | **MP** | **Total** |
| **D3310** | 3.72 | 3.28 | 0.77 | 7.77 |

| | FUD | Status | MUE | Modifiers | | | | IOM Reference |
|---|---|---|---|---|---|---|---|---|
| **D3310** | N/A | N | - | N/A | N/A | N/A | N/A | None |

* with documentation

# D3320

**D3320** endodontic therapy, premolar tooth (excluding final restoration)

## Explanation

Root canal therapy is performed on the primary or permanent bicuspid teeth. Bicuspids are teeth with to cusps (points), also called the premolars. Underneath each tooth is a soft tissue area, called the pulp, that contains nerves, veins, arteries, and lymph vessels. The pulp with its network of nerves, veins, arteries, and lymph vessels extends from the top of the tooth down to its root by way of a root canal. Each tooth has at least one root and one root canal, but some teeth have as many as four or five root and root canals. Root canal therapy is performed when the pulp becomes inflamed or infected due to deep decay, repeated dental procedures on the tooth, a crack or chip in the tooth, or an injury to the tooth with or without visible damage to the exterior tooth. After discussing treatment options with the patient, a plan for the root canal therapy is developed. The tooth is anesthetized. An opening is made in the tooth and the diseased pulp is removed. The root canal is thoroughly cleaned and enlarged. Temporary antibacterial filler is placed into the canal to prevent bacteria from reentering the canal. Once the infection has healed, the canal is permanently sealed and separately reportable restoration work such as a filling, crown, or bridgework is performed. Root canal therapy may be performed during a single visit or multiple visits. This code should be reported only once regardless of the number of visits required.

## Coding Tips

Local anesthesia is generally considered to be part of endodontic procedures. This code reports complete root canal therapy, including pulpectomy, intraoperative radiographs, and all appointments necessary to complete treatment. This code does not include final restoration. When performed on an anterior tooth, see D3310. When performed on a molar, see D3330. To report pulpotomy, see D3220–D3222.

## ICD-10-CM Diagnostic Codes

| | |
|---|---|
| K02.53 | Dental caries on pit and fissure surface penetrating into pulp |
| K02.61 | Dental caries on smooth surface limited to enamel |
| K02.62 | Dental caries on smooth surface penetrating into dentin |
| K02.63 | Dental caries on smooth surface penetrating into pulp |
| K02.7 | Dental root caries |
| K03.0 | Excessive attrition of teeth |
| K03.1 | Abrasion of teeth |
| K03.2 | Erosion of teeth |
| K03.81 | Cracked tooth |
| K03.89 | Other specified diseases of hard tissues of teeth |
| K04.01 | Reversible pulpitis |
| K04.02 | Irreversible pulpitis |
| K04.1 | Necrosis of pulp |
| K04.2 | Pulp degeneration |
| K04.3 | Abnormal hard tissue formation in pulp |
| K04.4 | Acute apical periodontitis of pulpal origin |
| K04.5 | Chronic apical periodontitis |
| K04.6 | Periapical abscess with sinus |
| K04.7 | Periapical abscess without sinus |
| K04.8 | Radicular cyst |
| K04.99 | Other diseases of pulp and periapical tissues |
| K05.00 | Acute gingivitis, plaque induced |
| K05.01 | Acute gingivitis, non-plaque induced |
| K05.10 | Chronic gingivitis, plaque induced |
| K05.11 | Chronic gingivitis, non-plaque induced |

| | |
|---|---|
| K05.211 | Aggressive periodontitis, localized, slight |
| K05.212 | Aggressive periodontitis, localized, moderate |
| K05.213 | Aggressive periodontitis, localized, severe |
| K05.222 | Aggressive periodontitis, generalized, moderate |
| K05.223 | Aggressive periodontitis, generalized, severe |
| K05.311 | Chronic periodontitis, localized, slight |
| K05.312 | Chronic periodontitis, localized, moderate |
| K05.313 | Chronic periodontitis, localized, severe |
| K05.321 | Chronic periodontitis, generalized, slight |
| K05.322 | Chronic periodontitis, generalized, moderate |
| K05.323 | Chronic periodontitis, generalized, severe |
| K05.4 | Periodontosis |
| K05.5 | Other periodontal diseases |
| K06.011 | Localized gingival recession, minimal |
| K06.012 | Localized gingival recession, moderate |
| K06.013 | Localized gingival recession, severe |
| K06.021 | Generalized gingival recession, minimal |
| K06.022 | Generalized gingival recession, moderate |
| K06.023 | Generalized gingival recession, severe |
| K06.1 | Gingival enlargement |
| K06.2 | Gingival and edentulous alveolar ridge lesions associated with trauma |
| K06.8 | Other specified disorders of gingiva and edentulous alveolar ridge |
| K08.0 | Exfoliation of teeth due to systemic causes |
| K08.51 | Open restoration margins of tooth |
| K08.52 | Unrepairable overhanging of dental restorative materials |
| K08.530 | Fractured dental restorative material without loss of material |
| K08.531 | Fractured dental restorative material with loss of material |
| K08.54 | Contour of existing restoration of tooth biologically incompatible with oral health |
| K08.55 | Allergy to existing dental restorative material |
| K08.56 | Poor aesthetic of existing restoration of tooth |
| K08.59 | Other unsatisfactory restoration of tooth |
| K08.81 | Primary occlusal trauma |
| K08.82 | Secondary occlusal trauma |

### Relative Value Units/Medicare Edits

| Non-Facility RVU | Work | PE | MP | Total |
|---|---|---|---|---|
| D3320 | 4.46 | 3.93 | 0.92 | 9.31 |
| **Facility RVU** | **Work** | **PE** | **MP** | **Total** |
| D3320 | 4.46 | 3.93 | 0.92 | 9.31 |

| | FUD | Status | MUE | Modifiers | | | | IOM Reference |
|---|---|---|---|---|---|---|---|---|
| D3320 | N/A | N | - | N/A | N/A | N/A | N/A | None |

* with documentation

# D3330

**D3330** endodontic therapy, molar tooth (excluding final restoration)

## Explanation

Root canal therapy is performed on the primary or permanent molars, which include the posterior teeth. Underneath each tooth is a soft tissue area, called the pulp, that contains nerves, veins, arteries, and lymph vessels. The pulp with its network of nerves, veins, arteries, and lymph vessels extends from the top of the tooth down to its root by way of a root canal. Each tooth has at least one root and one root canal, but some teeth have as many as four or five roots and root canals. Root canal therapy is performed when the pulp becomes inflamed or infected due to deep decay, repeated dental procedures on the tooth, a crack or chip in the tooth, or an injury to the tooth with or without visible damage to the exterior tooth. After discussing treatment options with the patient, a plan for the root canal therapy is developed. The tooth is anesthetized. An opening is made in the tooth and the diseased pulp is removed. The root canal is thoroughly cleaned and enlarged. Temporary antibacterial filler is placed into the canal to prevent bacteria from reentering the canal. Once the infection has healed, the canal is permanently sealed and separately reportable restoration work such as a filling, crown, or bridgework is performed. Root canal therapy may be performed during a single visit or multiple visits. This code should be reported only once regardless of the number of visits required.

## Coding Tips

Local anesthesia is generally considered to be part of endodontic procedures. This code reports complete root canal therapy, including pulpectomy, intraoperative radiographs, and all appointments necessary to complete treatment. This code does not include final restoration. When performed on an anterior tooth, see D3310. When performed on a premolar (bicuspid) tooth, see D3320. To report pulpotomy, see D3220–D3222.

## ICD-10-CM Diagnostic Codes

| | |
|---|---|
| K02.53 | Dental caries on pit and fissure surface penetrating into pulp |
| K02.61 | Dental caries on smooth surface limited to enamel |
| K02.62 | Dental caries on smooth surface penetrating into dentin |
| K02.63 | Dental caries on smooth surface penetrating into pulp |
| K02.7 | Dental root caries |
| K03.0 | Excessive attrition of teeth |
| K03.1 | Abrasion of teeth |
| K03.2 | Erosion of teeth |
| K03.81 | Cracked tooth |
| K03.89 | Other specified diseases of hard tissues of teeth |
| K04.01 | Reversible pulpitis |
| K04.02 | Irreversible pulpitis |
| K04.1 | Necrosis of pulp |
| K04.2 | Pulp degeneration |
| K04.3 | Abnormal hard tissue formation in pulp |
| K04.4 | Acute apical periodontitis of pulpal origin |
| K04.5 | Chronic apical periodontitis |
| K04.6 | Periapical abscess with sinus |
| K04.7 | Periapical abscess without sinus |
| K04.8 | Radicular cyst |
| K04.99 | Other diseases of pulp and periapical tissues |
| K05.00 | Acute gingivitis, plaque induced |
| K05.01 | Acute gingivitis, non-plaque induced |
| K05.10 | Chronic gingivitis, plaque induced |
| K05.11 | Chronic gingivitis, non-plaque induced |

K05.211 Aggressive periodontitis, localized, slight
K05.212 Aggressive periodontitis, localized, moderate
K05.213 Aggressive periodontitis, localized, severe
K05.221 Aggressive periodontitis, generalized, slight
K05.222 Aggressive periodontitis, generalized, moderate
K05.223 Aggressive periodontitis, generalized, severe
K05.311 Chronic periodontitis, localized, slight
K05.312 Chronic periodontitis, localized, moderate
K05.313 Chronic periodontitis, localized, severe
K05.321 Chronic periodontitis, generalized, slight
K05.322 Chronic periodontitis, generalized, moderate
K05.323 Chronic periodontitis, generalized, severe
K05.4 Periodontosis
K05.5 Other periodontal diseases
K06.011 Localized gingival recession, minimal
K06.012 Localized gingival recession, moderate
K06.013 Localized gingival recession, severe
K06.021 Generalized gingival recession, minimal
K06.022 Generalized gingival recession, moderate
K06.023 Generalized gingival recession, severe
K06.1 Gingival enlargement
K06.2 Gingival and edentulous alveolar ridge lesions associated with trauma
K06.8 Other specified disorders of gingiva and edentulous alveolar ridge
K08.0 Exfoliation of teeth due to systemic causes
K08.51 Open restoration margins of tooth
K08.52 Unrepairable overhanging of dental restorative materials
K08.530 Fractured dental restorative material without loss of material
K08.531 Fractured dental restorative material with loss of material
K08.54 Contour of existing restoration of tooth biologically incompatible with oral health
K08.55 Allergy to existing dental restorative material
K08.56 Poor aesthetic of existing restoration of tooth
K08.59 Other unsatisfactory restoration of tooth
K08.81 Primary occlusal trauma
K08.82 Secondary occlusal trauma

## Relative Value Units/Medicare Edits

| Non-Facility RVU | Work | PE | MP | Total |
|---|---|---|---|---|
| D3330 | 5.50 | 4.86 | 1.13 | 11.49 |
| **Facility RVU** | **Work** | **PE** | **MP** | **Total** |
| D3330 | 5.50 | 4.86 | 1.13 | 11.49 |

| | FUD | Status | MUE | Modifiers | | | | IOM Reference |
|---|---|---|---|---|---|---|---|---|
| D3330 | N/A | N | - | N/A | N/A | N/A | N/A | None |

* with documentation

## Terms To Know

**endodontics.** Subspecialty of dentistry that deals primarily with the pulp of the tooth or the dentine complex.

**molars.** Posterior teeth used for grinding.

# D3331

**D3331** treatment of root canal obstruction; non-surgical access

*In lieu of surgery, the formation of a pathway to achieve an apical seal without surgical intervention because of a non-negotiable root canal blocked by foreign bodies, including but not limited to separated instruments, broken posts or calcification of 50% or more of the length of the tooth root.*

## Explanation

Non-surgical root canal therapy for treatment of a root canal obstruction is performed. Occasionally during endodontic therapy, a complication occurs. One such complication is obstruction of the root canal by a broken instrument, dental materials, or dentin shavings. The ability to non-surgically access the obstruction is dependent on diameter, length, and position of the obstruction, as well as the anatomy (diameter, length, curvature) of the root canal. Once the anatomy has been surveyed using preoperative and working dental x-rays and the site of the obstruction determined, a variety of instruments may be required to access the obstruction. Coronal access is first required. Using a high speed, surgical length bur, access is established to all canal orifices. Radicular access is the next step and may be accomplished by the use of hand files followed by GG drills. Radicular access involves enlarging and shaping the canal. When the canal has been optimally shaped, it is flushed and dried. At this point the obstruction should be visible. Ultrasonic or microsonic techniques are then employed to remove the obstruction.

## Coding Tips

Local anesthesia is generally considered to be part of endodontic procedures. According to the ADA, codes D3330 and D3331 may be reported on the same date of service.

## Documentation Tips

Documentation should include the medical necessity of both procedures when D3330 and D3331 are reported together.

## Reimbursement Tips

Third-party payers may require clinical documentation and/or x-rays before making payment determination.

## ICD-10-CM Diagnostic Codes

K02.53 Dental caries on pit and fissure surface penetrating into pulp
K02.61 Dental caries on smooth surface limited to enamel
K02.62 Dental caries on smooth surface penetrating into dentin
K02.63 Dental caries on smooth surface penetrating into pulp
K02.7 Dental root caries
K03.0 Excessive attrition of teeth
K03.1 Abrasion of teeth
K03.2 Erosion of teeth
K03.81 Cracked tooth
K03.89 Other specified diseases of hard tissues of teeth
K04.01 Reversible pulpitis
K04.02 Irreversible pulpitis
K04.1 Necrosis of pulp
K04.2 Pulp degeneration
K04.3 Abnormal hard tissue formation in pulp
K04.4 Acute apical periodontitis of pulpal origin
K04.5 Chronic apical periodontitis
K04.6 Periapical abscess with sinus
K04.7 Periapical abscess without sinus
K04.8 Radicular cyst

| | |
|---|---|
| K04.99 | Other diseases of pulp and periapical tissues |
| K05.00 | Acute gingivitis, plaque induced |
| K05.01 | Acute gingivitis, non-plaque induced |
| K05.10 | Chronic gingivitis, plaque induced |
| K05.11 | Chronic gingivitis, non-plaque induced |
| K05.211 | Aggressive periodontitis, localized, slight |
| K05.212 | Aggressive periodontitis, localized, moderate |
| K05.213 | Aggressive periodontitis, localized, severe |
| K05.221 | Aggressive periodontitis, generalized, slight |
| K05.222 | Aggressive periodontitis, generalized, moderate |
| K05.223 | Aggressive periodontitis, generalized, severe |
| K05.311 | Chronic periodontitis, localized, slight |
| K05.312 | Chronic periodontitis, localized, moderate |
| K05.313 | Chronic periodontitis, localized, severe |
| K05.321 | Chronic periodontitis, generalized, slight |
| K05.322 | Chronic periodontitis, generalized, moderate |
| K05.323 | Chronic periodontitis, generalized, severe |
| K05.4 | Periodontosis |
| K05.5 | Other periodontal diseases |
| K06.011 | Localized gingival recession, minimal |
| K06.012 | Localized gingival recession, moderate |
| K06.013 | Localized gingival recession, severe |
| K06.021 | Generalized gingival recession, minimal |
| K06.022 | Generalized gingival recession, moderate |
| K06.023 | Generalized gingival recession, severe |
| K06.1 | Gingival enlargement |
| K06.2 | Gingival and edentulous alveolar ridge lesions associated with trauma |
| K06.8 | Other specified disorders of gingiva and edentulous alveolar ridge |
| K08.0 | Exfoliation of teeth due to systemic causes |
| K08.51 | Open restoration margins of tooth |
| K08.52 | Unrepairable overhanging of dental restorative materials |
| K08.530 | Fractured dental restorative material without loss of material |
| K08.531 | Fractured dental restorative material with loss of material |
| K08.54 | Contour of existing restoration of tooth biologically incompatible with oral health |
| K08.55 | Allergy to existing dental restorative material |
| K08.56 | Poor aesthetic of existing restoration of tooth |
| K08.59 | Other unsatisfactory restoration of tooth |
| K08.81 | Primary occlusal trauma |
| K08.82 | Secondary occlusal trauma |

## Relative Value Units/Medicare Edits

| Non-Facility RVU | Work | PE | MP | Total |
|---|---|---|---|---|
| D3331 | 2.07 | 1.83 | 0.43 | 4.33 |
| **Facility RVU** | **Work** | **PE** | **MP** | **Total** |
| D3331 | 2.07 | 1.83 | 0.43 | 4.33 |

| | FUD | Status | MUE | Modifiers | | | | IOM Reference |
|---|---|---|---|---|---|---|---|---|
| D3331 | N/A | N | - | N/A | N/A | N/A | N/A | None |

* with documentation

# D3332

**D3332** incomplete endodontic therapy; inoperable, unrestorable or fractured tooth

*Considerable time is necessary to determine diagnosis and/or provide initial treatment before the fracture makes the tooth unretainable.*

## Explanation

Endodontic therapy is started but not completed due to an inoperable or unrestorable condition of the tooth. Endodontic therapy is initiated with a treatment plan. Local anesthesia is provided. Clinical procedures such as a pulp test, pulpotomy, pulpectomy, or extirpation of the pulp are initiated. However, after beginning the endodontic therapy it is discovered that an inoperable and unrestorable condition exists, such as calcification or fracture of the root.

## Coding Tips

Local anesthesia is generally considered to be part of endodontic procedures. Report separately any tooth extractions (D7140) or root amputations (D3450). This code is rarely reported when endodontic treatment (D3310, D3320 or D3330) has previously been submitted.

## Reimbursement Tips

Third-party payers may require clinical documentation and/or x-rays before making payment determination. Check with payers to determine their specific requirements.

## ICD-10-CM Diagnostic Codes

| | |
|---|---|
| K04.1 | Necrosis of pulp |
| K04.2 | Pulp degeneration |
| K04.3 | Abnormal hard tissue formation in pulp |
| K04.4 | Acute apical periodontitis of pulpal origin |
| K04.5 | Chronic apical periodontitis |
| K04.6 | Periapical abscess with sinus |
| K04.7 | Periapical abscess without sinus |
| K04.8 | Radicular cyst |
| K04.90 | Unspecified diseases of pulp and periapical tissues |
| K04.99 | Other diseases of pulp and periapical tissues |
| K05.00 | Acute gingivitis, plaque induced |
| K05.01 | Acute gingivitis, non-plaque induced |
| K05.10 | Chronic gingivitis, plaque induced |
| K05.11 | Chronic gingivitis, non-plaque induced |
| K05.20 | Aggressive periodontitis, unspecified |
| K05.211 | Aggressive periodontitis, localized, slight |
| K05.212 | Aggressive periodontitis, localized, moderate |
| K05.213 | Aggressive periodontitis, localized, severe |
| K05.221 | Aggressive periodontitis, generalized, slight |
| K05.222 | Aggressive periodontitis, generalized, moderate |
| K05.223 | Aggressive periodontitis, generalized, severe |
| K05.30 | Chronic periodontitis, unspecified |
| K05.311 | Chronic periodontitis, localized, slight |
| K05.312 | Chronic periodontitis, localized, moderate |
| K05.313 | Chronic periodontitis, localized, severe |
| K05.321 | Chronic periodontitis, generalized, slight |
| K05.322 | Chronic periodontitis, generalized, moderate |
| K05.323 | Chronic periodontitis, generalized, severe |
| K05.4 | Periodontosis |
| K05.5 | Other periodontal diseases |

| | |
|---|---|
| K05.6 | Periodontal disease, unspecified |
| K06.010 | Localized gingival recession, unspecified |
| K06.011 | Localized gingival recession, minimal |
| K06.012 | Localized gingival recession, moderate |
| K06.013 | Localized gingival recession, severe |
| K06.020 | Generalized gingival recession, unspecified |
| K06.021 | Generalized gingival recession, minimal |
| K06.022 | Generalized gingival recession, moderate |
| K06.023 | Generalized gingival recession, severe |
| K06.1 | Gingival enlargement |
| K06.2 | Gingival and edentulous alveolar ridge lesions associated with trauma |
| K06.8 | Other specified disorders of gingiva and edentulous alveolar ridge |
| K06.9 | Disorder of gingiva and edentulous alveolar ridge, unspecified |
| K08.0 | Exfoliation of teeth due to systemic causes |
| K08.81 | Primary occlusal trauma |
| K08.82 | Secondary occlusal trauma |
| S02.81XA | Fracture of other specified skull and facial bones, right side, initial encounter for closed fracture ☑ |
| S02.81XB | Fracture of other specified skull and facial bones, right side, initial encounter for open fracture ☑ |

## Relative Value Units/Medicare Edits

| Non-Facility RVU | Work | PE | MP | Total |
|---|---|---|---|---|
| D3332 | 2.55 | 2.25 | 0.53 | 5.33 |
| Facility RVU | Work | PE | MP | Total |
| D3332 | 2.55 | 2.25 | 0.53 | 5.33 |

| | FUD | Status | MUE | Modifiers | | | | IOM Reference |
|---|---|---|---|---|---|---|---|---|
| D3332 | N/A | N | - | N/A | N/A | N/A | N/A | None |

* with documentation

## Terms To Know

**endodontics.** Subspecialty of dentistry that deals primarily with the pulp of the tooth or the dentine complex.

# D3333

**D3333** internal root repair of perforation defects

*Non-surgical seal of perforation caused by resorption and/or decay but not iatrogenic by provider filing claim.*

## Explanation

The dentist performs internal root repair of perforation defects. Occasionally during endodontic therapy, a complication occurs. One such complication is perforation of the root canal during mechanical debridement. Treatment of the perforation may be performed surgically or non-surgically and is dependent on the size and location of the perforation. Repair involves sealing the perforation to prevent bacteria and other noxious elements from escaping and causing damage to the associated periodontal tissues. Surgical repair is as follows. The mouth is rinsed with chlorhexidine and local anesthesia administered. An incision is made exposing the perforation site and the surrounding tissue is debrided. Following acid etching and bonding of the root surface, a restorative seal is placed. After allowing the seal to cure, it is contoured. The operative site is rinsed with normal saline and the incision sutured closed.

## Coding Tips

Local anesthesia is generally considered to be part of endodontic procedures.

## Reimbursement Tips

Third-party payers may require clinical documentation and/or x-rays before making payment determination. Check with payers to determine their specific requirements

## ICD-10-CM Diagnostic Codes

| | |
|---|---|
| K08.3 | Retained dental root |
| M27.51 | Perforation of root canal space due to endodontic treatment |
| M27.59 | Other periradicular pathology associated with previous endodontic treatment |

## Relative Value Units/Medicare Edits

| Non-Facility RVU | Work | PE | MP | Total |
|---|---|---|---|---|
| D3333 | 1.33 | 1.17 | 0.27 | 2.77 |
| Facility RVU | Work | PE | MP | Total |
| D3333 | 1.33 | 1.17 | 0.27 | 2.77 |

| | FUD | Status | MUE | Modifiers | | | | IOM Reference |
|---|---|---|---|---|---|---|---|---|
| D3333 | N/A | N | - | N/A | N/A | N/A | N/A | None |

* with documentation

## Terms To Know

**endodontics.** Subspecialty of dentistry that deals primarily with the pulp of the tooth or the dentine complex.

**perforation.** Hole in an object, organ, or tissue, or the act of punching or boring holes through a part.

**periodontal.** Relating to the tissues that support and surround the teeth.

# D3346-D3348

**D3346** retreatment of previous root canal therapy - anterior
**D3347** retreatment of previous root canal therapy - premolar
**D3348** retreatment of previous root canal therapy - molar

## Explanation

Root canal retreatment is performed on the primary or permanent teeth. Underneath each tooth is a soft tissue area, called the pulp, that contains nerves, veins, arteries, and lymph vessels. The pulp extends from the top of the tooth down to its root by way of a root canal. Each tooth has at least one root and one root canal, but some teeth have as many as four or five root and root canals. Retreatment of previously performed root canal therapy is sometimes necessary due to reinfection. Reinfection can occur due to decay or failure to treat all affected areas during a previous root canal procedure. After discussing treatment options with the patient, a plan for the retreatment is developed. The tooth is anesthetized. An opening is made in the tooth and the previous root canal material is removed. This may require removing a crown, post, and core material. Sometimes it is possible to make a small hole in the restoration work and work through that opening without removing the restoration work. The canal or canals are then cleaned, enlarged, and shaped for placement of gutta percha in the distal portion of the root canal. It can be molded to fit the root canal and acts as a sealer. The central portion and top of the canal is covered with a sterile cotton pellet and a small temporary filling placed in the opening made in the tooth. Once the infection has healed, the canal is permanently sealed and separately reportable restoration work such as a filling, crown, or bridgework is performed. Root canal retreatment may be performed during a single visit or multiple visits. This code should be reported only once regardless of the number of visits required. Report D3346 for anterior teeth (upper and lower incisors or cuspids); D3347 for bicuspids; or D3348 for molars.

## Coding Tips

Many payers have specific time frames in which additional payment for this type of treatment will not be considered. When reporting code D3346, third-party payers may require clinical documentation and/or x-rays before making payment determination.

## ICD-10-CM Diagnostic Codes

K08.3 Retained dental root
M27.51 Perforation of root canal space due to endodontic treatment
M27.59 Other periradicular pathology associated with previous endodontic treatment

## Relative Value Units/Medicare Edits

| Non-Facility RVU | Work | PE | MP | Total |
|---|---|---|---|---|
| D3346 | 4.70 | 4.15 | 0.97 | 9.82 |
| D3347 | 5.57 | 4.92 | 1.15 | 11.64 |
| D3348 | 6.89 | 6.08 | 1.42 | 14.39 |
| **Facility RVU** | **Work** | **PE** | **MP** | **Total** |
| D3346 | 4.70 | 4.15 | 0.97 | 9.82 |
| D3347 | 5.57 | 4.92 | 1.15 | 11.64 |
| D3348 | 6.89 | 6.08 | 1.42 | 14.39 |

| | FUD | Status | MUE | Modifiers | | | | IOM Reference |
|---|---|---|---|---|---|---|---|---|
| D3346 | N/A | N | - | N/A | N/A | N/A | N/A | None |
| D3347 | N/A | N | - | N/A | N/A | N/A | N/A | |
| D3348 | N/A | N | - | N/A | N/A | N/A | N/A | |

* with documentation

## Terms To Know

**anterior.** Situated in the front area or toward the belly surface of the body.

**molars.** Posterior teeth used for grinding.

**posterior.** Located in the back part or caudal end of the body.

**root.** Part of the tooth located in the socket, covered by cementum, and attached by the periodontal structures.

**root canal.** Inner soft tissue, or pulp, of the tooth containing the lymph vessels, veins, arteries, and nerves of the tooth within small channels (up to five) running from the top of the tooth down to the tip of the root. When the tooth is cracked or decayed, bacteria enter the pulp and infect it, causing damage or death to the pulpal tissue and possibly an abscess that can infect bone. Root canal therapy repairs the root canal by removing the damaged pulp and cleaning out bacteria to prevent further damage and save the tooth.

# D3351-D3353

**D3351** apexification/recalcification - initial visit (apical closure / calcific repair of perforations, root resorption, etc.)

*Includes opening tooth, preparation of canal spaces, first placement of medication and necessary radiographs. (This procedure may include first phase of complete root canal therapy.)*

**D3352** apexification/recalcification - interim medication replacement

*For visits in which the intra-canal medication is replaced with new medication. Includes any necessary radiographs.*

**D3353** apexification/recalcification - final visit (includes completed root canal therapy - apical closure/calcific repair of perforations, root resorption, etc.)

*Includes removal of intra-canal medication and procedures necessary to place final root canal filling material including necessary radiographs. (This procedure includes last phase of complete root canal therapy.)*

## Explanation

Apexification and recalcification are required when traumatic injury to the tooth has occurred resulting in incomplete root formation. These types of injuries occur in childhood and are often the result of a fall or other accident. At the time of the injury, visible damage to the tooth may not be present. However, the injury may cause damage to the internal tooth structure resulting in incomplete root formation. Incomplete root formation can cause dental problems later such as pulpal necrosis and discoloration of the tooth or fistula formation. Apexification and recalcification require multiple visits and involve stimulating the root apex to close and recalcify by the use of medications, such as calcium hydroxide. On the initial visit (D3351), the tooth is opened. The necrotic pulp is removed (pulpectomy), and the canal spaces prepared. Medication that will stimulate apical closure and recalcification is placed. Any necessary radiographs are obtained. In D3352, the tooth is opened and prepared and the intracanal medication is replaced with new medication. Radiographs may also be obtained to assess the progress of apexification and recalcification during the interim visits. The final phase of treatment, reported with D3353, involves removal of the intracanal medication and the procedures necessary to place the final root canal filling material. On the final visit, apexification is confirmed by clinical evaluation and the use of radiographs. The root canal is filled with gutta percha and cement. Final restorations, such as a filling, crown, or bridgework, is reported separately.

## Coding Tips

Local anesthesia is generally considered to be part of endodontic procedures. Necessary radiographs are included and should not be reported separately. To report pulpal regeneration, see D3355-D3357.

## Reimbursement Tips

The third-party payer may include any radiographs performed during the endodontic retreatment as part of the procedure and, therefore, are not separately reportable. Check with payers for their specific guidelines.

## ICD-10-CM Diagnostic Codes

| | |
|---|---|
| K04.01 | Reversible pulpitis |
| K04.02 | Irreversible pulpitis |
| K04.1 | Necrosis of pulp |
| K04.2 | Pulp degeneration |
| K04.3 | Abnormal hard tissue formation in pulp |
| K04.4 | Acute apical periodontitis of pulpal origin |
| K04.5 | Chronic apical periodontitis |
| K04.6 | Periapical abscess with sinus |
| K04.7 | Periapical abscess without sinus |
| K04.8 | Radicular cyst |
| K04.99 | Other diseases of pulp and periapical tissues |
| S02.81XA | Fracture of other specified skull and facial bones, right side, initial encounter for closed fracture ☑ |
| S02.81XB | Fracture of other specified skull and facial bones, right side, initial encounter for open fracture ☑ |

## Relative Value Units/Medicare Edits

| Non-Facility RVU | Work | PE | MP | Total |
|---|---|---|---|---|
| **D3351** | 2.03 | 1.80 | 0.42 | 4.25 |
| **D3352** | 1.07 | 0.94 | 0.22 | 2.23 |
| **D3353** | 2.92 | 2.57 | 0.60 | 6.09 |
| **Facility RVU** | **Work** | **PE** | **MP** | **Total** |
| **D3351** | 2.03 | 1.80 | 0.42 | 4.25 |
| **D3352** | 1.07 | 0.94 | 0.22 | 2.23 |
| **D3353** | 2.92 | 2.57 | 0.60 | 6.09 |

| | FUD | Status | MUE | Modifiers | | | | IOM Reference |
|---|---|---|---|---|---|---|---|---|
| **D3351** | N/A | N | - | N/A | N/A | N/A | N/A | None |
| **D3352** | N/A | N | - | N/A | N/A | N/A | N/A | |
| **D3353** | N/A | N | - | N/A | N/A | N/A | N/A | |

* with documentation

## Terms To Know

**apex.** Highest point of a root end of a tooth, or the end of any organ.

**apexification.** In dentistry, a method of bringing about root development.

**necrosis.** Death of cells or tissue within a living organ or structure.

**pulp.** Living connective tissue within the tooth's root canal space that supplies blood vessels and nerves to the tooth.

**pulpectomy.** In dentistry, complete excision of both vital and devitalized pulp from a tooth's root canal space.

**root.** Part of the tooth located in the socket, covered by cementum, and attached by the periodontal structures.

# D3355-D3357

**D3355** pulpal regeneration - initial visit

*Includes opening tooth, preparation of canal spaces, placement of medication.*

**D3356** pulpal regeneration - interim medication replacement

**D3357** pulpal regeneration - completion of treatment

*Does not include final restoration.*

## Explanation

Pulpal regeneration is performed to remove necrotic pulp and place medication [adjacent] to healthy pulp tissue inside of an immature (developing) permanent tooth allowing the tooth to continue to develop and grow. At the time of the initial visit (D3355) the provider administers local anesthesia, places a rubber dam to isolate the tooth and access the pulp. Copious irrigation is gently performed. The canal is then dried. Antibiotic paste or calcium hydroxide is inserted. The canal is sealed with a temporary material. At the time of a subsequent visit (D3356), the antibiotic paste is removed and the response to the initial treatment is assessed. When there is persistent infection, additional antibiotic paste is prescribed. At the time of the completion of the procedure (D3357) and after local anesthesia and isolation the area is copious irrigated and dried. Bleeding into the canal is induced by over-instrumentation using an endo file or endo explorer. The bleeding is stopped. It may be necessary to place a CollaPlug/Collacote at the orifice. Permanent restoration is then placed.

## Coding Tips

Code D3356 includes the removal of intracanal medication and any procedures performed to continue root development. Radiographs used during the performance of the procedure are included and should not be reported separately. Placement of a seal at the coronal portion of the root canal is included; however, final restorations may be billed separately. When pulpal regeneration is performed on a tooth other than an immature permanent tooth, see codes D3351-D3353.

## ICD-10-CM Diagnostic Codes

| | |
|---|---|
| K04.01 | Reversible pulpitis |
| K04.02 | Irreversible pulpitis |
| K04.1 | Necrosis of pulp |
| K04.2 | Pulp degeneration |
| K04.3 | Abnormal hard tissue formation in pulp |
| K04.4 | Acute apical periodontitis of pulpal origin |
| K04.5 | Chronic apical periodontitis |
| K04.6 | Periapical abscess with sinus |
| K04.7 | Periapical abscess without sinus |
| K04.8 | Radicular cyst |
| K04.99 | Other diseases of pulp and periapical tissues |
| S02.81XA | Fracture of other specified skull and facial bones, right side, initial encounter for closed fracture ☑ |
| S0_81XB | Fracture of other specified skull and facial bones, right side, initial encounter for open fracture ☑ |

## Relative Value Units/Medicare Edits

| Non-Facility RVU | Work | PE | MP | Total |
|---|---|---|---|---|
| D3355 | 1.93 | 1.71 | 0.40 | 4.04 |
| D3356 | 1.39 | 1.23 | 0.29 | 2.91 |
| D3357 | 1.39 | 1.23 | 0.29 | 2.91 |
| **Facility RVU** | **Work** | **PE** | **MP** | **Total** |
| D3355 | 1.93 | 1.71 | 0.40 | 4.04 |
| D3356 | 1.39 | 1.23 | 0.29 | 2.91 |
| D3357 | 1.39 | 1.23 | 0.29 | 2.91 |

| | FUD | Status | MUE | Modifiers | | | | IOM Reference |
|---|---|---|---|---|---|---|---|---|
| D3355 | N/A | N | - | N/A | N/A | N/A | N/A | None |
| D3356 | N/A | N | - | N/A | N/A | N/A | N/A | |
| D3357 | N/A | N | - | N/A | N/A | N/A | N/A | |

* with documentation

## Terms To Know

**direct restoration.** In dentistry, restoration produced inside of the mouth.

**irrigation.** To wash out or cleanse a body cavity, wound, or tissue with water or other fluid.

**pulp.** Living connective tissue within the tooth's root canal space that supplies blood vessels and nerves to the tooth.

**regeneration.** Process of reproducing or regrowing tissue.

Dental - Endodontics

# D3410-D3426

**D3410** apicoectomy - anterior

*For surgery on root of anterior tooth. Does not include placement of retrograde filling material.*

**D3421** apicoectomy - premolar (first root)

*For surgery on one root of a premolar. Does not include placement of retrograde filling material. If more than one root is treated, see D3426.*

**D3425** apicoectomy - molar (first root)

*For surgery on one root of a molar tooth. Does not include placement of retrograde filling material. If more than one root is treated, see D3426.*

**D3426** apicoectomy (each additional root)

*Typically used for premolar and molar surgeries when more than one root is treated during the same procedure. This does not include retrograde filling material placement.*

## Explanation

An apicoectomy is performed. An apicoectomy involves removal of the root tip and the surrounding infected tissue of an abscessed tooth. Apicoectomy may be necessary when inflammation and infection persists in the area around the root tip following root canal therapy. The tooth is numbed and the gum is reflected (lifted) to expose the underlying bone and tooth root. The root end and all infected tissue are excised. Root end filler is used to seal the root. The gum is repositioned and repaired with dissolvable sutures. The apicectomy affects incisors or cuspids in D3410; bicuspids in D3421; or molars in D3425. Each additional root is reported using D3426.

## Coding Tips

Local anesthesia is generally considered to be part of endodontic procedures. Code D3246 should be reported for each additional root treated. Payers may require that the tooth/root number be reported on the claim. Code D3426 should not be reported alone but should be reported in conjunction with D3421 or D3425.

## Reimbursement Tips

When reporting code D3410, third-party payers may require clinical documentation and/or x-rays before making payment determination. Check with payers to determine their specific requirements.

## ICD-10-CM Diagnostic Codes

| | |
|---|---|
| K04.1 | Necrosis of pulp |
| K04.2 | Pulp degeneration |
| K04.3 | Abnormal hard tissue formation in pulp |
| K04.4 | Acute apical periodontitis of pulpal origin |
| K04.5 | Chronic apical periodontitis |
| K04.6 | Periapical abscess with sinus |
| K04.7 | Periapical abscess without sinus |
| K04.8 | Radicular cyst |
| K04.99 | Other diseases of pulp and periapical tissues |
| S02.81XA | Fracture of other specified skull and facial bones, right side, initial encounter for closed fracture ☑ |
| S02.81XB | Fracture of other specified skull and facial bones, right side, initial encounter for open fracture ☑ |

## Relative Value Units/Medicare Edits

| Non-Facility RVU | Work | PE | MP | Total |
|---|---|---|---|---|
| **D3410** | 3.95 | 3.49 | 0.81 | 8.25 |
| **D3421** | 4.44 | 3.92 | 0.91 | 9.27 |
| **D3425** | 5.01 | 4.42 | 1.03 | 10.46 |
| **D3426** | 1.80 | 1.58 | 0.37 | 3.75 |
| **Facility RVU** | **Work** | **PE** | **MP** | **Total** |
| **D3410** | 3.95 | 3.49 | 0.81 | 8.25 |
| **D3421** | 4.44 | 3.92 | 0.91 | 9.27 |
| **D3425** | 5.01 | 4.42 | 1.03 | 10.46 |
| **D3426** | 1.80 | 1.58 | 0.37 | 3.75 |

| | FUD | Status | MUE | Modifiers | | | | IOM Reference |
|---|---|---|---|---|---|---|---|---|
| **D3410** | N/A | N | - | N/A | N/A | N/A | N/A | None |
| **D3421** | N/A | N | - | N/A | N/A | N/A | N/A | |
| **D3425** | N/A | N | - | N/A | N/A | N/A | N/A | |
| **D3426** | N/A | N | - | N/A | N/A | N/A | N/A | |

* with documentation

## Terms To Know

**anterior teeth.** Six upper and six lower front teeth; the upper and lower incisors and cuspids.

**apex.** Highest point of a root end of a tooth, or the end of any organ.

**apicoectomy.** In dentistry, amputation of the end of the root portion of a tooth.

**endodontics.** Subspecialty of dentistry that deals primarily with the pulp of the tooth or the dentine complex.

**periradicular.** Surrounding part of the tooth's root.

**root canal.** Inner soft tissue, or pulp, of the tooth containing the lymph vessels, veins, arteries, and nerves of the tooth within small channels (up to five) running from the top of the tooth down to the tip of the root. When the tooth is cracked or decayed, bacteria enter the pulp and infect it, causing damage or death to the pulpal tissue and possibly an abscess that can infect bone. Root canal therapy repairs the root canal by removing the damaged pulp and cleaning out bacteria to prevent further damage and save the tooth.

# D3430

**D3430** retrograde filling - per root

*For placement of retrograde filling material during periradicular surgery procedures. If more than one filling is placed in one root - report as D3999 and describe.*

## Explanation

Retrograde filling of the root canal is performed. Retrograde filling is a method of sealing the root canal by preparing and filling it from the root tip. This is generally done at the completion of an apicoectomy (excision of the root tip). The tooth is numbed and the gum is reflected (lifted) to expose the site of the previously excised root tip. Root end filler is used to seal the root. This procedure may be reported multiple times when more than one root of a single tooth requires retrograde filling.

## Coding Tips

Local anesthesia is generally considered to be part of endodontic procedures. This code is reported once per root. According to the ADA, when more than one filling is placed in one root, code D3999 should be reported.

## Reimbursement Tips

Third-party payers may require clinical documentation and/or x-rays before making payment determination. Check with payers to determine their specific requirements.

## ICD-10-CM Diagnostic Codes

| | |
|---|---|
| K04.01 | Reversible pulpitis |
| K04.1 | Necrosis of pulp |
| K04.2 | Pulp degeneration |
| K04.3 | Abnormal hard tissue formation in pulp |
| K04.4 | Acute apical periodontitis of pulpal origin |
| K04.5 | Chronic apical periodontitis |
| K04.6 | Periapical abscess with sinus |
| K04.7 | Periapical abscess without sinus |
| K04.8 | Radicular cyst |
| K04.99 | Other diseases of pulp and periapical tissues |
| S02.80XA | Fracture of other specified skull and facial bones, unspecified side, initial encounter for closed fracture |
| S02.80XB | Fracture of other specified skull and facial bones, unspecified side, initial encounter for open fracture |
| S02.81XA | Fracture of other specified skull and facial bones, right side, initial encounter for closed fracture ☑ |
| S02.81XB | Fracture of other specified skull and facial bones, right side, initial encounter for open fracture ☑ |

## Relative Value Units/Medicare Edits

| Non-Facility RVU | Work | PE | MP | Total |
|---|---|---|---|---|
| **D3430** | 1.25 | 1.11 | 0.26 | 2.62 |
| **Facility RVU** | **Work** | **PE** | **MP** | **Total** |
| **D3430** | 1.25 | 1.11 | 0.26 | 2.62 |

| | FUD | Status | MUE | Modifiers | | | | IOM Reference |
|---|---|---|---|---|---|---|---|---|
| **D3430** | N/A | N | - | N/A | N/A | N/A | N/A | None |

* with documentation

## Terms To Know

**apicoectomy.** In dentistry, amputation of the end of the root portion of a tooth.

**endodontics.** Subspecialty of dentistry that deals primarily with the pulp of the tooth or the dentine complex.

**local anesthesia.** Induced loss of feeling or sensation restricted to a certain area of the body, including topical, local tissue infiltration, field block, or nerve block methods.

**retrograde filling.** Filling of a root canal by sealing it from the root apex.

**root.** Part of the tooth located in the socket, covered by cementum, and attached by the periodontal structures.

**root canal.** Inner soft tissue, or pulp, of the tooth containing the lymph vessels, veins, arteries, and nerves of the tooth within small channels (up to five) running from the top of the tooth down to the tip of the root. When the tooth is cracked or decayed, bacteria enter the pulp and infect it, causing damage or death to the pulpal tissue and possibly an abscess that can infect bone. Root canal therapy repairs the root canal by removing the damaged pulp and cleaning out bacteria to prevent further damage and save the tooth.

# D3450

**D3450** root amputation - per root

*Root resection of a multi-rooted tooth while leaving the crown. If the crown is sectioned, see D3920.*

## Explanation

Root amputation is performed, which is the surgical removal of one or more roots in a tooth that has multiple roots. Root amputation is performed when there is a persistent endodontic failure (failed root canal surgery) in a root of a tooth that must be kept or if there is significant bone loss around a root due to periodontal (gum) disease. Root amputation may be done as a permanent or temporary procedure. It is done as a temporary procedure to allow bone healing so that an implant can be placed at a later date. This procedure may be reported multiple times when more than one root of a single tooth requires amputation.

## Coding Tips

Local anesthesia is generally considered to be part of endodontic procedures. This code reports root resection while the crown remains. For sectioning of the crown, see D3920. This code is reported once per root. Necessary radiographs are included and should not be reported separately. The tooth/root number should be indicated on the claim.

## ICD-10-CM Diagnostic Codes

| | |
|---|---|
| K04.01 | Reversible pulpitis |
| K04.02 | Irreversible pulpitis |
| K04.2 | Pulp degeneration |
| K04.3 | Abnormal hard tissue formation in pulp |
| K04.4 | Acute apical periodontitis of pulpal origin |
| K04.5 | Chronic apical periodontitis |
| K04.6 | Periapical abscess with sinus |
| K04.7 | Periapical abscess without sinus |
| K04.8 | Radicular cyst |
| K04.99 | Other diseases of pulp and periapical tissues |
| S02.81XA | Fracture of other specified skull and facial bones, right side, initial encounter for closed fracture ☑ |
| S02.81XB | Fracture of other specified skull and facial bones, right side, initial encounter for open fracture ☑ |

## Relative Value Units/Medicare Edits

| Non-Facility RVU | Work | PE | MP | Total |
|---|---|---|---|---|
| D3450 | 2.48 | 2.19 | 0.51 | 5.18 |
| Facility RVU | Work | PE | MP | Total |
| D3450 | 2.48 | 2.19 | 0.51 | 5.18 |

| | FUD | Status | MUE | Modifiers | | | | IOM Reference |
|---|---|---|---|---|---|---|---|---|
| D3450 | N/A | N | - | N/A | N/A | N/A | N/A | None |

* with documentation

# D3460

**D3460** endodontic endosseous implant

*Placement of implant material, which extends from a pulpal space into the bone beyond the end of the root.*

## Explanation

A tooth that has lost its alveolar support is stabilized and maintained using an endodontic endosseous implant. This consists of a metal post that obliterates the pulpal chamber of the tooth and extends through the root canal into the periapical bone.

## Coding Tips

Many payers require that x-rays or x-ray interpretations be submitted with the claim.

## ICD-10-CM Diagnostic Codes

| | |
|---|---|
| K04.01 | Reversible pulpitis |
| K04.02 | Irreversible pulpitis |
| K04.1 | Necrosis of pulp |
| K04.2 | Pulp degeneration |
| K04.3 | Abnormal hard tissue formation in pulp |
| K04.4 | Acute apical periodontitis of pulpal origin |
| K04.5 | Chronic apical periodontitis |
| K04.6 | Periapical abscess with sinus |
| K04.7 | Periapical abscess without sinus |
| K04.8 | Radicular cyst |
| K04.90 | Unspecified diseases of pulp and periapical tissues |
| K04.99 | Other diseases of pulp and periapical tissues |
| S02.80XA | Fracture of other specified skull and facial bones, unspecified side, initial encounter for closed fracture |
| S02.80XB | Fracture of other specified skull and facial bones, unspecified side, initial encounter for open fracture |
| S02.81XA | Fracture of other specified skull and facial bones, right side, initial encounter for closed fracture ☑ |
| S02.81XB | Fracture of other specified skull and facial bones, right side, initial encounter for open fracture ☑ |

## Relative Value Units/Medicare Edits

| Non-Facility RVU | Work | PE | MP | Total |
|---|---|---|---|---|
| D3460 | 8.96 | 7.91 | 1.84 | 18.71 |
| Facility RVU | Work | PE | MP | Total |
| D3460 | 8.96 | 7.91 | 1.84 | 18.71 |

| | FUD | Status | MUE | Modifiers | | | | IOM Reference |
|---|---|---|---|---|---|---|---|---|
| D3460 | N/A | R | - | N/A | N/A | N/A | 80* | 100-02,1,70; 100-04,4,20.5 |

* with documentation

Dental - Endodontics

# D3470

**D3470** intentional reimplantation (including necessary splinting)

*For the intentional removal, inspection and treatment of the root and replacement of a tooth into its own socket. This does not include necessary retrograde filling material placement.*

## Explanation

Intentional reimplantation of a tooth is used when traditional root canal therapy is not a viable option. The mouth is rinsed with chlorhexidine mouthwash and the surgical field is disinfected. The tooth to be reimplanted is extracted and immersed in sterile saline solution. The extracted tooth is then inspected to determine whether reimplantation is a possible option. If it is determined that any injury or disease, such as a root fracture, can be repaired, the tooth is reconstructed. The alveolus is then cleaned with antibacterial solution and irradiated to provide the necessary aseptic environment. The extracted tooth is reimplanted into the alveolus and sutures are placed to stabilize the tooth. The patient returns for a follow-up a week to 10 days later and the sutures are removed.

## Coding Tips

Local anesthesia is generally considered to be part of endodontic procedures. This code does not include placement of any necessary retrograde filling material.

## Reimbursement Tips

Many payers have limited coverage policies for this service. Contact payers for their specific guidelines.

## ICD-10-CM Diagnostic Codes

| | |
|---|---|
| K04.01 | Reversible pulpitis |
| K04.02 | Irreversible pulpitis |
| K04.1 | Necrosis of pulp |
| K04.2 | Pulp degeneration |
| K04.3 | Abnormal hard tissue formation in pulp |
| K04.4 | Acute apical periodontitis of pulpal origin |
| K04.5 | Chronic apical periodontitis |
| K04.6 | Periapical abscess with sinus |
| K04.7 | Periapical abscess without sinus |
| K04.8 | Radicular cyst |
| K04.99 | Other diseases of pulp and periapical tissues |
| S02.80XA | Fracture of other specified skull and facial bones, unspecified side, initial encounter for closed fracture |
| S02.80XB | Fracture of other specified skull and facial bones, unspecified side, initial encounter for open fracture |
| S02.81XA | Fracture of other specified skull and facial bones, right side, initial encounter for closed fracture ☑ |
| S02.81XB | Fracture of other specified skull and facial bones, right side, initial encounter for open fracture ☑ |

## Relative Value Units/Medicare Edits

| Non-Facility RVU | Work | PE | MP | Total |
|---|---|---|---|---|
| D3470 | 4.78 | 4.22 | 0.99 | 9.99 |
| **Facility RVU** | **Work** | **PE** | **MP** | **Total** |
| D3470 | 4.78 | 4.22 | 0.99 | 9.99 |

| | FUD | Status | MUE | Modifiers | | | | IOM Reference |
|---|---|---|---|---|---|---|---|---|
| D3470 | N/A | N | - | N/A | N/A | N/A | N/A | None |

* with documentation

## Terms To Know

**endodontics.** Subspecialty of dentistry that deals primarily with the pulp of the tooth or the dentine complex.

**retrograde filling.** Filling of a root canal by sealing it from the root apex.

**root canal.** Inner soft tissue, or pulp, of the tooth containing the lymph vessels, veins, arteries, and nerves of the tooth within small channels (up to five) running from the top of the tooth down to the tip of the root. When the tooth is cracked or decayed, bacteria enter the pulp and infect it, causing damage or death to the pulpal tissue and possibly an abscess that can infect bone. Root canal therapy repairs the root canal by removing the damaged pulp and cleaning out bacteria to prevent further damage and save the tooth.

# D3471-D3473

**D3471** surgical repair of root resorption - anterior

*For surgery on root of anterior tooth. Does not include placement of restoration.*

**D3472** surgical repair of root resorption - premolar

*For surgery on root of premolar tooth. Does not include placement of restoration.*

**D3473** surgical repair of root resorption - molar

*For surgery on root of molar tooth. Does not include placement of restoration.*

## Explanation

The coronal part of the pulp near the dentinocemental junction is removed and leaves the radicular pulp tissue. The root canal is instrumented, irrigated, and treated with medicaments such as sodium hypochlorite preparations. When the canal has no more vital or necrotic pulp tissue, an interappointment dressing, such as calcium hydroxide, is used to control bleeding, necrotize any residual pulp tissue, and disinfect the canal. At this point, the canal may be temporarily sealed. Medicament, usually gutta percha, is placed into the canal space. A permanent sealant is applied. If the root wall has been perforated, treatment must include any openings into the root. Severe cases may also involve exposure of the root tip and treatment with possible removal. Report D3471 for a tooth in the anterior portion of the mouth, D3472 for a premolar tooth, and D3473 for a molar tooth.

## Coding Tips

Do not use this code to report root canal therapy, see D3310-D3330. Local anesthesia is included in this service. Any evaluation, radiograph, or restoration service is reported separately. For pulpal debridement, see D3221.

## ICD-10-CM Diagnostic Codes

K03.3 Pathological resorption of teeth

## Relative Value Units/Medicare Edits

| Non-Facility RVU | Work | PE | MP | Total |
|---|---|---|---|---|
| D3471 | | | | |
| D3472 | | | | |
| D3473 | | | | |
| **Facility RVU** | **Work** | **PE** | **MP** | **Total** |
| D3471 | | | | |
| D3472 | | | | |
| D3473 | | | | |

| | FUD | Status | MUE | Modifiers | | | | IOM Reference |
|---|---|---|---|---|---|---|---|---|
| D3471 | N/A | | - | N/A | N/A | N/A | N/A | |
| D3472 | N/A | | - | N/A | N/A | N/A | N/A | |
| D3473 | N/A | | - | N/A | N/A | N/A | N/A | |

* with documentation

## Terms To Know

**resorption.** Asymptomatic intra-radicular pathologic process where transforming pulp cells resorb dentinal walls inside the root canal space of permanent teeth, usually discovered on routine dental x-ray exams.

# D3501-D3503

**D3501** surgical exposure of root surface without apicoectomy or repair of root resorption - anterior

*Exposure of root surface followed by observation and surgical closure of the exposed area. Not to be used for or in conjunction with apicoectomy or repair of root resorption.*

**D3502** surgical exposure of root surface without apicoectomy or repair of root resorption - premolar

*Exposure of root surface followed by observation and surgical closure of the exposed area. Not to be used for or in conjunction with apicoectomy or repair of root resorption.*

**D3503** surgical exposure of root surface without apicoectomy or repair of root resorption - molar

*Exposure of root surface followed by observation and surgical closure of the exposed area. Not to be used for or in conjunction with apicoectomy or repair of root resorption.*

## Explanation

The provider exposes the tooth root for evaluation. Based upon the findings the exposure is closed. This procedure is for evaluation and examination of the exposed root. Report D3501 for a tooth in the anterior portion of the mouth, D3502 for a premolar tooth, and D3503 for a molar tooth.

## Coding Tips

To report apicoectomy, see D3410-D3426. To report treatment of root resorption, see D3471-D3473. To report bone graft done with periradicular surgery, see D3428-D3429. To report the insertion of biologic materials used to increase soft and boney tissue regeneration at the time of periradicular procedures, see D3431. To report guided tissue regeneration or resorbable barrier performed at the time of periradicular procedures, see D3432.

## ICD-10-CM Diagnostic Codes

K00.4 Disturbances in tooth formation
K00.5 Hereditary disturbances in tooth structure, not elsewhere classified
K00.8 Other disorders of tooth development
K02.7 Dental root caries
K03.2 Erosion of teeth
K03.89 Other specified diseases of hard tissues of teeth
K04.6 Periapical abscess with sinus
K04.7 Periapical abscess without sinus
K04.8 Radicular cyst
K04.99 Other diseases of pulp and periapical tissues

## Relative Value Units/Medicare Edits

| Non-Facility RVU | Work | PE | MP | Total |
|---|---|---|---|---|
| D3501 | | | | |
| D3502 | | | | |
| D3503 | | | | |
| **Facility RVU** | **Work** | **PE** | **MP** | **Total** |
| D3501 | | | | |
| D3502 | | | | |
| D3503 | | | | |

| | FUD | Status | MUE | Modifiers | | | | IOM Reference |
|---|---|---|---|---|---|---|---|---|
| D3501 | N/A | | - | N/A | N/A | N/A | N/A | |
| D3502 | N/A | | - | N/A | N/A | N/A | N/A | |
| D3503 | N/A | | - | N/A | N/A | N/A | N/A | |

* with documentation

Dental - Endodontics

# D3910

**D3910** surgical procedure for isolation of tooth with rubber dam

## Explanation

A rubber dam is placed to provide isolation for better visibility and access to the tooth, moisture and environment control, and airway protection for procedures such as root canal therapy or acid-etch technique. Cotton wool is placed in the sulcus beside the tooth. While rubber dam is stretched, the tooth position is marked and a hole is punched to indicate tooth size. The clamp is tried-in and a lubricant is applied to the dam. The clamp is fitted into the hole and the clamp and dam are placed on the tooth and positioned. The dam must be secured to the tooth either with dam clamps, floss ligatures, wedges, pieces of dam or rubber band worked or pinched into a tight contact point. The dam is removed after the procedure by removing the clamps or ligatures, stretching it, and carefully cutting with scissors.

## Coding Tips

This service must be performed prior to many procedures to provide environmental control. Local anesthesia is included in this service. Any evaluation, radiograph, root canal, core buildup, or post or preparation service is reported separately.

## Reimbursement Tips

Many third-party payers consider this to be an integral part of a more intense service and should not be billed separately

## ICD-10-CM Diagnostic Codes

The application of this code is too broad to adequately present ICD-10-CM diagnostic code links here. Refer to your ICD-10-CM book.

## Relative Value Units/Medicare Edits

| Non-Facility RVU | Work | PE | MP | Total |
|---|---|---|---|---|
| D3910 | 0.79 | 0.70 | 0.16 | 1.65 |
| **Facility RVU** | **Work** | **PE** | **MP** | **Total** |
| D3910 | 0.79 | 0.70 | 0.16 | 1.65 |

| | FUD | Status | MUE | Modifiers | | | | IOM Reference |
|---|---|---|---|---|---|---|---|---|
| D3910 | N/A | N | - | N/A | N/A | N/A | N/A | None |

* with documentation

## Terms To Know

**bonding.** In dentistry, two or more components connected by chemical adhesion or mechanical means.

**clamp.** Tool used to grip, compress, join, or fasten body parts.

**endodontics.** Subspecialty of dentistry that deals primarily with the pulp of the tooth or the dentine complex.

# D3911

- **D3911** intraorifice barrier

  *Not to be used as a final restoration.*

## Explanation

After completion of a primary root canal and placement of the gutta-percha, the provider places an intraorifice barrier, usually glass ionomer cement (GIC), within the root orifice of the tooth. The barrier is followed by placement of a composite resin restoration. The barrier aids in the healing of apical periodontitis and prevention of infection due to microleakage.

## Coding Tips

Report D3911 separately in addition to a root canal service that includes placement of the composite resin restoration. Preparation of tooth for crown is not included and may be reported separately.

## Documentation Tips

Placement of an intraorifice barrier is not required for all root canals and placement must be documented in the patient record.

## ICD-10-CM Diagnostic Codes

K02.53 Dental caries on pit and fissure surface penetrating into pulp
K02.61 Dental caries on smooth surface limited to enamel
K02.62 Dental caries on smooth surface penetrating into dentin
K02.63 Dental caries on smooth surface penetrating into pulp
K02.7 Dental root caries
K03.0 Excessive attrition of teeth
K03.1 Abrasion of teeth
K03.2 Erosion of teeth
K03.3 Pathological resorption of teeth
K03.4 Hypercementosis
K03.5 Ankylosis of teeth
K03.6 Deposits [accretions] on teeth
K03.7 Posteruptive color changes of dental hard tissues
K03.81 Cracked tooth
K03.89 Other specified diseases of hard tissues of teeth
K04.01 Reversible pulpitis
K04.02 Irreversible pulpitis
K04.1 Necrosis of pulp
K04.2 Pulp degeneration
K04.3 Abnormal hard tissue formation in pulp
K04.4 Acute apical periodontitis of pulpal origin
K04.5 Chronic apical periodontitis
K04.6 Periapical abscess with sinus
K04.7 Periapical abscess without sinus
K04.8 Radicular cyst
K05.00 Acute gingivitis, plaque induced
K05.01 Acute gingivitis, non-plaque induced
K05.10 Chronic gingivitis, plaque induced
K05.11 Chronic gingivitis, non-plaque induced
K05.211 Aggressive periodontitis, localized, slight
K05.212 Aggressive periodontitis, localized, moderate
K05.213 Aggressive periodontitis, localized, severe
K05.221 Aggressive periodontitis, generalized, slight
K05.222 Aggressive periodontitis, generalized, moderate
K05.223 Aggressive periodontitis, generalized, severe
K05.311 Chronic periodontitis, localized, slight
K05.312 Chronic periodontitis, localized, moderate
K05.313 Chronic periodontitis, localized, severe
K05.321 Chronic periodontitis, generalized, slight
K05.322 Chronic periodontitis, generalized, moderate
K05.323 Chronic periodontitis, generalized, severe
K05.4 Periodontosis
K06.010 Localized gingival recession, unspecified
K06.011 Localized gingival recession, minimal
K06.012 Localized gingival recession, moderate
K06.013 Localized gingival recession, severe
K06.021 Generalized gingival recession, minimal
K06.022 Generalized gingival recession, moderate
K06.023 Generalized gingival recession, severe
K06.1 Gingival enlargement
K06.2 Gingival and edentulous alveolar ridge lesions associated with trauma
K08.0 Exfoliation of teeth due to systemic causes
K08.3 Retained dental root
K08.51 Open restoration margins of tooth
K08.52 Unrepairable overhanging of dental restorative materials
K08.530 Fractured dental restorative material without loss of material
K08.531 Fractured dental restorative material with loss of material
K08.54 Contour of existing restoration of tooth biologically incompatible with oral health
K08.55 Allergy to existing dental restorative material
K08.56 Poor aesthetic of existing restoration of tooth
K08.81 Primary occlusal trauma
K08.82 Secondary occlusal trauma
M27.51 Perforation of root canal space due to endodontic treatment
M27.59 Other periradicular pathology associated with previous endodontic treatment
S02.5XXA Fracture of tooth (traumatic), initial encounter for closed fracture
S02.5XXB Fracture of tooth (traumatic), initial encounter for open fracture

## Relative Value Units/Medicare Edits

| Non-Facility RVU | Work | PE | MP | Total |
|---|---|---|---|---|
| D3911 | | | | |
| **Facility RVU** | **Work** | **PE** | **MP** | **Total** |
| D3911 | | | | |

| | FUD | Status | MUE | Modifiers | | | | IOM Reference |
|---|---|---|---|---|---|---|---|---|
| D3911 | N/A | | - | N/A | N/A | N/A | N/A | |

* with documentation

Dental - Endodontics

# D3920

**D3920** hemisection (including any root removal), not including root canal therapy

*Includes separation of a multi-rooted tooth into separate sections containing the root and the overlying portion of the crown. It may also include the removal of one or more of those sections.*

## Explanation

Hemisection involves removal of one-half of a tooth and one of the roots (root amputation) in a multi-rooted tooth. A local anesthetic is administered. An incision is made exposing the bone and the root that is to be removed. Any inflamed tissue is debrided. Using a long, shank tapered fissure carbide bur, a vertical cut is made in the crown of the tooth and the crown is resected. A fine probe is passed through the cut to ensure separation. The distal root is extracted and the surgical site flushed with sterile saline to remove any bony chips or amalgam. The remaining half of the tooth is restored with the remaining roots. The resected tooth may be attached or anchored to an adjacent tooth for additional support and stability.

## Coding Tips

Root canal therapy on the remaining root is not included and should be reported separately. Local anesthesia is generally considered to be part of endodontic procedures. This code does not include root canal therapy.

## Reimbursement Tips

Coverage of this procedure may vary by payer and patient contract. Check with payers for their specific coverage guidelines.

## ICD-10-CM Diagnostic Codes

| | |
|---|---|
| K04.01 | Reversible pulpitis |
| K04.02 | Irreversible pulpitis |
| K04.1 | Necrosis of pulp |
| K04.2 | Pulp degeneration |
| K04.3 | Abnormal hard tissue formation in pulp |
| K04.4 | Acute apical periodontitis of pulpal origin |
| K04.5 | Chronic apical periodontitis |
| K04.6 | Periapical abscess with sinus |
| K04.7 | Periapical abscess without sinus |
| K04.8 | Radicular cyst |
| K04.99 | Other diseases of pulp and periapical tissues |
| S02.81XA | Fracture of other specified skull and facial bones, right side, initial encounter for closed fracture ☑ |
| S02.81XB | Fracture of other specified skull and facial bones, right side, initial encounter for open fracture ☑ |

## Relative Value Units/Medicare Edits

| Non-Facility RVU | Work | PE | MP | Total |
|---|---|---|---|---|
| D3920 | 2.14 | 1.88 | 0.44 | 4.46 |
| **Facility RVU** | **Work** | **PE** | **MP** | **Total** |
| D3920 | 2.14 | 1.88 | 0.44 | 4.46 |

| | FUD | Status | MUE | Modifiers | | | | IOM Reference |
|---|---|---|---|---|---|---|---|---|
| D3920 | N/A | N | - | N/A | N/A | N/A | N/A | None |

* with documentation

# D3921

● **D3921** decoronation or submergence of an erupted tooth

*Intentional removal of coronal tooth structure for preservation of the root and surrounding bone.*

## Explanation

An erupted tooth is decoronated or suberged. Local anesthesia is placed. An intrasulcular incision is made and full thickness mucoperiosteal flap is elevated. The tooth and root are exposed. The crown of the tooth is decoronated with removal of the root canal filling. After rinsing, blood from the surrounding tissue is allowed to fill in the root canal. Porous deproteinized bone mineral may be applied to the defect around the decoronated embedded root and alveolar bone followed by occlusive absorbable collagen membrane. The flap is released and sutured without tension.

## Coding Tips

Root canal is included in this service and is not reported separately.

## ICD-10-CM Diagnostic Codes

| | |
|---|---|
| K00.6 | Disturbances in tooth eruption |
| K01.0 | Embedded teeth |
| K01.1 | Impacted teeth |
| K03.5 | Ankylosis of teeth |
| M26.30 | Unspecified anomaly of tooth position of fully erupted tooth or teeth |
| M26.33 | Horizontal displacement of fully erupted tooth or teeth |
| M26.34 | Vertical displacement of fully erupted tooth or teeth |
| M26.39 | Other anomalies of tooth position of fully erupted tooth or teeth |

## Relative Value Units/Medicare Edits

| Non-Facility RVU | Work | PE | MP | Total |
|---|---|---|---|---|
| D3921 | | | | |
| **Facility RVU** | **Work** | **PE** | **MP** | **Total** |
| D3921 | | | | |

| | FUD | Status | MUE | Modifiers | | | | IOM Reference |
|---|---|---|---|---|---|---|---|---|
| D3921 | N/A | | - | N/A | N/A | N/A | N/A | |

* with documentation

## Terms To Know

**decoronation.** Surgical removal of the crown and root filling of a tooth to allow root resorption or retaining of alveolar bone.

# D3950

**D3950** canal preparation and fitting of preformed dowel or post

*Should not be reported in conjunction with D2952, D2953, D2954 or D2957 by the same practitioner.*

## Explanation

The root canal is prepared and fitted with a preformed (prefabricated) dowel or post. Preformed dowels or posts may be cylindrical or conical in shape or a combination of both. The surface of the preformed dowel or post may be smooth, rough, or equipped with retention devices such as grooves or taps. The root canal is prepared by first removing any gutta percha placed during previous root canal therapy. Next, drills, in increasing diameters, are used interchangeably with reamers to create an opening in the root. Drilling is continued until the drill is in contact with dentine over the entire length of the canal where the dowel or post will be placed. The dowel or post drill is then used to place the dowel or post in the canal. The dowel or post is luted into place. This type of procedure is necessary when there is not sufficient coronal tooth structure to support reconstruction with a crown.

## Coding Tips

Local anesthesia is generally considered to be part of endodontic procedures. This code is not to be reported in conjunction with the following codes when performed by the same practitioner: D2952, D2953, D2954, or D2957.

## Reimbursement Tips

Coverage of this procedure may vary by payer and patient contract. Check with payers for specific coverage guidelines.

## ICD-10-CM Diagnostic Codes

This/these CPT code(s) are add-on code(s). See the primary procedure code that this code is performed with for your ICD-10-CM code selections.

## Relative Value Units/Medicare Edits

| Non-Facility RVU | Work | PE | MP | Total |
|---|---|---|---|---|
| D3950 | 0.99 | 0.87 | 0.20 | 2.06 |
| **Facility RVU** | **Work** | **PE** | **MP** | **Total** |
| D3950 | 0.99 | 0.87 | 0.20 | 2.06 |

| | FUD | Status | MUE | Modifiers | | | | IOM Reference |
|---|---|---|---|---|---|---|---|---|
| D3950 | N/A | N | - | N/A | N/A | N/A | N/A | None |

* with documentation

## Terms To Know

**coronal.** Relating to the top of a tooth or the crown of the head.

Dental - Endodontics

# D4210-D4211

**D4210** gingivectomy or gingivoplasty - four or more contiguous teeth or tooth bounded spaces per quadrant

*It is performed to eliminate suprabony pockets or to restore normal architecture when gingival enlargements or asymmetrical or unaesthetic topography is evident with normal bony configuration.*

**D4211** gingivectomy or gingivoplasty - one to three contiguous teeth or tooth bounded spaces per quadrant

*It is performed to eliminate suprabony pockets or to restore normal architecture when gingival enlargements or asymmetrical or unaesthetic topography is evident with normal bony configuration.*

## Explanation

The dentist performs a gingivectomy or gingivoplasty to reshape damaged gingivae or excise excess tissue into a better contour for restorative treatment and/or a more esthetic look. Pockets of gingiva are marked for the line of incision, which is then made with the blade angled to the long axis of the tooth. Supragingival pockets are thereby excised and recontouring of the gums is accomplished using the beveled incision. The strip of remaining gingiva is released, the root surfaces are curetted, and the area is packed and left to heal by granulation. Report D4210 for a gingivectomy or gingivoplasty performed in each quadrant on four or more contiguous teeth or bounded teeth spaces and D4211 for one to three teeth per quadrant.

## Coding Tips

Local anesthesia is included in these services. Any evaluation or radiograph is reported separately. Pathology exam of tissue with interpretation is reported separately. These codes are reported once per quadrant. Usual postoperative care is included in these services. These codes include frenulectomy. Report D4212 when the gingival surgery is performed to allow access for a restorative service.

## Documentation Tips

Payers may require periodontal charting. Periodontal charting should include the identification of the quadrants and sites involved, a minimum of three pocket measurements per tooth involved, indication of recession, furcation involvement, mobility and mucogingival defects, and identification of missing teeth.

## Reimbursement Tips

When selecting the procedure or service that accurately identifies the service performed, dentists must use the most accurate code. If the CDT code more accurately identifies the service, this should be used rather than the CPT codes. Many payers will not separately reimburse the following services when performed by the same provider, on the same date of service, and at the same surgical site: biopsy (D7285–D7286), frenulectomy (D7960), and/or excision of hard and soft tissue lesions (D7410–D7411, D7450–D7451). When one or more of the above services are provided on a different date of service, a narrative indicating the medical necessity of separating the services should be provided; otherwise, payers may deny those services.

## Associated CPT Codes

41820 Gingivectomy, excision gingiva, each quadrant
41872 Gingivoplasty, each quadrant (specify)

## ICD-10-CM Diagnostic Codes

K06.011 Localized gingival recession, minimal
K06.012 Localized gingival recession, moderate
K06.013 Localized gingival recession, severe
K06.021 Generalized gingival recession, minimal
K06.022 Generalized gingival recession, moderate
K06.023 Generalized gingival recession, severe
K06.1 Gingival enlargement
K06.2 Gingival and edentulous alveolar ridge lesions associated with trauma
K06.8 Other specified disorders of gingiva and edentulous alveolar ridge

## Relative Value Units/Medicare Edits

| Non-Facility RVU | Work | PE | MP | Total |
|---|---|---|---|---|
| **D4210** | 3.15 | 2.78 | 0.65 | 6.58 |
| **D4211** | 1.34 | 1.18 | 0.28 | 2.80 |
| **Facility RVU** | **Work** | **PE** | **MP** | **Total** |
| **D4210** | 3.15 | 2.78 | 0.65 | 6.58 |
| **D4211** | 1.34 | 1.18 | 0.28 | 2.80 |

| | FUD | Status | MUE | Modifiers | | | | IOM Reference |
|---|---|---|---|---|---|---|---|---|
| **D4210** | N/A | I | - | N/A | N/A | N/A | N/A | None |
| **D4211** | N/A | I | - | N/A | N/A | N/A | N/A | |

* with documentation

## Terms To Know

**gingivectomy.** Surgical excision or trimming of overgrown gum tissue back to normal contours using a scalpel, electrocautery, or a laser.

**gingivitis.** Inflamed gingiva (oral mucosa) that surrounds the teeth.

**gingivoplasty.** Repair or reconstruction of the gum tissue, altering the gingival contours by excising areas of gum tissue or making incisions through the gingiva to create a gingival flap.

**tooth bounded space.** Empty space in the mouth due to a missing tooth that is surrounded by a tooth on each side.

# D4212

**D4212** gingivectomy or gingivoplasty to allow access for restorative procedure, per tooth

## Explanation

The provider excises gingivae or excessive tissue to allow access for restorative procedures. Pockets of gingiva are marked for the line of incision, which is then made with the blade angled to the long axis of the tooth. Supragingival pockets are thereby excised and recontouring of the gums is accomplished using the beveled incision. The strip of remaining gingiva is released, the root surfaces are curetted, and the area is packed and left to heal by granulation.

## Coding Tips

When performed to restore normal architecture due to gingival enlargements or asymmetrical or unaesthetic gum lines, report D4210 for a gingivectomy or gingivoplasty performed in each quadrant on four or more contiguous teeth or bounded teeth spaces and D4211 for one to three teeth per quadrant. Payers may require documentation on the claim form indicating the tooth space on which the procedure was performed.

## Documentation Tips

Treatment plan documentation should reflect any treatment failure or change in diagnosis and/or a change in treatment plan. There should also be evidence of any initiation or reinstatement of a drug regime, which requires close and continuous skilled medical observation. The following information can be documented on a tooth chart: treatment/location of caries, endodontic procedures, prosthetic services, preventive services, treatment of lesions and dental disease, or other special procedures. A tooth chart may also be used to identify structure and rationale of disease process and the type of service performed on intraoral structures other than teeth.

## Reimbursement Tips

When selecting the procedure or service that accurately identifies the service performed, dentists must use the most accurate code. If the CDT code more accurately identifies the service, this should be used rather than the CPT codes. This procedure may be covered by the patient's medical insurance. When covered by medical insurance, the payer may require that the appropriate CPT code be reported on the CMS-1500 claim form. Many payers will not separately reimburse the following services when performed by the same provider, on the same date of service, and at the same surgical site: biopsy (D7285–D7286), frenulectomy (D7960), and/or excision of hard and soft tissue lesions (D7410–D7411, D7450–D7451). When one or more of the above services are provided on a different date of service, a narrative indicating the medical necessity of separating the services should be provided; otherwise, payers may deny those services.

## Associated CPT Codes

41820 Gingivectomy, excision gingiva, each quadrant
41872 Gingivoplasty, each quadrant (specify)

## ICD-10-CM Diagnostic Codes

K06.010 Localized gingival recession, unspecified
K06.011 Localized gingival recession, minimal
K06.012 Localized gingival recession, moderate
K06.013 Localized gingival recession, severe
K06.020 Generalized gingival recession, unspecified
K06.021 Generalized gingival recession, minimal
K06.022 Generalized gingival recession, moderate
K06.023 Generalized gingival recession, severe
K06.1 Gingival enlargement
K06.2 Gingival and edentulous alveolar ridge lesions associated with trauma
K06.8 Other specified disorders of gingiva and edentulous alveolar ridge

## Relative Value Units/Medicare Edits

| Non-Facility RVU | Work | PE | MP | Total |
|---|---|---|---|---|
| **D4212** | 0.80 | 0.71 | 0.16 | 1.67 |
| **Facility RVU** | **Work** | **PE** | **MP** | **Total** |
| **D4212** | 0.80 | 0.71 | 0.16 | 1.67 |

| | FUD | Status | MUE | Modifiers | | | | IOM Reference |
|---|---|---|---|---|---|---|---|---|
| **D4212** | N/A | I | - | N/A | N/A | N/A | N/A | None |

* with documentation

## Terms To Know

**excise.** Remove or cut out.

**gingivectomy.** Surgical excision or trimming of overgrown gum tissue back to normal contours using a scalpel, electrocautery, or a laser.

**gingivitis.** Inflamed gingiva (oral mucosa) that surrounds the teeth.

**gingivoplasty.** Repair or reconstruction of the gum tissue, altering the gingival contours by excising areas of gum tissue or making incisions through the gingiva to create a gingival flap.

# D4230-D4231

**D4230** anatomical crown exposure - four or more contiguous teeth or tooth bounded spaces per quadrant

*This procedure is utilized in an otherwise periodontally healthy area to remove enlarged gingival tissue and supporting bone (ostectomy) to provide an anatomically correct gingival relationship.*

**D4231** anatomical crown exposure - one to three teeth or tooth bounded spaces per quadrant

*This procedure is utilized in an otherwise periodontally healthy area to remove enlarged gingival tissue and supporting bone (ostectomy) to provide an anatomically correct gingival relationship.*

## Explanation

The dentist removes enlarged gingival tissue and supporting bone to improve the health and cosmetic appearance of the teeth and gums. Incisions are made that allow the gums to be retracted from around the teeth. Some bone may be removed using a combination of hand instruments or rotary burrs. The retracted flap is sutured back in place after some soft tissue has been removed. This will result in more tooth or teeth being exposed once the gum incisions have healed. Report D4230 when four our more contiguous teeth are treated or D4231 for up to three teeth in a single quadrant.

## Coding Tips

Local anesthesia is generally considered part of restorative procedures. For crown lengthening focused upon hard tissue, see D4249.

## Reimbursement Tips

When selecting the procedure or service that accurately identifies the service performed, dentists must use the most accurate code. If the CDT code more accurately identifies the service, this should be used rather than the CPT codes. Payers often require documentation before covering these procedures. Check with the specific payer to determine coverage. These procedures are often performed for cosmetic reasons and may not be covered by third-party payers. Many payers will not separately reimburse the following services when performed by the same provider, on the same date of service, and at the same surgical site: biopsy (D7285–D7286), frenulectomy (D7960), and/or excision of hard and soft tissue lesions (D7410–D7411, D7450–D7451). When one or more of the above services are provided on a different date of service, a narrative indicating the medical necessity of separating the services should be provided; otherwise, payers may deny those services.

## Associated CPT Codes

41820 Gingivectomy, excision gingiva, each quadrant

41821 Operculectomy, excision pericoronal tissues

## ICD-10-CM Diagnostic Codes

K06.1 Gingival enlargement

K06.2 Gingival and edentulous alveolar ridge lesions associated with trauma

K06.8 Other specified disorders of gingiva and edentulous alveolar ridge

## Relative Value Units/Medicare Edits

| Non-Facility RVU | Work | PE | MP | Total |
|---|---|---|---|---|
| D4230 | 4.08 | 3.60 | 0.84 | 8.52 |
| D4231 | 2.25 | 1.98 | 0.46 | 4.69 |
| **Facility RVU** | **Work** | **PE** | **MP** | **Total** |
| D4230 | 4.08 | 3.60 | 0.84 | 8.52 |
| D4231 | 2.25 | 1.98 | 0.46 | 4.69 |

| | FUD | Status | MUE | Modifiers | | | | IOM Reference |
|---|---|---|---|---|---|---|---|---|
| D4230 | N/A | N | - | N/A | N/A | N/A | N/A | None |
| D4231 | N/A | N | - | N/A | N/A | N/A | N/A | |

* with documentation

## Terms To Know

**clinical crown.** Part of the tooth that is not covered by any supporting structures such as the gums.

**flap graft.** Mass of flesh and skin partially excised from its location but retaining its blood supply, grafted onto another site to repair adjacent or distant defects.

**gingiva.** Soft tissues surrounding the crowns of unerupted teeth and necks of erupted teeth.

**gingivectomy.** Surgical excision or trimming of overgrown gum tissue back to normal contours using a scalpel, electrocautery, or a laser.

**periodontal.** Relating to the tissues that support and surround the teeth.

# D4240-D4241

**D4240** gingival flap procedure, including root planing - four or more contiguous teeth or tooth bounded spaces per quadrant

*A soft tissue flap is reflected or resected to allow debridement of the root surface and the removal of granulation tissue. Osseous recontouring is not accomplished in conjunction with this procedure. May include open flap curettage, reverse bevel flap surgery, modified Kirkland flap procedure, and modified Widman surgery. This procedure is performed in the presence of moderate to deep probing depths, loss of attachment, need to maintain esthetics, need for increased access to the root surface and alveolar bone, or to determine the presence of a cracked tooth, fractured root, or external root resorption. Other procedures may be required concurrent to D4240 and should be reported separately using their own unique codes*

**D4241** gingival flap procedure, including root planing - one to three contiguous teeth or tooth bounded spaces per quadrant

*A soft tissue flap is reflected or resected to allow debridement of the root surface and the removal of granulation tissue. Osseous recontouring is not accomplished in conjunction with this procedure. May include open flap curettage, reverse bevel flap surgery, modified Kirkland flap procedure, and modified Widman surgery. This procedure is performed in the presence of moderate to deep probing depths, loss of attachment, need to maintain esthetics, need for increased access to the root surface and alveolar bone, or to determine the presence of a cracked tooth, fractured root, or external root resorption. Other procedures may be required concurrent to D4241 and should be reported separately using their own unique codes.*

## Explanation

A gingival flap procedure is done to alter the contours of the gums and carry out root planing or scaling of the root surface. The flap is designed and a scalloped incision is made parallel to the long axis of the teeth and extended interproximally to separate the underlying pocket of epithelium from the flap to be raised, and distally enough to raise the flap like an envelope, without cutting definitive sides squared at the ends. A second intracrevicular incision is made to release the collar of pocket epithelium and expose the alveolar bone a few millimeters. The superficial collar of tissue is removed. The root surface is thoroughly scaled and planed, the flaps are returned to position, all exposed bone is covered, and the flap is sutured in place. Periodontal packing is placed. Report D4240 for a gingival flap procedure with root planing performed in each quadrant on four or more contiguous teeth or bounded teeth spaces and D4241 for one to three teeth per quadrant.

## Coding Tips

Use these codes to report gingival curettage. Local anesthesia is included in these services. Any evaluation or radiograph is reported separately. Pathology exam of tissue with interpretation is reported separately. Usual postoperative care is included in these services.

## Documentation Tips

Third-party payers may require periodontal charting. Periodontal charting should include the identification of the quadrants and sites involved, a minimum of three pocket measurements per tooth involved, indication of recession, furcation involvement, mobility and mucogingival defects, and identification of missing teeth.

## Reimbursement Tips

When selecting the procedure or service that accurately identifies the service performed, dentists must use the most accurate code. If the CDT code more accurately identifies the service, this should be used rather than the CPT codes. Many payers will not separately reimburse the following services when performed by the same provider, on the same date of service, and at the same surgical site: biopsy (D7285–D7286), frenulectomy (D7960), and/or excision of hard and soft tissue lesions (D7410–D7411, D7450–D7451). When one or more of the above services are provided on a different date of service, a narrative indicating the medical necessity of separating the services should be provided; otherwise, payers may deny those services.

## Associated CPT Codes

41870 Periodontal mucosal grafting

## ICD-10-CM Diagnostic Codes

| | |
|---|---|
| K05.00 | Acute gingivitis, plaque induced |
| K05.01 | Acute gingivitis, non-plaque induced |
| K05.10 | Chronic gingivitis, plaque induced |
| K05.11 | Chronic gingivitis, non-plaque induced |
| K06.011 | Localized gingival recession, minimal |
| K06.012 | Localized gingival recession, moderate |
| K06.013 | Localized gingival recession, severe |
| K06.021 | Generalized gingival recession, minimal |
| K06.022 | Generalized gingival recession, moderate |
| K06.023 | Generalized gingival recession, severe |
| K06.1 | Gingival enlargement |
| K06.2 | Gingival and edentulous alveolar ridge lesions associated with trauma |
| K06.8 | Other specified disorders of gingiva and edentulous alveolar ridge |

## Relative Value Units/Medicare Edits

| Non-Facility RVU | Work | PE | MP | Total |
|---|---|---|---|---|
| **D4240** | 3.90 | 3.44 | 0.80 | 8.14 |
| **D4241** | 2.46 | 2.17 | 0.51 | 5.14 |
| **Facility RVU** | **Work** | **PE** | **MP** | **Total** |
| **D4240** | 3.90 | 3.44 | 0.80 | 8.14 |
| **D4241** | 2.46 | 2.17 | 0.51 | 5.14 |

| | FUD | Status | MUE | Modifiers | | | | IOM Reference |
|---|---|---|---|---|---|---|---|---|
| **D4240** | N/A | N | - | N/A | N/A | N/A | N/A | None |
| **D4241** | N/A | N | - | N/A | N/A | N/A | N/A | |

* with documentation

# D4245

**D4245** apically positioned flap

*Procedure is used to preserve keratinized gingiva in conjunction with osseous resection and second stage implant procedure. Procedure may also be used to preserve keratinized/attached gingiva during surgical exposure of labially impacted teeth, and may be used during treatment of peri-implantitis.*

## Explanation

An apically positioned flap procedure can be done to remodel the gum line and/or hard tissue for crown lengthening, for root surface debridement, or possible osseous surgery. This flap procedure is designed to deliberately expose alveolar bone, as opposed to other flap procedures, and reposition the flap with post-operative exposure of the root surfaces. It allows for a flap that can be repositioned. An angled, reverse bevel incision is made in the gingiva and the ends are vertically squared with another incision. A split thickness flap converted to full thickness at the bone is created, the flap elevated, and the residual collar of pocket epithelium and granulation tissue around the root surfaces is removed. Some root scaling or planing may be done. The flap is apically repositioned and sutured primarily.

## Coding Tips

Local anesthesia is included in this service. Any evaluation or radiograph is reported separately. Pathology exam of tissue with interpretation is reported separately.

## Documentation Tips

Third-party payers may require periodontal charting. Periodontal charting should include the identification of the quadrants and sites involved, a minimum of three pocket measurements per tooth involved, indication of recession, furcation involvement, mobility and mucogingival defects, and identification of missing teeth.

## Reimbursement Tips

When selecting the procedure or service that accurately identifies the service performed, dentists must use the most accurate code. If the CDT code more accurately identifies the service, this should be used rather than the CPT codes. Many payers will not separately reimburse the following services when performed by the same provider, on the same date of service, and at the same surgical site: biopsy (D7285–D7286), frenulectomy (D7960), and/or excision of hard and soft tissue lesions (D7410–D7411, D7450–D7451). When one or more of the above services are provided on a different date of service, a narrative indicating the medical necessity of separating the services should be provided; otherwise, payers may deny those services.

## Associated CPT Codes

41870 Periodontal mucosal grafting

## ICD-10-CM Diagnostic Codes

K05.00 Acute gingivitis, plaque induced
K05.01 Acute gingivitis, non-plaque induced
K05.10 Chronic gingivitis, plaque induced
K05.11 Chronic gingivitis, non-plaque induced
K06.011 Localized gingival recession, minimal
K06.012 Localized gingival recession, moderate
K06.013 Localized gingival recession, severe
K06.021 Generalized gingival recession, minimal
K06.022 Generalized gingival recession, moderate
K06.023 Generalized gingival recession, severe
K06.1 Gingival enlargement
K06.2 Gingival and edentulous alveolar ridge lesions associated with trauma
K06.8 Other specified disorders of gingiva and edentulous alveolar ridge

## Relative Value Units/Medicare Edits

| Non-Facility RVU | Work | PE | MP | Total |
|---|---|---|---|---|
| D4245 | 3.27 | 2.88 | 0.67 | 6.82 |
| **Facility RVU** | **Work** | **PE** | **MP** | **Total** |
| D4245 | 3.27 | 2.88 | 0.67 | 6.82 |

| | FUD | Status | MUE | Modifiers | | | | IOM Reference |
|---|---|---|---|---|---|---|---|---|
| D4245 | N/A | N | - | N/A | N/A | N/A | N/A | None |

* with documentation

## Terms To Know

**anatomical crown.** Portion of a tooth covered by enamel.

**clinical crown.** Part of the tooth that is not covered by any supporting structures such as the gums.

**flap graft.** Mass of flesh and skin partially excised from its location but retaining its blood supply, grafted onto another site to repair adjacent or distant defects.

**gingiva.** Soft tissues surrounding the crowns of unerupted teeth and necks of erupted teeth.

**gingivitis.** Inflamed gingiva (oral mucosa) that surrounds the teeth.

**gingivoplasty.** Repair or reconstruction of the gum tissue, altering the gingival contours by excising areas of gum tissue or making incisions through the gingiva to create a gingival flap.

# D4249

**D4249** clinical crown lengthening - hard tissue

*This procedure is employed to allow a restorative procedure on a tooth with little or no tooth structure exposed to the oral cavity. Crown lengthening requires reflection of a full thickness flap and removal of bone, altering the crown to root ratio. It is performed in a healthy periodontal environment, as opposed to osseous surgery, which is performed in the presence of periodontal disease.*

## Explanation

Crown lengthening is performed, which involves reshaping the underlying bone tissue so that more of the hard tissue of the natural tooth is exposed. A local anesthetic is administered. An incision is made around the tooth that requires lengthening. The gum tissue is peeled back from the tooth. The length of the exposed tooth is evaluated to determine whether it is long enough to perform the necessary restorative procedure. If there is not enough healthy tooth available, the bone around the tooth is removed until the dentist achieves the necessary length. The gums are placed over the remaining bone and sutured closed. The gums are allowed to heal for approximately six weeks before beginning the restorative work. Crown lengthening may be required if a tooth is decayed or broken below the gum line or has insufficient tooth structure for restoration with a crown or bridge.

## Coding Tips

Local anesthesia is generally considered to be part of periodontal procedures. This code reports the procedure, as well as the usual postoperative care. For crown lengthening focused upon removal of soft tissue, see D4231. This procedure includes distal wedge performed in the same area on the same date of service.

## Reimbursement Tips

Some payers may require that x-rays and/or x-ray reports be submitted with the claim.

## ICD-10-CM Diagnostic Codes

| | |
|---|---|
| K00.2 | Abnormalities of size and form of teeth |
| K00.4 | Disturbances in tooth formation |
| K00.5 | Hereditary disturbances in tooth structure, not elsewhere classified |
| K00.8 | Other disorders of tooth development |
| K01.0 | Embedded teeth |
| K01.1 | Impacted teeth |
| K02.53 | Dental caries on pit and fissure surface penetrating into pulp |
| K02.63 | Dental caries on smooth surface penetrating into pulp |
| K02.7 | Dental root caries |
| K03.0 | Excessive attrition of teeth |
| K03.1 | Abrasion of teeth |
| K03.2 | Erosion of teeth |
| K03.3 | Pathological resorption of teeth |
| K03.5 | Ankylosis of teeth |

## Relative Value Units/Medicare Edits

| Non-Facility RVU | Work | PE | MP | Total |
|---|---|---|---|---|
| **D4249** | 4.13 | 3.65 | 0.85 | 8.63 |
| **Facility RVU** | **Work** | **PE** | **MP** | **Total** |
| **D4249** | 4.13 | 3.65 | 0.85 | 8.63 |

| | FUD | Status | MUE | Modifiers | | | | IOM Reference |
|---|---|---|---|---|---|---|---|---|
| **D4249** | N/A | N | - | N/A | N/A | N/A | N/A | None |

* with documentation

## Terms To Know

**clinical crown.** Part of the tooth that is not covered by any supporting structures such as the gums.

**flap.** Mass of flesh and skin partially excised from its location but retaining its blood supply that is moved to another site to repair adjacent or distant defects.

**flap rotation.** Flap of skin is incised in a circular manner, leaving the existing blood flow to the skin intact, and then turned to cover the defect area or wound.

# D4260-D4261

**D4260** osseous surgery (including elevation of a full thickness flap and closure) - four or more contiguous teeth or tooth bounded spaces per quadrant

*This procedure modifies the bony support of the teeth by reshaping the alveolar process to achieve a more physiologic form during the surgical procedure. This must include the removal of supporting bone (ostectomy) and/or non-supporting bone (osteoplasty). Other procedures may be required concurrent to D4260 and should be reported using their own unique codes.*

**D4261** osseous surgery (including elevation of a full thickness flap and closure) - one to three contiguous teeth or tooth bounded spaces per quadrant

*This procedure modifies the bony support of the teeth by reshaping the alveolar process to achieve a more physiologic form during the surgical procedure. This must include the removal of supporting bone (ostectomy) and/or non-supporting bone (osteoplasty). Other procedures may be required concurrent to D4261 and should be reported using their own unique codes.*

## Explanation

When osseous surgery, such as bone margin recontouring, remodeling of the alveolar crest, or bone excision (ostectomy), is done, a full-thickness flap, such as an apically repositioned flap deliberately designed to expose alveolar bone, is first made in the gingiva to gain access to the bone. A beveled incision is made along the gum line and relieved with vertical incisions at the ends. The flap in incised down toward the bone and elevated. Any pocket epithelium to be removed is excised and the osseous part of the procedure is then performed on the exposed bone. The flap is repositioned as desired and sutured for primary closure. The flap entry and closure is included in these osseous surgery codes. Report D4260 for four or more contiguous teeth or bounded teeth spaces per quadrant and D4261 for one to three teeth per quadrant.

## Coding Tips

Local anesthesia is included in these services. Any evaluation or radiograph is reported separately. Pathology exam of tissue with interpretation is reported separately. Check with payers for their specific requirements. These codes include postoperative care. These codes include frenulectomy, root planing and scaling, osseous contouring, distal or proximal wedge surgery, soft tissue grafts, gingivectomy, and flap procedures.

## Documentation Tips

Third-party payers may require periodontal charting. Periodontal charting should include the identification of the quadrants and sites involved, a minimum of three pocket measurements per tooth involved, indication of recession, furcation involvement, mobility and mucogingival defects, and identification of missing teeth.

## Reimbursement Tips

Many payers will not separately reimburse the following services when performed by the same provider, on the same date of service, and at the same surgical site: biopsy (D7285–D7286), frenulectomy (D7960), and/or excision of hard and soft tissue lesions (D7410–D7411, D7450–D7451). When one or more of the above services are provided on a different date of service, a narrative indicating the medical necessity of separating the services should be provided; otherwise, payers may deny those services.

## Associated CPT Codes

41823 Excision of osseous tuberosities, dentoalveolar structures

## ICD-10-CM Diagnostic Codes

| | |
|---|---|
| K08.21 | Minimal atrophy of the mandible |
| K08.22 | Moderate atrophy of the mandible |
| K08.23 | Severe atrophy of the mandible |
| K08.24 | Minimal atrophy of maxilla |
| K08.25 | Moderate atrophy of the maxilla |
| K08.26 | Severe atrophy of the maxilla |
| Q38.6 | Other congenital malformations of mouth |
| Q78.2 | Osteopetrosis |
| S02.5XXA | Fracture of tooth (traumatic), initial encounter for closed fracture |
| S02.5XXB | Fracture of tooth (traumatic), initial encounter for open fracture |
| S03.2XXA | Dislocation of tooth, initial encounter |

## Relative Value Units/Medicare Edits

| Non-Facility RVU | Work | PE | MP | Total |
|---|---|---|---|---|
| **D4260** | 6.32 | 5.58 | 1.30 | 13.20 |
| **D4261** | 3.70 | 3.27 | 0.76 | 7.73 |
| **Facility RVU** | **Work** | **PE** | **MP** | **Total** |
| **D4260** | 6.32 | 5.58 | 1.30 | 13.20 |
| **D4261** | 3.70 | 3.27 | 0.76 | 7.73 |

| | FUD | Status | MUE | Modifiers | | | | IOM Reference |
|---|---|---|---|---|---|---|---|---|
| **D4260** | N/A | R | - | N/A | N/A | N/A | 80* | None |
| **D4261** | N/A | N | - | N/A | N/A | N/A | N/A | |

* with documentation

## Terms To Know

**flap graft.** Mass of flesh and skin partially excised from its location but retaining its blood supply, grafted onto another site to repair adjacent or distant defects.

**ostectomy.** Excision of bone.

**tooth bounded space.** Empty space in the mouth due to a missing tooth that is surrounded by a tooth on each side.

# D4263-D4264

**D4263** bone replacement graft - retained natural tooth - first site in quadrant

*This procedure involves the use of grafts to stimulate periodontal regeneration when the disease process has led to a deformity of the bone. This procedure does not include flap entry and closure, wound debridement, osseous contouring, or the placement of biologic materials to aid in osseous tissue regeneration or barrier membranes. Other separate procedures delivered concurrently are documented with their own codes. Not to be reported for an edentulous space or an extraction site.*

**D4264** bone replacement graft - retained natural tooth - each additional site in quadrant

*This procedure involves the use of grafts to stimulate periodontal regeneration when the disease process has led to a deformity of the bone. This procedure does not include flap entry and closure, wound debridement, osseous contouring, or the placement of biologic materials to aid in osseous tissue regeneration or barrier membranes. This procedure is performed concurrently with one or more bone replacement grafts to document the number of sites involved. Not to be reported for an edentulous space or an extraction site.*

## Explanation

A bone replacement graft is used to replace damaged, atrophic, or excised bone. Incisions are made down through the soft tissue to expose the recipient site for the bone replacement graft and the graft is placed into position. The graft may be packed firmly into position or secured by other methods. The incisions are then sutured closed. Report D4263 for the first site in a quadrant and D4264 for each additional site in the quadrant on the same day of service.

## Coding Tips

Any radiograph is reported separately. Report D4264 in addition to D4263 as it cannot be reported alone. These codes include postoperative care.

## Documentation Tips

Periodontal charting should include the identification of the quadrants and sites involved, a minimum of three pocket measurements per tooth involved, indication of recession, furcation involvement, mobility and mucogingival defects, and identification of missing teeth. Check with payers for their specific requirements.

## Reimbursement Tips

When selecting the procedure or service that accurately identifies the service performed, dentists must use the most accurate code. If the CDT code more accurately identifies the service, this should be used rather than the CPT codes. Third-party payers may require submission of x-rays or x-ray reports and periodontal charting. Many payers will not separately reimburse the following services when performed by the same provider, on the same date of service, and at the same surgical site: biopsy (D7285–D7286), frenulectomy (D7960), and/or excision of hard and soft tissue lesions (D7410–D7411, D7450–D7451). When one or more of the above services are provided on a different date of service, a narrative indicating the medical necessity of separating the services should be provided; otherwise, payers may deny those services.

## Associated CPT Codes

| | |
|---|---|
| 21210 | Graft, bone; nasal, maxillary or malar areas (includes obtaining graft) |
| 21215 | Graft, bone; mandible (includes obtaining graft) |

## ICD-10-CM Diagnostic Codes

| | |
|---|---|
| K08.51 | Open restoration margins of tooth |
| K08.530 | Fractured dental restorative material without loss of material |
| K08.531 | Fractured dental restorative material with loss of material |
| K08.54 | Contour of existing restoration of tooth biologically incompatible with oral health |
| K08.55 | Allergy to existing dental restorative material |
| K08.56 | Poor aesthetic of existing restoration of tooth |
| M27.1 | Giant cell granuloma, central |
| M27.2 | Inflammatory conditions of jaws |
| M27.61 | Osseointegration failure of dental implant |
| M27.62 | Post-osseointegration biological failure of dental implant |
| M27.63 | Post-osseointegration mechanical failure of dental implant |
| S02.5XXA | Fracture of tooth (traumatic), initial encounter for closed fracture |
| S02.5XXB | Fracture of tooth (traumatic), initial encounter for open fracture |
| T85.79XA | Infection and inflammatory reaction due to other internal prosthetic devices, implants and grafts, initial encounter |

## Relative Value Units/Medicare Edits

| Non-Facility RVU | Work | PE | MP | Total |
|---|---|---|---|---|
| **D4263** | 2.57 | 2.27 | 0.53 | 5.37 |
| **D4264** | 2.16 | 1.91 | 0.45 | 4.52 |
| **Facility RVU** | **Work** | **PE** | **MP** | **Total** |
| **D4263** | 2.57 | 2.27 | 0.53 | 5.37 |
| **D4264** | 2.16 | 1.91 | 0.45 | 4.52 |

| | FUD | Status | MUE | Modifiers | | | | IOM Reference |
|---|---|---|---|---|---|---|---|---|
| **D4263** | N/A | R | - | N/A | N/A | N/A | 80* | 100-02,1,70; 100-04,4,20.5 |
| **D4264** | N/A | R | - | N/A | N/A | N/A | 80* | |

* with documentation

## Terms To Know

**contour.** Act of shaping along desired lines.

**flap graft.** Mass of flesh and skin partially excised from its location but retaining its blood supply, grafted onto another site to repair adjacent or distant defects.

**ostectomy.** Excision of bone.

Dental - Periodontics

# D4265

▲ **D4265** biologic materials to aid in soft and osseous tissue regeneration, per site

*Biologic materials may be used alone or with other regenerative substrates such as bone and barrier membranes, depending upon their formulation and the presentation of the periodontal defect. This procedure does not include surgical entry and closure, wound debridement, osseous contouring, or the placement of graft materials and/or barrier membranes. Other separate procedures may be required concurrent to D4265 and should be reported using their own unique codes.*

## Explanation

Biological materials that aid in soft tissue and osseous tissue regeneration are used as an adjunct to periodontal surgery. One type of biological material approved for this purpose is enamel matrix derivative (EMD). EMD contains a variety of hydrophobic enamel matrix proteins that have been extracted from the developing embryonic enamel of porcine teeth. EMD is applied topically onto exposed root surfaces to treat infrabony defects resulting from the loss of tooth support due to moderate or severe periodontitis. EMD or other biologic materials may be used alone or in combination with autografts, allografts, xenografts, or guided tissue regeneration (GTR). Other regenerative substrates, such as bone and barrier membranes, may also be used in conjunction with biologic materials.

## Coding Tips

Local anesthesia is generally considered to be part of periodontal procedures. This procedure does not include surgical entry and closure, wound debridement, osseous contouring, or the placement of graft materials and/or barrier membranes, which may be reported separately as appropriate with D4240, D4241, D4260, D4261, D4263, D4264, D4266, and/or D4267. These codes include postoperative care.

## Documentation Tips

Periodontal charting should include the identification of the quadrants and sites involved, a minimum of three pocket measurements per tooth involved, indication of recession, furcation involvement, mobility and mucogingival defects, and identification of missing teeth. Check with payers for their specific requirements.

## Reimbursement Tips

Many payers will not separately reimburse the following services when performed by the same provider, on the same date of service, and at the same surgical site: biopsy (D7285–D7286), frenulectomy (D7960), and/or excision of hard and soft tissue lesions (D7410–D7411, D7450–D7451). When one or more of the above services are provided on a different date of service, a narrative indicating the medical necessity of separating the services should be provided; otherwise, payers may deny those services.

## ICD-10-CM Diagnostic Codes

K08.51 Open restoration margins of tooth
K08.530 Fractured dental restorative material without loss of material
K08.531 Fractured dental restorative material with loss of material
K08.54 Contour of existing restoration of tooth biologically incompatible with oral health
K08.55 Allergy to existing dental restorative material
K08.56 Poor aesthetic of existing restoration of tooth
K08.59 Other unsatisfactory restoration of tooth
M27.1 Giant cell granuloma, central
M27.2 Inflammatory conditions of jaws
M27.61 Osseointegration failure of dental implant
M27.62 Post-osseointegration biological failure of dental implant
M27.63 Post-osseointegration mechanical failure of dental implant
S02.5XXA Fracture of tooth (traumatic), initial encounter for closed fracture
S02.5XXB Fracture of tooth (traumatic), initial encounter for open fracture
T85.79XA Infection and inflammatory reaction due to other internal prosthetic devices, implants and grafts, initial encounter

## Relative Value Units/Medicare Edits

| Non-Facility RVU | Work | PE | MP | Total |
|---|---|---|---|---|
| D4265 | 1.50 | 1.33 | 0.31 | 3.14 |
| Facility RVU | Work | PE | MP | Total |
| D4265 | 1.50 | 1.33 | 0.31 | 3.14 |

| | FUD | Status | MUE | Modifiers | | | | IOM Reference |
|---|---|---|---|---|---|---|---|---|
| D4265 | N/A | N | - | N/A | N/A | N/A | N/A | None |

* with documentation

## Terms To Know

**osseous.** Related to, consisting of, or resembling bone.

**periodontal.** Relating to the tissues that support and surround the teeth.

**regeneration.** Process of reproducing or regrowing tissue.

**tissue.** Group of similar cells with a similar function that form definite structures and organs. Tissue types include epithelial tissue, which lines the outside of the body and the inner surface of internal organs; muscle tissue, which can be voluntary (found in skeletal muscle) or involuntary (found in the heart and digestive system); connective tissue, such as fat, cartilage, bone, or blood; and nervous tissue.

# D4266-D4267

**D4266** guided tissue regeneration - resorbable barrier, per site

*This procedure does not include flap entry and closure, or, when indicated, wound debridement, osseous contouring, bone replacement grafts, and placement of biologic materials to aid in osseous regeneration. This procedure can be used for periodontal and peri-implant defects.*

**D4267** guided tissue regeneration - nonresorbable barrier, per site (includes membrane removal)

*This procedure does not include flap entry and closure, or, when indicated, wound debridement, osseous contouring, bone replacement grafts, and placement of biologic materials to aid in osseous regeneration. This procedure can be used for periodontal and peri-implant defects.*

## Explanation

After periodontal surgery, new connective tissue attachment is prevented by epithelial tissue migration along the root surface. To prevent the epithelium from migrating, a barrier is put in place before completing the procedure. Guided tissue regeneration is placement of this barrier. Gortex membranes are commonly used for a nonresorbable barrier in D4267. After the particular defect has been infilled, the membrane is placed to cover the infill material. The Gortex must be removed after a few weeks. In D4266, biocompatible resorbable materials, such as Vicryl or Resolute (lyophilized collagen), are used as the barrier and require only one operation. Biological materials that aid in soft and osseous tissue regeneration (D4265) may also be placed. Tissue growth factor and bone morphogenic protein can stimulate the deposition of new connective tissue and bone. Emdogain is a solution that contains enamel matrix derivative proteins and helps form acellular cementum. After surgical access to the root surface is gained and the cementum is cleaned, the solution containing the enamel matrix derivative proteins is applied before the flaps are repositioned and sutured.

## Coding Tips

These codes may be reported for the treatment of periodontal and peri-implant defects. Local anesthesia is included in these services. Any radiograph is reported separately. Removal of tissue for examination is reported separately. These codes include postoperative care. Flap entry, closure, wound debridement, osseous contouring, bone replacement grafts, and placement of biologic materials to aid in osseous regeneration are not included and may be reported separately.

## Documentation Tips

Periodontal charting should include the identification of the quadrants and sites involved, a minimum of three pocket measurements per tooth involved, indication of recession, furcation involvement, mobility and mucogingival defects, and identification of missing teeth. Check with payers for their specific requirements.

## Reimbursement Tips

Third-party payers may require submission of x-rays or x-ray reports and periodontal charting.

## ICD-10-CM Diagnostic Codes

| | |
|---|---|
| K08.51 | Open restoration margins of tooth |
| K08.530 | Fractured dental restorative material without loss of material |
| K08.531 | Fractured dental restorative material with loss of material |
| K08.54 | Contour of existing restoration of tooth biologically incompatible with oral health |
| K08.55 | Allergy to existing dental restorative material |
| K08.56 | Poor aesthetic of existing restoration of tooth |
| M27.1 | Giant cell granuloma, central |
| M27.2 | Inflammatory conditions of jaws |
| M27.61 | Osseointegration failure of dental implant |
| M27.62 | Post-osseointegration biological failure of dental implant |
| M27.63 | Post-osseointegration mechanical failure of dental implant |
| S02.5XXA | Fracture of tooth (traumatic), initial encounter for closed fracture |
| S02.5XXB | Fracture of tooth (traumatic), initial encounter for open fracture |
| T85.79XA | Infection and inflammatory reaction due to other internal prosthetic devices, implants and grafts, initial encounter |

## Relative Value Units/Medicare Edits

| Non-Facility RVU | Work | PE | MP | Total |
|---|---|---|---|---|
| **D4266** | 2.98 | 2.63 | 0.61 | 6.22 |
| **D4267** | 3.68 | 3.25 | 0.76 | 7.69 |
| **Facility RVU** | **Work** | **PE** | **MP** | **Total** |
| **D4266** | 2.98 | 2.63 | 0.61 | 6.22 |
| **D4267** | 3.68 | 3.25 | 0.76 | 7.69 |

| | FUD | Status | MUE | Modifiers | | | | IOM Reference |
|---|---|---|---|---|---|---|---|---|
| **D4266** | N/A | N | - | N/A | N/A | N/A | N/A | None |
| **D4267** | N/A | N | - | N/A | N/A | N/A | N/A | |

* with documentation

## Terms To Know

**connective tissue.** Body tissue made from fibroblasts, collagen, and elastic fibrils that connects, supports, and holds together other tissues and cells and includes cartilage, collagenous, fibrous, elastic, and osseous tissue.

**regeneration.** Process of reproducing or regrowing tissue.

# D4268

**D4268** surgical revision procedure, per tooth

*This procedure is to refine the results of a previously provided surgical procedure. This may require a surgical procedure to modify the irregular contours of hard or soft tissue. A mucoperiosteal flap may be elevated to allow access to reshape alveolar bone. The flaps are replaced or repositioned and sutured.*

## Explanation

A surgical revision procedure is performed to refine the results of a previous periodontal surgical intervention. The exact nature of the surgical procedure performed is determined by the current problem, as well as the type of previous surgical intervention. One example of a revision that would be reported with D4268 is a surgical procedure to modify the irregular contours of hard or soft tissue. Another example would be elevation of a mucoperiosteal flap for reshaping of the alveolar bone. Because the exact nature of the procedure may vary significantly, documentation should be submitted to describe the procedure and to support medical necessity. This code is reported per tooth.

## Coding Tips

Local anesthesia is generally considered to be part of periodontal procedures. This code is reported once per tooth. These codes include postoperative care.

## Documentation Tips

Periodontal charting should include the identification of the quadrants and sites involved, a minimum of three pocket measurements per tooth involved, indication of recession, furcation involvement, mobility and mucogingival defects, and identification of missing teeth. Check with payers for their specific requirements.

## Reimbursement Tips

Many payers will not separately reimburse the following services when performed by the same provider, on the same date of service, and at the same surgical site: biopsy (D7285–D7286), frenulectomy (D7960), and/or excision of hard and soft tissue lesions (D7410–D7411, D7450–D7451). When one or more of the above services are provided on a different date of service, a narrative indicating the medical necessity of separating the services should be provided; otherwise, payers may deny those services.

## ICD-10-CM Diagnostic Codes

| | |
|---|---|
| K08.51 | Open restoration margins of tooth |
| K08.530 | Fractured dental restorative material without loss of material |
| K08.531 | Fractured dental restorative material with loss of material |
| K08.54 | Contour of existing restoration of tooth biologically incompatible with oral health |
| K08.55 | Allergy to existing dental restorative material |
| K08.56 | Poor aesthetic of existing restoration of tooth |
| M27.1 | Giant cell granuloma, central |
| M27.2 | Inflammatory conditions of jaws |
| M27.61 | Osseointegration failure of dental implant |
| M27.62 | Post-osseointegration biological failure of dental implant |
| M27.63 | Post-osseointegration mechanical failure of dental implant |
| S02.5XXA | Fracture of tooth (traumatic), initial encounter for closed fracture |
| S02.5XXB | Fracture of tooth (traumatic), initial encounter for open fracture |
| T85.79XA | Infection and inflammatory reaction due to other internal prosthetic devices, implants and grafts, initial encounter |

## Relative Value Units/Medicare Edits

| Non-Facility RVU | Work | PE | MP | Total |
|---|---|---|---|---|
| **D4268** | 3.03 | 2.68 | 0.62 | 6.33 |
| **Facility RVU** | **Work** | **PE** | **MP** | **Total** |
| **D4268** | 3.03 | 2.68 | 0.62 | 6.33 |

| | FUD | Status | MUE | Modifiers | | | | IOM Reference |
|---|---|---|---|---|---|---|---|---|
| **D4268** | N/A | R | - | N/A | N/A | N/A | N/A | 100-02,1,70; 100-04,4,20.5 |

* with documentation

## Terms To Know

**alveolar process.** Bony part of the maxilla or mandible that supports the tooth roots and into which the teeth are implanted.

**periodontal.** Relating to the tissues that support and surround the teeth.

# D4270

**D4270** pedicle soft tissue graft procedure

*A pedicle flap of gingiva can be raised from an edentulous ridge, adjacent teeth, or from the existing gingiva on the tooth and moved laterally or coronally to replace alveolar mucosa as marginal tissue. The procedure can be used to cover an exposed root or to eliminate a gingival defect if the root is not too prominent in the arch.*

## Explanation

A pedicle soft tissue graft procedure is done in the mouth. The dentist uses a pedicle flap to reconstruct defects. A flap is developed in the donor area and rotated to the defect area while the pedicle of the flap remains attached to retain its supporting blood vessels. The flap is sutured to the recipient bed. The dentist repairs the harvest region as needed. Once the recipient site has healed, a second surgery will detach the pedicle and return any unused flap to its anatomic location.

## Coding Tips

Local anesthesia is included in this service. Any radiographs are reported separately. Preparation of recipient site is included. This code includes postoperative care. This code includes frenulectomy and any distal wedge procedure done on the same area on the same date of service.

## Documentation Tips

Third-party payers may require periodontal charting. Periodontal charting should include the identification of the quadrants and sites involved, a minimum of three pocket measurements per tooth involved, indication of recession, furcation involvement, mobility and mucogingival defects, and identification of missing teeth. Check with payers for their specific requirements.

## Reimbursement Tips

When selecting the procedure or service that accurately identifies the service performed, dentists must use the most accurate code. If the CDT code more accurately identifies the service, this should be used rather than the CPT codes. Many payers will not separately reimburse the following services when performed by the same provider, on the same date of service, and at the same surgical site: biopsy (D7285–D7286), frenulectomy (D7960), and/or excision of hard and soft tissue lesions (D7410–D7411, D7450–D7451). When one or more of the above services are provided on a different date of service, a narrative indicating the medical necessity of separating the services should be provided; otherwise, payers may deny those services.

## Associated CPT Codes

15574 Formation of direct or tubed pedicle, with or without transfer; forehead, cheeks, chin, mouth, neck, axillae, genitalia, hands or feet

## ICD-10-CM Diagnostic Codes

C03.0 Malignant neoplasm of upper gum
C03.1 Malignant neoplasm of lower gum
C04.0 Malignant neoplasm of anterior floor of mouth
C04.1 Malignant neoplasm of lateral floor of mouth
C04.8 Malignant neoplasm of overlapping sites of floor of mouth
C05.0 Malignant neoplasm of hard palate
C05.1 Malignant neoplasm of soft palate
C05.2 Malignant neoplasm of uvula
C05.8 Malignant neoplasm of overlapping sites of palate
C06.0 Malignant neoplasm of cheek mucosa
C06.1 Malignant neoplasm of vestibule of mouth
C06.2 Malignant neoplasm of retromolar area
C07 Malignant neoplasm of parotid gland
C08.0 Malignant neoplasm of submandibular gland
C08.1 Malignant neoplasm of sublingual gland
K12.0 Recurrent oral aphthae
K12.2 Cellulitis and abscess of mouth
K13.21 Leukoplakia of oral mucosa, including tongue
K13.22 Minimal keratinized residual ridge mucosa
K13.23 Excessive keratinized residual ridge mucosa
K13.24 Leukokeratosis nicotina palati
K13.3 Hairy leukoplakia
K13.4 Granuloma and granuloma-like lesions of oral mucosa
K13.5 Oral submucous fibrosis
K13.6 Irritative hyperplasia of oral mucosa
K13.79 Other lesions of oral mucosa
K14.0 Glossitis
K14.1 Geographic tongue
K14.2 Median rhomboid glossitis
K14.3 Hypertrophy of tongue papillae
K14.4 Atrophy of tongue papillae
K14.5 Plicated tongue
K14.6 Glossodynia

## Relative Value Units/Medicare Edits

| Non-Facility RVU | Work | PE | MP | Total |
|---|---|---|---|---|
| **D4270** | 4.56 | 4.03 | 0.94 | 9.53 |
| **Facility RVU** | **Work** | **PE** | **MP** | **Total** |
| **D4270** | 4.56 | 4.03 | 0.94 | 9.53 |

| | FUD | Status | MUE | Modifiers | | | | IOM Reference |
|---|---|---|---|---|---|---|---|---|
| **D4270** | N/A | R | - | N/A | N/A | N/A | 80* | 100-02,1,70; 100-04,4,20.5 |

* with documentation

## Terms To Know

**oral reconstruction.** Reforming, recreating, or rebuilding tissues or structures within the mouth following an injury or disease.

**oral soft tissue.** Subcutaneous fat layers beneath oral mucosa or gingiva; excludes bone and teeth.

**pedicle.** Stem-like, narrow base or stalk attached to a new growth.

# D4273, D4283

**D4273** autogenous connective tissue graft procedure (including donor and recipient surgical sites) first tooth, implant, or edentulous tooth position in graft

*There are two surgical sites. The recipient site utilizes a split thickness incision, retaining the overlapping flap of gingiva and/or mucosa. The connective tissue is dissected from a separate donor site leaving an epithelialized flap for closure.*

**D4283** autogenous connective tissue graft procedure (including donor and recipient surgical sites) - each additional contiguous tooth, implant or edentulous tooth position in same graft site

*Used in conjunction with D4273.*

## Explanation

A subepithelial connective tissue graft procedure is performed to create or augment gingiva to obtain root coverage thereby eliminating sensitivity and preventing root caries, to eliminate frenulum pull, to extend the vestibular fornix, to augment collapsed ridges, to provide an adequate gingival interface with a restoration, or to cover bone or ridge regeneration sites when adequate gingival tissues are not available for effective closure. The graft procedure utilizes two surgical sites: the recipient site where the graft will be placed and the donor site where the graft will be harvested. At the recipient site, a split thickness incision is made and the overlying flap of gingiva and mucosa retained. At the donor site, connective tissue is dissected free leaving an epithelialized flap for closure. The graft is placed on the recipient site and covered with the retained overlying flap, which is sutured into place. The donor site is also sutured closed. Report D4273 for the first tooth, implant, or edentulous tooth space and D4283 for each additional contiguous space.

## Coding Tips

Code D4283 is an "out of sequence" code and will not display in numeric order in the CDT manual. Local anesthesia is generally considered to be part of periodontal procedures. Local anesthesia is included in this service. Any radiographs are reported separately. Preparation of recipient site is included. These codes include postoperative care. These codes include frenulectomy, distal wedge procedure(s), and stenting done on the same area on the same date of service.

## Documentation Tips

Periodontal charting should include the identification of the quadrants and sites involved, a minimum of three pocket measurements per tooth involved, indication of recession, furcation involvement, mobility and mucogingival defects, and identification of missing teeth. Check with payers for their specific requirements.

## Reimbursement Tips

When selecting the procedure or service that accurately identifies the service performed, dentists must use the most accurate code. If the CDT code more accurately identifies the service, this should be used rather than the CPT codes. These codes include frenulectomy, distal wedge procedure(s), and stenting done on the same area on the same date of service.

## Associated CPT Codes

41870 Periodontal mucosal grafting

## ICD-10-CM Diagnostic Codes

K05.10 Chronic gingivitis, plaque induced
K05.11 Chronic gingivitis, non-plaque induced
K06.011 Localized gingival recession, minimal
K06.012 Localized gingival recession, moderate
K06.013 Localized gingival recession, severe
K06.021 Generalized gingival recession, minimal
K06.022 Generalized gingival recession, moderate
K06.023 Generalized gingival recession, severe
K06.1 Gingival enlargement
K06.2 Gingival and edentulous alveolar ridge lesions associated with trauma
K08.0 Exfoliation of teeth due to systemic causes
S02.42XA Fracture of alveolus of maxilla, initial encounter for closed fracture
S02.42XB Fracture of alveolus of maxilla, initial encounter for open fracture
S02.5XXA Fracture of tooth (traumatic), initial encounter for closed fracture
S02.5XXB Fracture of tooth (traumatic), initial encounter for open fracture
S07.0XXA Crushing injury of face, initial encounter
S07.1XXA Crushing injury of skull, initial encounter

## Relative Value Units/Medicare Edits

| Non-Facility RVU | Work | PE | MP | Total |
|---|---|---|---|---|
| **D4273** | 5.70 | 5.03 | 1.17 | 11.90 |
| **D4283** | 1.89 | 1.67 | 0.39 | 3.95 |
| **Facility RVU** | **Work** | **PE** | **MP** | **Total** |
| **D4273** | 5.70 | 5.03 | 1.17 | 11.90 |
| **D4283** | 1.89 | 1.67 | 0.39 | 3.95 |

| | FUD | Status | MUE | Modifiers | | | | IOM Reference |
|---|---|---|---|---|---|---|---|---|
| **D4273** | N/A | R | - | N/A | N/A | N/A | 80* | 100-02,1,70; 100-04,4,20.5; None |
| **D4283** | N/A | N | - | N/A | N/A | N/A | N/A | |

* with documentation

## Terms To Know

**gingiva.** Soft tissues surrounding the crowns of unerupted teeth and necks of erupted teeth.

**periodontal.** Relating to the tissues that support and surround the teeth.

# D4274

**D4274** mesial/distal wedge procedure, single tooth (when not performed in conjunction with surgical procedures in the same anatomical area)

*This procedure is performed in an edentulous area adjacent to a tooth, allowing removal of a tissue wedge to gain access for debridement, permit close flap adaptation, and reduce pocket depths.*

## Explanation

A distal or proximal wedge procedure is performed in an edentulous area adjacent to the periodontally involved tooth. An anesthetic is administered. The dentist makes a gingival incision and removes a tissue wedge to gain access to the underlying osseous defect. The osseous defect is corrected and the gingival tissue closed with sutures.

## Coding Tips

Local anesthesia is generally considered to be part of periodontal procedures. Most payers feel that this procedure is included in more complex services and when performed at the time of a more complex procedure is not separately reimbursed. Check with individual payers for their specific guidelines.

## Documentation Tips

Periodontal charting should include the identification of the quadrants and sites involved, a minimum of three pocket measurements per tooth involved, indication of recession, furcation involvement, mobility and mucogingival defects, and identification of missing teeth.

## Reimbursement Tips

Coverage may be available through the patient's medical insurance for this service. Check with third-party payers for specific coverage information. Services submitted to the medical coverage will require that the service be reported with the appropriate CPT code on a CMS-1500 claim form.

## ICD-10-CM Diagnostic Codes

K05.00 Acute gingivitis, plaque induced
K05.01 Acute gingivitis, non-plaque induced
K05.10 Chronic gingivitis, plaque induced
K05.11 Chronic gingivitis, non-plaque induced
K05.221 Aggressive periodontitis, generalized, slight
K05.222 Aggressive periodontitis, generalized, moderate
K05.223 Aggressive periodontitis, generalized, severe
K05.311 Chronic periodontitis, localized, slight
K05.312 Chronic periodontitis, localized, moderate
K05.313 Chronic periodontitis, localized, severe
K05.321 Chronic periodontitis, generalized, slight
K05.322 Chronic periodontitis, generalized, moderate
K05.323 Chronic periodontitis, generalized, severe
K05.4 Periodontosis
K05.5 Other periodontal diseases
K05.6 Periodontal disease, unspecified
K06.011 Localized gingival recession, minimal
K06.012 Localized gingival recession, moderate
K06.013 Localized gingival recession, severe
K06.021 Generalized gingival recession, minimal
K06.022 Generalized gingival recession, moderate
K06.023 Generalized gingival recession, severe
K06.1 Gingival enlargement
K06.2 Gingival and edentulous alveolar ridge lesions associated with trauma
K06.8 Other specified disorders of gingiva and edentulous alveolar ridge
S02.42XA Fracture of alveolus of maxilla, initial encounter for closed fracture
S02.42XB Fracture of alveolus of maxilla, initial encounter for open fracture
S02.5XXA Fracture of tooth (traumatic), initial encounter for closed fracture
S02.5XXB Fracture of tooth (traumatic), initial encounter for open fracture
S07.0XXA Crushing injury of face, initial encounter
S07.1XXA Crushing injury of skull, initial encounter

## Relative Value Units/Medicare Edits

| Non-Facility RVU | Work | PE | MP | Total |
|---|---|---|---|---|
| **D4274** | 3.30 | 2.92 | 0.68 | 6.90 |
| **Facility RVU** | **Work** | **PE** | **MP** | **Total** |
| **D4274** | 3.30 | 2.92 | 0.68 | 6.90 |

| | FUD | Status | MUE | Modifiers | | | | IOM Reference |
|---|---|---|---|---|---|---|---|---|
| **D4274** | N/A | N | - | N/A | N/A | N/A | N/A | None |

* with documentation

## Terms To Know

**gingiva.** Soft tissues surrounding the crowns of unerupted teeth and necks of erupted teeth.

**osseous.** Related to, consisting of, or resembling bone.

**periodontal.** Relating to the tissues that support and surround the teeth.

# D4275, D4285

**D4275** non-autogenous connective tissue graft (including recipient site and donor material) first tooth, implant, or edentulous tooth position in graft

*There is only a recipient surgical site utilizing split thickness incision, retaining the overlaying flap of gingiva and/or mucosa. A donor surgical site is not present.*

**D4285** non-autogenous connective tissue graft procedure (including recipient surgical site and donor material) - each additional contiguous tooth, implant or edentulous tooth position in same graft site

*Used in conjunction with D4275.*

## Explanation

The surgeon performs a soft tissue allograft procedure and takes soft tissue harvested from a suitable donor or cadaver, not from the patient, and grafts it to the recipient area in the patient's mouth (i.e., around the teeth to repair areas of gingival recession). After preparing the recipient site, the dentist sutures the free allograft in the area needing repair.

## Coding Tips

Code D4285 is an "out of sequence" code and will not display in numeric order in the CDT manual. Local anesthesia is generally considered to be part of periodontal procedures. Local anesthesia is included in this service. Any radiographs are reported separately. Preparation of recipient site is included. These codes include postoperative care. These codes include frenulectomy, distal wedge procedure(s), and stenting done on the same area on the same date of service. Report D4275 for the first tooth, implant or edentulous tooth space and D4285 for each contiguous space.

## Documentation Tips

Periodontal charting should include the identification of the quadrants and sites involved, a minimum of three pocket measurements per tooth involved, indication of recession, furcation involvement, mobility and mucogingival defects, and identification of missing teeth. Check with payers for their specific requirements.

## Reimbursement Tips

When selecting the procedure or service that accurately identifies the service performed, dentists must use the most accurate code. If the CDT code more accurately identifies the service, this should be used rather than the CPT codes. This procedure may be covered by the patient's medical insurance. When covered by medical insurance, the payer may require that the appropriate CPT code be reported on the CMS-1500 claim form. Many payers will not separately reimburse the following services when performed by the same provider, on the same date of service, and at the same surgical site: biopsy (D7285–D7286), frenulectomy (D7960), and/or excision of hard and soft tissue lesions (D7410–D7411, D7450–D7451). When one or more of the above services are provided on a different date of service, a narrative indicating the medical necessity of separating the services should be provided; otherwise; payers may deny those services.

## Associated CPT Codes

41870 Periodontal mucosal grafting

## ICD-10-CM Diagnostic Codes

C03.0 Malignant neoplasm of upper gum
C03.1 Malignant neoplasm of lower gum
C04.0 Malignant neoplasm of anterior floor of mouth
C04.1 Malignant neoplasm of lateral floor of mouth
C04.8 Malignant neoplasm of overlapping sites of floor of mouth
C05.0 Malignant neoplasm of hard palate
C05.1 Malignant neoplasm of soft palate
C05.2 Malignant neoplasm of uvula
C05.8 Malignant neoplasm of overlapping sites of palate
C06.0 Malignant neoplasm of cheek mucosa
C06.1 Malignant neoplasm of vestibule of mouth
C06.2 Malignant neoplasm of retromolar area
C07 Malignant neoplasm of parotid gland
C08.0 Malignant neoplasm of submandibular gland
C08.1 Malignant neoplasm of sublingual gland
K05.00 Acute gingivitis, plaque induced
K05.01 Acute gingivitis, non-plaque induced
K05.10 Chronic gingivitis, plaque induced
K05.11 Chronic gingivitis, non-plaque induced
K05.221 Aggressive periodontitis, generalized, slight
K05.222 Aggressive periodontitis, generalized, moderate
K05.223 Aggressive periodontitis, generalized, severe
K05.311 Chronic periodontitis, localized, slight
K05.312 Chronic periodontitis, localized, moderate
K05.313 Chronic periodontitis, localized, severe
K05.321 Chronic periodontitis, generalized, slight
K05.322 Chronic periodontitis, generalized, moderate
K05.323 Chronic periodontitis, generalized, severe
K05.4 Periodontosis
K06.011 Localized gingival recession, minimal
K06.012 Localized gingival recession, moderate
K06.013 Localized gingival recession, severe
K06.021 Generalized gingival recession, minimal
K06.022 Generalized gingival recession, moderate
K06.023 Generalized gingival recession, severe
K06.1 Gingival enlargement
K06.2 Gingival and edentulous alveolar ridge lesions associated with trauma
K12.0 Recurrent oral aphthae
K13.3 Hairy leukoplakia
K13.4 Granuloma and granuloma-like lesions of oral mucosa
K13.5 Oral submucous fibrosis
K13.6 Irritative hyperplasia of oral mucosa
K14.0 Glossitis
K14.1 Geographic tongue
K14.2 Median rhomboid glossitis
K14.5 Plicated tongue
K14.6 Glossodynia
S02.42XA Fracture of alveolus of maxilla, initial encounter for closed fracture
S02.42XB Fracture of alveolus of maxilla, initial encounter for open fracture
S02.5XXA Fracture of tooth (traumatic), initial encounter for closed fracture
S02.5XXB Fracture of tooth (traumatic), initial encounter for open fracture
S07.0XXA Crushing injury of face, initial encounter
S07.1XXA Crushing injury of skull, initial encounter

## Relative Value Units/Medicare Edits

| Non-Facility RVU | Work | PE | MP | Total |
|---|---|---|---|---|
| D4275 | 4.43 | 3.91 | 0.91 | 9.25 |
| D4285 | 1.62 | 1.43 | 0.33 | 3.38 |
| **Facility RVU** | **Work** | **PE** | **MP** | **Total** |
| D4275 | 4.43 | 3.91 | 0.91 | 9.25 |
| D4285 | 1.62 | 1.43 | 0.33 | 3.38 |

| | FUD | Status | MUE | Modifiers | | | | IOM Reference |
|---|---|---|---|---|---|---|---|---|
| D4275 | N/A | N | - | N/A | N/A | N/A | N/A | None |
| D4285 | N/A | N | - | N/A | N/A | N/A | N/A | |

* with documentation

## Terms To Know

**allograft.** Graft from one individual to another of the same species.

**harvest.** Removal of cells or tissue from their native site to be used as a graft or transplant to another part of the donor's body or placed into another person.

**oral reconstruction.** Reforming, recreating, or rebuilding tissues or structures within the mouth following an injury or disease.

**oral soft tissue.** Subcutaneous fat layers beneath oral mucosa or gingiva; excludes bone and teeth.

# D4276

▲ **D4276** combined connective tissue and pedicle graft, per tooth

*Advanced gingival recession often cannot be corrected with a single procedure. Combined tissue grafting procedures are needed to achieve the desired outcome.*

## Explanation

When advanced gingival recession is present, a combined connective tissue and double pedicle graft procedure may be needed to achieve the desired outcome. There are a number of different grafting techniques that can be employed. One technique is to first root plane and eliminate any convexities in the exposed tooth. A split thickness double pedicle graft is then created around the defect. Two vertical releasing incisions are made following the plane of the tooth along the mesial (toward the dental arch) and distal edges of the gingival recession. A sulcular incision is made to create the coronal margin of the flap. The interproximal papillae are left intact. The flap is extended past the mucogingival line to allow adequate mobilization. Next, a connective tissue graft is harvested from the palate by cutting two parallel incisions, 1.5 to 2 mm apart. This graft contains a band of epithelium at its top and a deep band of connective tissue as its main component. The donor site in the palate is closed by suturing the parallel edges together. The connective tissue graft is trimmed as necessary and placed in the prepared recipient site and sutured into place. The partial thickness pedicle graft is positioned coronally over the connective tissue graft to cover as much of it as possible without creating tension and sutured into place. This code is reported per tooth.

## Coding Tips

Local anesthesia is generally considered to be part of periodontal procedures. Local anesthesia is included in this service. Any radiographs are reported separately. Preparation of the recipient site is included.

## Documentation Tips

Third-party payers may require periodontal charting. Periodontal charting should include the identification of the quadrants and sites involved, a minimum of three pocket measurements per tooth involved, indication of recession, furcation involvement, mobility and mucogingival defects, and identification of missing teeth. Check with payers for their specific requirements.

## Reimbursement Tips

When selecting the procedure or service that accurately identifies the service performed, dentists must use the most accurate code. If the CDT code more accurately identifies the service, this should be used rather than the CPT codes. Third-party payers may require periodontal charting. This procedure may be covered by the patient's medical insurance. When covered by medical insurance, the payer may require that the appropriate CPT code be reported on the CMS-1500 claim form. Many payers will not separately reimburse the following services when performed by the same provider, on the same date of service, and at the same surgical site: biopsy (D7285–D7286), frenulectomy (D7960), and/or excision of hard and soft tissue lesions (D7410–D7411, D7450–D7451). When one or more of the above services are provided on a different date of service, a narrative indicating the medical necessity of separating the services should be provided; otherwise, payers may deny those services.

## Associated CPT Codes

41870 Periodontal mucosal grafting

## ICD-10-CM Diagnostic Codes

| | |
|---|---|
| C03.0 | Malignant neoplasm of upper gum |
| C03.1 | Malignant neoplasm of lower gum |
| C04.0 | Malignant neoplasm of anterior floor of mouth |
| C04.1 | Malignant neoplasm of lateral floor of mouth |
| C04.8 | Malignant neoplasm of overlapping sites of floor of mouth |
| C05.0 | Malignant neoplasm of hard palate |
| C05.1 | Malignant neoplasm of soft palate |
| C05.2 | Malignant neoplasm of uvula |
| C05.8 | Malignant neoplasm of overlapping sites of palate |
| C06.0 | Malignant neoplasm of cheek mucosa |
| C06.1 | Malignant neoplasm of vestibule of mouth |
| C06.2 | Malignant neoplasm of retromolar area |
| C07 | Malignant neoplasm of parotid gland |
| C08.0 | Malignant neoplasm of submandibular gland |
| C08.1 | Malignant neoplasm of sublingual gland |
| K05.00 | Acute gingivitis, plaque induced |
| K05.01 | Acute gingivitis, non-plaque induced |
| K05.10 | Chronic gingivitis, plaque induced |
| K05.11 | Chronic gingivitis, non-plaque induced |
| K05.221 | Aggressive periodontitis, generalized, slight |
| K05.222 | Aggressive periodontitis, generalized, moderate |
| K05.223 | Aggressive periodontitis, generalized, severe |
| K05.311 | Chronic periodontitis, localized, slight |
| K05.312 | Chronic periodontitis, localized, moderate |
| K05.313 | Chronic periodontitis, localized, severe |
| K05.321 | Chronic periodontitis, generalized, slight |
| K05.322 | Chronic periodontitis, generalized, moderate |
| K05.323 | Chronic periodontitis, generalized, severe |
| K05.4 | Periodontosis |
| K06.011 | Localized gingival recession, minimal |
| K06.012 | Localized gingival recession, moderate |
| K06.013 | Localized gingival recession, severe |
| K06.021 | Generalized gingival recession, minimal |
| K06.022 | Generalized gingival recession, moderate |
| K06.023 | Generalized gingival recession, severe |
| K06.1 | Gingival enlargement |
| K06.2 | Gingival and edentulous alveolar ridge lesions associated with trauma |
| K12.0 | Recurrent oral aphthae |
| K12.2 | Cellulitis and abscess of mouth |
| K13.3 | Hairy leukoplakia |
| K13.4 | Granuloma and granuloma-like lesions of oral mucosa |
| K13.5 | Oral submucous fibrosis |
| K13.6 | Irritative hyperplasia of oral mucosa |
| K14.0 | Glossitis |
| K14.1 | Geographic tongue |
| K14.2 | Median rhomboid glossitis |
| K14.3 | Hypertrophy of tongue papillae |
| K14.4 | Atrophy of tongue papillae |
| K14.5 | Plicated tongue |
| K14.6 | Glossodynia |
| S02.42XA | Fracture of alveolus of maxilla, initial encounter for closed fracture |
| S02.42XB | Fracture of alveolus of maxilla, initial encounter for open fracture |
| S02.5XXA | Fracture of tooth (traumatic), initial encounter for closed fracture |
| S02.5XXB | Fracture of tooth (traumatic), initial encounter for open fracture |
| S07.0XXA | Crushing injury of face, initial encounter |
| S07.1XXA | Crushing injury of skull, initial encounter |

## Relative Value Units/Medicare Edits

| Non-Facility RVU | Work | PE | MP | Total |
|---|---|---|---|---|
| **D4276** | 6.19 | 5.46 | 1.27 | 12.92 |
| **Facility RVU** | **Work** | **PE** | **MP** | **Total** |
| **D4276** | 6.19 | 5.46 | 1.27 | 12.92 |

| | FUD | Status | MUE | Modifiers | | | | IOM Reference |
|---|---|---|---|---|---|---|---|---|
| **D4276** | N/A | N | - | N/A | N/A | N/A | N/A | None |

* with documentation

## Terms To Know

**gingiva.** Soft tissues surrounding the crowns of unerupted teeth and necks of erupted teeth.

**mesial.** In dentistry, toward the dental arch's midline.

**periodontal.** Relating to the tissues that support and surround the teeth.

**periodontitis.** Inflammation of the tissue structures supporting the teeth leading to a loss of connective tissue attachments.

**submandibular gland.** Salivary gland located beneath the floor of the mouth.

**vestibule of the mouth.** Mucosal and submucosal tissue of the lips and cheeks within the oral cavity, not including the dentoalveolar structures.

# D4277-D4278

**D4277** free soft tissue graft procedure (including recipient and donor surgical sites) first tooth, implant or edentulous tooth position in graft

**D4278** free soft tissue graft procedure (including recipient and donor surgical sites) each additional contiguous tooth, implant or edentulous tooth position in same graft site

*Used in conjunction with D4277.*

## Explanation

The surgeon performs a free soft tissue graft procedure and takes mucosa from one area of the mouth and grafts it to another part in the mouth (i.e., around the teeth to repair areas of gingival recession). The physician uses a scalpel to remove a small piece of mucosa, such as from the hard palate. After preparing the recipient site, the physician sutures the free graft in the area needing repair. This code includes harvesting the graft from the donor site and any donor site closure needed. Code D4277 is used for the first tooth or edentulous tooth position; D4278 is used for each additional tooth or edentulous tooth position.

## Coding Tips

Code D4278 must be reported in conjunction with code D4277. Local anesthesia is included in these services. Any radiographs are reported separately. Preparation of recipient site is included. These codes include postoperative care.

## Documentation Tips

Periodontal charting should include the identification of the quadrants and sites involved, a minimum of three pocket measurements per tooth involved, indication of recession, furcation involvement, mobility and mucogingival defects, and identification of missing teeth. Check with payers for their specific requirements. These codes include frenulectomy, distal wedge procedure, and stenting done on the same area on the same date of service.

## Reimbursement Tips

Third-party payers may require periodontal charting. This procedure may be covered by the patient's medical insurances. When covered by medical insurance, the payer may require that the appropriate CPT code be reported on the CMS-1500 claim form.

## Associated CPT Codes

15120 Split-thickness autograft, face, scalp, eyelids, mouth, neck, ears, orbits, genitalia, hands, feet, and/or multiple digits; first 100 sq cm or less, or 1% of body area of infants and children (except 15050)

15121 Split-thickness autograft, face, scalp, eyelids, mouth, neck, ears, orbits, genitalia, hands, feet, and/or multiple digits; each additional 100 sq cm, or each additional 1% of body area of infants and children, or part thereof (List separately in addition to code for primary procedure)

15240 Full thickness graft, free, including direct closure of donor site, forehead, cheeks, chin, mouth, neck, axillae, genitalia, hands, and/or feet; 20 sq cm or less

15241 Full thickness graft, free, including direct closure of donor site, forehead, cheeks, chin, mouth, neck, axillae, genitalia, hands, and/or feet; each additional 20 sq cm, or part thereof (List separately in addition to code for primary procedure)

## ICD-10-CM Diagnostic Codes

C03.0 Malignant neoplasm of upper gum
C03.1 Malignant neoplasm of lower gum
C04.0 Malignant neoplasm of anterior floor of mouth
C04.1 Malignant neoplasm of lateral floor of mouth
C04.8 Malignant neoplasm of overlapping sites of floor of mouth
C05.0 Malignant neoplasm of hard palate
C05.1 Malignant neoplasm of soft palate
C05.2 Malignant neoplasm of uvula
C05.8 Malignant neoplasm of overlapping sites of palate
C06.0 Malignant neoplasm of cheek mucosa
C06.1 Malignant neoplasm of vestibule of mouth
C06.2 Malignant neoplasm of retromolar area
C07 Malignant neoplasm of parotid gland
C08.0 Malignant neoplasm of submandibular gland
C08.1 Malignant neoplasm of sublingual gland
K05.00 Acute gingivitis, plaque induced
K05.01 Acute gingivitis, non-plaque induced
K05.10 Chronic gingivitis, plaque induced
K05.11 Chronic gingivitis, non-plaque induced
K05.211 Aggressive periodontitis, localized, slight
K05.212 Aggressive periodontitis, localized, moderate
K05.213 Aggressive periodontitis, localized, severe
K05.221 Aggressive periodontitis, generalized, slight
K05.222 Aggressive periodontitis, generalized, moderate
K05.223 Aggressive periodontitis, generalized, severe
K05.311 Chronic periodontitis, localized, slight
K05.312 Chronic periodontitis, localized, moderate
K05.313 Chronic periodontitis, localized, severe
K05.321 Chronic periodontitis, generalized, slight
K05.322 Chronic periodontitis, generalized, moderate
K05.323 Chronic periodontitis, generalized, severe
K05.4 Periodontosis
K05.5 Other periodontal diseases
K06.011 Localized gingival recession, minimal
K06.012 Localized gingival recession, moderate
K06.013 Localized gingival recession, severe
K06.021 Generalized gingival recession, minimal
K06.022 Generalized gingival recession, moderate
K06.023 Generalized gingival recession, severe
K06.1 Gingival enlargement
K06.2 Gingival and edentulous alveolar ridge lesions associated with trauma
K12.0 Recurrent oral aphthae
K12.1 Other forms of stomatitis
K12.2 Cellulitis and abscess of mouth
K12.31 Oral mucositis (ulcerative) due to antineoplastic therapy
K12.32 Oral mucositis (ulcerative) due to other drugs
K12.33 Oral mucositis (ulcerative) due to radiation
K12.39 Other oral mucositis (ulcerative)
K13.21 Leukoplakia of oral mucosa, including tongue
K13.22 Minimal keratinized residual ridge mucosa
K13.23 Excessive keratinized residual ridge mucosa
K13.24 Leukokeratosis nicotina palati
K13.29 Other disturbances of oral epithelium, including tongue
K13.3 Hairy leukoplakia
K13.4 Granuloma and granuloma-like lesions of oral mucosa
K13.5 Oral submucous fibrosis
K13.6 Irritative hyperplasia of oral mucosa

| | |
|---|---|
| K14.0 | Glossitis |
| K14.1 | Geographic tongue |
| K14.2 | Median rhomboid glossitis |
| K14.3 | Hypertrophy of tongue papillae |
| K14.4 | Atrophy of tongue papillae |
| K14.5 | Plicated tongue |
| K14.6 | Glossodynia |

## Relative Value Units/Medicare Edits

| Non-Facility RVU | Work | PE | MP | Total |
|---|---|---|---|---|
| **D4277** | 6.84 | 6.04 | 1.41 | 14.29 |
| **D4278** | 2.28 | 2.01 | 0.47 | 4.76 |
| **Facility RVU** | **Work** | **PE** | **MP** | **Total** |
| **D4277** | 6.84 | 6.04 | 1.41 | 14.29 |
| **D4278** | 2.28 | 2.01 | 0.47 | 4.76 |

| | FUD | Status | MUE | Modifiers | | | | IOM Reference |
|---|---|---|---|---|---|---|---|---|
| **D4277** | N/A | R | - | N/A | N/A | N/A | N/A | None |
| **D4278** | N/A | R | - | N/A | N/A | N/A | N/A | |

* with documentation

## Terms To Know

**autograft.** Any tissue harvested from one anatomical site of a person and grafted to another anatomical site of the same person. Most commonly, blood vessels, skin, tendons, fascia, and bone are used as autografts.

**graft.** Tissue implant from another part of the body or another person.

**mucosa.** Moist tissue lining the mouth (buccal mucosa), stomach (gastric mucosa), intestines, and respiratory tract.

# D4322-D4323

- **D4322** splint - intra-coronal; natural teeth or prosthetic crowns

  *Additional procedure that physically links individual teeth or prosthetic crowns to provide stabilization and additional strength.*

- **D4323** splint - extra-coronal; natural teeth or prosthetic crowns

  *Additional procedure that physically links individual teeth or prosthetic crowns to provide stabilization and additional strength.*

## Explanation

Splinting is performed to stabilize tooth position to preserve the tooth for as long as possible. Periodontal disease and injury may cause tooth mobility; the type of splinting required depends on the type of tooth, the injury, or the severity of the periodontal disease. Examples of extracoronal splinting include etching the tooth with phosphoric acid with application of the splint, utilization of crowns or dental attachments, or application of composite resin. In intracoronal splinting, the affected tooth is connected to neighboring teeth using a variety of appliances and/or methods, such as reinforcing with metal wires or glass-reinforced fibers or pins bonded to the neighboring teeth. Report D4322 for intracoronal splinting and D4323 for extracoronal splinting.

## Coding Tips

Local anesthesia is included in these services. Any evaluation or radiograph is reported separately.

## ICD-10-CM Diagnostic Codes

| | |
|---|---|
| K05.00 | Acute gingivitis, plaque induced |
| K05.01 | Acute gingivitis, non-plaque induced |
| K05.10 | Chronic gingivitis, plaque induced |
| K05.11 | Chronic gingivitis, non-plaque induced |
| K05.221 | Aggressive periodontitis, generalized, slight |
| K05.222 | Aggressive periodontitis, generalized, moderate |
| K05.223 | Aggressive periodontitis, generalized, severe |
| K05.311 | Chronic periodontitis, localized, slight |
| K05.312 | Chronic periodontitis, localized, moderate |
| K05.313 | Chronic periodontitis, localized, severe |
| K05.321 | Chronic periodontitis, generalized, slight |
| K05.322 | Chronic periodontitis, generalized, moderate |
| K05.323 | Chronic periodontitis, generalized, severe |
| K05.4 | Periodontosis |
| K05.5 | Other periodontal diseases |
| K06.011 | Localized gingival recession, minimal |
| K06.012 | Localized gingival recession, moderate |
| K06.013 | Localized gingival recession, severe |
| K06.021 | Generalized gingival recession, minimal |
| K06.022 | Generalized gingival recession, moderate |
| K06.023 | Generalized gingival recession, severe |
| K06.1 | Gingival enlargement |
| K06.2 | Gingival and edentulous alveolar ridge lesions associated with trauma |
| K06.8 | Other specified disorders of gingiva and edentulous alveolar ridge |
| S02.5XXA | Fracture of tooth (traumatic), initial encounter for closed fracture |
| S02.5XXB | Fracture of tooth (traumatic), initial encounter for open fracture |

## Relative Value Units/Medicare Edits

| Non-Facility RVU | Work | PE | MP | Total |
|---|---|---|---|---|
| D4322 | | | | |
| D4323 | | | | |
| **Facility RVU** | **Work** | **PE** | **MP** | **Total** |
| D4322 | | | | |
| D4323 | | | | |

| | FUD | Status | MUE | Modifiers | | | | IOM Reference |
|---|---|---|---|---|---|---|---|---|
| D4322 | N/A | | - | N/A | N/A | N/A | N/A | |
| D4323 | N/A | | - | N/A | N/A | N/A | N/A | |

* with documentation

## Terms To Know

**coronal.** Relating to the top of a tooth or the crown of the head.

**extracoronal.** Portion of the tooth outside the corona or crown.

**intracoronal.** In dentistry, portion of the tooth inside the corona or crown.

**splint.** Brace or support.

# D4341-D4342

**D4341** periodontal scaling and root planing - four or more teeth per quadrant

*This procedure involves instrumentation of the crown and root surfaces of the teeth to remove plaque and calculus from these surfaces. It is indicated for patients with periodontal disease and is therapeutic, not prophylactic, in nature. Root planing is the definitive procedure designed for the removal of cementum and dentin that is rough, and/or permeated by calculus or contaminated with toxins or microorganisms. Some soft tissue removal occurs. This procedure may be used as a definitive treatment in some stages of periodontal disease and/or as a part of pre-surgical procedures in others.*

**D4342** periodontal scaling and root planing - one to three teeth per quadrant

*This procedure involves instrumentation of the crown and root surfaces of the teeth to remove plaque and calculus from these surfaces. It is indicated for patients with periodontal disease and is therapeutic, not prophylactic, in nature. Root planing is the definitive procedure designed for the removal of cementum and dentin that is rough, and/or permeated by calculus or contaminated with toxins or microorganisms. Some soft tissue removal occurs. This procedure may be used as a definitive treatment in some stages of periodontal disease and/or as a part of pre-surgical procedures in others.*

## Explanation

Scaling is removing the plaque and calculus from the tooth surface. Root planing is removing damaged dentin and cementum that is endotoxin-contaminated from microorganisms and/or permeated by calcification from the root surface by scraping the root. The same instruments are used for both and when deep scaling is done on the root surface, they are practically indistinguishable as the root surface is simply debrided. Deep scaling and root planing are done under local anesthesia, as removing plaque, calculus, and damaged cementum from the root surface is painful and must be done meticulously. Hand instruments are chosen by personal preference. Ultrasonic scalers may also be used. Report D4341 for scaling and root planing done in each quadrant on four or more contiguous teeth or bounded teeth spaces and D4342 for one to three teeth per quadrant. This is intended as therapeutic treatment for those with periodontal disease.

## Coding Tips

Local anesthesia is included in these services. Any evaluation or radiograph is reported separately. Irrigation with chlorhexidine is reported separately with D4999. For prophylactic treatment of plaque, calculus and stains, see D1110. To report scaling in generalized moderate or severe gingival inflammation following an oral evaluation see code D4346.

## Documentation Tips

Periodontal charting should include the identification of the quadrants and sites involved, a minimum of three pocket measurements per tooth involved, indication of recession, furcation involvement, mobility and mucogingival defects, and identification of missing teeth. Check with payers for their specific requirements.

## Reimbursement Tips

Third-party payers may require periodontal charting. Payers may require documentation on the claim form indicating the quadrant on which the procedure was performed.

## ICD-10-CM Diagnostic Codes

| | |
|---|---|
| K05.00 | Acute gingivitis, plaque induced |
| K05.01 | Acute gingivitis, non-plaque induced |
| K05.10 | Chronic gingivitis, plaque induced |

| | |
|---|---|
| K05.11 | Chronic gingivitis, non-plaque induced |
| K05.211 | Aggressive periodontitis, localized, slight |
| K05.212 | Aggressive periodontitis, localized, moderate |
| K05.213 | Aggressive periodontitis, localized, severe |
| K05.221 | Aggressive periodontitis, generalized, slight |
| K05.222 | Aggressive periodontitis, generalized, moderate |
| K05.223 | Aggressive periodontitis, generalized, severe |
| K05.311 | Chronic periodontitis, localized, slight |
| K05.312 | Chronic periodontitis, localized, moderate |
| K05.313 | Chronic periodontitis, localized, severe |
| K05.321 | Chronic periodontitis, generalized, slight |
| K05.322 | Chronic periodontitis, generalized, moderate |
| K05.323 | Chronic periodontitis, generalized, severe |
| K05.4 | Periodontosis |
| K05.5 | Other periodontal diseases |

## Relative Value Units/Medicare Edits

| Non-Facility RVU | Work | PE | MP | Total |
|---|---|---|---|---|
| **D4341** | 1.41 | 1.25 | 0.29 | 2.95 |
| **D4342** | 0.80 | 0.71 | 0.16 | 1.67 |
| **Facility RVU** | **Work** | **PE** | **MP** | **Total** |
| **D4341** | 1.41 | 1.25 | 0.29 | 2.95 |
| **D4342** | 0.80 | 0.71 | 0.16 | 1.67 |

| | FUD | Status | MUE | Modifiers | | | | IOM Reference |
|---|---|---|---|---|---|---|---|---|
| **D4341** | N/A | N | - | N/A | N/A | N/A | N/A | None |
| **D4342** | N/A | N | - | N/A | N/A | N/A | N/A | |

* with documentation

## Terms To Know

**dental calculus.** Concretion of calcium, cholesterol, salts, or other substances that forms around the tooth supragingivally or subgingivally.

**dental plaque.** Thin film composed of organic and inorganic deposits from food and epithelial cells that adheres to the tooth surface and is not readily removed, providing a medium for bacterial growth.

**root planing.** Smoothing a root surface by abrasion or filing of the exposed root surface.

**scaling.** Removal of plaque, calculus, and stains from teeth.

Dental - Periodontics

# D4346

**D4346** scaling in presence of generalized moderate or severe gingival inflammation - full mouth, after oral evaluation

*The removal of plaque, calculus and stains from supra- and sub-gingival tooth surfaces when there is generalized moderate or severe gingival inflammation in the absence of periodontitis. It is indicated for patients who have swollen, inflamed gingiva, generalized suprabony pockets, and moderate to severe bleeding on probing. Should not be reported in conjunction with prophylaxis, scaling and root planing, or debridement procedures.*

## Explanation

This code reports the removing of stains, plaque, and calculus from the tooth surface and subgingival tooth surface (scaling) when moderate to severe gingival inflammation is present without periodontitis after oral examination. Under local anesthesia the removal of plaque, calculus, and damaged cementum is removed using hand instruments chosen by personal preference. Ultrasonic scalers may also be used.

## Coding Tips

To report periodontal scaling and root planing, see D4341–D4342. For prophylactic treatment of plaque, calculus, and stains, see D1110.

## Documentation Tips

Documentation will indicate the presence of swollen, inflamed gingiva accompanied by generalized suprabony pockets with moderate to severe bleeding when the gum is probed.

## Reimbursement Tips

Periodontal charting may be required by payers.

## ICD-10-CM Diagnostic Codes

| | |
|---|---|
| K05.00 | Acute gingivitis, plaque induced |
| K05.01 | Acute gingivitis, non-plaque induced |
| K05.10 | Chronic gingivitis, plaque induced |
| K05.11 | Chronic gingivitis, non-plaque induced |

## Relative Value Units/Medicare Edits

| Non-Facility RVU | Work | PE | MP | Total |
|---|---|---|---|---|
| **D4346** | 2.05 | 1.81 | 0.42 | 4.28 |
| **Facility RVU** | **Work** | **PE** | **MP** | **Total** |
| **D4346** | 2.05 | 1.81 | 0.42 | 4.28 |

| | FUD | Status | MUE | Modifiers | | | | IOM Reference |
|---|---|---|---|---|---|---|---|---|
| **D4346** | N/A | N | - | N/A | N/A | N/A | N/A | None |

* with documentation

## Terms To Know

**gingivitis.** Inflamed gingiva (oral mucosa) that surrounds the teeth.

**scaling.** Removal of plaque, calculus, and stains from teeth.

# D4355

**D4355** full mouth debridement to enable a comprehensive oral evaluation and diagnosis on a subsequent visit

*Full mouth debridement involves the preliminary removal of plaque and calculus that interferes with the ability of the dentist to perform a comprehensive oral evaluation. Not to be completed on the same day as D0150, D0160, or D0180.*

## Explanation

A full mouth debridement is carried out to enable comprehensive evaluation and diagnosis. This includes both supra- and subgingival removal of plaque, calculus, and damaged cementum from the tooth surfaces and affected roots through the entire mouth. Deep scaling and root planing is done under local anesthesia, as removing plaque, calculus, and damaged cementum from the root surface is painful and must be done meticulously. Hand instruments are chosen by personal preference. Ultrasonic scalers may also be used. This code does not preclude the need for any other procedures or services.

## Coding Tips

This procedure is reported only at the time of a subsequent encounter. Local anesthesia is included in this service. Any evaluation or radiograph is reported separately. For prophylactic treatment of plaque, calculus, and stains, see D1110. For the removal of plaque and calculus from the tooth surface or removal of damaged dentin and cementum from the root surface (scaling and root planing), see D4341–D4342. Local anesthesia is included in this service. Any radiographs are reported separately. Preparation of recipient site is included. These codes include postoperative care. These codes include frenulectomy, distal wedge procedure, and stenting done on the same area on the same date of service.

## Documentation Tips

Periodontal charting should include the identification of the quadrants and sites involved, a minimum of three pocket measurements per tooth involved, indication of recession, furcation involvement, mobility and mucogingival defects, and identification of missing teeth. Check with payers for their specific requirements.

## Reimbursement Tips

This procedure is covered by Medicare if its purpose is to identify a patient's existing infections prior to kidney transplantation. Third-party payers may require periodontal charting be submitted with the claim.

## ICD-10-CM Diagnostic Codes

| | |
|---|---|
| K03.4 | Hypercementosis |
| K03.5 | Ankylosis of teeth |
| K03.6 | Deposits [accretions] on teeth |
| K03.89 | Other specified diseases of hard tissues of teeth |
| K04.3 | Abnormal hard tissue formation in pulp |
| K04.4 | Acute apical periodontitis of pulpal origin |
| K04.5 | Chronic apical periodontitis |
| K04.6 | Periapical abscess with sinus |
| K04.7 | Periapical abscess without sinus |
| K04.8 | Radicular cyst |
| K04.99 | Other diseases of pulp and periapical tissues |
| K05.00 | Acute gingivitis, plaque induced |
| K05.01 | Acute gingivitis, non-plaque induced |
| K05.10 | Chronic gingivitis, plaque induced |
| K05.11 | Chronic gingivitis, non-plaque induced |
| K05.211 | Aggressive periodontitis, localized, slight |
| K05.212 | Aggressive periodontitis, localized, moderate |
| K05.213 | Aggressive periodontitis, localized, severe |
| K05.221 | Aggressive periodontitis, generalized, slight |
| K05.222 | Aggressive periodontitis, generalized, moderate |
| K05.223 | Aggressive periodontitis, generalized, severe |
| K05.311 | Chronic periodontitis, localized, slight |
| K05.312 | Chronic periodontitis, localized, moderate |
| K05.313 | Chronic periodontitis, localized, severe |
| K05.321 | Chronic periodontitis, generalized, slight |
| K05.322 | Chronic periodontitis, generalized, moderate |
| K05.323 | Chronic periodontitis, generalized, severe |
| K05.4 | Periodontosis |
| K05.5 | Other periodontal diseases |
| K06.011 | Localized gingival recession, minimal |
| K06.012 | Localized gingival recession, moderate |
| K06.013 | Localized gingival recession, severe |
| K06.021 | Generalized gingival recession, minimal |
| K06.022 | Generalized gingival recession, moderate |
| K06.023 | Generalized gingival recession, severe |

## Relative Value Units/Medicare Edits

| Non-Facility RVU | Work | PE | MP | Total |
|---|---|---|---|---|
| D4355 | | | | |
| **Facility RVU** | **Work** | **PE** | **MP** | **Total** |
| D4355 | | | | |

| | FUD | Status | MUE | Modifiers | | | | IOM Reference |
|---|---|---|---|---|---|---|---|---|
| D4355 | N/A | | - | N/A | N/A | N/A | N/A | |

* with documentation

## Terms To Know

**dental calculus.** Concretion of calcium, cholesterol, salts, or other substances that forms around the tooth supragingivally or subgingivally.

**dental plaque.** Thin film composed of organic and inorganic deposits from food and epithelial cells that adheres to the tooth surface and is not readily removed, providing a medium for bacterial growth.

**root planing.** Smoothing a root surface by abrasion or filing of the exposed root surface.

**scaling.** Removal of plaque, calculus, and stains from teeth.

# D4381

**D4381** localized delivery of antimicrobial agents via a controlled release vehicle into diseased crevicular tissue, per tooth

*FDA approved subgingival delivery devices containing antimicrobial medication(s) are inserted into periodontal pockets to suppress the pathogenic microbiota. These devices slowly release the pharmacological agents so they can remain at the intended site of action in a therapeutic concentration for a sufficient length of time.*

## Explanation

A controlled-release antimicrobial agent also known as a localized delivery of antimicrobial agent (LDAA) is delivered through an approved device such as Arestin®, PerioChip®, and Atridox® into specific sites of diseased tissue through implantation in a periodontal pocket. This is an additional short-term therapeutic procedure for areas not responding to conventional therapy to reduce subgingival flora or when current systemic disease rules out other surgical therapy. Pertinent documentation to evaluate medical appropriateness should be included when this code is reported.

## Coding Tips

This service should be reported once per tooth treated. To report periodontal medicament carrier to the entire upper and lower jaw such as a Perio Protect®, see D5994. To report the provision of drugs and/or medicaments by the provider, such as oral antibiotics, oral analgesics, or topical fluoride, see D9360.

## Documentation Tips

Treatment plan documentation should reflect any treatment failure or change in diagnosis and/or a change in treatment plan. There should also be evidence of any initiation or reinstatement of a drug regime, which requires close and continuous skilled medical observation.

## Reimbursement Tips

The tooth/root number should be indicated on the claim. Coverage of this procedure varies by payer and patient contract. Check with the payer for specific coverage guidelines.

## ICD-10-CM Diagnostic Codes

| | |
|---|---|
| K05.222 | Aggressive periodontitis, generalized, moderate |
| K05.223 | Aggressive periodontitis, generalized, severe |
| K05.229 | Aggressive periodontitis, generalized, unspecified severity |
| K05.312 | Chronic periodontitis, localized, moderate |
| K05.313 | Chronic periodontitis, localized, severe |
| K05.319 | Chronic periodontitis, localized, unspecified severity |
| K05.322 | Chronic periodontitis, generalized, moderate |
| K05.323 | Chronic periodontitis, generalized, severe |
| K05.329 | Chronic periodontitis, generalized, unspecified severity |

## Relative Value Units/Medicare Edits

| Non-Facility RVU | Work | PE | MP | Total |
|---|---|---|---|---|
| D4381 | 0.78 | 0.68 | 0.16 | 1.62 |
| **Facility RVU** | **Work** | **PE** | **MP** | **Total** |
| D4381 | 0.78 | 0.68 | 0.16 | 1.62 |

| | FUD | Status | MUE | Modifiers | | | | IOM Reference |
|---|---|---|---|---|---|---|---|---|
| D4381 | N/A | R | - | N/A | N/A | N/A | 80* | 100-02,1,70; 100-04,4,20.5 |

* with documentation

# D4910

**D4910** periodontal maintenance

*This procedure is instituted following periodontal therapy and continues at varying intervals, determined by the clinical evaluation of the dentist, for the life of the dentition or any implant replacements. It includes removal of the bacterial plaque and calculus from supragingival and subgingival regions, site specific scaling and root planing where indicated, and polishing the teeth. If new or recurring periodontal disease appears, additional diagnostic and treatment procedures must be considered.*

## Explanation

Use this code to report periodontal maintenance on patients who have already been treated for periodontal disease. Maintenance is considered as the period that starts after the completion of surgical or nonsurgical active treatment. Periodontal maintenance is continued through the life of the dentition, at the dentist's discretion. During a maintenance check-up, the dentist may remove supra- and subgingival flora and areas of calculus, carrying out site-specific scaling and/or root planing, and polishing the teeth.

## Coding Tips

To report gingival irrigation with a medicinal substance, see D4921. Local anesthesia is included in this service. This service may include scaling, planing, or other services. Any evaluation or radiograph is reported separately.

## ICD-10-CM Diagnostic Codes

| | |
|---|---|
| K04.01 | Reversible pulpitis |
| K04.02 | Irreversible pulpitis |
| K04.1 | Necrosis of pulp |
| K04.2 | Pulp degeneration |
| K04.3 | Abnormal hard tissue formation in pulp |
| K04.4 | Acute apical periodontitis of pulpal origin |
| K04.5 | Chronic apical periodontitis |
| K04.90 | Unspecified diseases of pulp and periapical tissues |
| K04.99 | Other diseases of pulp and periapical tissues |
| K05.00 | Acute gingivitis, plaque induced |
| K05.01 | Acute gingivitis, non-plaque induced |
| K05.10 | Chronic gingivitis, plaque induced |
| K05.11 | Chronic gingivitis, non-plaque induced |
| K05.20 | Aggressive periodontitis, unspecified |
| K05.211 | Aggressive periodontitis, localized, slight |
| K05.212 | Aggressive periodontitis, localized, moderate |
| K05.213 | Aggressive periodontitis, localized, severe |
| K05.221 | Aggressive periodontitis, generalized, slight |
| K05.222 | Aggressive periodontitis, generalized, moderate |
| K05.223 | Aggressive periodontitis, generalized, severe |
| K05.30 | Chronic periodontitis, unspecified |
| K05.311 | Chronic periodontitis, localized, slight |
| K05.312 | Chronic periodontitis, localized, moderate |
| K05.313 | Chronic periodontitis, localized, severe |
| K05.321 | Chronic periodontitis, generalized, slight |
| K05.322 | Chronic periodontitis, generalized, moderate |
| K05.323 | Chronic periodontitis, generalized, severe |
| K05.4 | Periodontosis |
| K05.5 | Other periodontal diseases |
| K05.6 | Periodontal disease, unspecified |
| K06.010 | Localized gingival recession, unspecified |
| K06.011 | Localized gingival recession, minimal |

| | |
|---|---|
| K06.012 | Localized gingival recession, moderate |
| K06.013 | Localized gingival recession, severe |
| K06.020 | Generalized gingival recession, unspecified |
| K06.021 | Generalized gingival recession, minimal |
| K06.022 | Generalized gingival recession, moderate |
| K06.023 | Generalized gingival recession, severe |
| K06.1 | Gingival enlargement |
| K06.2 | Gingival and edentulous alveolar ridge lesions associated with trauma |
| K06.8 | Other specified disorders of gingiva and edentulous alveolar ridge |
| K06.9 | Disorder of gingiva and edentulous alveolar ridge, unspecified |

## Relative Value Units/Medicare Edits

| Non-Facility RVU | Work | PE | MP | Total |
|---|---|---|---|---|
| **D4910** | 0.78 | 0.69 | 0.16 | 1.63 |
| **Facility RVU** | **Work** | **PE** | **MP** | **Total** |
| **D4910** | 0.78 | 0.69 | 0.16 | 1.63 |

| | FUD | Status | MUE | Modifiers | | | | IOM Reference |
|---|---|---|---|---|---|---|---|---|
| **D4910** | N/A | N | - | N/A | N/A | N/A | N/A | None |

* with documentation

## Terms To Know

**gingivitis.** Inflamed gingiva (oral mucosa) that surrounds the teeth.

**periodontal.** Relating to the tissues that support and surround the teeth.

**periodontitis.** Inflammation of the tissue structures supporting the teeth leading to a loss of connective tissue attachments.

**scaling.** Removal of plaque, calculus, and stains from teeth.

# D4920

**D4920** unscheduled dressing change (by someone other than treating dentist or their staff)

## Explanation

This code is used by an oral care giver, who has not been the treating dentist or a member of their staff, for a currently healing problem that requires the professional attention of another available dentist for removing the old dressing and placing a new one.

## Coding Tips

Local anesthesia is included in this service. Any radiographs are reported separately.

## Reimbursement Tips

Medicare considers surgical dressings part of the health care provider's service. Third-party payers may require clinical documentation and/or x-rays before making payment determination. Check with payers to determine their specific requirements.

## ICD-10-CM Diagnostic Codes

| | |
|---|---|
| S01.502A | Unspecified open wound of oral cavity, initial encounter |
| S01.512A | Laceration without foreign body of oral cavity, initial encounter |
| S01.532A | Puncture wound without foreign body of oral cavity, initial encounter |
| S01.552A | Open bite of oral cavity, initial encounter |
| Z48.89 | Encounter for other specified surgical aftercare |

## Relative Value Units/Medicare Edits

| Non-Facility RVU | Work | PE | MP | Total |
|---|---|---|---|---|
| **D4920** | 0.56 | 0.49 | 0.11 | 1.16 |
| **Facility RVU** | **Work** | **PE** | **MP** | **Total** |
| **D4920** | 0.56 | 0.49 | 0.11 | 1.16 |

| | FUD | Status | MUE | Modifiers | | | | IOM Reference |
|---|---|---|---|---|---|---|---|---|
| **D4920** | N/A | N | - | N/A | N/A | N/A | N/A | None |

* with documentation

## Terms To Know

**dressing.** Material applied to a wound or surgical site for protection, absorption, or drainage of the area.

**health care provider.** Entity that administers diagnostic and therapeutic services.

**laceration.** Tearing injury; a torn, ragged-edged wound.

# D4921

**D4921** gingival irrigation - per quadrant

*Irrigation of gingival pockets with medicinal agent. Not to be used to report use of mouth rinses or non-invasive chemical debridement.*

## Explanation

The dental professional irrigates gingival pockets using standard irrigation tips. When using a standard tip, the tip is held at a 90-degree angle at the neck of the tooth near the gingival margin. The gingiva is then irrigated with a medicinal solution. A subgingival tip allows the antimicrobial agent to penetrate deeper into a pocket and is recommended for areas with deep pockets, furcation or dental implants as well as areas that are difficult to reach with the standard tip. The subgingival tip is held at a 45-degree angle and placed at the gingival margin or slightly beneath the gingival margin and the gingiva is then irrigated with the medicinal solution.

## Coding Tips

Local anesthesia is inlcuded and should not be reported separately.

## Documentation Tips

Periodontal charting should include the identification of the quadrants and sites involved, a minimum of three pocket measurements per tooth involved, indication of recession, furcation involvement, mobility and mucogingival defects, and identification of missing teeth.

## Reimbursement Tips

Payers may require periodontal charting to determine the medical necessity of the procedure.

## ICD-10-CM Diagnostic Codes

K04.01 Reversible pulpitis
K04.02 Irreversible pulpitis
K04.1 Necrosis of pulp
K04.2 Pulp degeneration
K04.3 Abnormal hard tissue formation in pulp
K04.4 Acute apical periodontitis of pulpal origin
K04.5 Chronic apical periodontitis
K04.90 Unspecified diseases of pulp and periapical tissues
K04.99 Other diseases of pulp and periapical tissues
K05.00 Acute gingivitis, plaque induced
K05.01 Acute gingivitis, non-plaque induced
K05.10 Chronic gingivitis, plaque induced
K05.11 Chronic gingivitis, non-plaque induced
K05.20 Aggressive periodontitis, unspecified
K05.211 Aggressive periodontitis, localized, slight
K05.212 Aggressive periodontitis, localized, moderate
K05.213 Aggressive periodontitis, localized, severe
K05.221 Aggressive periodontitis, generalized, slight
K05.222 Aggressive periodontitis, generalized, moderate
K05.223 Aggressive periodontitis, generalized, severe
K05.30 Chronic periodontitis, unspecified
K05.311 Chronic periodontitis, localized, slight
K05.312 Chronic periodontitis, localized, moderate
K05.313 Chronic periodontitis, localized, severe
K05.321 Chronic periodontitis, generalized, slight
K05.322 Chronic periodontitis, generalized, moderate
K05.323 Chronic periodontitis, generalized, severe
K05.4 Periodontosis
K05.5 Other periodontal diseases
K05.6 Periodontal disease, unspecified
K06.010 Localized gingival recession, unspecified
K06.011 Localized gingival recession, minimal
K06.012 Localized gingival recession, moderate
K06.013 Localized gingival recession, severe
K06.020 Generalized gingival recession, unspecified
K06.021 Generalized gingival recession, minimal
K06.022 Generalized gingival recession, moderate
K06.023 Generalized gingival recession, severe
K06.1 Gingival enlargement
K06.2 Gingival and edentulous alveolar ridge lesions associated with trauma
K06.8 Other specified disorders of gingiva and edentulous alveolar ridge
K06.9 Disorder of gingiva and edentulous alveolar ridge, unspecified

## Relative Value Units/Medicare Edits

| Non-Facility RVU | Work | PE | MP | Total |
|---|---|---|---|---|
| D4921 | 0.23 | 0.20 | 0.05 | 0.48 |
| **Facility RVU** | **Work** | **PE** | **MP** | **Total** |
| D4921 | 0.23 | 0.20 | 0.05 | 0.48 |

| | FUD | Status | MUE | Modifiers | | | | IOM Reference |
|---|---|---|---|---|---|---|---|---|
| D4921 | N/A | N | - | N/A | N/A | N/A | N/A | None |

* with documentation

## Terms To Know

**furcation.** In dentistry, the area where roots separate in a multirooted tooth.

**gingiva.** Soft tissues surrounding the crowns of unerupted teeth and necks of erupted teeth.

**irrigation.** To wash out or cleanse a body cavity, wound, or tissue with water or other fluid.

# D5110-D5120

**D5110** complete denture - maxillary
**D5120** complete denture - mandibular

## Explanation

These codes report complete dentures. Complete dentures cover the entire jaw, upper or lower. Complete dentures are classified as conventional or immediate. Conventional dentures are made and inserted after the teeth have been extracted and the gums have healed, leaving the patient without teeth while the denture is being made. Immediate dentures are made prior to extraction and placed during the same appointment that the teeth are removed. A conventional denture requires approximately six appointments over one to two months. At the first appointment, a dental exam is performed and denture treatment options are presented. At subsequent visits, impressions of the mouth are taken to determine the bite (the way your teeth come together) and the teeth are extracted. Next, the dentist assists the patient in selecting the appropriate teeth. The size, shape, and color of the teeth selected depend on a variety of factors including anatomical variations in the mouth, skin tone, and the shape of the skull. The next appointment will be a trial fitting. The teeth that are held in the base with wax are tried on to determine how they look and feel in the mouth. If the fit and look of the teeth are acceptable to the patient, the denture is completed and the patient returns for another appointment to receive the completed denture. The dentist again checks the denture for fit and instructs the patient on denture care and oral hygiene. Over the next few weeks or months, the patient returns for follow-up visits to monitor the fit and comfort of the denture. Report D5110 for a complete upper denture or D5120 for a complete lower denture.

## Coding Tips

Local anesthesia is generally considered to be part of removable prosthodontic procedures. The type of material used to fabricate the denture does not affect code assignment. When the denture is placed at during the same encounter as extraction, see D5130-D5140.

## Documentation Tips

Documentation should indicate the location and number of missing teeth.

## ICD-10-CM Diagnostic Codes

K00.0 Anodontia
K08.101 Complete loss of teeth, unspecified cause, class I
K08.102 Complete loss of teeth, unspecified cause, class II
K08.103 Complete loss of teeth, unspecified cause, class III
K08.104 Complete loss of teeth, unspecified cause, class IV
K08.109 Complete loss of teeth, unspecified cause, unspecified class
K08.111 Complete loss of teeth due to trauma, class I
K08.112 Complete loss of teeth due to trauma, class II
K08.113 Complete loss of teeth due to trauma, class III
K08.114 Complete loss of teeth due to trauma, class IV
K08.119 Complete loss of teeth due to trauma, unspecified class
K08.121 Complete loss of teeth due to periodontal diseases, class I
K08.122 Complete loss of teeth due to periodontal diseases, class II
K08.123 Complete loss of teeth due to periodontal diseases, class III
K08.124 Complete loss of teeth due to periodontal diseases, class IV
K08.129 Complete loss of teeth due to periodontal diseases, unspecified class
K08.131 Complete loss of teeth due to caries, class I
K08.132 Complete loss of teeth due to caries, class II
K08.133 Complete loss of teeth due to caries, class III
K08.134 Complete loss of teeth due to caries, class IV
K08.139 Complete loss of teeth due to caries, unspecified class
K08.191 Complete loss of teeth due to other specified cause, class I
K08.192 Complete loss of teeth due to other specified cause, class II
K08.193 Complete loss of teeth due to other specified cause, class III
K08.194 Complete loss of teeth due to other specified cause, class IV
K08.199 Complete loss of teeth due to other specified cause, unspecified class
K08.401 Partial loss of teeth, unspecified cause, class I
K08.402 Partial loss of teeth, unspecified cause, class II
K08.403 Partial loss of teeth, unspecified cause, class III
K08.404 Partial loss of teeth, unspecified cause, class IV
K08.409 Partial loss of teeth, unspecified cause, unspecified class
K08.411 Partial loss of teeth due to trauma, class I
K08.412 Partial loss of teeth due to trauma, class II
K08.413 Partial loss of teeth due to trauma, class III
K08.414 Partial loss of teeth due to trauma, class IV
K08.419 Partial loss of teeth due to trauma, unspecified class
K08.421 Partial loss of teeth due to periodontal diseases, class I
K08.422 Partial loss of teeth due to periodontal diseases, class II
K08.423 Partial loss of teeth due to periodontal diseases, class III
K08.424 Partial loss of teeth due to periodontal diseases, class IV
K08.429 Partial loss of teeth due to periodontal diseases, unspecified class
K08.431 Partial loss of teeth due to caries, class I
K08.432 Partial loss of teeth due to caries, class II
K08.433 Partial loss of teeth due to caries, class III
K08.434 Partial loss of teeth due to caries, class IV
K08.439 Partial loss of teeth due to caries, unspecified class
K08.491 Partial loss of teeth due to other specified cause, class I
K08.492 Partial loss of teeth due to other specified cause, class II
K08.493 Partial loss of teeth due to other specified cause, class III
K08.494 Partial loss of teeth due to other specified cause, class IV
K08.499 Partial loss of teeth due to other specified cause, unspecified class

## Relative Value Units/Medicare Edits

| Non-Facility RVU | Work | PE | MP | Total |
|---|---|---|---|---|
| **D5110** | 8.38 | 7.40 | 1.73 | 17.51 |
| **D5120** | 8.38 | 7.40 | 1.73 | 17.51 |
| **Facility RVU** | **Work** | **PE** | **MP** | **Total** |
| **D5110** | 8.38 | 7.40 | 1.73 | 17.51 |
| **D5120** | 8.38 | 7.40 | 1.73 | 17.51 |

| | FUD | Status | MUE | Modifiers | | | | IOM Reference |
|---|---|---|---|---|---|---|---|---|
| **D5110** | N/A | N | - | N/A | N/A | N/A | N/A | None |
| **D5120** | N/A | N | - | N/A | N/A | N/A | N/A | |

* with documentation

Dental - Removable Prosthodontics

# D5130-D5140

**D5130** immediate denture - maxillary

*Includes limited follow-up care only; does not include required future rebasing/relining procedure(s).*

**D5140** immediate denture - mandibular

*Includes limited follow-up care only; does not include required future rebasing/relining procedure(s).*

## Explanation

These codes report immediate dentures. Conventional dentures are made and inserted after the teeth have been extracted and the gums have healed, leaving the patient without teeth while the denture is being made. Immediate dentures are made prior to extraction of the teeth using an impression obtained prior to extraction. When the denture is ready, the teeth are extracted and the denture inserted. The patient is instructed not to remove the denture for one or two days and nights, except to rinse. Two days after receiving the denture, a follow-up exam is performed to make sure the denture fits properly and the bite is correct. After this visit, the patient is instructed to remove the denture at night and treat it like a conventional denture. Disadvantages of immediate dentures include an inability to see and test the denture before it is inserted; potential shrinkage of bones and gums following extraction of the teeth requiring that the denture be refitted (relined) after several months; and the possibility that an entirely new denture may be required due to bone and gum shrinkage. However, immediate fitting does have the advantage of reducing postoperative swelling. Report D5130 for intermediate denture of the upper jaw or D5140 for intermediate denture of the lower jaw.

## Coding Tips

Local anesthesia is generally considered to be part of removable prosthodontic procedures. The type of material used to fabricate the denture does not affect code assignment. When extraction is performed at a previous visit and then the denture is fabricated and inserted during a separate encounter, see D5110-D5120.

## Documentation Tips

Documentation should indicate the location and number of missing teeth.

## ICD-10-CM Diagnostic Codes

K00.0 Anodontia
K08.101 Complete loss of teeth, unspecified cause, class I
K08.102 Complete loss of teeth, unspecified cause, class II
K08.103 Complete loss of teeth, unspecified cause, class III
K08.104 Complete loss of teeth, unspecified cause, class IV
K08.109 Complete loss of teeth, unspecified cause, unspecified class
K08.111 Complete loss of teeth due to trauma, class I
K08.112 Complete loss of teeth due to trauma, class II
K08.113 Complete loss of teeth due to trauma, class III
K08.114 Complete loss of teeth due to trauma, class IV
K08.119 Complete loss of teeth due to trauma, unspecified class
K08.121 Complete loss of teeth due to periodontal diseases, class I
K08.122 Complete loss of teeth due to periodontal diseases, class II
K08.123 Complete loss of teeth due to periodontal diseases, class III
K08.124 Complete loss of teeth due to periodontal diseases, class IV
K08.129 Complete loss of teeth due to periodontal diseases, unspecified class
K08.131 Complete loss of teeth due to caries, class I
K08.132 Complete loss of teeth due to caries, class II
K08.133 Complete loss of teeth due to caries, class III
K08.134 Complete loss of teeth due to caries, class IV
K08.139 Complete loss of teeth due to caries, unspecified class
K08.191 Complete loss of teeth due to other specified cause, class I
K08.192 Complete loss of teeth due to other specified cause, class II
K08.193 Complete loss of teeth due to other specified cause, class III
K08.194 Complete loss of teeth due to other specified cause, class IV
K08.199 Complete loss of teeth due to other specified cause, unspecified class
K08.401 Partial loss of teeth, unspecified cause, class I
K08.402 Partial loss of teeth, unspecified cause, class II
K08.403 Partial loss of teeth, unspecified cause, class III
K08.404 Partial loss of teeth, unspecified cause, class IV
K08.409 Partial loss of teeth, unspecified cause, unspecified class
K08.411 Partial loss of teeth due to trauma, class I
K08.412 Partial loss of teeth due to trauma, class II
K08.413 Partial loss of teeth due to trauma, class III
K08.414 Partial loss of teeth due to trauma, class IV
K08.419 Partial loss of teeth due to trauma, unspecified class
K08.421 Partial loss of teeth due to periodontal diseases, class I
K08.422 Partial loss of teeth due to periodontal diseases, class II
K08.423 Partial loss of teeth due to periodontal diseases, class III
K08.424 Partial loss of teeth due to periodontal diseases, class IV
K08.429 Partial loss of teeth due to periodontal diseases, unspecified class
K08.431 Partial loss of teeth due to caries, class I
K08.432 Partial loss of teeth due to caries, class II
K08.433 Partial loss of teeth due to caries, class III
K08.434 Partial loss of teeth due to caries, class IV
K08.439 Partial loss of teeth due to caries, unspecified class
K08.491 Partial loss of teeth due to other specified cause, class I
K08.492 Partial loss of teeth due to other specified cause, class II
K08.493 Partial loss of teeth due to other specified cause, class III
K08.494 Partial loss of teeth due to other specified cause, class IV
K08.499 Partial loss of teeth due to other specified cause, unspecified class

## Relative Value Units/Medicare Edits

| Non-Facility RVU | Work | PE | MP | Total |
|---|---|---|---|---|
| **D5130** | 9.16 | 8.08 | 1.89 | 19.13 |
| **D5140** | 9.16 | 8.08 | 1.89 | 19.13 |
| **Facility RVU** | **Work** | **PE** | **MP** | **Total** |
| **D5130** | 9.16 | 8.08 | 1.89 | 19.13 |
| **D5140** | 9.16 | 8.08 | 1.89 | 19.13 |

| | FUD | Status | MUE | Modifiers | | | | IOM Reference |
|---|---|---|---|---|---|---|---|---|
| **D5130** | N/A | N | - | N/A | N/A | N/A | N/A | None |
| **D5140** | N/A | N | - | N/A | N/A | N/A | N/A | |

* with documentation

# D5211-D5214

**D5211** maxillary partial denture - resin base (including any conventional clasps, rests and teeth)

**D5212** mandibular partial denture - resin base (including any conventional clasps, rests and teeth)

**D5213** maxillary partial denture - cast metal framework with resin denture bases (including retentive/clasping materials, rests and teeth)

**D5214** mandibular partial denture - cast metal framework with resin denture bases (including retentive/clasping materials, rests and teeth)

## Explanation

The dentist applies an acrylic resin base partial denture to the upper jaw in D5211 and the lower jaw in D5212. Tooth preparation is done to accommodate the rest seats, modify unfavorable lines, and increase retention by adding composite and creating undercuts. Second impressions are taken. The framework is tried in to check extension, adaptation, and positioning of the clasps and rests, check occlusion, and identify any faults. Minor faults are adjusted. Major faults require repeat second impressions. The tooth mould and shade are selected. The waxed denture is tried and all points verified again before proceeding. The dentures are tried in, adjusting undercuts and contacts, if necessary, and then adjusting the extension, occlusion, and articulation as needed. Report D5213 and D5214 for a partial denture of the upper and lower jaw, respectively, that is cast metal framework with resin bases. Report D5225 for a maxillary partial denture with a flexible base and D5226 for a flexible based mandibular partial denture.

## Coding Tips

Local anesthesia is included in these services. Any evaluation, radiograph, core buildup, or post or preparation service is reported separately. These services include routine postdelivery care. Report D5282–D5283 for a one piece cast metal unilateral partial denture. For flexible-base partial denture, see D5225–D5226. For complete dentures, see D5110–D5140. To ensure proper code assignment particular attention to the type of material used to fabricate the denture is required. When reporting codes D5211 or D5212, third-party payers may require clinical documentation and/or x-rays before making payment determination. Check with payers to determine their specific requirements.

## Documentation Tips

The following information can be documented on a tooth chart: treatment/location of caries, endodontic procedures, prosthetic services, preventive services, treatment of lesions and dental disease, or other special procedures. A tooth chart may also be used to identify structure and rationale of disease process and the type of service performed on intraoral structures other than teeth.

## Reimbursement Tips

Most payers require that missing teeth be indicated on the dental claim form. Coverage guidelines vary by payer and by patient contract. Patients are often responsible for copayments or may reach contract limitations. Check with the payer to determine coverage policies and patient responsibility.

## ICD-10-CM Diagnostic Codes

K08.401 Partial loss of teeth, unspecified cause, class I
K08.402 Partial loss of teeth, unspecified cause, class II
K08.403 Partial loss of teeth, unspecified cause, class III
K08.404 Partial loss of teeth, unspecified cause, class IV
K08.409 Partial loss of teeth, unspecified cause, unspecified class
K08.411 Partial loss of teeth due to trauma, class I
K08.412 Partial loss of teeth due to trauma, class II
K08.413 Partial loss of teeth due to trauma, class III
K08.414 Partial loss of teeth due to trauma, class IV
K08.419 Partial loss of teeth due to trauma, unspecified class
K08.421 Partial loss of teeth due to periodontal diseases, class I
K08.422 Partial loss of teeth due to periodontal diseases, class II
K08.423 Partial loss of teeth due to periodontal diseases, class III
K08.424 Partial loss of teeth due to periodontal diseases, class IV
K08.429 Partial loss of teeth due to periodontal diseases, unspecified class
K08.431 Partial loss of teeth due to caries, class I
K08.432 Partial loss of teeth due to caries, class II
K08.433 Partial loss of teeth due to caries, class III
K08.434 Partial loss of teeth due to caries, class IV
K08.439 Partial loss of teeth due to caries, unspecified class
K08.491 Partial loss of teeth due to other specified cause, class I
K08.492 Partial loss of teeth due to other specified cause, class II
K08.493 Partial loss of teeth due to other specified cause, class III
K08.494 Partial loss of teeth due to other specified cause, class IV
K08.499 Partial loss of teeth due to other specified cause, unspecified class

## Relative Value Units/Medicare Edits

| Non-Facility RVU | Work | PE | MP | Total |
|---|---|---|---|---|
| **D5211** | 6.65 | 5.87 | 1.37 | 13.89 |
| **D5212** | 7.51 | 6.63 | 1.55 | 15.69 |
| **D5213** | 9.50 | 8.38 | 1.96 | 19.84 |
| **D5214** | 9.50 | 8.38 | 1.96 | 19.84 |
| **Facility RVU** | **Work** | **PE** | **MP** | **Total** |
| **D5211** | 6.65 | 5.87 | 1.37 | 13.89 |
| **D5212** | 7.51 | 6.63 | 1.55 | 15.69 |
| **D5213** | 9.50 | 8.38 | 1.96 | 19.84 |
| **D5214** | 9.50 | 8.38 | 1.96 | 19.84 |

| | FUD | Status | MUE | Modifiers | | | | IOM Reference |
|---|---|---|---|---|---|---|---|---|
| **D5211** | N/A | N | - | N/A | N/A | N/A | N/A | None |
| **D5212** | N/A | N | - | N/A | N/A | N/A | N/A | |
| **D5213** | N/A | N | - | N/A | N/A | N/A | N/A | |
| **D5214** | N/A | N | - | N/A | N/A | N/A | N/A | |

* with documentation

## Terms To Know

**denture.** Manmade substitution of natural teeth and neighboring structures.

# D5221-D5222

**D5221** immediate maxillary partial denture - resin base (including retentive/clasping materials, rests and teeth)

*Includes limited follow-up care only; does not include future rebasing/relining procedure(s).*

**D5222** immediate mandibular partial denture - resin base (including retentive/clasping materials, rests and teeth)

*Includes limited follow-up care only; does not include future rebasing/relining procedure(s).*

## Explanation

The dentist provides a partial denture immediately following the extraction of the natural teeth. Immediate dentures are made prior to extraction of the teeth using an impression obtained prior to extraction. When the denture is ready, the teeth are extracted and the denture inserted. The patient is instructed not to remove the denture for one or two days and nights, except to rinse. Two days after receiving the denture, a follow-up exam is performed to make sure the denture fits properly and the bite is correct. After this visit, the patient is instructed to remove the denture at night and treat it like a conventional denture. Disadvantages of immediate dentures include an inability to see and test the denture before it is inserted, potential shrinkage of bones and gums following extraction of the teeth requiring that the denture be refitted (relined) after several months, and the possibility that an entirely new denture may be required due to bone and gum shrinkage. However, immediate fitting does have the advantage of reducing postoperative swelling. Report D5221 for immediate partial denture of the upper jaw or D5222 for immediate partial denture of the lower jaw.

## Coding Tips

These codes are used to report immediate partial dentures that are resin based. To report immediate partial dentures that have a cast metal framework see D5223–D5224. To report immediate full denture see D5130–D5140.

## Documentation Tips

The following information can be documented on a tooth chart: treatment/location of caries, endodontic procedures, prosthetic services, preventive services, treatment of lesions and dental disease, or other special procedures. A tooth chart may also be used to identify structure and rationale of disease process and the type of service performed on intraoral structures other than teeth.

## Reimbursement Tips

Most payers require that missing teeth be indicated on the dental claim form. Coverage guidelines vary by payer and by patient contract. Patients are often responsible for copayments or may reach contract limitations. Check with the payer to determine coverage policies and patient responsibility.

## ICD-10-CM Diagnostic Codes

K08.411 Partial loss of teeth due to trauma, class I
K08.412 Partial loss of teeth due to trauma, class II
K08.413 Partial loss of teeth due to trauma, class III
K08.414 Partial loss of teeth due to trauma, class IV
K08.419 Partial loss of teeth due to trauma, unspecified class
K08.421 Partial loss of teeth due to periodontal diseases, class I
K08.422 Partial loss of teeth due to periodontal diseases, class II
K08.423 Partial loss of teeth due to periodontal diseases, class III
K08.424 Partial loss of teeth due to periodontal diseases, class IV
K08.429 Partial loss of teeth due to periodontal diseases, unspecified class
K08.431 Partial loss of teeth due to caries, class I
K08.432 Partial loss of teeth due to caries, class II
K08.433 Partial loss of teeth due to caries, class III
K08.434 Partial loss of teeth due to caries, class IV
K08.439 Partial loss of teeth due to caries, unspecified class
K08.491 Partial loss of teeth due to other specified cause, class I
K08.492 Partial loss of teeth due to other specified cause, class II
K08.493 Partial loss of teeth due to other specified cause, class III
K08.494 Partial loss of teeth due to other specified cause, class IV
K08.499 Partial loss of teeth due to other specified cause, unspecified class

## Relative Value Units/Medicare Edits

| Non-Facility RVU | Work | PE | MP | Total |
|---|---|---|---|---|
| **D5221** | 5.76 | 5.08 | 1.19 | 12.03 |
| **D5222** | 5.99 | 5.29 | 1.23 | 12.51 |
| **Facility RVU** | **Work** | **PE** | **MP** | **Total** |
| **D5221** | 5.76 | 5.08 | 1.19 | 12.03 |
| **D5222** | 5.99 | 5.29 | 1.23 | 12.51 |

| | FUD | Status | MUE | Modifiers | | | | IOM Reference |
|---|---|---|---|---|---|---|---|---|
| **D5221** | N/A | N | - | N/A | N/A | N/A | N/A | None |
| **D5222** | N/A | N | - | N/A | N/A | N/A | N/A | |

* with documentation

## Terms To Know

**denture.** Manmade substitution of natural teeth and neighboring structures.

# D5223-D5224

**D5223** immediate maxillary partial denture - cast metal framework with resin denture bases (including retentive/clasping materials, rests and teeth)

*Includes limited follow-up care only; does not include future rebasing/relining procedure(s).*

**D5224** immediate mandibular partial denture - cast metal framework with resin denture bases (including retentive/clasping materials, rests and teeth)

*Includes limited follow-up care only; does not include future rebasing/relining procedure(s).*

## Explanation

Immediate dentures are made prior to extraction of the teeth using an impression obtained prior to extraction. When the denture is ready, the teeth are extracted and the denture inserted. The patient is instructed not to remove the denture for one or two days and nights, except to rinse. Two days after receiving the denture, a follow-up exam is performed to make sure the denture fits properly and the bite is correct. After this visit, the patient is instructed to remove the denture at night and treat it like a conventional denture. Disadvantages of immediate dentures include an inability to see and test the denture before it is inserted; potential shrinkage of bones and gums following extraction of the teeth requiring that the denture be refitted (relined) after several months; and the possibility that an entirely new denture may be required due to bone and gum shrinkage. However, immediate fitting does have the advantage of reducing postoperative swelling. Report D5223 for immediate partial denture of the upper jaw or D5224 for immediate partial denture of the lower jaw.

## Coding Tips

These codes are used to report immediate partial dentures that are on a metal framework. To report resin-based dentures, see D5221–D5222. For immediate flexible base partial dentures, see D5227-D5228.

## Documentation Tips

The following information can be documented on a tooth chart: treatment/location of caries, endodontic procedures, prosthetic services, preventive services, treatment of lesions and dental disease, or other special procedures. A tooth chart may also be used to identify structure and rationale of disease process and the type of service performed on intraoral structures other than teeth.

## Reimbursement Tips

Most payers require that missing teeth be indicated on the dental claim form. Coverage guidelines vary by payer and by patient contract. Patients are often responsible for copayments or may reach contract limitations. Check with the payer to determine coverage policies and patient responsibility.

## ICD-10-CM Diagnostic Codes

K08.401 Partial loss of teeth, unspecified cause, class I
K08.402 Partial loss of teeth, unspecified cause, class II
K08.403 Partial loss of teeth, unspecified cause, class III
K08.404 Partial loss of teeth, unspecified cause, class IV
K08.409 Partial loss of teeth, unspecified cause, unspecified class
K08.411 Partial loss of teeth due to trauma, class I
K08.412 Partial loss of teeth due to trauma, class II
K08.413 Partial loss of teeth due to trauma, class III
K08.414 Partial loss of teeth due to trauma, class IV
K08.419 Partial loss of teeth due to trauma, unspecified class
K08.421 Partial loss of teeth due to periodontal diseases, class I
K08.422 Partial loss of teeth due to periodontal diseases, class II
K08.423 Partial loss of teeth due to periodontal diseases, class III
K08.424 Partial loss of teeth due to periodontal diseases, class IV
K08.429 Partial loss of teeth due to periodontal diseases, unspecified class
K08.431 Partial loss of teeth due to caries, class I
K08.432 Partial loss of teeth due to caries, class II
K08.433 Partial loss of teeth due to caries, class III
K08.434 Partial loss of teeth due to caries, class IV
K08.439 Partial loss of teeth due to caries, unspecified class
K08.491 Partial loss of teeth due to other specified cause, class I
K08.492 Partial loss of teeth due to other specified cause, class II
K08.493 Partial loss of teeth due to other specified cause, class III
K08.494 Partial loss of teeth due to other specified cause, class IV
K08.499 Partial loss of teeth due to other specified cause, unspecified class

## Relative Value Units/Medicare Edits

| Non-Facility RVU | Work | PE | MP | Total |
|---|---|---|---|---|
| **D5223** | 10.15 | 8.96 | 2.09 | 21.20 |
| **D5224** | 10.15 | 8.96 | 2.09 | 21.20 |
| **Facility RVU** | **Work** | **PE** | **MP** | **Total** |
| **D5223** | 10.15 | 8.96 | 2.09 | 21.20 |
| **D5224** | 10.15 | 8.96 | 2.09 | 21.20 |

| | FUD | Status | MUE | Modifiers | | | | IOM Reference |
|---|---|---|---|---|---|---|---|---|
| **D5223** | N/A | N | - | N/A | N/A | N/A | N/A | None |
| **D5224** | N/A | N | - | N/A | N/A | N/A | N/A | |

* with documentation

## Terms To Know

**partial dentures.** In dentistry, artificial teeth composed of a framework with plastic teeth and gum area replacing part but not all of the natural teeth. The framework can either be formed from an acrylic resin base, cast metal or may be made more flexible using thermoplastics.

Dental - Removable Prosthodontics

# D5225-D5226

**D5225** maxillary partial denture - flexible base (including retentive/clasping materials, rests, and teeth)

**D5226** mandibular partial denture - flexible base (including retentive/clasping materials, rests, and teeth)

## Explanation

Partial dentures are composed of a metal framework with plastic teeth and gum areas. The framework contains retentive or clasping materials and rests that hold the denture in place. Two types of attachments are available: metal clasps and precision attachments. Metal clasps consist of C-shaped pieces of denture framework that fit around adjacent natural teeth. The adjacent teeth sometimes require shaping to hold the clasps and keep the denture securely in place. A precision attachment uses a receptacle created within a remaining tooth. The receptacle typically is covered with a crown. The precision attachment extends into the receptacle securing the partial denture. Precision attachments have no visible clasps and the forces of chewing usually are better distributed along the teeth. However, precision attachments are more expensive than retentive clasps, so most partial dentures still use retentive clasps. Both types of dentures are easily removed for cleaning. Report D5225 for a maxillary partial denture; report D5226 for a mandibular partial denture.

## Coding Tips

Local anesthesia is generally considered to be part of removable prosthodontic procedures. For a resin based partial denture, see D5211-D5212. For a cast metal partial denture, see D5213-D5214. For immediate flexible base partial denture, see D5227-D5228.

## Documentation Tips

Dentists should be certain that sufficient documentation is provided in the dental records to accurately verify and describe the services rendered. Additionally, records should be legible and signed with the appropriate name and title of the provider of the service.

## Reimbursement Tips

Coverage guidelines vary by payer and by patient contract. Patients are often responsible for copayments or may reach contract limitations. Check with the payer to determine coverage policies and patient responsibility.

## ICD-10-CM Diagnostic Codes

K08.401 Partial loss of teeth, unspecified cause, class I
K08.402 Partial loss of teeth, unspecified cause, class II
K08.403 Partial loss of teeth, unspecified cause, class III
K08.404 Partial loss of teeth, unspecified cause, class IV
K08.409 Partial loss of teeth, unspecified cause, unspecified class
K08.411 Partial loss of teeth due to trauma, class I
K08.412 Partial loss of teeth due to trauma, class II
K08.413 Partial loss of teeth due to trauma, class III
K08.414 Partial loss of teeth due to trauma, class IV
K08.419 Partial loss of teeth due to trauma, unspecified class
K08.421 Partial loss of teeth due to periodontal diseases, class I
K08.422 Partial loss of teeth due to periodontal diseases, class II
K08.423 Partial loss of teeth due to periodontal diseases, class III
K08.424 Partial loss of teeth due to periodontal diseases, class IV
K08.429 Partial loss of teeth due to periodontal diseases, unspecified class
K08.431 Partial loss of teeth due to caries, class I
K08.432 Partial loss of teeth due to caries, class II
K08.433 Partial loss of teeth due to caries, class III
K08.434 Partial loss of teeth due to caries, class IV
K08.439 Partial loss of teeth due to caries, unspecified class
K08.491 Partial loss of teeth due to other specified cause, class I
K08.492 Partial loss of teeth due to other specified cause, class II
K08.493 Partial loss of teeth due to other specified cause, class III
K08.494 Partial loss of teeth due to other specified cause, class IV
K08.499 Partial loss of teeth due to other specified cause, unspecified class

## Relative Value Units/Medicare Edits

| Non-Facility RVU | Work | PE | MP | Total |
|---|---|---|---|---|
| D5225 | 7.09 | 6.26 | 1.46 | 14.81 |
| D5226 | 7.89 | 6.96 | 1.62 | 16.47 |
| **Facility RVU** | **Work** | **PE** | **MP** | **Total** |
| D5225 | 7.09 | 6.26 | 1.46 | 14.81 |
| D5226 | 7.89 | 6.96 | 1.62 | 16.47 |

| | FUD | Status | MUE | Modifiers | | | | IOM Reference |
|---|---|---|---|---|---|---|---|---|
| D5225 | N/A | N | - | N/A | N/A | N/A | N/A | None |
| D5226 | N/A | N | - | N/A | N/A | N/A | N/A | |

* with documentation

## Terms To Know

**denture.** Manmade substitution of natural teeth and neighboring structures.

**partial dentures.** In dentistry, artificial teeth composed of a framework with plastic teeth and gum area replacing part but not all of the natural teeth. The framework can either be formed from an acrylic resin base, cast metal or may be made more flexible using thermoplastics.

**prosthodontics.** Branch of dentistry that specializes in the replacement of missing or damaged teeth.

# D5227-D5228

- ● **D5227** immediate maxillary partial denture - flexible base (including any clasps, rests and teeth)
- ● **D5228** immediate mandibular partial denture - flexible base (including any clasps, rests and teeth)

## Explanation

Immediate dentures are made prior to extraction of the teeth using an impression obtained prior to extraction. When the flexible base denture is ready, the teeth are extracted and the denture inserted at the same session. The patient is instructed not to remove the denture for one or two days and nights, except to rinse. Two days after receiving the denture, a follow-up exam is performed to make sure the denture fits properly and the bite is correct. After this visit, the patient is instructed to remove the denture at night and treat it like a conventional denture. Disadvantages of immediate dentures include the inability to see and test the denture before it is inserted; potential shrinkage of bones and gums following extraction of the teeth requiring that the denture be refitted (relined) after several months; and the possibility that an entirely new denture may be required due to bone and gum shrinkage. However, immediate fitting does have the advantage of reducing postoperative swelling. Report D5227 for immediate partial flexible base denture of the upper jaw or D5228 for immediate partial flexible base denture of the lower jaw.

## Coding Tips

Local anesthesia is generally considered to be part of removable prosthodontic procedures. For an immediate cast metal partial denture, see D5223-D5224. For a flexible base partial denture, see D5225-D5226.

## Documentation Tips

Most payers require that missing teeth be indicated on the dental claim form.

## Reimbursement Tips

Coverage guidelines vary by payer and by patient contract.

## ICD-10-CM Diagnostic Codes

K08.401 Partial loss of teeth, unspecified cause, class I
K08.402 Partial loss of teeth, unspecified cause, class II
K08.403 Partial loss of teeth, unspecified cause, class III
K08.404 Partial loss of teeth, unspecified cause, class IV
K08.411 Partial loss of teeth due to trauma, class I
K08.412 Partial loss of teeth due to trauma, class II
K08.413 Partial loss of teeth due to trauma, class III
K08.414 Partial loss of teeth due to trauma, class IV
K08.421 Partial loss of teeth due to periodontal diseases, class I
K08.422 Partial loss of teeth due to periodontal diseases, class II
K08.423 Partial loss of teeth due to periodontal diseases, class III
K08.424 Partial loss of teeth due to periodontal diseases, class IV
K08.431 Partial loss of teeth due to caries, class I
K08.432 Partial loss of teeth due to caries, class II
K08.433 Partial loss of teeth due to caries, class III
K08.434 Partial loss of teeth due to caries, class IV
K08.491 Partial loss of teeth due to other specified cause, class I
K08.492 Partial loss of teeth due to other specified cause, class II
K08.493 Partial loss of teeth due to other specified cause, class III
K08.494 Partial loss of teeth due to other specified cause, class IV

## Relative Value Units/Medicare Edits

| Non-Facility RVU | Work | PE | MP | Total |
|---|---|---|---|---|
| D5227 | | | | |
| D5228 | | | | |
| **Facility RVU** | **Work** | **PE** | **MP** | **Total** |
| D5227 | | | | |
| D5228 | | | | |

| | FUD | Status | MUE | Modifiers | | | | IOM Reference |
|---|---|---|---|---|---|---|---|---|
| D5227 | N/A | | - | N/A | N/A | N/A | N/A | |
| D5228 | N/A | | - | N/A | N/A | N/A | N/A | |

* with documentation

## Terms To Know

**caries.** Localized section of tooth decay that begins on the tooth surface with destruction of the calcified enamel, allowing bacterial destruction to continue and form cavities and may extend to the dentin and pulp.

**denture.** Manmade substitution of natural teeth and neighboring structures.

**periodontal.** Relating to the tissues that support and surround the teeth.

Dental - Removable Prosthodontics

# D5282-D5283

**D5282** removable unilateral partial denture - one piece cast metal (including retentive/clasping materials, rests, and teeth), maxillary

**D5283** removable unilateral partial denture - one piece cast metal (including rentative/clasping materials, rests, and teeth), mandibular

## Explanation

Partial dentures are composed of a metal framework with plastic teeth and gum areas. The cast framework contains retentive/clasping material, rests, or other attachments that hold the denture in place. Two types of attachments are available: retentive clasps and precision attachments. Retentive clasps consist of C-shaped pieces of denture framework that fit around adjacent natural teeth. The adjacent teeth sometimes require shaping to hold the clasps and keep the denture securely in place. A precision attachment uses a receptacle created within a remaining tooth. The receptacle typically is covered with a crown. The precision attachment extends into the receptacle securing the partial denture. Precision attachments have no visible clasps and the forces of chewing usually are better distributed along the teeth. However, precision attachments are more expensive than retentive clasps, so most partial dentures still use retentive clasps. Both types of dentures are easily removed for cleaning. Report D5282 for a maxillary partial denture; report D5283 for a mandibular partial denture.

## Coding Tips

To report resin based partial dentures, see D5211–D5212. To report cast metal framework with resin denture bases, see D5213–D5214. To report immediate partial denture, see D5221–D5224. To report flexible unilateral partial denture, see D5284. To report partial dentures consist of a flexible denture base and clasps, see D5286.

## Reimbursement Tips

Most payers require that the missing teeth be indicated on the dental claim form. Coverage guidelines vary by payer and by patient contract. Patients are often responsible for copayments or may reach contract limitations. Check with the payer to determine coverage policies and patient responsibility.

## ICD-10-CM Diagnostic Codes

K08.401 Partial loss of teeth, unspecified cause, class I
K08.402 Partial loss of teeth, unspecified cause, class II
K08.403 Partial loss of teeth, unspecified cause, class III
K08.404 Partial loss of teeth, unspecified cause, class IV
K08.409 Partial loss of teeth, unspecified cause, unspecified class
K08.411 Partial loss of teeth due to trauma, class I
K08.412 Partial loss of teeth due to trauma, class II
K08.413 Partial loss of teeth due to trauma, class III
K08.414 Partial loss of teeth due to trauma, class IV
K08.419 Partial loss of teeth due to trauma, unspecified class
K08.421 Partial loss of teeth due to periodontal diseases, class I
K08.422 Partial loss of teeth due to periodontal diseases, class II
K08.423 Partial loss of teeth due to periodontal diseases, class III
K08.424 Partial loss of teeth due to periodontal diseases, class IV
K08.429 Partial loss of teeth due to periodontal diseases, unspecified class
K08.431 Partial loss of teeth due to caries, class I
K08.432 Partial loss of teeth due to caries, class II
K08.433 Partial loss of teeth due to caries, class III
K08.434 Partial loss of teeth due to caries, class IV
K08.439 Partial loss of teeth due to caries, unspecified class
K08.491 Partial loss of teeth due to other specified cause, class I
K08.492 Partial loss of teeth due to other specified cause, class II
K08.493 Partial loss of teeth due to other specified cause, class III
K08.494 Partial loss of teeth due to other specified cause, class IV
K08.499 Partial loss of teeth due to other specified cause, unspecified class

## Relative Value Units/Medicare Edits

| Non-Facility RVU | Work | PE | MP | Total |
|---|---|---|---|---|
| **D5282** | 4.53 | 4.00 | 0.93 | 9.46 |
| **D5283** | 4.53 | 4.00 | 0.93 | 9.46 |
| **Facility RVU** | **Work** | **PE** | **MP** | **Total** |
| **D5282** | 4.53 | 4.00 | 0.93 | 9.46 |
| **D5283** | 4.53 | 4.00 | 0.93 | 9.46 |

| | FUD | Status | MUE | Modifiers | | | | IOM Reference |
|---|---|---|---|---|---|---|---|---|
| **D5282** | N/A | N | - | N/A | N/A | N/A | N/A | None |
| **D5283** | N/A | N | - | N/A | N/A | N/A | N/A | |

* with documentation

## Terms To Know

**partial dentures.** In dentistry, artificial teeth composed of a framework with plastic teeth and gum area replacing part but not all of the natural teeth. The framework can either be formed from an acrylic resin base, cast metal or may be made more flexible using thermoplastics.

**unilateral.** Located on or affecting one side.

# D5284-D5286

**D5284** removable unilateral partial denture - one piece flexible base (including retentive/clasping materials, rests, and teeth) - per quadrant

**D5286** removable unilateral partial denture - one piece resin (including retentive/clasping materials, rests, and teeth) - per quadrant

## Explanation

A flexible unilateral partial denture for the replacement of missing natural teeth is provided to a patient. Code D5284 is a flexible base with retentive/clasping material and rests; the teeth are created using thin thermoplastic materials such as nylon. Flexible base dentures are thinner than other types of dentures and are flexible; however, the cost is higher. Code D5286 describes types of partial dentures consisting of a flexible denture base and retentive/clasping material and rests consisting of C-shaped pieces of acrylic resin denture framework that fit around adjacent natural teeth. The adjacent teeth sometimes require shaping to hold the clasps and keep the denture securely in place. Resin-based, partial dentures are more lightweight than other types of dentures and are easily adjusted in the provider's office. These codes are reported once per quadrant.

## Coding Tips

To report resin-based, partial dentures, see D5211–D5212. To report cast metal framework with resin denture bases, see D5213–D5214. To report immediate partial denture, see D5221–D5224. To report one-piece, cast metal, removable, unilateral partial dentures, see D5282–D5283.

## Reimbursement Tips

Most payers require that the missing teeth be indicated on the dental claim form. Coverage guidelines vary by payer and by patient contract. Patients are often responsible for copayments or may reach contract limitations. Check with the payer to determine coverage policies and patient responsibility.

## ICD-10-CM Diagnostic Codes

K08.401 Partial loss of teeth, unspecified cause, class I
K08.402 Partial loss of teeth, unspecified cause, class II
K08.403 Partial loss of teeth, unspecified cause, class III
K08.404 Partial loss of teeth, unspecified cause, class IV
K08.409 Partial loss of teeth, unspecified cause, unspecified class
K08.411 Partial loss of teeth due to trauma, class I
K08.412 Partial loss of teeth due to trauma, class II
K08.413 Partial loss of teeth due to trauma, class III
K08.414 Partial loss of teeth due to trauma, class IV
K08.419 Partial loss of teeth due to trauma, unspecified class
K08.421 Partial loss of teeth due to periodontal diseases, class I
K08.422 Partial loss of teeth due to periodontal diseases, class II
K08.423 Partial loss of teeth due to periodontal diseases, class III
K08.424 Partial loss of teeth due to periodontal diseases, class IV
K08.429 Partial loss of teeth due to periodontal diseases, unspecified class
K08.431 Partial loss of teeth due to caries, class I
K08.432 Partial loss of teeth due to caries, class II
K08.433 Partial loss of teeth due to caries, class III
K08.434 Partial loss of teeth due to caries, class IV
K08.439 Partial loss of teeth due to caries, unspecified class
K08.491 Partial loss of teeth due to other specified cause, class I
K08.492 Partial loss of teeth due to other specified cause, class II
K08.493 Partial loss of teeth due to other specified cause, class III
K08.494 Partial loss of teeth due to other specified cause, class IV
K08.499 Partial loss of teeth due to other specified cause, unspecified class

## Relative Value Units/Medicare Edits

| Non-Facility RVU | Work | PE | MP | Total |
|---|---|---|---|---|
| **D5284** | 4.53 | 4.00 | 0.93 | 9.46 |
| **D5286** | 4.53 | 4.00 | 0.93 | 9.46 |
| **Facility RVU** | **Work** | **PE** | **MP** | **Total** |
| **D5284** | 4.53 | 4.00 | 0.93 | 9.46 |
| **D5286** | 4.53 | 4.00 | 0.93 | 9.46 |

| | FUD | Status | MUE | Modifiers | | | | IOM Reference |
|---|---|---|---|---|---|---|---|---|
| **D5284** | N/A | N | - | N/A | N/A | N/A | N/A | None |
| **D5286** | N/A | N | - | N/A | N/A | N/A | N/A | |

* with documentation

## Terms To Know

**partial dentures.** In dentistry, artificial teeth composed of a framework with plastic teeth and gum area replacing part but not all of the natural teeth. The framework can either be formed from an acrylic resin base, cast metal or may be made more flexible using thermoplastics.

**unilateral.** Located on or affecting one side.

Dental - Removable Prosthodontics

# D5410-D5411

**D5410** adjust complete denture - maxillary
**D5411** adjust complete denture - mandibular

## Explanation

A previously constructed complete denture is adjusted for fit usually due to shrinkage of bones and gums following extraction of the teeth. The inner surface of the denture is relined or resized to fit the changes that have occurred in the bones and gums. Report D5410 for an adjustment to a complete maxillary denture; report D5411 for an adjustment to a complete mandibular denture.

## Coding Tips

Local anesthesia is generally considered to be part of removable prosthodontic procedures. Adjustment of a partial denture is reported using D5421–D5422. For repair of denture base, see D5511–D5512. For replacement of missing tooth, see D5520.

## Reimbursement Tips

Many payers consider adjustment made within a specified time frame (for example, six months) of placement to be included in the price of the denture. Check with payers for their specific guidelines.

## ICD-10-CM Diagnostic Codes

Z46.3 Encounter for fitting and adjustment of dental prosthetic device

## Relative Value Units/Medicare Edits

| Non-Facility RVU | Work | PE | MP | Total |
|---|---|---|---|---|
| D5410 | 0.44 | 0.39 | 0.09 | 0.92 |
| D5411 | 0.44 | 0.39 | 0.09 | 0.92 |
| **Facility RVU** | **Work** | **PE** | **MP** | **Total** |
| D5410 | 0.44 | 0.39 | 0.09 | 0.92 |
| D5411 | 0.44 | 0.39 | 0.09 | 0.92 |

| | FUD | Status | MUE | Modifiers | | | | IOM Reference |
|---|---|---|---|---|---|---|---|---|
| D5410 | N/A | N | - | N/A | N/A | N/A | N/A | None |
| D5411 | N/A | N | - | N/A | N/A | N/A | N/A | |

* with documentation

## Terms To Know

**denture.** Manmade substitution of natural teeth and neighboring structures.

**denture base.** Portion of the artificial substitute for natural teeth that makes contact with the soft tissue of the mouth and serves as the anchor for the artificial teeth.

**mandibular.** Having to do with the lower jaw.

**maxillary.** Located between the eyes and the upper teeth.

**prosthodontics.** Branch of dentistry that specializes in the replacement of missing or damaged teeth.

# D5421-D5422

**D5421** adjust partial denture - maxillary
**D5422** adjust partial denture - mandibular

## Explanation

A previously constructed partial denture is adjusted for fit usually due to shrinkage of bones and gums following extraction of the teeth. The inner surface of the denture is relined or resized to fit the changes that have occurred in the bones and gums. Report D5421 for an adjustment to a partial maxillary denture; report D5422 for an adjustment to a partial mandibular denture.

## Coding Tips

Local anesthesia is generally considered to be part of removable prosthodontic procedures. For adjustments to complete dentures, see D5410-D5411.

## Reimbursement Tips

Many payers consider adjustment made within a specified time frame (for example, six months) of placement to be included in the price of the denture. Check with payers for their specific guidelines.

## ICD-10-CM Diagnostic Codes

Z46.3 Encounter for fitting and adjustment of dental prosthetic device

## Relative Value Units/Medicare Edits

| Non-Facility RVU | Work | PE | MP | Total |
|---|---|---|---|---|
| D5421 | 0.44 | 0.39 | 0.09 | 0.92 |
| D5422 | 0.44 | 0.39 | 0.09 | 0.92 |
| **Facility RVU** | **Work** | **PE** | **MP** | **Total** |
| D5421 | 0.44 | 0.39 | 0.09 | 0.92 |
| D5422 | 0.44 | 0.39 | 0.09 | 0.92 |

| | FUD | Status | MUE | Modifiers | | | | IOM Reference |
|---|---|---|---|---|---|---|---|---|
| D5421 | N/A | N | - | N/A | N/A | N/A | N/A | None |
| D5422 | N/A | N | - | N/A | N/A | N/A | N/A | |

* with documentation

## Terms To Know

**denture base.** Portion of the artificial substitute for natural teeth that makes contact with the soft tissue of the mouth and serves as the anchor for the artificial teeth.

**mandibular.** Having to do with the lower jaw.

**maxillary.** Located between the eyes and the upper teeth.

**partial dentures.** In dentistry, artificial teeth composed of a framework with plastic teeth and gum area replacing part but not all of the natural teeth. The framework can either be formed from an acrylic resin base, cast metal or may be made more flexible using thermoplastics.

**prosthodontics.** Branch of dentistry that specializes in the replacement of missing or damaged teeth.

# D5511-D5512

**D5511** repair broken complete denture base, mandibular
**D5512** repair broken complete denture base, maxillary

## Explanation

A cracked or broken complete denture base is repaired. Depending on the nature of the break, different repair techniques may be required. If the fractured base can be accurately positioned outside of the mouth, the dentist will unite them with a wire held in place by sticky wax or by applying an adhesive to the fracture surfaces. The assembled denture will then be fitted in the mouth prior to repair. If the fractured denture pieces cannot be positioned accurately outside of the mouth, they are placed in the best position possible and a cold-curing acrylic resin is applied. While the resin is still pliable, the denture is placed into the mouth and the broken pieces held in place until the resin hardens. The denture is then sent to a laboratory for completion of the repair. It is sometimes possible to repair dentures in the office (chair side) using a cold-curing acrylic or heat-curing resin. Cold-curing resins will cure in six to nine minutes. Heat-curing resins require approximately 15 minutes. Report D5511 when performed on a mandibular (upper) denture or D5512 when performed on a maxillary (lower) denture.

## Coding Tips

To report the repair of a resin denture base, see D5611–D5612.

## Reimbursement Tips

Coverage guidelines vary by payer and by patient contract. Patients are often responsible for copayments or may reach contract limitations. Check with the payer to determine coverage policies and patient responsibility.

## ICD-10-CM Diagnostic Codes

Z46.3 Encounter for fitting and adjustment of dental prosthetic device

## Relative Value Units/Medicare Edits

| Non-Facility RVU | Work | PE | MP | Total |
|---|---|---|---|---|
| **D5511** | 1.02 | 0.90 | 0.21 | 2.13 |
| **D5512** | 1.02 | 0.90 | 0.21 | 2.13 |
| **Facility RVU** | **Work** | **PE** | **MP** | **Total** |
| **D5511** | 1.02 | 0.90 | 0.21 | 2.13 |
| **D5512** | 1.02 | 0.90 | 0.21 | 2.13 |

| | FUD | Status | MUE | Modifiers | | | | IOM Reference |
|---|---|---|---|---|---|---|---|---|
| **D5511** | N/A | N | - | N/A | N/A | N/A | N/A | None |
| **D5512** | N/A | N | - | N/A | N/A | N/A | N/A | |

* with documentation

## Terms To Know

**denture.** Manmade substitution of natural teeth and neighboring structures.

**denture base.** Portion of the artificial substitute for natural teeth that makes contact with the soft tissue of the mouth and serves as the anchor for the artificial teeth.

**prosthodontics.** Branch of dentistry that specializes in the replacement of missing or damaged teeth.

# D5520

**D5520** replace missing or broken teeth - complete denture (each tooth)

## Explanation

A missing or broken tooth is replaced on a complete denture. The broken or lost tooth is replaced with a custom-fabricated tooth or a pre-fabricated tooth. If the tooth is broken, it must first be extracted from the denture base. This is done using a tooth extractor. The area is then filed and sanded to allow placement of the new tooth. The replacement tooth is cemented into place using a bonding adhesive. Alternatively, it may be possible to build up a broken tooth by direct additions of tooth-colored, cold-curing acrylic resin to the denture at the chair side. Report D5520 per tooth.

## Coding Tips

Local anesthesia is generally considered to be part of removable prosthodontic procedures.

## Reimbursement Tips

Coverage guidelines vary by payer and by patient contract. Patients are often responsible for copayments or may reach contract limitations. Check with the payer to determine coverage policies and patient responsibility.

## ICD-10-CM Diagnostic Codes

Z46.3 Encounter for fitting and adjustment of dental prosthetic device

## Relative Value Units/Medicare Edits

| Non-Facility RVU | Work | PE | MP | Total |
|---|---|---|---|---|
| **D5520** | 0.74 | 0.65 | 0.15 | 1.54 |
| **Facility RVU** | **Work** | **PE** | **MP** | **Total** |
| **D5520** | 0.74 | 0.65 | 0.15 | 1.54 |

| | FUD | Status | MUE | Modifiers | | | | IOM Reference |
|---|---|---|---|---|---|---|---|---|
| **D5520** | N/A | N | - | N/A | N/A | N/A | N/A | None |

* with documentation

## Terms To Know

**denture.** Manmade substitution of natural teeth and neighboring structures.

**denture base.** Portion of the artificial substitute for natural teeth that makes contact with the soft tissue of the mouth and serves as the anchor for the artificial teeth.

**prosthodontics.** Branch of dentistry that specializes in the replacement of missing or damaged teeth.

# D5611-D5612

**D5611** repair resin partial denture base, mandibular
**D5612** repair resin partial denture base, maxillary

## Explanation

A cracked or broken complete denture base is repaired. Depending on the nature of the break, different repair techniques may be required. If the fractured base can be accurately positioned outside of the mouth, the dentist will unite them with a wire held in place by sticky wax or by applying an adhesive to the fracture surfaces. The assembled denture will then be fitted in the mouth prior to repair. If the fractured denture pieces cannot be positioned accurately outside of the mouth, they are placed in the best position possible and a cold-curing acrylic resin is applied. While the resin is still pliable, the denture is placed into the mouth and the broken pieces held in place until the resin hardens. The denture is then sent to a laboratory for completion of the repair. It is sometimes possible to repair dentures in the office (chair side) using a cold-curing acrylic or heat-curing resin. Cold-curing resins will cure in six to nine minutes. Heat-curing resins require approximately 15 minutes. Report D5511 when performed on a mandibular (upper) denture or D5512 when performed on a maxillary (lower) denture.

## Coding Tips

To report the repair of a denture base other than resin, see D5511–D5512.

## Reimbursement Tips

Providers should be certain that sufficient documentation is provided in the record to accurately verify and describe the service rendered (i.e., the repair provided and the type of denture base).

## ICD-10-CM Diagnostic Codes

Z46.3 Encounter for fitting and adjustment of dental prosthetic device

## Relative Value Units/Medicare Edits

| Non-Facility RVU | Work | PE | MP | Total |
|---|---|---|---|---|
| D5611 | 1.02 | 0.90 | 0.21 | 2.13 |
| D5612 | 1.02 | 0.90 | 0.21 | 2.13 |
| **Facility RVU** | **Work** | **PE** | **MP** | **Total** |
| D5611 | 1.02 | 0.90 | 0.21 | 2.13 |
| D5612 | 1.02 | 0.90 | 0.21 | 2.13 |

| | FUD | Status | MUE | Modifiers | | | | IOM Reference |
|---|---|---|---|---|---|---|---|---|
| D5611 | N/A | N | - | N/A | N/A | N/A | N/A | None |
| D5612 | N/A | N | - | N/A | N/A | N/A | N/A | |

* with documentation

## Terms To Know

**denture base.** Portion of the artificial substitute for natural teeth that makes contact with the soft tissue of the mouth and serves as the anchor for the artificial teeth.

**partial dentures.** In dentistry, artificial teeth composed of a framework with plastic teeth and gum area replacing part but not all of the natural teeth. The framework can either be formed from an acrylic resin base, cast metal or may be made more flexible using thermoplastics.

**prosthodontics.** Branch of dentistry that specializes in the replacement of missing or damaged teeth.

# D5621-D5630

**D5621** repair cast partial framework, mandibular
**D5622** repair cast partial framework, maxillary
**D5630** repair or replace broken retentive clasping materials - per tooth

## Explanation

Partial dentures are composed of a framework with plastic teeth and gum areas. The framework contains clasps or other attachments that hold the denture in place. Two types of attachments are available: clasps and precision attachments. Clasps consist of C-shaped pieces of denture framework that fit around adjacent natural teeth. A precision attachment uses a receptacle created within a remaining tooth. The receptacle typically is covered with a crown. The precision attachment extends into the receptacle securing the partial denture. If the framework, clasps, or precision attachments break they are repaired in the dentist's office or sent to a dental laboratory. To repair cast framework or replace a fractured clasp or precision attachment, an alginate impression in a stock tray is made of the denture with the patient wearing the denture. Care must be taken to ensure the impression material does not displace the denture from its correct position. The new framework, clasp, or precision attachment is fabricated and attached to the existing denture using the impression to correctly align and place the required part. Repair of the cast framework is reported with D5621 (mandibular or upper) or D5622 (maxillary or lower). Repair of a clasp or precision attachment is reported with D5630.

## Coding Tips

To report the repair of a denture base other than resin, see D5511–D5512; for resin, see D5611–D5612.

## Reimbursement Tips

Coverage of this procedure varies by payer. Check with the payer for specific coverage guidelines.

## ICD-10-CM Diagnostic Codes

Z46.3 Encounter for fitting and adjustment of dental prosthetic device

## Relative Value Units/Medicare Edits

| Non-Facility RVU | Work | PE | MP | Total |
|---|---|---|---|---|
| D5621 | 1.39 | 1.23 | 0.29 | 2.91 |
| D5622 | 1.39 | 1.23 | 0.29 | 2.91 |
| D5630 | 1.28 | 1.13 | 0.26 | 2.67 |
| **Facility RVU** | **Work** | **PE** | **MP** | **Total** |
| D5621 | 1.39 | 1.23 | 0.29 | 2.91 |
| D5622 | 1.39 | 1.23 | 0.29 | 2.91 |
| D5630 | 1.28 | 1.13 | 0.26 | 2.67 |

| | FUD | Status | MUE | Modifiers | | | | IOM Reference |
|---|---|---|---|---|---|---|---|---|
| D5621 | N/A | N | - | N/A | N/A | N/A | N/A | None |
| D5622 | N/A | N | - | N/A | N/A | N/A | N/A | |
| D5630 | N/A | N | - | N/A | N/A | N/A | N/A | |

* with documentation

## Terms To Know

**conventional dentures.** Dentures made and inserted after the teeth have been extracted and the gums have healed. The patient is edentulous while the denture is being made.

# D5640-D5650

**D5640** replace broken teeth - per tooth
**D5650** add tooth to existing partial denture

## Explanation

Partial dentures are composed of a metal framework with plastic teeth and gum areas. The framework contains metal clasps or other attachments that hold the denture in place. Two types of attachments are available: metal clasps and precision attachments. Metal clasps consist of C-shaped pieces of denture framework that fit around adjacent natural teeth. A precision attachment uses a receptacle created within a remaining tooth. The receptacle typically is covered with a crown. The precision attachment extends into the receptacle securing the partial denture. If the framework, clasps, or precision attachments break they are repaired in the dentist's office or sent to a dental laboratory. To repair cast framework or replace a fractured clasp or precision attachment, an alginate impression in a stock tray is made of the denture with the patient wearing the denture. Care must be taken to ensure the impression material does not displace the denture from its correct position. The new framework, clasp, or precision attachment is fabricated and attached to the existing denture using the impression to correctly align and place the required part. Repair of the cast framework is reported with D5621 (mandibular or upper) or D5622 (maxillary or lower). Repair of a metal clasp or precision attachment is reported with D5630.

## Coding Tips

Local anesthesia is generally considered to be part of removable prosthodontic procedures.

## Reimbursement Tips

Third-party payers may not reimburse separately for this service. Check with the payer for specific guidelines.

## ICD-10-CM Diagnostic Codes

Z46.3 Encounter for fitting and adjustment of dental prosthetic device

## Relative Value Units/Medicare Edits

| Non-Facility RVU | Work | PE | MP | Total |
|---|---|---|---|---|
| D5640 | 0.89 | 0.79 | 0.18 | 1.86 |
| D5650 | 1.10 | 0.97 | 0.23 | 2.30 |
| **Facility RVU** | **Work** | **PE** | **MP** | **Total** |
| D5640 | 0.89 | 0.79 | 0.18 | 1.86 |
| D5650 | 1.10 | 0.97 | 0.23 | 2.30 |

| | FUD | Status | MUE | Modifiers | | | | IOM Reference |
|---|---|---|---|---|---|---|---|---|
| D5640 | N/A | N | - | N/A | N/A | N/A | N/A | None |
| D5650 | N/A | N | - | N/A | N/A | N/A | N/A | |

* with documentation

## Terms To Know

**denture base.** Portion of the artificial substitute for natural teeth that makes contact with the soft tissue of the mouth and serves as the anchor for the artificial teeth.

**partial dentures.** In dentistry, artificial teeth composed of a framework with plastic teeth and gum area replacing part but not all of the natural teeth. The framework can either be formed from an acrylic resin base, cast metal or may be made more flexible using thermoplastics.

# D5660

**D5660** add clasp to existing partial denture - per tooth

## Explanation

A clasp is added to an existing partial denture. To add a clasp to a denture, an alginate impression in a stock tray is made of the denture with the patient wearing the denture. Care must be taken to ensure that the impression material does not displace the denture from its correct position. An impression of the opposing dentition is also made if the component to be added is affected by the occlusion (bite), as this will influence the design and position of the component. If the casts cannot be placed by hand into the intercuspal position, an interocclusal record will be obtained to allow the casts to be mounted on an articulator. A new clasp arm is then produced by adapting a wrought stainless steel wire to the tooth on the cast and attaching the wire to the existing denture base.

## Coding Tips

Local anesthesia is generally considered to be part of removable prosthodontic procedures.

## Reimbursement Tips

Third-party payers may not reimburse separately for this service. Check with the payer for specific guidelines.

## ICD-10-CM Diagnostic Codes

Z46.3 Encounter for fitting and adjustment of dental prosthetic device

## Relative Value Units/Medicare Edits

| Non-Facility RVU | Work | PE | MP | Total |
|---|---|---|---|---|
| D5660 | 1.47 | 1.30 | 0.30 | 3.07 |
| **Facility RVU** | **Work** | **PE** | **MP** | **Total** |
| D5660 | 1.47 | 1.30 | 0.30 | 3.07 |

| | FUD | Status | MUE | Modifiers | | | | IOM Reference |
|---|---|---|---|---|---|---|---|---|
| D5660 | N/A | N | - | N/A | N/A | N/A | N/A | None |

* with documentation

## Terms To Know

**partial dentures.** In dentistry, artificial teeth composed of a framework with plastic teeth and gum area replacing part but not all of the natural teeth. The framework can either be formed from an acrylic resin base, cast metal or may be made more flexible using thermoplastics.

**prosthodontics.** Branch of dentistry that specializes in the replacement of missing or damaged teeth.

# D5670-D5671

**D5670** replace all teeth and acrylic on cast metal framework (maxillary)
**D5671** replace all teeth and acrylic on cast metal framework (mandibular)

## Explanation

All teeth and acrylic on a cast metal framework partial denture are replaced. Partial dentures are composed of a metal framework with plastic teeth and gum areas. The framework contains metal clasps or other attachments that hold the denture in place. Metal clasps consist of C-shaped pieces of denture framework that fit around adjacent natural teeth. The adjacent teeth sometimes require shaping to hold the clasps and keep the denture securely in place. Replacement of all teeth and acrylic on a cast metal framework requires several dental appointments that begin with new dental impressions. An alginate impression in a stock tray is made. An impression of the opposing dentition is also made, as replacement of teeth and acrylic is affected by the occlusion (bite) and will influence the fabrication replacement components. The impressions are sent to the dental laboratory for fabrication of the replacement teeth and acrylic using the existing metal framework. The next appointment will be a trial fitting. The teeth that are held in the base with wax are tried on to determine how they look and feel in the mouth. If the fit and look of the teeth are acceptable to the patient, the denture work is completed and the patient returns for another appointment to receive the completed denture. The dentist again checks the denture for fit and instructs the patient on denture care and oral hygiene. Over the next few weeks or months, the patient returns for follow-up visits to monitor the fit and comfort of the denture. Use D5670 to report replacement of all teeth and acrylic in a maxillary denture and D5671 for a mandibular denture.

## Coding Tips

Local anesthesia is generally considered to be part of removable prosthodontic procedures.

## Reimbursement Tips

Coverage of this procedure varies by payer. Check with the payer for specific coverage guidelines.

## ICD-10-CM Diagnostic Codes

Z46.3 Encounter for fitting and adjustment of dental prosthetic device

## Relative Value Units/Medicare Edits

| Non-Facility RVU | Work | PE | MP | Total |
|---|---|---|---|---|
| **D5670** | 3.86 | 3.41 | 0.80 | 8.07 |
| **D5671** | 3.86 | 3.41 | 0.80 | 8.07 |
| **Facility RVU** | **Work** | **PE** | **MP** | **Total** |
| **D5670** | 3.86 | 3.41 | 0.80 | 8.07 |
| **D5671** | 3.86 | 3.41 | 0.80 | 8.07 |

| | FUD | Status | MUE | Modifiers | | | | IOM Reference |
|---|---|---|---|---|---|---|---|---|
| **D5670** | N/A | N | - | N/A | N/A | N/A | N/A | None |
| **D5671** | N/A | N | - | N/A | N/A | N/A | N/A | |

* with documentation

## Terms To Know

**denture.** Manmade substitution of natural teeth and neighboring structures.

# D5710-D5721

**D5710** rebase complete maxillary denture
**D5711** rebase complete mandibular denture
**D5720** rebase maxillary partial denture
**D5721** rebase mandibular partial denture

## Explanation

Rebasing is replacing most or all of the denture base (pink part) when the entire fitting surface requires improvement. Rebase materials can be either hard or soft, self- or heat-cure. Heat cure is the preferred choice but the patient is without the denture while the rebase addition is done. The heat-cure rebase requires an impression of the inside of the denture. The impression material is applied, the denture is inserted to take the impression, and the patient bites into closing contact. The impression is removed and examined and repeated until satisfactory and sent with the denture piece to the lab. The heat-cure material is applied to rebuild the base of the denture, and made to fit the patient's mouth from the impression taken. The rebuilt denture is then finished with polishing before being returned. Report codes D5710 and D5711 for rebasing a complete upper and lower denture, respectively, and report codes D5720 and D5721 for a partial denture, upper and lower, respectively.

## Coding Tips

To report reline denture, see D5730–D5741. For rebasing of a hybrid prosthesis, see D5725.

## Reimbursement Tips

Coverage of this procedure varies by payer. Check with the payer for specific coverage guidelines.

## ICD-10-CM Diagnostic Codes

Z46.3 Encounter for fitting and adjustment of dental prosthetic device

## Relative Value Units/Medicare Edits

| Non-Facility RVU | Work | PE | MP | Total |
|---|---|---|---|---|
| **D5710** | 3.39 | 2.99 | 0.70 | 7.08 |
| **D5711** | 3.28 | 2.89 | 0.68 | 6.85 |
| **D5720** | 3.05 | 2.69 | 0.63 | 6.37 |
| **D5721** | 3.05 | 2.69 | 0.63 | 6.37 |
| **Facility RVU** | **Work** | **PE** | **MP** | **Total** |
| **D5710** | 3.39 | 2.99 | 0.70 | 7.08 |
| **D5711** | 3.28 | 2.89 | 0.68 | 6.85 |
| **D5720** | 3.05 | 2.69 | 0.63 | 6.37 |
| **D5721** | 3.05 | 2.69 | 0.63 | 6.37 |

| | FUD | Status | MUE | Modifiers | | | | IOM Reference |
|---|---|---|---|---|---|---|---|---|
| **D5710** | N/A | N | - | N/A | N/A | N/A | N/A | None |
| **D5711** | N/A | N | - | N/A | N/A | N/A | N/A | |
| **D5720** | N/A | N | - | N/A | N/A | N/A | N/A | |
| **D5721** | N/A | N | - | N/A | N/A | N/A | N/A | |

* with documentation

## Terms To Know

**rebase.** In dentistry, refitting of a denture by replacement of the base materials.

# D5725

- **D5725** rebase hybrid prosthesis

  *Replacing the base material connected to the framework.*

## Explanation

A hybrid prosthesis is an acrylic resin dental prosthesis that is supported by implants into the gum and bone. Over time the prosthesis may require changes to the fitting surface by replacing some or all of the denture base (rebasing). Rebase materials can be either hard or soft, self- or heat-cure. The heat-cure rebase requires an impression of the inside of the denture and the patient may be without the prosthesis while the rebasing is completed. The impression material is applied, the denture is inserted to take the impression, and the patient bites into closing contact. The impression is removed and examined and repeated until satisfactory and sent with the denture piece to the lab. The heat-cure material is applied to rebuild the base of the denture and made to fit the patient's mouth from the impression taken. The rebuilt denture is then finished with polishing before being returned and reattached to the patient's implants.

## Coding Tips

To report rebase of dentures, see D5710-D5721.

## Reimbursement Tips

Most third-party payers will only cover rebase services on a prescribed frequency. For example, payers may only pay a rebase service once every two years. Preauthorization may be required.

## ICD-10-CM Diagnostic Codes

Z46.3 Encounter for fitting and adjustment of dental prosthetic device

## Relative Value Units/Medicare Edits

| Non-Facility RVU | Work | PE | MP | Total |
|---|---|---|---|---|
| D5725 | | | | |
| **Facility RVU** | **Work** | **PE** | **MP** | **Total** |
| D5725 | | | | |

| | FUD | Status | MUE | Modifiers | | | | IOM Reference |
|---|---|---|---|---|---|---|---|---|
| D5725 | N/A | | - | N/A | N/A | N/A | N/A | |

* with documentation

## Terms To Know

**denture.** Manmade substitution of natural teeth and neighboring structures.

**hybrid prosthesis.** Fixed acrylic resin dental prosthesis support by metallic implants.

# D5730-D5741

**D5730** reline complete maxillary denture (direct)
**D5731** reline complete mandibular denture (direct)
**D5740** reline maxillary partial denture (direct)
**D5741** reline mandibular partial denture (direct)

## Explanation

Acrylic dentures can be relined directly (chairside) with self-cure materials. Relining is replacing the fitting surface of the denture. Relining materials can be hard or soft, self- or heat-cure. Self-cure materials are used at chairside. The denture is thoroughly cleaned and dried and the inside surface is roughened. The acrylic self-cure relining material is applied. The gingivae are coated for protection and the denture is inserted as for taking an impression. The patient closes to biting position, the denture is removed, and excess material is trimmed. The denture is reinserted and normal biting position is maintained for a few minutes. The denture is removed and allowed to cure or is pressurized in a hot water bath. The acrylic denture is finished by polishing with sandpaper discs or cones. Report D5730 and D5731 for relining a complete upper and lower denture, respectively, and D5740 and D5741 for a partial denture, upper and lower, respectively.

## Coding Tips

Local anesthesia is included in these services. Any evaluation or radiograph is reported separately.

## Reimbursement Tips

Coverage of this procedure varies by payer. Check with the payer for specific coverage guidelines.

## ICD-10-CM Diagnostic Codes

Z46.3 Encounter for fitting and adjustment of dental prosthetic device

## Relative Value Units/Medicare Edits

| Non-Facility RVU | Work | PE | MP | Total |
|---|---|---|---|---|
| D5730 | 1.95 | 1.72 | 0.40 | 4.07 |
| D5731 | 1.95 | 1.72 | 0.40 | 4.07 |
| D5740 | 1.73 | 1.53 | 0.36 | 3.62 |
| D5741 | 1.73 | 1.53 | 0.36 | 3.62 |
| **Facility RVU** | **Work** | **PE** | **MP** | **Total** |
| D5730 | 1.95 | 1.72 | 0.40 | 4.07 |
| D5731 | 1.95 | 1.72 | 0.40 | 4.07 |
| D5740 | 1.73 | 1.53 | 0.36 | 3.62 |
| D5741 | 1.73 | 1.53 | 0.36 | 3.62 |

| | FUD | Status | MUE | Modifiers | | | | IOM Reference |
|---|---|---|---|---|---|---|---|---|
| D5730 | N/A | N | - | N/A | N/A | N/A | N/A | None |
| D5731 | N/A | N | - | N/A | N/A | N/A | N/A | |
| D5740 | N/A | N | - | N/A | N/A | N/A | N/A | |
| D5741 | N/A | N | - | N/A | N/A | N/A | N/A | |

* with documentation

## Terms To Know

**mandible.** Lower jawbone giving structure to the floor of the oral cavity.

**maxillary.** Located between the eyes and the upper teeth.

# D5750-D5761

**D5750** reline complete maxillary denture (indirect)
**D5751** reline complete mandibular denture (indirect)
**D5760** reline maxillary partial denture (indirect)
**D5761** reline mandibular partial denture (indirect)

## Explanation

Relining is replacing the fitting surface of the denture, but not replacing the whole base (pink part) of the denture. Relining materials can be hard or soft, self- or heat-cure. Indirect relining is completed in the laboratory. Heat cure methods and materials are used, and the patient is without the denture while the relining is done. The heat-cure reline requires an impression of the inside of the denture. The impression material is applied, the denture is inserted to take the impression, and the patient bites into closing contact. The impression is removed and examined and repeated until satisfactory and sent with the denture piece to the lab. The heat-cure material is applied to reline the fitting surface of the denture and made to fit the patient's mouth from the impression taken. The relined denture is then finished with polishing before being returned.

## Coding Tips

Local anesthesia is included in these services. Any evaluation or radiograph is reported separately. When direct relining of the denture is performed at the chairside, see D5730-D5741. To report rebase services, see D5710-D5721

## Reimbursement Tips

Coverage of this procedure varies by payer. Check with the payer for specific coverage guidelines.

## ICD-10-CM Diagnostic Codes

Z46.3 Encounter for fitting and adjustment of dental prosthetic device

## Relative Value Units/Medicare Edits

| Non-Facility RVU | Work | PE | MP | Total |
|---|---|---|---|---|
| D5750 | 2.60 | 2.29 | 0.54 | 5.43 |
| D5751 | 2.60 | 2.29 | 0.54 | 5.43 |
| D5760 | 2.57 | 2.27 | 0.53 | 5.37 |
| D5761 | 2.57 | 2.27 | 0.53 | 5.37 |
| **Facility RVU** | **Work** | **PE** | **MP** | **Total** |
| D5750 | 2.60 | 2.29 | 0.54 | 5.43 |
| D5751 | 2.60 | 2.29 | 0.54 | 5.43 |
| D5760 | 2.57 | 2.27 | 0.53 | 5.37 |
| D5761 | 2.57 | 2.27 | 0.53 | 5.37 |

| | FUD | Status | MUE | Modifiers | | | | IOM Reference |
|---|---|---|---|---|---|---|---|---|
| D5750 | N/A | N | - | N/A | N/A | N/A | N/A | None |
| D5751 | N/A | N | - | N/A | N/A | N/A | N/A | |
| D5760 | N/A | N | - | N/A | N/A | N/A | N/A | |
| D5761 | N/A | N | - | N/A | N/A | N/A | N/A | |

* with documentation

## Terms To Know

**denture.** Manmade substitution of natural teeth and neighboring structures.

# D5765

● **D5765** soft liner for complete or partial removable denture - indirect

*A discrete procedure provided when the dentist determines placement of the soft liner is clinically indicated.*

## Explanation

A soft liner is replacing the fitting surface of the denture. A soft liner is an alternative to a reline for patients who may have had changes to their gum tissue, pain, or may not tolerate an acrylic reline. The soft liner is made of soft polymer or silicone and is applied to the denture surface next to the gums and acts as a cushion between the gums and denture. The denture is thoroughly cleaned and dried and the inside surface may be roughened. The soft liner material is applied. The gingivae are coated for protection and the denture is inserted as for taking an impression. The patient closes to biting position, the denture is removed, and excess material is trimmed. The denture is reinserted, and normal biting position is maintained for a few minutes.

## Coding Tips

To report reline of dentures chairside, see D5730–D5734. Report reline of dentures by a laboratory, see D5750-D5761. To report rebase services, see D5710–D5721.

## ICD-10-CM Diagnostic Codes

Z46.3 Encounter for fitting and adjustment of dental prosthetic device

## Relative Value Units/Medicare Edits

| Non-Facility RVU | Work | PE | MP | Total |
|---|---|---|---|---|
| D5765 | | | | |
| **Facility RVU** | **Work** | **PE** | **MP** | **Total** |
| D5765 | | | | |

| | FUD | Status | MUE | Modifiers | | | | IOM Reference |
|---|---|---|---|---|---|---|---|---|
| D5765 | N/A | | - | N/A | N/A | N/A | N/A | |

* with documentation

## Terms To Know

**denture.** Manmade substitution of natural teeth and neighboring structures.

**soft liner.** Soft polymer or silicone replacement of the fitting surface of a denture.

# D5810-D5821

**D5810** interim complete denture (maxillary)
**D5811** interim complete denture (mandibular)
**D5820** interim partial denture (including retentive/clasping materials, rests, and teeth), maxillary

*Includes any necessary clasps and rests.*

**D5821** interim partial denture (including retentive/clasping materials, rests, and teeth), mandibular

## Explanation

An interim denture is a temporary prosthetic device that may be provided prior to manufacture of a more permanent denture to allow the patient to experience and adjust to denture use. Interim dentures are also provided to modify jaw and occlusal relationships prior to restorative work or other prosthetic work such as implants. Jaw and occlusal relationships may need to be modified when loss of teeth or the congenital absence of teeth causes the remaining teeth to shift. An interim denture is used before restorative treatment or fabrication of a permanent denture to facilitate progressive occlusal adjustment until the optimum occlusal relationship is achieved. An interim prosthesis may also be used for severely worn teeth when there is uncertainty regarding the increase in occlusal vertical dimension necessary to accommodate the required restoration's patient toleration. For worn teeth, an interim denture is constructed and the occlusal height increased slightly. The interim denture may be progressively adjusted over several appointments to allow the patient to gradually adapt to progressive, modest increases in occlusal height until the desired occlusal height is reached. Interim dentures are sometimes used in patients with gingival trauma resulting from a deep incisal overbite. An interim denture with a palatal table can provide relief while a decision is being made on a more permanent solution, whether it be orthodontic, restorative, periodontal, or surgical. An interim complete denture for the maxillary jaw is reported with D5810; the mandibular jaw is reported with D5811. An interim partial denture for the maxillary jaw is reported with D5820; and one for the mandibular jaw is reported with D5821

## Coding Tips

Local anesthesia is generally considered to be part of removable prosthodontic procedures.

## Reimbursement Tips

Many payers do not provide coverage for interim dentures.

## ICD-10-CM Diagnostic Codes

K08.101 Complete loss of teeth, unspecified cause, class I
K08.102 Complete loss of teeth, unspecified cause, class II
K08.103 Complete loss of teeth, unspecified cause, class III
K08.104 Complete loss of teeth, unspecified cause, class IV
K08.111 Complete loss of teeth due to trauma, class I
K08.112 Complete loss of teeth due to trauma, class II
K08.113 Complete loss of teeth due to trauma, class III
K08.114 Complete loss of teeth due to trauma, class IV
K08.121 Complete loss of teeth due to periodontal diseases, class I
K08.122 Complete loss of teeth due to periodontal diseases, class II
K08.123 Complete loss of teeth due to periodontal diseases, class III
K08.124 Complete loss of teeth due to periodontal diseases, class IV
K08.131 Complete loss of teeth due to caries, class I
K08.132 Complete loss of teeth due to caries, class II
K08.133 Complete loss of teeth due to caries, class III
K08.134 Complete loss of teeth due to caries, class IV
K08.191 Complete loss of teeth due to other specified cause, class I
K08.192 Complete loss of teeth due to other specified cause, class II
K08.193 Complete loss of teeth due to other specified cause, class III
K08.194 Complete loss of teeth due to other specified cause, class IV
K08.401 Partial loss of teeth, unspecified cause, class I
K08.402 Partial loss of teeth, unspecified cause, class II
K08.403 Partial loss of teeth, unspecified cause, class III
K08.404 Partial loss of teeth, unspecified cause, class IV
K08.411 Partial loss of teeth due to trauma, class I
K08.412 Partial loss of teeth due to trauma, class II
K08.413 Partial loss of teeth due to trauma, class III
K08.414 Partial loss of teeth due to trauma, class IV
K08.421 Partial loss of teeth due to periodontal diseases, class I
K08.422 Partial loss of teeth due to periodontal diseases, class II
K08.423 Partial loss of teeth due to periodontal diseases, class III
K08.424 Partial loss of teeth due to periodontal diseases, class IV
K08.431 Partial loss of teeth due to caries, class I
K08.432 Partial loss of teeth due to caries, class II
K08.433 Partial loss of teeth due to caries, class III
K08.434 Partial loss of teeth due to caries, class IV
K08.491 Partial loss of teeth due to other specified cause, class I
K08.492 Partial loss of teeth due to other specified cause, class II
K08.493 Partial loss of teeth due to other specified cause, class III
K08.494 Partial loss of teeth due to other specified cause, class IV

## Relative Value Units/Medicare Edits

| Non-Facility RVU | Work | PE | MP | Total |
|---|---|---|---|---|
| **D5810** | 4.04 | 3.57 | 0.83 | 8.44 |
| **D5811** | 4.25 | 3.75 | 0.88 | 8.88 |
| **D5820** | 3.20 | 2.82 | 0.66 | 6.68 |
| **D5821** | 3.33 | 2.94 | 0.69 | 6.96 |
| **Facility RVU** | **Work** | **PE** | **MP** | **Total** |
| **D5810** | 4.04 | 3.57 | 0.83 | 8.44 |
| **D5811** | 4.25 | 3.75 | 0.88 | 8.88 |
| **D5820** | 3.20 | 2.82 | 0.66 | 6.68 |
| **D5821** | 3.33 | 2.94 | 0.69 | 6.96 |

| | FUD | Status | MUE | Modifiers | | | | IOM Reference |
|---|---|---|---|---|---|---|---|---|
| **D5810** | N/A | N | - | N/A | N/A | N/A | N/A | None |
| **D5811** | N/A | N | - | N/A | N/A | N/A | N/A | |
| **D5820** | N/A | N | - | N/A | N/A | N/A | N/A | |
| **D5821** | N/A | N | - | N/A | N/A | N/A | N/A | |

* with documentation

## Terms To Know

**denture.** Manmade substitution of natural teeth and neighboring structures.

# D5850-D5851

**D5850** tissue conditioning, maxillary

*Treatment reline using materials designed to heal unhealthy ridges prior to more definitive final restoration.*

**D5851** tissue conditioning, mandibular

*Treatment reline using materials designed to heal unhealthy ridges prior to more definitive final restoration.*

## Explanation

Tissue conditioners are soft-lining, resilient materials that help heal unhealthy or inflamed tissues by more evenly distributing the loading, especially where dentures have caused trauma. The soft material is used to reline the fitting surface of dentures temporarily to allow the tissues to heal prior to impressions for replacement dentures, a rebase, or definitive final restorative treatment. Areas of pressure on the fitting surface are relieved and occlusion is adjusted, if needed, before placing the soft lining in the denture and fitting it. A liquid of esters and alcohol is added to a poly-ethylmethacrylate powder, which then softens into a gel that hardens over time. The material is not left for long periods, and repeat applications may be necessary every few days. Anti-infective agents may even be incorporated into the material before mixing. Report D5850 for maxillary tissue conditioning and D5851 for mandibular.

## Coding Tips

Local anesthesia is included in these services. Any evaluation or radiograph is reported separately.

## Reimbursement Tips

Third-party payers may not provide coverage for this procedure. Check with payers for specific guidelines.

## ICD-10-CM Diagnostic Codes

| | |
|---|---|
| K08.22 | Moderate atrophy of the mandible |
| K08.23 | Severe atrophy of the mandible |
| K08.24 | Minimal atrophy of maxilla |
| K08.25 | Moderate atrophy of the maxilla |
| K08.26 | Severe atrophy of the maxilla |

## Relative Value Units/Medicare Edits

| Non-Facility RVU | Work | PE | MP | Total |
|---|---|---|---|---|
| D5850 | 0.82 | 0.73 | 0.17 | 1.72 |
| D5851 | 0.82 | 0.73 | 0.17 | 1.72 |
| **Facility RVU** | **Work** | **PE** | **MP** | **Total** |
| D5850 | 0.82 | 0.73 | 0.17 | 1.72 |
| D5851 | 0.82 | 0.73 | 0.17 | 1.72 |

| | FUD | Status | MUE | Modifiers | | | | IOM Reference |
|---|---|---|---|---|---|---|---|---|
| D5850 | N/A | N | - | N/A | N/A | N/A | N/A | None |
| D5851 | N/A | N | - | N/A | N/A | N/A | N/A | |

* with documentation

## Terms To Know

**denture.** Manmade substitution of natural teeth and neighboring structures.

# D5862

▲ **D5862** precision attachment, by report

*Each pair of components is one precision attachment. Describe the type of attachment used.*

## Explanation

This code reports the custom fabrication of precision attachments. Overdentures and some types of partial dentures use precision attachments that hold the denture in place. A precision attachment in an overdenture uses a receptacle in a tooth root that has been saved or in a dental implant. Dental attachments in the overdenture clip into these receptacles and secure the overdenture. A precision attachment in a partial denture uses a receptacle created within a remaining tooth. The receptacle typically is covered with a crown. The precision attachment extends into the receptacle securing the partial denture. Because the exact nature of the precision attachment can vary, this code requires submission of a report.

## Coding Tips

Local anesthesia is generally considered to be part of removable prosthodontic procedures. This code reports one set of male and female components.

## Reimbursement Tips

Third-party payers may not reimburse separately for this service. Check with payers for specific guidelines.

## ICD-10-CM Diagnostic Codes

| | |
|---|---|
| Z46.3 | Encounter for fitting and adjustment of dental prosthetic device |

## Relative Value Units/Medicare Edits

| Non-Facility RVU | Work | PE | MP | Total |
|---|---|---|---|---|
| D5862 | 3.01 | 2.66 | 0.62 | 6.29 |
| **Facility RVU** | **Work** | **PE** | **MP** | **Total** |
| D5862 | 3.01 | 2.66 | 0.62 | 6.29 |

| | FUD | Status | MUE | Modifiers | | | | IOM Reference |
|---|---|---|---|---|---|---|---|---|
| D5862 | N/A | N | - | N/A | N/A | N/A | N/A | None |

* with documentation

## Terms To Know

**artificial crown.** In dentistry, a ceramic or metal restoration made to cover or replace a major part of the top of a tooth.

**overdenture.** In dentistry, prosthesis of artificial teeth that overlies and is supported by retained tooth roots or implants. It is removable.

**precision attachment.** In dentistry, an interlocking device in which one component is attached to an abutment and the other is incorporated into a prosthesis (fixed or removable) to stabilize or retain it.

**prosthodontics.** Branch of dentistry that specializes in the replacement of missing or damaged teeth.

# D5863-D5866

**D5863** overdenture - complete maxillary
**D5864** overdenture - partial maxillary
**D5865** overdenture - complete mandibular
**D5866** overdenture - partial mandibular

## Explanation

When most or all of the teeth are lost, there is nothing to hold a denture down while chewing. An overdenture solves this problem by fastening the denture to the jawbone, similar to the way natural teeth are anchored. An overdenture uses a combination of precision dental attachments placed into the resin base that connect to precision attachments placed in the tooth root or jawbone. When the tooth roots are used, a root canal is performed on each tooth and a metal post is inserted. When no tooth roots have been saved, a dental implant is placed in the jawbone. Two types of overdentures are available: bar joint dentures and telescopic dentures. Bar joint overdentures are partial dentures used when the patient still has some natural teeth. The remaining adjacent teeth are fitted with locking devices or connecting bars to ensure the denture fits properly. Implants in the tooth root or jawbone are also used to support the bars and attach the denture. When patients have lost all or most of their teeth and also have compromised bone density due to age or oral disease, a telescopic overdenture is used. The telescopic overdenture uses a double crown system, with inner metal crowns placed in the resin base and outer crowns in the remaining natural teeth or in the dental implants. Fabrication of telescopic dentures is extremely complicated and requires root canal therapy for each remaining natural tooth and the insertion of a metal post to ensure the root is strong enough. Report D5863 for a complete maxillary overdenture or D5861 for a partial maxillary overdenture. Report D5865 for a complete mandibular overdenture or D5866 for a partial mandibular overdenture

## Coding Tips

Local anesthesia is generally considered to be part of removable prosthodontic procedures. Report any adjunctive procedures, such as extractions, separately following payer guidelines. See D5211–D5283 for other types of the partial dentures. See D5110–D5120 for complete dentures. For precision attachments, see code D5862. To report the surgical placement of a mini-implant, see D6013.

## Reimbursement Tips

Third-party payers may require preauthorization and/or supporting documentation justifying the need for the procedure.

## ICD-10-CM Diagnostic Codes

K08.101 Complete loss of teeth, unspecified cause, class I
K08.102 Complete loss of teeth, unspecified cause, class II
K08.103 Complete loss of teeth, unspecified cause, class III
K08.104 Complete loss of teeth, unspecified cause, class IV
K08.111 Complete loss of teeth due to trauma, class I
K08.112 Complete loss of teeth due to trauma, class II
K08.113 Complete loss of teeth due to trauma, class III
K08.114 Complete loss of teeth due to trauma, class IV
K08.121 Complete loss of teeth due to periodontal diseases, class I
K08.122 Complete loss of teeth due to periodontal diseases, class II
K08.123 Complete loss of teeth due to periodontal diseases, class III
K08.124 Complete loss of teeth due to periodontal diseases, class IV
K08.131 Complete loss of teeth due to caries, class I
K08.132 Complete loss of teeth due to caries, class II
K08.133 Complete loss of teeth due to caries, class III
K08.134 Complete loss of teeth due to caries, class IV
K08.191 Complete loss of teeth due to other specified cause, class I
K08.192 Complete loss of teeth due to other specified cause, class II
K08.193 Complete loss of teeth due to other specified cause, class III
K08.194 Complete loss of teeth due to other specified cause, class IV
K08.401 Partial loss of teeth, unspecified cause, class I
K08.402 Partial loss of teeth, unspecified cause, class II
K08.403 Partial loss of teeth, unspecified cause, class III
K08.404 Partial loss of teeth, unspecified cause, class IV
K08.411 Partial loss of teeth due to trauma, class I
K08.412 Partial loss of teeth due to trauma, class II
K08.413 Partial loss of teeth due to trauma, class III
K08.414 Partial loss of teeth due to trauma, class IV
K08.421 Partial loss of teeth due to periodontal diseases, class I
K08.422 Partial loss of teeth due to periodontal diseases, class II
K08.423 Partial loss of teeth due to periodontal diseases, class III
K08.424 Partial loss of teeth due to periodontal diseases, class IV
K08.431 Partial loss of teeth due to caries, class I
K08.432 Partial loss of teeth due to caries, class II
K08.433 Partial loss of teeth due to caries, class III
K08.434 Partial loss of teeth due to caries, class IV
K08.491 Partial loss of teeth due to other specified cause, class I
K08.492 Partial loss of teeth due to other specified cause, class II
K08.493 Partial loss of teeth due to other specified cause, class III
K08.494 Partial loss of teeth due to other specified cause, class IV

## Relative Value Units/Medicare Edits

| Non-Facility RVU | Work | PE | MP | Total |
|---|---|---|---|---|
| **D5863** | 8.97 | 7.92 | 1.85 | 18.74 |
| **D5864** | 9.14 | 8.06 | 1.88 | 19.08 |
| **D5865** | 8.97 | 7.92 | 1.85 | 18.74 |
| **D5866** | 9.14 | 8.06 | 1.88 | 19.08 |
| **Facility RVU** | **Work** | **PE** | **MP** | **Total** |
| **D5863** | 8.97 | 7.92 | 1.85 | 18.74 |
| **D5864** | 9.14 | 8.06 | 1.88 | 19.08 |
| **D5865** | 8.97 | 7.92 | 1.85 | 18.74 |
| **D5866** | 9.14 | 8.06 | 1.88 | 19.08 |

| | FUD | Status | MUE | Modifiers | | | | IOM Reference |
|---|---|---|---|---|---|---|---|---|
| **D5863** | N/A | N | - | N/A | N/A | N/A | N/A | None |
| **D5864** | N/A | N | - | N/A | N/A | N/A | N/A | |
| **D5865** | N/A | N | - | N/A | N/A | N/A | N/A | |
| **D5866** | N/A | N | - | N/A | N/A | N/A | N/A | |

* with documentation

## Terms To Know

**mandible.** Lower jawbone giving structure to the floor of the oral cavity.

**maxilla.** Pyramidally-shaped bone forming the upper jaw, part of the eye orbit, nasal cavity, and palate and lodging the upper teeth.

**overdenture.** In dentistry, prosthesis of artificial teeth that overlies and is supported by retained tooth roots or implants. It is removable.

# D5867

▲ **D5867** replacement of replaceable part of semi-precision or precision attachment, per attachment

## Explanation

Overdentures and some types of partial dentures use semi-precious or precision attachments that hold the denture in place. A precision attachment in an overdenture uses a receptacle in a tooth root that has been saved or a dental implant to secure the prosthesis. A precision attachment in a partial denture uses a receptacle created with a remaining tooth; a crown typically covers the receptacle. The attachment extends into the receptacle to secure the partial denture. This code reports the removal and replacement of a damaged semi-precision or precision attachment.

## Coding Tips

Local anesthesia is generally considered part of restorative procedures.

## Reimbursement Tips

Many third-party payers do not provide coverage for this service. Check with individual payers to determine specific guidelines.

## ICD-10-CM Diagnostic Codes

Z46.3 Encounter for fitting and adjustment of dental prosthetic device

## Relative Value Units/Medicare Edits

| Non-Facility RVU | Work | PE | MP | Total |
|---|---|---|---|---|
| D5867 | 1.29 | 1.14 | 0.27 | 2.70 |
| **Facility RVU** | **Work** | **PE** | **MP** | **Total** |
| D5867 | 1.29 | 1.14 | 0.27 | 2.70 |

| | FUD | Status | MUE | Modifiers | | | | IOM Reference |
|---|---|---|---|---|---|---|---|---|
| D5867 | N/A | N | - | N/A | N/A | N/A | N/A | None |

* with documentation

## Terms To Know

**artificial crown.** In dentistry, a ceramic or metal restoration made to cover or replace a major part of the top of a tooth.

**partial dentures.** In dentistry, artificial teeth composed of a framework with plastic teeth and gum area replacing part but not all of the natural teeth. The framework can either be formed from an acrylic resin base, cast metal or may be made more flexible using thermoplastics.

**precision attachment.** In dentistry, an interlocking device in which one component is attached to an abutment and the other is incorporated into a prosthesis (fixed or removable) to stabilize or retain it.

**prosthodontics.** Branch of dentistry that specializes in the replacement of missing or damaged teeth.

# D5876

**D5876** add metal substructure to acrylic full denture (per arch)

## Explanation

Metal is added to strengthen or repair an acrylic full denture. Cast metal is used. The procedure varies depending upon the reason for performing the procedure. This code is reported once for each arch.

## Coding Tips

This procedure is reported as an additional procedure when the full denture is being fabricated. This procedure should not be reported as a repair of the denture. To report the repair of a full denture, see D5512.

## Reimbursement Tips

Most payers require that missing teeth be indicated on the dental claim form. Coverage guidelines vary by payer and by patient contract. Patients are often responsible for copayments or may reach contract limitations. Check with the payer to determine coverage policies and patient responsibility.

## ICD-10-CM Diagnostic Codes

K08.111 Complete loss of teeth due to trauma, class I
K08.112 Complete loss of teeth due to trauma, class II
K08.113 Complete loss of teeth due to trauma, class III
K08.114 Complete loss of teeth due to trauma, class IV
K08.121 Complete loss of teeth due to periodontal diseases, class I
K08.122 Complete loss of teeth due to periodontal diseases, class II
K08.123 Complete loss of teeth due to periodontal diseases, class III
K08.124 Complete loss of teeth due to periodontal diseases, class IV
K08.131 Complete loss of teeth due to caries, class I
K08.132 Complete loss of teeth due to caries, class II
K08.133 Complete loss of teeth due to caries, class III
K08.134 Complete loss of teeth due to caries, class IV
K08.191 Complete loss of teeth due to other specified cause, class I
K08.192 Complete loss of teeth due to other specified cause, class II
K08.193 Complete loss of teeth due to other specified cause, class III
K08.194 Complete loss of teeth due to other specified cause, class IV
K08.401 Partial loss of teeth, unspecified cause, class I
K08.402 Partial loss of teeth, unspecified cause, class II
K08.403 Partial loss of teeth, unspecified cause, class III
K08.404 Partial loss of teeth, unspecified cause, class IV
K08.411 Partial loss of teeth due to trauma, class I
K08.412 Partial loss of teeth due to trauma, class II
K08.413 Partial loss of teeth due to trauma, class III
K08.414 Partial loss of teeth due to trauma, class IV
K08.421 Partial loss of teeth due to periodontal diseases, class I
K08.422 Partial loss of teeth due to periodontal diseases, class II
K08.423 Partial loss of teeth due to periodontal diseases, class III
K08.424 Partial loss of teeth due to periodontal diseases, class IV
K08.431 Partial loss of teeth due to caries, class I
K08.432 Partial loss of teeth due to caries, class II
K08.433 Partial loss of teeth due to caries, class III
K08.434 Partial loss of teeth due to caries, class IV
K08.491 Partial loss of teeth due to other specified cause, class I
K08.492 Partial loss of teeth due to other specified cause, class II
K08.493 Partial loss of teeth due to other specified cause, class III
K08.494 Partial loss of teeth due to other specified cause, class IV
Z46.3 Encounter for fitting and adjustment of dental prosthetic device

## Relative Value Units/Medicare Edits

| Non-Facility RVU | Work | PE | MP | Total |
|---|---|---|---|---|
| **D5876** | 1.15 | 1.01 | 0.24 | 2.40 |
| **Facility RVU** | **Work** | **PE** | **MP** | **Total** |
| **D5876** | 1.15 | 1.01 | 0.24 | 2.40 |

| | FUD | Status | MUE | Modifiers | | | | IOM Reference |
|---|---|---|---|---|---|---|---|---|
| **D5876** | N/A | N | - | N/A | N/A | N/A | N/A | None |

* with documentation

## Terms To Know

**caries.** Localized section of tooth decay that begins on the tooth surface with destruction of the calcified enamel, allowing bacterial destruction to continue and form cavities and may extend to the dentin and pulp.

**denture.** Manmade substitution of natural teeth and neighboring structures.

**denture base.** Portion of the artificial substitute for natural teeth that makes contact with the soft tissue of the mouth and serves as the anchor for the artificial teeth.

**periodontal.** Relating to the tissues that support and surround the teeth.

# D5991

**D5991** vesiculobullous disease medicament carrier

*A custom fabricated carrier that covers the teeth and alveolar mucosa, or alveolar mucosa alone, and is used to deliver prescription medicaments for treatment of immunologically mediated vesiculobullous disease.*

## Explanation

This device is used for treating desquamative diseases of the gingival and oral mucosa, which are characterized by diffuse gingival erythema and various degrees of sloughing and erosion of the mucosa.

## Coding Tips

This is an out-of-sequence code and will not display in numeric order in the CDT book. For periodontal medicament carrier with a peripheral seal, see D5994.

## ICD-10-CM Diagnostic Codes

K05.00 Acute gingivitis, plaque induced
K05.01 Acute gingivitis, non-plaque induced
K05.10 Chronic gingivitis, plaque induced
K05.11 Chronic gingivitis, non-plaque induced
K05.211 Aggressive periodontitis, localized, slight
K05.212 Aggressive periodontitis, localized, moderate
K05.213 Aggressive periodontitis, localized, severe
K05.219 Aggressive periodontitis, localized, unspecified severity
K05.221 Aggressive periodontitis, generalized, slight
K05.222 Aggressive periodontitis, generalized, moderate
K05.223 Aggressive periodontitis, generalized, severe
K05.229 Aggressive periodontitis, generalized, unspecified severity
K05.30 Chronic periodontitis, unspecified
K05.311 Chronic periodontitis, localized, slight
K05.312 Chronic periodontitis, localized, moderate
K05.313 Chronic periodontitis, localized, severe
K05.319 Chronic periodontitis, localized, unspecified severity
K05.321 Chronic periodontitis, generalized, slight
K05.322 Chronic periodontitis, generalized, moderate
K05.323 Chronic periodontitis, generalized, severe
K05.329 Chronic periodontitis, generalized, unspecified severity
K06.010 Localized gingival recession, unspecified
K06.011 Localized gingival recession, minimal
K06.012 Localized gingival recession, moderate
K06.013 Localized gingival recession, severe
K06.020 Generalized gingival recession, unspecified
K06.021 Generalized gingival recession, minimal
K06.022 Generalized gingival recession, moderate
K06.023 Generalized gingival recession, severe
K06.1 Gingival enlargement
K06.2 Gingival and edentulous alveolar ridge lesions associated with trauma
K12.31 Oral mucositis (ulcerative) due to antineoplastic therapy
K12.32 Oral mucositis (ulcerative) due to other drugs
K12.33 Oral mucositis (ulcerative) due to radiation

## Relative Value Units/Medicare Edits

| Non-Facility RVU | Work | PE | MP | Total |
|---|---|---|---|---|
| D5991 | 0.89 | 0.78 | 0.18 | 1.85 |
| **Facility RVU** | **Work** | **PE** | **MP** | **Total** |
| D5991 | 0.89 | 0.78 | 0.18 | 1.85 |

| | FUD | Status | MUE | Modifiers | | | | IOM Reference |
|---|---|---|---|---|---|---|---|---|
| D5991 | N/A | N | - | N/A | N/A | N/A | N/A | None |

* with documentation

## Terms To Know

**alveolar process.** Bony part of the maxilla or mandible that supports the tooth roots and into which the teeth are implanted.

**gingivitis.** Inflamed gingiva (oral mucosa) that surrounds the teeth.

**medicament.** Medical and therapeutic compound, drug, substance, or remedy.

**periodontitis.** Inflammation of the tissue structures supporting the teeth leading to a loss of connective tissue attachments.

# D5992-D5993

**D5992** adjust maxillofacial prosthetic appliance, by report
**D5993** maintenance and cleaning of a maxillofacial prosthesis (extra- or intra-oral) other than required adjustments, by report

## Explanation

Prostheses are used to replace something either removed or congenitally missing and include prosthesis to replace tissues removed by surgical treatment of malignancies or cysts, or for the treatment of congenital defects such a cleft lip or palate deformities. For example, a prosthodontist may build a soft palate obturator or speech and feeding aid to block openings in the palate or to lift the soft palate. These types of prostheses replace missing muscle(s) and/or fill any defects. A palatal lift prosthesis aids in repositioning the soft palate. Both of these types of prostheses aid in swallowing and/or speech; however, some prostheses may be for aesthetic purposes only. Code D5992 is used to report changes made to correct for fitting and/or fabrication inaccuracies. Code D5993 is used to report the maintenance and/or cleaning of the prosthesis.

## Coding Tips

When reporting code D5992, documentation should be submitted with the claim.

## Reimbursement Tips

Many third-party payers consider initial adjustments to the prosthesis for fitting and/or fabrication to be included in the fee for the placement and will not reimburse separately for these services.

## ICD-10-CM Diagnostic Codes

Z46.3 Encounter for fitting and adjustment of dental prosthetic device

## Relative Value Units/Medicare Edits

| Non-Facility RVU | Work | PE | MP | Total |
|---|---|---|---|---|
| D5992 | 1.46 | 1.28 | 0.30 | 3.04 |
| D5993 | 2.57 | 2.27 | 0.53 | 5.37 |
| **Facility RVU** | **Work** | **PE** | **MP** | **Total** |
| D5992 | 1.46 | 1.28 | 0.30 | 3.04 |
| D5993 | 2.57 | 2.27 | 0.53 | 5.37 |

| | FUD | Status | MUE | Modifiers | | | | IOM Reference |
|---|---|---|---|---|---|---|---|---|
| D5992 | N/A | I | - | N/A | N/A | N/A | N/A | None |
| D5993 | N/A | I | - | N/A | N/A | N/A | N/A | |

* with documentation

## Terms To Know

**prosthesis.** Man-made substitute for a missing body part.

**prosthodontics.** Branch of dentistry that specializes in the replacement of missing or damaged teeth.

# D5995-D5996

**D5995** periodontal medicament carrier with peripheral seal - laboratory processed - maxillary

*A custom fabricated, laboratory processed carrier for the maxillary arch that covers the teeth and alveolar mucosa. Used as a vehicle to deliver prescribed medicaments for sustained contact with the gingiva, alveolar mucosa, and into the periodontal sulcus or pocket.*

**D5996** periodontal medicament carrier with peripheral seal - laboratory processed - mandibular

*A custom fabricated, laboratory processed carrier for the mandibular arch that covers the teeth and alveolar mucosa. Used as a vehicle to deliver prescribed medicaments for sustained contact with the gingiva, alveolar mucosa, and into the periodontal sulcus or pocket.*

## Explanation

The dental professional provides the patient with a laboratory processed, custom-fabricated medication carrier that covers the teeth, gingiva, alveolar mucosa, and extends into the periodontal sulcus or pocket and prevents leakage of the medication by incorporating a peripheral seal. This carrier is used to deliver prescribed medication that must be in sustained contact with affected periodontal condition and is used for the treatment of periodontal pathogens.

## Coding Tips

To report the localized delivery of antimicrobial agents using a controlled release vehicle, see D4381 or D5991. To report the provision of drugs and/or medicaments by the provider, see D9630.

## Documentation Tips

Treatment plan documentation should reflect any treatment failure or change in diagnosis and/or a change in treatment plan. There should also be evidence of any initiation or reinstatement of a drug regime, which requires close and continuous skilled medical observation.

## ICD-10-CM Diagnostic Codes

The application of this code is too broad to adequately present ICD-10-CM diagnostic code links here. Refer to your ICD-10-CM book.

## Relative Value Units/Medicare Edits

| Non-Facility RVU | Work | PE | MP | Total |
|---|---|---|---|---|
| D5995 | | | | |
| D5996 | | | | |
| **Facility RVU** | **Work** | **PE** | **MP** | **Total** |
| D5995 | | | | |
| D5996 | | | | |

| | FUD | Status | MUE | Modifiers | | | | IOM Reference |
|---|---|---|---|---|---|---|---|---|
| D5995 | N/A | | - | N/A | N/A | N/A | N/A | |
| D5996 | N/A | | - | N/A | N/A | N/A | N/A | |

* with documentation

## Terms To Know

**alveolar process.** Bony part of the maxilla or mandible that supports the tooth roots and into which the teeth are implanted.

**periodontal.** Relating to the tissues that support and surround the teeth.

Dental - Maxillofacial Prosthetics

# D6010, D6012

**D6010** surgical placement of implant body: endosteal implant
▲ **D6012** surgical placement of interim implant body for transitional prosthesis: endosteal implant

## Explanation

Surgical placement of an endosteal implant body requires two to three surgical sessions. At the first surgical session (D6010), a local anesthetic is administered. An incision is made to expose the bone at the site where the implant will be placed. The bone is prepared using a drill and a screw-like implant is twisted into position. The incision is closed and the implant site allowed to heal. Approximately three to six months later, whenever osteointegration of the implant is confirmed, a second surgery is performed (D6011). A local anesthetic is administered and a small incision is made over the implant site. At this time either a healing abutment or a permanent abutment is placed. If a healing abutment is placed, the gum grows over the abutment and a third procedure (D6012) is required about two to three weeks later to remove the healing abutment and to place the permanent abutment. Once the permanent abutment is in place, teeth are fabricated and attached to the implant. Dental implants can be made of a variety of materials, such as titanium, aluminum oxide, and surgical stainless steel.

## Coding Tips

To report placement of endosteal implant body, see D6010. To report the surgical placement of an eposteal implant, see D6040. Report a transosteal implant with D6050. To report removal of an implant, see D6100. To report the surgical placement of a mini-implant, see D6013. Debridement of peri-implant defects is reported with codes D6101–D6102.

## Reimbursement Tips

When selecting the procedure or service that accurately identifies the service performed, dentists must use the most accurate code. If the CDT code more accurately identifies the service, this should be used rather than the CPT codes. When the condition is the result of an accident, the dental insurer may require that the medical insurance be billed first. When covered by medical insurance, the payer may require that the appropriate CPT code be reported on the CMS-1500 claim form.

## Associated CPT Codes

21248 Reconstruction of mandible or maxilla, endosteal implant (eg, blade, cylinder); partial
21249 Reconstruction of mandible or maxilla, endosteal implant (eg, blade, cylinder); complete

## ICD-10-CM Diagnostic Codes

K08.111 Complete loss of teeth due to trauma, class I
K08.112 Complete loss of teeth due to trauma, class II
K08.113 Complete loss of teeth due to trauma, class III
K08.114 Complete loss of teeth due to trauma, class IV
K08.121 Complete loss of teeth due to periodontal diseases, class I
K08.122 Complete loss of teeth due to periodontal diseases, class II
K08.123 Complete loss of teeth due to periodontal diseases, class III
K08.124 Complete loss of teeth due to periodontal diseases, class IV
K08.131 Complete loss of teeth due to caries, class I
K08.132 Complete loss of teeth due to caries, class II
K08.133 Complete loss of teeth due to caries, class III
K08.134 Complete loss of teeth due to caries, class IV
K08.191 Complete loss of teeth due to other specified cause, class I
K08.192 Complete loss of teeth due to other specified cause, class II
K08.193 Complete loss of teeth due to other specified cause, class III
K08.194 Complete loss of teeth due to other specified cause, class IV
K08.21 Minimal atrophy of the mandible
K08.22 Moderate atrophy of the mandible
K08.23 Severe atrophy of the mandible
K08.24 Minimal atrophy of maxilla
K08.25 Moderate atrophy of the maxilla
K08.26 Severe atrophy of the maxilla
K08.411 Partial loss of teeth due to trauma, class I
K08.412 Partial loss of teeth due to trauma, class II
K08.413 Partial loss of teeth due to trauma, class III
K08.414 Partial loss of teeth due to trauma, class IV
K08.421 Partial loss of teeth due to periodontal diseases, class I
K08.422 Partial loss of teeth due to periodontal diseases, class II
K08.423 Partial loss of teeth due to periodontal diseases, class III
K08.424 Partial loss of teeth due to periodontal diseases, class IV
K08.431 Partial loss of teeth due to caries, class I
K08.432 Partial loss of teeth due to caries, class II
K08.433 Partial loss of teeth due to caries, class III
K08.434 Partial loss of teeth due to caries, class IV
K08.491 Partial loss of teeth due to other specified cause, class I
K08.492 Partial loss of teeth due to other specified cause, class II
K08.493 Partial loss of teeth due to other specified cause, class III
K08.494 Partial loss of teeth due to other specified cause, class IV

## Relative Value Units/Medicare Edits

| Non-Facility RVU | Work | PE | MP | Total |
|---|---|---|---|---|
| **D6010** | 12.43 | 10.97 | 2.56 | 25.96 |
| **D6012** | 11.24 | 9.92 | 2.31 | 23.47 |
| **Facility RVU** | **Work** | **PE** | **MP** | **Total** |
| **D6010** | 12.43 | 10.97 | 2.56 | 25.96 |
| **D6012** | 11.24 | 9.92 | 2.31 | 23.47 |

| | FUD | Status | MUE | Modifiers | | | | IOM Reference |
|---|---|---|---|---|---|---|---|---|
| **D6010** | N/A | I | - | N/A | N/A | N/A | N/A | None |
| **D6012** | N/A | N | - | N/A | N/A | N/A | N/A | |

* with documentation

## Terms To Know

**abutment.** Tooth or implant fixture supporting a prosthesis.

**endosteal implant.** Metal implants that are cylindrical or blade-like in structure, placed into the maxillary or mandibular bone. Metal posts that protrude through the mucosa into the mouth are attached to the implants so that artificial teeth or dentures can be attached to the roots to replace missing teeth.

**implant.** Material or device inserted or placed within the body for therapeutic, reconstructive, or diagnostic purposes.

# D6013

**D6013** surgical placement of mini implant

## Explanation

The dental health care provider surgically places a mini-implant. Mini-implants are generally 1.8-2.9 mm in diameter and of various lengths. After local anesthesia the provider marks the location of the implant. The soft tissue is punctured and pilot holes are drilled into the center of the bony ridge. The implant is then positioned into place using the drill. An O-ring is placed over the implant and the denture is prepared with manufacturer recommended adhesive and placed over the O-ring and held in place for 3-4 minutes. This transfers the O-ring onto the denture. The denture is snapped out, cleaned and polished and the fit is evaluated. Any adjustments to the denture are made.

## Coding Tips

To report surgical placement of an endosteal implant, see D6010; eposteal implant D6040; or transosteal implant D6050. Report the denture separately.

## ICD-10-CM Diagnostic Codes

| | |
|---|---|
| K08.401 | Partial loss of teeth, unspecified cause, class I |
| K08.402 | Partial loss of teeth, unspecified cause, class II |
| K08.403 | Partial loss of teeth, unspecified cause, class III |
| K08.404 | Partial loss of teeth, unspecified cause, class IV |
| K08.411 | Partial loss of teeth due to trauma, class I |
| K08.412 | Partial loss of teeth due to trauma, class II |
| K08.413 | Partial loss of teeth due to trauma, class III |
| K08.414 | Partial loss of teeth due to trauma, class IV |
| K08.421 | Partial loss of teeth due to periodontal diseases, class I |
| K08.422 | Partial loss of teeth due to periodontal diseases, class II |
| K08.423 | Partial loss of teeth due to periodontal diseases, class III |
| K08.424 | Partial loss of teeth due to periodontal diseases, class IV |
| K08.431 | Partial loss of teeth due to caries, class I |
| K08.432 | Partial loss of teeth due to caries, class II |
| K08.433 | Partial loss of teeth due to caries, class III |
| K08.434 | Partial loss of teeth due to caries, class IV |
| K08.491 | Partial loss of teeth due to other specified cause, class I |
| K08.492 | Partial loss of teeth due to other specified cause, class II |
| K08.493 | Partial loss of teeth due to other specified cause, class III |
| K08.494 | Partial loss of teeth due to other specified cause, class IV |

## Relative Value Units/Medicare Edits

| Non-Facility RVU | Work | PE | MP | Total |
|---|---|---|---|---|
| D6013 | 6.02 | 5.31 | 1.24 | 12.57 |
| **Facility RVU** | **Work** | **PE** | **MP** | **Total** |
| D6013 | 6.02 | 5.31 | 1.24 | 12.57 |

| | FUD | Status | MUE | Modifiers | | | | IOM Reference |
|---|---|---|---|---|---|---|---|---|
| D6013 | N/A | N | - | N/A | N/A | N/A | N/A | None |

* with documentation

## Terms To Know

**implant.** Material or device inserted or placed within the body for therapeutic, reconstructive, or diagnostic purposes.

# D6040

**D6040** surgical placement: eposteal implant

*An eposteal (subperiosteal) framework of a biocompatible material designed and fabricated to fit on the surface of the bone of the mandible or maxilla with permucosal extensions which provide support and attachment of a prosthesis. This may be a complete arch or unilateral appliance. Eposteal implants rest upon the bone and under the periosteum.*

## Explanation

An eposteal (subperiosteal) implant is used when the bone underlying the teeth has atrophied and the jaw structure is not sufficient to support an endosteal implant. An eposteal implant consists of a metal framework that fits over the bone with an implant between the periosteum and the alveolar bone; the posts project through the gum (gingiva) and into the oral cavity. Eposteal implants may be used on a limited area or to replace all the teeth if the patient is edentulous. Eposteal implants are custom fabricated, and two techniques are currently available for obtaining the information required for fabrication. The first method requires that an impression be made of the jawbone. A local anesthetic Is administered, the jawbone exposed, and an impression made. The impression is sent to a dental laboratory for the custom-fabrication of the implant. The second method involves use of a CT scan. Using computer modeling, the dental laboratory then constructs the implant. When the custom-fabricated implant is ready, a procedure is performed to expose your jawbone and place the implant. The gums are closed with stitches and replacement teeth are installed. Dental implants can be made of a variety of materials, such as titanium, aluminum oxide, and surgical stainless steel.

## Coding Tips

Local anesthesia is generally considered part of restorative procedures. For endosteal implant, see D6010–D6012; for transosteal implant, see D6050. To report endodontic endosseous implants, see D3460.

## Reimbursement Tips

When selecting the procedure or service that accurately identifies the service performed, dentists must use the most accurate code. If the CDT code more accurately identifies the service, this should be used rather than the CPT codes. The third-party payer may require an x-ray or x-ray report. Coverage of this implant procedure varies by payer and by individual contract. Check with payers for specific coverage guidelines.

## Associated CPT Codes

| | |
|---|---|
| 21248 | Reconstruction of mandible or maxilla, endosteal implant (eg, blade, cylinder); partial |

## ICD-10-CM Diagnostic Codes

| | |
|---|---|
| K08.101 | Complete loss of teeth, unspecified cause, class I |
| K08.102 | Complete loss of teeth, unspecified cause, class II |
| K08.103 | Complete loss of teeth, unspecified cause, class III |
| K08.104 | Complete loss of teeth, unspecified cause, class IV |
| K08.111 | Complete loss of teeth due to trauma, class I |
| K08.112 | Complete loss of teeth due to trauma, class II |
| K08.113 | Complete loss of teeth due to trauma, class III |
| K08.114 | Complete loss of teeth due to trauma, class IV |
| K08.121 | Complete loss of teeth due to periodontal diseases, class I |
| K08.122 | Complete loss of teeth due to periodontal diseases, class II |
| K08.123 | Complete loss of teeth due to periodontal diseases, class III |
| K08.124 | Complete loss of teeth due to periodontal diseases, class IV |

K08.131 Complete loss of teeth due to caries, class I
K08.132 Complete loss of teeth due to caries, class II
K08.133 Complete loss of teeth due to caries, class III
K08.134 Complete loss of teeth due to caries, class IV
K08.191 Complete loss of teeth due to other specified cause, class I
K08.192 Complete loss of teeth due to other specified cause, class II
K08.193 Complete loss of teeth due to other specified cause, class III
K08.194 Complete loss of teeth due to other specified cause, class IV
K08.21 Minimal atrophy of the mandible
K08.22 Moderate atrophy of the mandible
K08.23 Severe atrophy of the mandible
K08.24 Minimal atrophy of maxilla
K08.25 Moderate atrophy of the maxilla
K08.26 Severe atrophy of the maxilla
K08.401 Partial loss of teeth, unspecified cause, class I
K08.402 Partial loss of teeth, unspecified cause, class II
K08.403 Partial loss of teeth, unspecified cause, class III
K08.404 Partial loss of teeth, unspecified cause, class IV
K08.411 Partial loss of teeth due to trauma, class I
K08.412 Partial loss of teeth due to trauma, class II
K08.413 Partial loss of teeth due to trauma, class III
K08.414 Partial loss of teeth due to trauma, class IV
K08.421 Partial loss of teeth due to periodontal diseases, class I
K08.422 Partial loss of teeth due to periodontal diseases, class II
K08.423 Partial loss of teeth due to periodontal diseases, class III
K08.424 Partial loss of teeth due to periodontal diseases, class IV
K08.431 Partial loss of teeth due to caries, class I
K08.432 Partial loss of teeth due to caries, class II
K08.433 Partial loss of teeth due to caries, class III
K08.434 Partial loss of teeth due to caries, class IV
K08.491 Partial loss of teeth due to other specified cause, class I
K08.492 Partial loss of teeth due to other specified cause, class II
K08.493 Partial loss of teeth due to other specified cause, class III
K08.494 Partial loss of teeth due to other specified cause, class IV

## Relative Value Units/Medicare Edits

| Non-Facility RVU | Work | PE | MP | Total |
|---|---|---|---|---|
| **D6040** | 43.24 | 38.17 | 8.90 | 90.31 |
| **Facility RVU** | **Work** | **PE** | **MP** | **Total** |
| **D6040** | 43.24 | 38.17 | 8.90 | 90.31 |

| | FUD | Status | MUE | Modifiers | | | | IOM Reference |
|---|---|---|---|---|---|---|---|---|
| **D6040** | N/A | I | - | N/A | N/A | N/A | N/A | None |

* with documentation

## Terms To Know

**eposteal implant.** Dental implant receiving bone support by leaning on residual mandibular bone.

**mandible.** Lower jawbone giving structure to the floor of the oral cavity.

# D6050

**D6050** surgical placement: transosteal implant

*A transosteal (transosseous) biocompatible device with threaded posts penetrating both the superior and inferior cortical bone plates of the mandibular symphysis and exiting through the permucosa providing support and attachment for a dental prosthesis. Transosteal implants are placed completely through the bone and into the oral cavity from extraoral or intraoral.*

## Explanation

A transosteal implant is used only in the mandible (lower jaw). It uses a metal plate that lies under the jaw. The plate contains posts that pass completely through the bone and extend through the gingiva (gum) and into the oral cavity. A dental prosthesis is attached to the posts. Surgical placement of the transosteal implant is accomplished through a skin incision under the chin. This procedure includes the mandibular staple implant.

## Coding Tips

Local anesthesia is generally considered part of restorative procedures. For endosteal implant, see D6010–D6012; for eposteal implant, see D6040. To report endodontic endosseous implants, see D3460.

## Reimbursement Tips

When selecting the procedure or service that accurately identifies the service performed, dentists must use the most accurate code. If the CDT code more accurately identifies the service, this should be used rather than the CPT codes. The third-party payer may require an x-ray or x-ray report. Coverage of this implant procedure varies by payer and by individual contract. Check with payers for their specific coverage guidelines. This procedure may be covered by the patient's medical insurance. When covered by medical insurance, the payer may require that the appropriate CPT code be reported on the CMS-1500 claim form.

## Associated CPT Codes

21248 Reconstruction of mandible or maxilla, endosteal implant (eg, blade, cylinder); partial

## ICD-10-CM Diagnostic Codes

K08.101 Complete loss of teeth, unspecified cause, class I
K08.102 Complete loss of teeth, unspecified cause, class II
K08.103 Complete loss of teeth, unspecified cause, class III
K08.104 Complete loss of teeth, unspecified cause, class IV
K08.111 Complete loss of teeth due to trauma, class I
K08.112 Complete loss of teeth due to trauma, class II
K08.113 Complete loss of teeth due to trauma, class III
K08.114 Complete loss of teeth due to trauma, class IV
K08.121 Complete loss of teeth due to periodontal diseases, class I
K08.122 Complete loss of teeth due to periodontal diseases, class II
K08.123 Complete loss of teeth due to periodontal diseases, class III
K08.124 Complete loss of teeth due to periodontal diseases, class IV
K08.131 Complete loss of teeth due to caries, class I
K08.132 Complete loss of teeth due to caries, class II
K08.133 Complete loss of teeth due to caries, class III
K08.134 Complete loss of teeth due to caries, class IV
K08.191 Complete loss of teeth due to other specified cause, class I
K08.192 Complete loss of teeth due to other specified cause, class II
K08.193 Complete loss of teeth due to other specified cause, class III
K08.194 Complete loss of teeth due to other specified cause, class IV

| | |
|---|---|
| K08.21 | Minimal atrophy of the mandible |
| K08.22 | Moderate atrophy of the mandible |
| K08.23 | Severe atrophy of the mandible |
| K08.24 | Minimal atrophy of maxilla |
| K08.25 | Moderate atrophy of the maxilla |
| K08.26 | Severe atrophy of the maxilla |
| K08.401 | Partial loss of teeth, unspecified cause, class I |
| K08.402 | Partial loss of teeth, unspecified cause, class II |
| K08.403 | Partial loss of teeth, unspecified cause, class III |
| K08.404 | Partial loss of teeth, unspecified cause, class IV |
| K08.411 | Partial loss of teeth due to trauma, class I |
| K08.412 | Partial loss of teeth due to trauma, class II |
| K08.413 | Partial loss of teeth due to trauma, class III |
| K08.414 | Partial loss of teeth due to trauma, class IV |
| K08.421 | Partial loss of teeth due to periodontal diseases, class I |
| K08.422 | Partial loss of teeth due to periodontal diseases, class II |
| K08.423 | Partial loss of teeth due to periodontal diseases, class III |
| K08.424 | Partial loss of teeth due to periodontal diseases, class IV |
| K08.431 | Partial loss of teeth due to caries, class I |
| K08.432 | Partial loss of teeth due to caries, class II |
| K08.433 | Partial loss of teeth due to caries, class III |
| K08.434 | Partial loss of teeth due to caries, class IV |
| K08.491 | Partial loss of teeth due to other specified cause, class I |
| K08.492 | Partial loss of teeth due to other specified cause, class II |
| K08.493 | Partial loss of teeth due to other specified cause, class III |
| K08.494 | Partial loss of teeth due to other specified cause, class IV |

## Relative Value Units/Medicare Edits

| Non-Facility RVU | Work | PE | MP | Total |
|---|---|---|---|---|
| D6050 | 32.77 | 28.93 | 6.75 | 68.45 |
| **Facility RVU** | **Work** | **PE** | **MP** | **Total** |
| D6050 | 32.77 | 28.93 | 6.75 | 68.45 |

| | FUD | Status | MUE | Modifiers | | | | IOM Reference |
|---|---|---|---|---|---|---|---|---|
| D6050 | N/A | I | - | N/A | N/A | N/A | N/A | None |

* with documentation

## Terms To Know

**eposteal implant.** Dental implant receiving bone support by leaning on residual mandibular bone.

**mandible.** Lower jawbone giving structure to the floor of the oral cavity.

**transosteal implant.** Dental implant composed of a plate and retentive pins or posts that are affixed to the mandible.

# D6051, D6056-D6057

▲ **D6051** interim implant abutment placement

*A healing cap is not an interim abutment.*

**D6056** prefabricated abutment - includes modification and placement

*Modification of a prefabricated abutment may be necessary.*

**D6057** custom fabricated abutment - includes placement

*Created by a laboratory process, specific for an individual application.*

## Explanation

An implant replaces lost teeth with a nonremovable restoration to help restore function, aesthetics, and speech. Most implant treatment consists of a two-stage procedure. After treatment planning, the bone is surgically exposed and is placed. The implant is left buried in the bone and unloaded, usually for three months in the mandible and six months in the maxilla. After the healing period, the implant is uncovered. The second step of the procedure is necessary to uncover the implant and attach an extension. This small metal post, called an abutment, completes the foundation on which the tooth will be placed. A prefabricated abutment is purchased and does not require casting. A custom abutment is typically fabricated using a casting process and usually is made of noble or high noble metal. The abutment is screwed into the implant using a screwdriver and ratchet and fixed to the implant. A prefabricated abutment may need to be modified. Before cementing the crown, the screw channel is sealed off with wax or gutta-percha to allow release of the screw if required. A transfer coping at the impression stage is given to the laboratory to assist in the crown manufacture. The code includes placement. Appropriate code selection depends upon the type of crown attached to the abutment. For placement of a prefabricated abutment, see D6056; customized is reported with D6057. An interim abutment is reported using D6051.

## Coding Tips

These codes are out-of-sequence codes and will not display in numeric order in the CDT manual. Local anesthesia is generally considered part of restorative procedures. For removal of an interim abutment, see D6198.

## Reimbursement Tips

The third-party payer may require an x-ray or x-ray report. Coverage of implant procedures varies by payer and by individual contract. Check with payers for specific coverage guidelines. This procedure may be covered by the patient's medical insurance. When covered by medical insurance, the payer may require that the appropriate CPT code be reported on the CMS-1500 claim form.

## ICD-10-CM Diagnostic Codes

| | |
|---|---|
| K08.101 | Complete loss of teeth, unspecified cause, class I |
| K08.102 | Complete loss of teeth, unspecified cause, class II |
| K08.103 | Complete loss of teeth, unspecified cause, class III |
| K08.104 | Complete loss of teeth, unspecified cause, class IV |
| K08.111 | Complete loss of teeth due to trauma, class I |
| K08.112 | Complete loss of teeth due to trauma, class II |
| K08.113 | Complete loss of teeth due to trauma, class III |
| K08.114 | Complete loss of teeth due to trauma, class IV |
| K08.121 | Complete loss of teeth due to periodontal diseases, class I |
| K08.122 | Complete loss of teeth due to periodontal diseases, class II |
| K08.123 | Complete loss of teeth due to periodontal diseases, class III |
| K08.124 | Complete loss of teeth due to periodontal diseases, class IV |
| K08.131 | Complete loss of teeth due to caries, class I |
| K08.132 | Complete loss of teeth due to caries, class II |
| K08.133 | Complete loss of teeth due to caries, class III |

| | |
|---|---|
| K08.134 | Complete loss of teeth due to caries, class IV |
| K08.191 | Complete loss of teeth due to other specified cause, class I |
| K08.192 | Complete loss of teeth due to other specified cause, class II |
| K08.193 | Complete loss of teeth due to other specified cause, class III |
| K08.194 | Complete loss of teeth due to other specified cause, class IV |
| K08.21 | Minimal atrophy of the mandible |
| K08.22 | Moderate atrophy of the mandible |
| K08.23 | Severe atrophy of the mandible |
| K08.24 | Minimal atrophy of maxilla |
| K08.25 | Moderate atrophy of the maxilla |
| K08.26 | Severe atrophy of the maxilla |
| K08.401 | Partial loss of teeth, unspecified cause, class I |
| K08.402 | Partial loss of teeth, unspecified cause, class II |
| K08.403 | Partial loss of teeth, unspecified cause, class III |
| K08.404 | Partial loss of teeth, unspecified cause, class IV |
| K08.411 | Partial loss of teeth due to trauma, class I |
| K08.412 | Partial loss of teeth due to trauma, class II |
| K08.413 | Partial loss of teeth due to trauma, class III |
| K08.414 | Partial loss of teeth due to trauma, class IV |
| K08.421 | Partial loss of teeth due to periodontal diseases, class I |
| K08.422 | Partial loss of teeth due to periodontal diseases, class II |
| K08.423 | Partial loss of teeth due to periodontal diseases, class III |
| K08.424 | Partial loss of teeth due to periodontal diseases, class IV |
| K08.431 | Partial loss of teeth due to caries, class I |
| K08.432 | Partial loss of teeth due to caries, class II |
| K08.433 | Partial loss of teeth due to caries, class III |
| K08.434 | Partial loss of teeth due to caries, class IV |
| K08.491 | Partial loss of teeth due to other specified cause, class I |
| K08.492 | Partial loss of teeth due to other specified cause, class II |
| K08.493 | Partial loss of teeth due to other specified cause, class III |
| K08.494 | Partial loss of teeth due to other specified cause, class IV |

## Relative Value Units/Medicare Edits

| Non-Facility RVU | Work | PE | MP | Total |
|---|---|---|---|---|
| D6051 | 1.36 | 1.20 | 0.28 | 2.84 |
| D6056 | 2.89 | 2.55 | 0.60 | 6.04 |
| D6057 | 3.72 | 3.28 | 0.77 | 7.77 |
| **Facility RVU** | **Work** | **PE** | **MP** | **Total** |
| D6051 | 1.36 | 1.20 | 0.28 | 2.84 |
| D6056 | 2.89 | 2.55 | 0.60 | 6.04 |
| D6057 | 3.72 | 3.28 | 0.77 | 7.77 |

| | FUD | Status | MUE | Modifiers | | | | IOM Reference |
|---|---|---|---|---|---|---|---|---|
| D6051 | N/A | N | - | N/A | N/A | N/A | N/A | None |
| D6056 | N/A | N | - | N/A | N/A | N/A | N/A | |
| D6057 | N/A | N | - | N/A | N/A | N/A | N/A | |

* with documentation

### Terms To Know

**abutment.** Tooth or implant fixture supporting a prosthesis.

**implant.** Material or device inserted or placed within the body for therapeutic, reconstructive, or diagnostic purposes.

# D6055

**D6055** connecting bar - implant supported or abutment supported

*Utilized to stabilize and anchor a prosthesis.*

### Explanation

A fixed bar connects two or more premucosal extensions. In the case of the ramus frame or subperiosteal implant, it can be an integral part of the substructure. The dentist attaches a device to transmucosal abutments to stabilize and anchor a removable overdenture prosthesis. This procedure is for a cast, fixed framework connected to the implant(s) to provide firm support for a separate prosthesis.

### Coding Tips

This is an out-of-sequence code and will not display in numeric order in the CDT manual. Local anesthesia is generally considered part of restorative procedures.

### Documentation Tips

Documentation should indicate the location and number of missing teeth.

### Reimbursement Tips

The third-party payer may require an x-ray or x-ray report. Coverage of implant procedures varies by payer and by individual contract. Check with payers for specific coverage guidelines.

### ICD-10-CM Diagnostic Codes

| | |
|---|---|
| Z46.3 | Encounter for fitting and adjustment of dental prosthetic device |

### Relative Value Units/Medicare Edits

| Non-Facility RVU | Work | PE | MP | Total |
|---|---|---|---|---|
| D6055 | 6.03 | 5.32 | 1.24 | 12.59 |
| **Facility RVU** | **Work** | **PE** | **MP** | **Total** |
| D6055 | 6.03 | 5.32 | 1.24 | 12.59 |

| | FUD | Status | MUE | Modifiers | | | | IOM Reference |
|---|---|---|---|---|---|---|---|---|
| D6055 | N/A | I | - | N/A | N/A | N/A | N/A | None |

* with documentation

### Terms To Know

**denture base.** Portion of the artificial substitute for natural teeth that makes contact with the soft tissue of the mouth and serves as the anchor for the artificial teeth.

**fixed.** Not able to be removed easily.

**overdenture.** In dentistry, prosthesis of artificial teeth that overlies and is supported by retained tooth roots or implants. It is removable.

**transmucosal.** Through or across the oral mucosa.

# D6058

**D6058** abutment supported porcelain/ceramic crown

*A single crown restoration that is retained, supported and stabilized by an abutment on an implant.*

## Explanation

An implant replaces lost teeth with a nonremovable restoration to help restore function, aesthetics, and speech. Most implant treatment consists of a two-stage procedure. After treatment planning, the bone is surgically exposed and is placed. The implant is left buried in the bone and unloaded, usually for three months in the mandible and six months in the maxilla. After the healing period, the implant is uncovered. The second step of the procedure is necessary to uncover the implant and attach an extension. This small metal post, called an abutment, completes the foundation on which the tooth will be placed. The prosthesis (abutment) is screwed into the implant using a screwdriver and ratchet and fixed to the implant. Before cementing the crown, the screw channel is sealed off with wax or gutta-percha to allow release of the screw if required. A transfer coping at the impression stage is given to the laboratory to assist in the crown manufacture. During this time, a temporary tooth replacement option can be worn over the implant site. Appropriate code selection depends upon the type of crown. The porcelain/ceramic dental materials include porcelain, ceramic or glasslike fillings, and crowns. The crown is cemented to the implant once completed.

## Coding Tips

Local anesthesia is generally considered part of restorative procedures. The third-party payer may require an x-ray or x-ray report.

## Documentation Tips

The following information can be documented on a tooth chart: treatment/location of caries, endodontic procedures, prosthetic services, preventive services, treatment of lesions and dental disease, or other special procedures. A tooth chart may also be used to identify structure and rationale of disease process and the type of service performed on intraoral structures other than teeth.

## Reimbursement Tips

Coverage of implant procedures varies by payer and by individual contract. Check with payers for specific coverage guidelines.

## ICD-10-CM Diagnostic Codes

| | |
|---|---|
| K02.51 | Dental caries on pit and fissure surface limited to enamel |
| K02.52 | Dental caries on pit and fissure surface penetrating into dentin |
| K02.53 | Dental caries on pit and fissure surface penetrating into pulp |
| K02.61 | Dental caries on smooth surface limited to enamel |
| K02.62 | Dental caries on smooth surface penetrating into dentin |
| K02.63 | Dental caries on smooth surface penetrating into pulp |
| K02.7 | Dental root caries |
| K03.0 | Excessive attrition of teeth |
| K03.1 | Abrasion of teeth |
| K03.2 | Erosion of teeth |
| K03.3 | Pathological resorption of teeth |
| K03.4 | Hypercementosis |
| K03.5 | Ankylosis of teeth |
| K03.6 | Deposits [accretions] on teeth |
| K03.7 | Posteruptive color changes of dental hard tissues |
| K03.81 | Cracked tooth |
| K03.89 | Other specified diseases of hard tissues of teeth |
| K03.9 | Disease of hard tissues of teeth, unspecified |
| K04.01 | Reversible pulpitis |
| K04.02 | Irreversible pulpitis |
| K04.1 | Necrosis of pulp |
| K04.2 | Pulp degeneration |
| K04.3 | Abnormal hard tissue formation in pulp |
| K08.50 | Unsatisfactory restoration of tooth, unspecified |
| K08.51 | Open restoration margins of tooth |
| K08.52 | Unrepairable overhanging of dental restorative materials |
| K08.530 | Fractured dental restorative material without loss of material |
| K08.531 | Fractured dental restorative material with loss of material |
| K08.539 | Fractured dental restorative material, unspecified |
| K08.55 | Allergy to existing dental restorative material |
| K08.56 | Poor aesthetic of existing restoration of tooth |
| K08.59 | Other unsatisfactory restoration of tooth |
| K08.81 | Primary occlusal trauma |
| K08.82 | Secondary occlusal trauma |

## Relative Value Units/Medicare Edits

| Non-Facility RVU | Work | PE | MP | Total |
|---|---|---|---|---|
| **D6058** | 7.25 | 6.40 | 1.49 | 15.14 |
| **Facility RVU** | **Work** | **PE** | **MP** | **Total** |
| **D6058** | 7.25 | 6.40 | 1.49 | 15.14 |

| | FUD | Status | MUE | Modifiers | | | | IOM Reference |
|---|---|---|---|---|---|---|---|---|
| **D6058** | N/A | N | - | N/A | N/A | N/A | N/A | None |

* with documentation

## Terms To Know

**abutment.** Tooth or implant fixture supporting a prosthesis.

**crown.** Dental restoration that completely caps or encircles a tooth or dental implant.

Dental - Implant Services

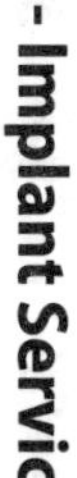

# D6059-D6061

**D6059** abutment supported porcelain fused to metal crown (high noble metal)

*A single metal-ceramic crown restoration that is retained, supported and stabilized by an abutment on an implant.*

**D6060** abutment supported porcelain fused to metal crown (predominantly base metal)

*A single metal-ceramic crown restoration that is retained, supported and stabilized by an abutment on an implant.*

**D6061** abutment supported porcelain fused to metal crown (noble metal)

*A single metal-ceramic crown restoration that is retained, supported and stabilized by an abutment on an implant.*

## Explanation

An implant replaces lost teeth with a nonremovable restoration to help restore function, aesthetics, and speech. Most implant treatment consists of a two-stage procedure. After treatment planning, the bone is surgically exposed and is placed. The implant is left buried in the bone and unloaded, usually for three months in the mandible and six months in the maxilla. After the healing period, the implant is uncovered. The second step of the procedure is necessary to uncover the implant and attach an extension. This small metal post, called an abutment, completes the foundation on which the tooth will be placed. The prosthesis (abutment) is screwed into the implant using a screwdriver and ratchet and fixed to the implant. Before cementing the crown, the screw channel is sealed off with wax or gutta-percha to allow release of the screw if required. A transfer coping at the impression stage is given to the laboratory to assist in the crown manufacture. During this time, a temporary tooth replacement option can be worn over the implant site. Appropriate code selection depends upon the type of crown. Code D6059 reports porcelain fused to a metal crown that is made from a shell of a high noble metal (gold) that fits over the tooth. Code D6060 reports a porcelain fused to metal crown that is made from a shell of base metal alloy (non-noble metals with a silver appearance) that fits over the tooth. The porcelain fused to metal crown in D6061 is made from a shell of noble metal, usually a gold alloy containing gold, copper, and other metals, which fits over the tooth. A veneering of porcelain is fused over this metal, giving the crown a white tooth-like appearance. The porcelain veneer may cover the portion of the crown having a metal surface or be fully surfaced with porcelain. The crown is cemented to the abutment once completed.

## Coding Tips

Local anesthesia is generally considered part of restorative procedures. The third-party payer may require an x-ray or x-ray report.

## Documentation Tips

The following information can be documented on a tooth chart: treatment/location of caries, endodontic procedures, prosthetic services, preventive services, treatment of lesions and dental disease, or other special procedures. A tooth chart may also be used to identify structure and rationale of disease process and the type of service performed on intraoral structures other than teeth.

## Reimbursement Tips

Coverage of implant procedures varies by payer and by individual contract. Check with payers for specific coverage guidelines.

## ICD-10-CM Diagnostic Codes

K02.51 Dental caries on pit and fissure surface limited to enamel
K02.52 Dental caries on pit and fissure surface penetrating into dentin
K02.53 Dental caries on pit and fissure surface penetrating into pulp
K02.61 Dental caries on smooth surface limited to enamel
K02.62 Dental caries on smooth surface penetrating into dentin
K02.63 Dental caries on smooth surface penetrating into pulp
K02.7 Dental root caries
K03.0 Excessive attrition of teeth
K03.1 Abrasion of teeth
K03.2 Erosion of teeth
K03.3 Pathological resorption of teeth
K03.4 Hypercementosis
K03.5 Ankylosis of teeth
K03.6 Deposits [accretions] on teeth
K03.7 Posteruptive color changes of dental hard tissues
K03.81 Cracked tooth
K03.89 Other specified diseases of hard tissues of teeth
K03.9 Disease of hard tissues of teeth, unspecified
K04.01 Reversible pulpitis
K04.02 Irreversible pulpitis
K04.1 Necrosis of pulp
K04.2 Pulp degeneration
K04.3 Abnormal hard tissue formation in pulp
K08.50 Unsatisfactory restoration of tooth, unspecified
K08.51 Open restoration margins of tooth
K08.52 Unrepairable overhanging of dental restorative materials
K08.530 Fractured dental restorative material without loss of material
K08.531 Fractured dental restorative material with loss of material
K08.539 Fractured dental restorative material, unspecified
K08.55 Allergy to existing dental restorative material
K08.56 Poor aesthetic of existing restoration of tooth
K08.59 Other unsatisfactory restoration of tooth
K08.81 Primary occlusal trauma
K08.82 Secondary occlusal trauma

## Relative Value Units/Medicare Edits

| Non-Facility RVU | Work | PE | MP | Total |
|---|---|---|---|---|
| **D6059** | 7.13 | 6.30 | 1.47 | 14.90 |
| **D6060** | 6.71 | 5.92 | 1.38 | 14.01 |
| **D6061** | 6.85 | 6.04 | 1.41 | 14.30 |
| **Facility RVU** | **Work** | **PE** | **MP** | **Total** |
| **D6059** | 7.13 | 6.30 | 1.47 | 14.90 |
| **D6060** | 6.71 | 5.92 | 1.38 | 14.01 |
| **D6061** | 6.85 | 6.04 | 1.41 | 14.30 |

| | FUD | Status | MUE | Modifiers | | | | IOM Reference |
|---|---|---|---|---|---|---|---|---|
| **D6059** | N/A | N | - | N/A | N/A | N/A | N/A | None |
| **D6060** | N/A | N | - | N/A | N/A | N/A | N/A | |
| **D6061** | N/A | N | - | N/A | N/A | N/A | N/A | |

* with documentation

## Terms To Know

**abutment.** Tooth or implant fixture supporting a prosthesis.

Dental - Implant Services

# D6062-D6064

**D6062** abutment supported cast metal crown (high noble metal)

*A single cast metal crown restoration that is retained, supported and stabilized by an abutment on an implant.*

**D6063** abutment supported cast metal crown (predominantly base metal)

*A single cast metal crown restoration that is retained, supported and stabilized by an abutment on an implant.*

**D6064** abutment supported cast metal crown (noble metal)

*A single cast metal crown restoration that is retained, supported and stabilized by an abutment on an implant.*

## Explanation

An implant replaces lost teeth with a nonremovable restoration to help restore function, aesthetics, and speech. Most implant treatment consists of a two-stage procedure. After treatment planning, the bone is surgically exposed and is placed. The implant is left buried in the bone and unloaded, usually for three months in the mandible and six months in the maxilla. After the healing period, the implant is uncovered. The second step of the procedure is necessary to uncover the implant and attach an extension. This small metal post, called an abutment, completes the foundation on which the tooth will be placed. The prosthesis (abutment) is screwed into the implant using a screwdriver and ratchet and fixed to the implant. Before cementing the crown, the screw channel is sealed off with wax or gutta-percha to allow release of the screw if required. A transfer coping at the impression stage is given to the laboratory to assist in the crown manufacture. Appropriate code selection depends upon the type of crown attached to the abutment. The crown in D6062 is made entirely from high noble metal (gold). The crown in D6063 is made from a base metal alloy (non-noble metals with a silver appearance) that fits over the tooth. The crown in D6064 is made from a noble metal, usually a gold alloy containing gold, copper, and other metals, which fits over the tooth. The crown is cemented to the abutment once completed.

## Coding Tips

Local anesthesia is generally considered part of restorative procedures. High noble metals include gold, palladium, and platinum. The content must be ≥ 60 percent gold plus platinum and ≥ 40 percent gold. Noble metals include 25 percent or less gold plus platinum group. Predominantly base alloys contain a noble metal content of < 25 percent gold plus platinum group. The metals of the platinum group include platinum, palladium, rhodium, iridium, osmium, and ruthenium.

## Documentation Tips

The following information can be documented on a tooth chart: treatment/location of caries, endodontic procedures, prosthetic services, preventive services, treatment of lesions and dental disease, or other special procedures. A tooth chart may also be used to identify structure and rationale of disease process and the type of service performed on intraoral structures other than teeth.

## Reimbursement Tips

The third-party payer may require an x-ray or x-ray report. Coverage of implant procedures varies by payer and by individual contract. Check with payers for specific coverage guidelines.

## ICD-10-CM Diagnostic Codes

K02.51 Dental caries on pit and fissure surface limited to enamel
K02.52 Dental caries on pit and fissure surface penetrating into dentin
K02.53 Dental caries on pit and fissure surface penetrating into pulp
K02.61 Dental caries on smooth surface limited to enamel
K02.62 Dental caries on smooth surface penetrating into dentin
K02.63 Dental caries on smooth surface penetrating into pulp
K02.7 Dental root caries
K03.0 Excessive attrition of teeth
K03.1 Abrasion of teeth
K03.2 Erosion of teeth
K03.3 Pathological resorption of teeth
K03.4 Hypercementosis
K03.5 Ankylosis of teeth
K03.6 Deposits [accretions] on teeth
K03.7 Posteruptive color changes of dental hard tissues
K03.81 Cracked tooth
K03.89 Other specified diseases of hard tissues of teeth
K03.9 Disease of hard tissues of teeth, unspecified
K04.01 Reversible pulpitis
K04.02 Irreversible pulpitis
K04.1 Necrosis of pulp
K04.2 Pulp degeneration
K04.3 Abnormal hard tissue formation in pulp
K08.50 Unsatisfactory restoration of tooth, unspecified
K08.51 Open restoration margins of tooth
K08.52 Unrepairable overhanging of dental restorative materials
K08.530 Fractured dental restorative material without loss of material
K08.531 Fractured dental restorative material with loss of material
K08.539 Fractured dental restorative material, unspecified
K08.55 Allergy to existing dental restorative material
K08.56 Poor aesthetic of existing restoration of tooth
K08.59 Other unsatisfactory restoration of tooth
K08.81 Primary occlusal trauma
K08.82 Secondary occlusal trauma

## Relative Value Units/Medicare Edits

| Non-Facility RVU | Work | PE | MP | Total |
|---|---|---|---|---|
| **D6062** | 6.85 | 6.05 | 1.41 | 14.31 |
| **D6063** | 6.06 | 5.35 | 1.25 | 12.66 |
| **D6064** | 6.35 | 5.60 | 1.31 | 13.26 |
| **Facility RVU** | **Work** | **PE** | **MP** | **Total** |
| **D6062** | 6.85 | 6.05 | 1.41 | 14.31 |
| **D6063** | 6.06 | 5.35 | 1.25 | 12.66 |
| **D6064** | 6.35 | 5.60 | 1.31 | 13.26 |

| | FUD | Status | MUE | Modifiers | | | | IOM Reference |
|---|---|---|---|---|---|---|---|---|
| **D6062** | N/A | N | - | N/A | N/A | N/A | N/A | None |
| **D6063** | N/A | N | - | N/A | N/A | N/A | N/A | |
| **D6064** | N/A | N | - | N/A | N/A | N/A | N/A | |

* with documentation

## Terms To Know

**abutment.** Tooth or implant fixture supporting a prosthesis.

Dental - Implant Services

# D6065

**D6065** implant supported porcelain/ceramic crown

*A single crown restoration that is retained, supported and stabilized by an implant.*

## Explanation

An implant replaces lost teeth with a nonremovable restoration to help restore function, aesthetics, and speech. This is a one-stage procedure. The system already has the extension piece (abutment) attached. After treatment planning, the bone is surgically exposed and is placed. The implant is left buried in the bone and unloaded, usually for three months in the mandible and six months in the maxilla. After the healing period, the implant is uncovered. A transfer coping at the impression stage is given to the laboratory to assist in the crown manufacture. During this time, a temporary tooth replacement option can be worn over the implant site. Appropriate code selection depends upon the type of crown. The porcelain/ceramic dental materials include porcelain, ceramic or glasslike fillings, and crowns. The crown is cemented to the implant once completed.

## Coding Tips

Local anesthesia is generally considered part of restorative procedures.

## Documentation Tips

The following information can be documented on a tooth chart: treatment/location of caries, endodontic procedures, prosthetic services, preventive services, treatment of lesions and dental disease, or other special procedures. A tooth chart may also be used to identify structure and rationale of disease process and the type of service performed on intraoral structures other than teeth.

## Reimbursement Tips

The third-party payer may require an x-ray or x-ray report. Coverage of this implant procedure varies by payer and by individual contract. Check with payers for specific coverage guidelines.

## ICD-10-CM Diagnostic Codes

K02.51 Dental caries on pit and fissure surface limited to enamel
K02.52 Dental caries on pit and fissure surface penetrating into dentin
K02.53 Dental caries on pit and fissure surface penetrating into pulp
K02.61 Dental caries on smooth surface limited to enamel
K02.62 Dental caries on smooth surface penetrating into dentin
K02.63 Dental caries on smooth surface penetrating into pulp
K02.7 Dental root caries
K03.0 Excessive attrition of teeth
K03.1 Abrasion of teeth
K03.2 Erosion of teeth
K03.3 Pathological resorption of teeth
K03.4 Hypercementosis
K03.5 Ankylosis of teeth
K03.6 Deposits [accretions] on teeth
K03.7 Posteruptive color changes of dental hard tissues
K03.81 Cracked tooth
K03.89 Other specified diseases of hard tissues of teeth
K03.9 Disease of hard tissues of teeth, unspecified
K04.01 Reversible pulpitis
K04.02 Irreversible pulpitis
K04.1 Necrosis of pulp
K04.2 Pulp degeneration
K04.3 Abnormal hard tissue formation in pulp
K08.50 Unsatisfactory restoration of tooth, unspecified
K08.51 Open restoration margins of tooth
K08.52 Unrepairable overhanging of dental restorative materials
K08.530 Fractured dental restorative material without loss of material
K08.531 Fractured dental restorative material with loss of material
K08.539 Fractured dental restorative material, unspecified
K08.55 Allergy to existing dental restorative material
K08.56 Poor aesthetic of existing restoration of tooth
K08.59 Other unsatisfactory restoration of tooth
K08.81 Primary occlusal trauma
K08.82 Secondary occlusal trauma

## Relative Value Units/Medicare Edits

| Non-Facility RVU | Work | PE | MP | Total |
|---|---|---|---|---|
| D6065 | 7.57 | 6.68 | 1.56 | 15.81 |
| **Facility RVU** | **Work** | **PE** | **MP** | **Total** |
| D6065 | 7.57 | 6.68 | 1.56 | 15.81 |

| | FUD | Status | MUE | Modifiers | | | | IOM Reference |
|---|---|---|---|---|---|---|---|---|
| D6065 | N/A | N | - | N/A | N/A | N/A | N/A | None |

* with documentation

## Terms To Know

**abutment crown.** Artificial tooth cap for the retention and/or support of a dental prosthesis.

**dental implant.** Surgical implantation of a device within the mandible or maxilla for dental replacement.

Dental - Implant Services

# D6066-D6067

**D6066** implant supported crown - porcelain fused to high noble alloys

*A single metal-ceramic crown restoration that is retained, supported and stabilized by an implant.*

**D6067** implant supported crown - high noble alloys

*A single metal crown restoration that is retained, supported and stabilized by an implant.*

## Explanation

An implant replaces lost teeth with a nonremovable restoration to help restore function, aesthetics, and speech. This is a one-stage procedure. The system already has the extension piece (abutment) attached. After treatment planning, the bone is surgically exposed and is placed. The implant is left buried in the bone and unloaded, usually for three months in the mandible and six months in the maxilla. After the healing period, the implant is uncovered. A transfer coping at the impression stage is given to the laboratory to assist in the crown manufacture. During this time, a temporary tooth replacement option can be worn over the implant site. Appropriate code selection depends upon the type of crown. The porcelain fused to metal crown in code D6066 is made from a shell of high noble alloy that fits over the implant. A veneering of porcelain is fused over this metal, giving the crown a white tooth-like appearance. The porcelain veneer may cover the portion of the crown having a metal surface or be fully surfaced with porcelain. The metal crown in code D6067 is made from titanium, titanium alloy, or a high noble metal that fits over the implant. The crown is cemented to the implant once completed.

## Coding Tips

These codes are out-of-sequence codes and will not display in numeric order in the CDT book. Local anesthesia is generally considered part of restorative procedures. High noble metals include gold, palladium, and platinum. The content must be ≥ 60 percent gold plus platinum and ≥ 40 percent gold. Noble metals include 25 percent or less gold plus platinum group. Predominantly base alloys contain a noble metal content of < 25 percent gold plus platinum group. The metals of the platinum group include platinum, palladium, rhodium, iridium, osmium, and ruthenium.

## Documentation Tips

The following information can be documented on a tooth chart: treatment/location of caries, endodontic procedures, prosthetic services, preventive services, treatment of lesions and dental disease, or other special procedures. A tooth chart may also be used to identify structure and rationale of disease process and the type of service performed on intraoral structures other than teeth.

## Reimbursement Tips

The third-party payer may require an x-ray or x-ray report. Coverage of implant procedures varies by payer and by individual contract. Check with payers for specific coverage guidelines.

## ICD-10-CM Diagnostic Codes

| | |
|---|---|
| K02.51 | Dental caries on pit and fissure surface limited to enamel |
| K02.52 | Dental caries on pit and fissure surface penetrating into dentin |
| K02.53 | Dental caries on pit and fissure surface penetrating into pulp |
| K02.61 | Dental caries on smooth surface limited to enamel |
| K02.62 | Dental caries on smooth surface penetrating into dentin |
| K02.63 | Dental caries on smooth surface penetrating into pulp |
| K02.7 | Dental root caries |
| K03.0 | Excessive attrition of teeth |
| K03.1 | Abrasion of teeth |
| K03.2 | Erosion of teeth |
| K03.3 | Pathological resorption of teeth |
| K03.4 | Hypercementosis |
| K03.5 | Ankylosis of teeth |
| K03.6 | Deposits [accretions] on teeth |
| K03.7 | Posteruptive color changes of dental hard tissues |
| K03.81 | Cracked tooth |
| K03.89 | Other specified diseases of hard tissues of teeth |
| K03.9 | Disease of hard tissues of teeth, unspecified |
| K04.01 | Reversible pulpitis |
| K04.02 | Irreversible pulpitis |
| K04.1 | Necrosis of pulp |
| K04.2 | Pulp degeneration |
| K04.3 | Abnormal hard tissue formation in pulp |
| K08.50 | Unsatisfactory restoration of tooth, unspecified |
| K08.51 | Open restoration margins of tooth |
| K08.52 | Unrepairable overhanging of dental restorative materials |
| K08.530 | Fractured dental restorative material without loss of material |
| K08.531 | Fractured dental restorative material with loss of material |
| K08.539 | Fractured dental restorative material, unspecified |
| K08.55 | Allergy to existing dental restorative material |
| K08.56 | Poor aesthetic of existing restoration of tooth |
| K08.59 | Other unsatisfactory restoration of tooth |
| K08.81 | Primary occlusal trauma |
| K08.82 | Secondary occlusal trauma |

## Relative Value Units/Medicare Edits

| Non-Facility RVU | Work | PE | MP | Total |
|---|---|---|---|---|
| **D6066** | 7.43 | 6.55 | 1.53 | 15.51 |
| **D6067** | 7.26 | 6.41 | 1.50 | 15.17 |
| **Facility RVU** | **Work** | **PE** | **MP** | **Total** |
| **D6066** | 7.43 | 6.55 | 1.53 | 15.51 |
| **D6067** | 7.26 | 6.41 | 1.50 | 15.17 |

| | FUD | Status | MUE | Modifiers | | | | IOM Reference |
|---|---|---|---|---|---|---|---|---|
| **D6066** | N/A | N | - | N/A | N/A | N/A | N/A | None |
| **D6067** | N/A | N | - | N/A | N/A | N/A | N/A | |

* with documentation

## Terms To Know

**abutment crown.** Artificial tooth cap for the retention and/or support of a dental prosthesis.

# D6068

**D6068** abutment supported retainer for porcelain/ceramic FPD

*A ceramic retainer for a fixed partial denture that gains retention, support and stability from an abutment on an implant.*

## Explanation

A prosthodontic retainer is a part of a fixed partial denture (FPD) that attaches a bridge to an adjacent tooth, an implant abutment, or an implant. The retainer provides support, retention, and stability to the dental prosthesis. The type of retainer the dentist selects depends upon the retention required, the bridge design, the extent of existing restorations, and the amount of metal display the patient finds tolerable (aesthetics). The retainer is designed during the diagnostic wax-up of the bridge being made to replace the lost tooth. Code selection depends on the type of FPD as well as whether the abutment is implant supported. Code D6068 describes an abutment-supported retainer for a porcelain/ceramic FPD. The porcelain/ceramic dental materials include porcelain, ceramic or glasslike fillings, and crowns.

## Coding Tips

Local anesthesia is generally considered part of restorative procedures.

## Documentation Tips

The following information can be documented on a tooth chart: treatment/location of caries, endodontic procedures, prosthetic services, preventive services, treatment of lesions and dental disease, or other special procedures. A tooth chart may also be used to identify structure and rationale of disease process and the type of service performed on intraoral structures other than teeth.

## Reimbursement Tips

The third-party payer may require an x-ray or x-ray report. Coverage of implant procedures varies by payer and by individual contract. Check with payers for specific coverage guidelines.

## ICD-10-CM Diagnostic Codes

K02.51 Dental caries on pit and fissure surface limited to enamel
K02.52 Dental caries on pit and fissure surface penetrating into dentin
K02.53 Dental caries on pit and fissure surface penetrating into pulp
K02.61 Dental caries on smooth surface limited to enamel
K02.62 Dental caries on smooth surface penetrating into dentin
K02.63 Dental caries on smooth surface penetrating into pulp
K02.7 Dental root caries
K03.0 Excessive attrition of teeth
K03.1 Abrasion of teeth
K03.2 Erosion of teeth
K03.3 Pathological resorption of teeth
K03.4 Hypercementosis
K03.5 Ankylosis of teeth
K03.6 Deposits [accretions] on teeth
K03.7 Posteruptive color changes of dental hard tissues
K03.81 Cracked tooth
K03.89 Other specified diseases of hard tissues of teeth
K03.9 Disease of hard tissues of teeth, unspecified
K04.01 Reversible pulpitis
K04.02 Irreversible pulpitis
K04.1 Necrosis of pulp
K04.2 Pulp degeneration
K04.3 Abnormal hard tissue formation in pulp
K08.51 Open restoration margins of tooth
K08.52 Unrepairable overhanging of dental restorative materials
K08.530 Fractured dental restorative material without loss of material
K08.531 Fractured dental restorative material with loss of material
K08.539 Fractured dental restorative material, unspecified
K08.55 Allergy to existing dental restorative material
K08.56 Poor aesthetic of existing restoration of tooth
K08.59 Other unsatisfactory restoration of tooth
K08.81 Primary occlusal trauma
K08.82 Secondary occlusal trauma

## Relative Value Units/Medicare Edits

| Non-Facility RVU | Work | PE | MP | Total |
|---|---|---|---|---|
| **D6068** | 7.01 | 6.19 | 1.44 | 14.64 |
| **Facility RVU** | **Work** | **PE** | **MP** | **Total** |
| **D6068** | 7.01 | 6.19 | 1.44 | 14.64 |

| | FUD | Status | MUE | Modifiers | | | | IOM Reference |
|---|---|---|---|---|---|---|---|---|
| **D6068** | N/A | N | - | N/A | N/A | N/A | N/A | None |

* with documentation

## Terms To Know

**abutment.** Tooth or implant fixture supporting a prosthesis.

**dental implant.** Surgical implantation of a device within the mandible or maxilla for dental replacement.

**fixed partial denture.** Prosthetic replacement of one or more missing teeth attached to the abutment teeth or implant replacements.

Dental - Implant Services

# D6069-D6071

**D6069** abutment supported retainer for porcelain fused to metal FPD (high noble metal)

*A metal-ceramic retainer for a fixed partial denture that gains retention, support and stability from an abutment on an implant.*

**D6070** abutment supported retainer for porcelain fused to metal FPD (predominantly base metal)

*A metal-ceramic retainer for a fixed partial denture that gains retention, support and stability from an abutment on an implant.*

**D6071** abutment supported retainer for porcelain fused to metal FPD (noble metal)

*A metal-ceramic retainer for a fixed partial denture that gains retention, support and stability from an abutment on an implant.*

## Explanation

A prosthodontic retainer is a part of a fixed partial denture (FPD) that attaches a bridge to an adjacent tooth, an implant abutment, or an implant. The retainer provides support, retention, and stability to the dental prosthesis. The type of retainer the dentist selects depends upon the retention required, the bridge design, the extent of existing restorations, and the amount of metal display the patient finds tolerable (aesthetics). The retainer is designed during the diagnostic wax-up of the bridge being made to replace the lost tooth. Code selection depends on the type of FPD as well as whether the abutment is implant-supported. The metal crown in code D6067 is made from titanium, titanium alloy, or a high noble metal that fits over the implant. Code D6070 describes an abutment-supported retainer for a porcelain pontic fused to a base metal alloy (non-noble metals with a silver appearance) FPD. Code D6071 describes an abutment supported retainer for a porcelain pontic fused to a noble metal FPD. The noble metal FPD is usually a gold alloy containing gold, copper, and other metals.

## Coding Tips

Local anesthesia is generally considered part of restorative procedures. High noble metals include gold, palladium, and platinum. The content must be ≥ 60 percent gold plus platinum and ≥ 40 percent gold. Noble metals include 25 percent or less gold plus platinum group. Predominantly base alloys contain a noble metal content of < 25 percent gold plus platinum group. The metals of the platinum group include platinum, palladium, rhodium, iridium, osmium, and ruthenium.

## Reimbursement Tips

The third-party payer may require an x-ray or x-ray report. Coverage of implant procedures varies by payer and by individual contract. Check with payers for specific coverage guidelines.

## ICD-10-CM Diagnostic Codes

| | |
|---|---|
| K02.51 | Dental caries on pit and fissure surface limited to enamel |
| K02.52 | Dental caries on pit and fissure surface penetrating into dentin |
| K02.53 | Dental caries on pit and fissure surface penetrating into pulp |
| K02.61 | Dental caries on smooth surface limited to enamel |
| K02.62 | Dental caries on smooth surface penetrating into dentin |
| K02.63 | Dental caries on smooth surface penetrating into pulp |
| K02.7 | Dental root caries |
| K03.0 | Excessive attrition of teeth |
| K03.1 | Abrasion of teeth |
| K03.2 | Erosion of teeth |
| K03.3 | Pathological resorption of teeth |
| K03.4 | Hypercementosis |
| K03.5 | Ankylosis of teeth |
| K03.6 | Deposits [accretions] on teeth |
| K03.7 | Posteruptive color changes of dental hard tissues |
| K03.81 | Cracked tooth |
| K03.89 | Other specified diseases of hard tissues of teeth |
| K04.01 | Reversible pulpitis |
| K04.02 | Irreversible pulpitis |
| K04.1 | Necrosis of pulp |
| K04.2 | Pulp degeneration |
| K04.3 | Abnormal hard tissue formation in pulp |
| K08.51 | Open restoration margins of tooth |
| K08.52 | Unrepairable overhanging of dental restorative materials |
| K08.530 | Fractured dental restorative material without loss of material |
| K08.531 | Fractured dental restorative material with loss of material |
| K08.539 | Fractured dental restorative material, unspecified |
| K08.55 | Allergy to existing dental restorative material |
| K08.56 | Poor aesthetic of existing restoration of tooth |
| K08.59 | Other unsatisfactory restoration of tooth |
| K08.81 | Primary occlusal trauma |
| K08.82 | Secondary occlusal trauma |

## Relative Value Units/Medicare Edits

| Non-Facility RVU | Work | PE | MP | Total |
|---|---|---|---|---|
| **D6069** | 7.12 | 6.29 | 1.47 | 14.88 |
| **D6070** | 6.67 | 5.89 | 1.37 | 13.93 |
| **D6071** | 6.85 | 6.04 | 1.41 | 14.30 |
| **Facility RVU** | **Work** | **PE** | **MP** | **Total** |
| **D6069** | 7.12 | 6.29 | 1.47 | 14.88 |
| **D6070** | 6.67 | 5.89 | 1.37 | 13.93 |
| **D6071** | 6.85 | 6.04 | 1.41 | 14.30 |

| | FUD | Status | MUE | Modifiers | | | | IOM Reference |
|---|---|---|---|---|---|---|---|---|
| **D6069** | N/A | N | - | N/A | N/A | N/A | N/A | None |
| **D6070** | N/A | N | - | N/A | N/A | N/A | N/A | |
| **D6071** | N/A | N | - | N/A | N/A | N/A | N/A | |

* with documentation

## Terms To Know

**abutment.** Tooth or implant fixture supporting a prosthesis.

**fixed partial denture.** Prosthetic replacement of one or more missing teeth attached to the abutment teeth or implant replacements.

**retainer.** In dentistry, portion of a fixed partial denture that attaches an artificial tooth to the abutment tooth or implant.

# D6072-D6074

**D6072** abutment supported retainer for cast metal FPD (high noble metal)

*A cast metal retainer for a fixed partial denture that gains retention, support and stability from an abutment on an implant.*

**D6073** abutment supported retainer for cast metal FPD (predominantly base metal)

*A cast metal retainer for a fixed partial denture that gains retention, support and stability from an abutment on an implant.*

**D6074** abutment supported retainer for cast metal FPD (noble metal)

*A cast metal retainer for a fixed partial denture that gains retention, support and stability from an abutment on an implant.*

## Explanation

A prosthodontic retainer is a part of a fixed partial denture (FPD) that attaches a bridge to an adjacent tooth, an implant abutment, or an implant. The retainer provides support, retention, and stability to the dental prosthesis. The type of retainer the dentist selects depends upon the retention required, the bridge design, the extent of existing restorations, and the amount of metal display the patient finds tolerable (aesthetics). The retainer is designed during the diagnostic wax-up of the bridge being made to replace the lost tooth. Code selection depends on the type of FPD as well as whether the abutment is implant-supported. Code D6072 describes an abutment-supported retainer for a cast high noble metal (gold) FPD. Code D6073 describes an abutment-supported retainer for a base metal alloy (non-noble metals with a silver appearance) FPD. Code D6074 describes an abutment-supported retainer for a noble metal FPD. The noble metal FPD is usually a gold alloy containing gold, copper, and other metals.

## Coding Tips

Local anesthesia is generally considered part of restorative procedures. High noble metals include gold, palladium, and platinum. The content must be ≥ 60 percent gold plus platinum and ≥ 40 percent gold. Noble metals include 25 percent or less gold plus platinum group. Predominantly base alloys contain a noble metal content of < 25 percent gold plus platinum group. The metals of the platinum group include platinum, palladium, rhodium, iridium, osmium, and ruthenium.

## Reimbursement Tips

The third-party payer may require an x-ray or x-ray report. Coverage of implant procedures varies by payer and by individual contract. Check with payers for specific coverage guidelines.

## ICD-10-CM Diagnostic Codes

| | |
|---|---|
| K02.51 | Dental caries on pit and fissure surface limited to enamel |
| K02.52 | Dental caries on pit and fissure surface penetrating into dentin |
| K02.53 | Dental caries on pit and fissure surface penetrating into pulp |
| K02.61 | Dental caries on smooth surface limited to enamel |
| K02.62 | Dental caries on smooth surface penetrating into dentin |
| K02.63 | Dental caries on smooth surface penetrating into pulp |
| K02.7 | Dental root caries |
| K03.0 | Excessive attrition of teeth |
| K03.1 | Abrasion of teeth |
| K03.2 | Erosion of teeth |
| K03.3 | Pathological resorption of teeth |
| K03.4 | Hypercementosis |
| K03.5 | Ankylosis of teeth |
| K03.6 | Deposits [accretions] on teeth |
| K03.7 | Posteruptive color changes of dental hard tissues |
| K03.81 | Cracked tooth |
| K03.89 | Other specified diseases of hard tissues of teeth |
| K04.01 | Reversible pulpitis |
| K04.02 | Irreversible pulpitis |
| K04.1 | Necrosis of pulp |
| K04.2 | Pulp degeneration |
| K04.3 | Abnormal hard tissue formation in pulp |
| K08.51 | Open restoration margins of tooth |
| K08.52 | Unrepairable overhanging of dental restorative materials |
| K08.530 | Fractured dental restorative material without loss of material |
| K08.531 | Fractured dental restorative material with loss of material |
| K08.539 | Fractured dental restorative material, unspecified |
| K08.55 | Allergy to existing dental restorative material |
| K08.56 | Poor aesthetic of existing restoration of tooth |
| K08.59 | Other unsatisfactory restoration of tooth |
| K08.81 | Primary occlusal trauma |
| K08.82 | Secondary occlusal trauma |

## Relative Value Units/Medicare Edits

| Non-Facility RVU | Work | PE | MP | Total |
|---|---|---|---|---|
| **D6072** | 7.00 | 6.17 | 1.44 | 14.61 |
| **D6073** | 6.31 | 5.57 | 1.30 | 13.18 |
| **D6074** | 6.64 | 5.86 | 1.37 | 13.87 |
| **Facility RVU** | **Work** | **PE** | **MP** | **Total** |
| **D6072** | 7.00 | 6.17 | 1.44 | 14.61 |
| **D6073** | 6.31 | 5.57 | 1.30 | 13.18 |
| **D6074** | 6.64 | 5.86 | 1.37 | 13.87 |

| | FUD | Status | MUE | Modifiers | | | | IOM Reference |
|---|---|---|---|---|---|---|---|---|
| **D6072** | N/A | N | - | N/A | N/A | N/A | N/A | None |
| **D6073** | N/A | N | - | N/A | N/A | N/A | N/A | |
| **D6074** | N/A | N | - | N/A | N/A | N/A | N/A | |

* with documentation

## Terms To Know

**abutment.** Tooth or implant fixture supporting a prosthesis.

**fixed partial denture.** Prosthetic replacement of one or more missing teeth attached to the abutment teeth or implant replacements.

**retainer.** In dentistry, portion of a fixed partial denture that attaches an artificial tooth to the abutment tooth or implant.

# D6075

**D6075** implant supported retainer for ceramic FPD

*A ceramic retainer for a fixed partial denture that gains retention, support and stability from an implant.*

## Explanation

A prosthodontic retainer is a part of a fixed partial denture (FPD) that attaches a bridge to an adjacent tooth, an implant abutment, or an implant. The retainer provides support, retention, and stability to the dental prosthesis. The type of retainer the dentist selects depends upon the retention required, the bridge design, the extent of existing restorations, and the amount of metal display the patient finds tolerable (aesthetics). The retainer is designed during the diagnostic wax-up of the bridge being made to replace the lost tooth. Code selection depends on the type of FPD as well as whether the abutment is implant-supported. Code D6075 describes an implant-supported retainer for a ceramic FPD.

## Coding Tips

Local anesthesia is generally considered part of restorative procedures.

## Reimbursement Tips

The third-party payer may require an x-ray or x-ray report. Coverage of implant procedures varies by payer and by individual contract. Check with payers for specific coverage guidelines.

## ICD-10-CM Diagnostic Codes

| | |
|---|---|
| K02.51 | Dental caries on pit and fissure surface limited to enamel |
| K02.52 | Dental caries on pit and fissure surface penetrating into dentin |
| K02.53 | Dental caries on pit and fissure surface penetrating into pulp |
| K02.61 | Dental caries on smooth surface limited to enamel |
| K02.62 | Dental caries on smooth surface penetrating into dentin |
| K02.63 | Dental caries on smooth surface penetrating into pulp |
| K02.7 | Dental root caries |
| K03.0 | Excessive attrition of teeth |
| K03.1 | Abrasion of teeth |
| K03.2 | Erosion of teeth |
| K03.3 | Pathological resorption of teeth |
| K03.4 | Hypercementosis |
| K03.5 | Ankylosis of teeth |
| K03.6 | Deposits [accretions] on teeth |
| K03.7 | Posteruptive color changes of dental hard tissues |
| K03.81 | Cracked tooth |
| K03.89 | Other specified diseases of hard tissues of teeth |
| K04.01 | Reversible pulpitis |
| K04.02 | Irreversible pulpitis |
| K04.1 | Necrosis of pulp |
| K04.2 | Pulp degeneration |
| K04.3 | Abnormal hard tissue formation in pulp |
| K08.51 | Open restoration margins of tooth |
| K08.52 | Unrepairable overhanging of dental restorative materials |
| K08.530 | Fractured dental restorative material without loss of material |
| K08.531 | Fractured dental restorative material with loss of material |
| K08.55 | Allergy to existing dental restorative material |
| K08.56 | Poor aesthetic of existing restoration of tooth |
| K08.59 | Other unsatisfactory restoration of tooth |
| K08.81 | Primary occlusal trauma |
| K08.82 | Secondary occlusal trauma |

## Relative Value Units/Medicare Edits

| Non-Facility RVU | Work | PE | MP | Total |
|---|---|---|---|---|
| **D6075** | 7.17 | 6.33 | 1.48 | 14.98 |
| **Facility RVU** | **Work** | **PE** | **MP** | **Total** |
| **D6075** | 7.17 | 6.33 | 1.48 | 14.98 |

| | FUD | Status | MUE | Modifiers | | | | IOM Reference |
|---|---|---|---|---|---|---|---|---|
| **D6075** | N/A | N | - | N/A | N/A | N/A | N/A | None |

* with documentation

## Terms To Know

**dental implant.** Surgical implantation of a device within the mandible or maxilla for dental replacement.

**fixed partial denture.** Prosthetic replacement of one or more missing teeth attached to the abutment teeth or implant replacements.

**retainer.** In dentistry, portion of a fixed partial denture that attaches an artificial tooth to the abutment tooth or implant.



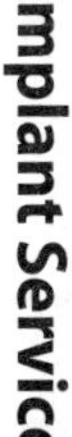

# D6076-D6077

**D6076** implant supported retainer for FPD - porcelain fused to high noble alloys

*A metal-ceramic retainer for a fixed partial denture that gains retention, support and stability from an implant.*

**D6077** implant supported retainer for metal FPD - high noble alloys

*A metal retainer for a fixed partial denture that gains retention, support and stability from an implant.*

## Explanation

A prosthodontic retainer is a part of a fixed partial denture (FPD) that attaches a bridge to an adjacent tooth, an implant abutment, or an implant. The retainer provides support, retention, and stability to the dental prosthesis. The type of retainer the dentist selects depends upon the retention required, the bridge design, the extent of existing restorations, and the amount of metal display the patient finds tolerable (aesthetics). The retainer is designed during the diagnostic wax-up of the bridge being made to replace the lost tooth. Code selection depends on the type of FPD as well as whether the abutment is implant-supported. Code D6076 describes an implant-supported retainer for porcelain fused to metal FPD. Code D6077 describes an implant-supported retainer for a cast metal FPD. The FPD is made from a high grade noble alloy.

## Coding Tips

These codes are out-of-sequence codes and will not display in numeric order in the CDT book. Local anesthesia is generally considered part of restorative procedures. High noble metals include gold, palladium, and platinum. The content must be ≥ 60 percent gold plus platinum and ≥ 40 percent gold. Noble metals include 25 percent or less gold plus platinum group. Predominantly base alloys contain a noble metal content of < 25 percent gold plus platinum group. The metals of the platinum group include platinum, palladium, rhodium, iridium, osmium, and ruthenium.

## Reimbursement Tips

The third-party payer may require an x-ray or x-ray report. Coverage of implant procedures varies by payer and by individual contract. Check with payers for specific coverage guidelines.

## ICD-10-CM Diagnostic Codes

K08.411 Partial loss of teeth due to trauma, class I
K08.412 Partial loss of teeth due to trauma, class II
K08.413 Partial loss of teeth due to trauma, class III
K08.414 Partial loss of teeth due to trauma, class IV
K08.421 Partial loss of teeth due to periodontal diseases, class I
K08.422 Partial loss of teeth due to periodontal diseases, class II
K08.423 Partial loss of teeth due to periodontal diseases, class III
K08.424 Partial loss of teeth due to periodontal diseases, class IV
K08.431 Partial loss of teeth due to caries, class I
K08.432 Partial loss of teeth due to caries, class II
K08.433 Partial loss of teeth due to caries, class III
K08.434 Partial loss of teeth due to caries, class IV
K08.491 Partial loss of teeth due to other specified cause, class I
K08.492 Partial loss of teeth due to other specified cause, class II
K08.493 Partial loss of teeth due to other specified cause, class III
K08.494 Partial loss of teeth due to other specified cause, class IV

## Relative Value Units/Medicare Edits

| Non-Facility RVU | Work | PE | MP | Total |
|---|---|---|---|---|
| **D6076** | 6.98 | 6.16 | 1.44 | 14.58 |
| **D6077** | 7.00 | 6.18 | 1.44 | 14.62 |
| **Facility RVU** | **Work** | **PE** | **MP** | **Total** |
| **D6076** | 6.98 | 6.16 | 1.44 | 14.58 |
| **D6077** | 7.00 | 6.18 | 1.44 | 14.62 |

| | FUD | Status | MUE | Modifiers | | | | IOM Reference |
|---|---|---|---|---|---|---|---|---|
| **D6076** | N/A | N | - | N/A | N/A | N/A | N/A | None |
| **D6077** | N/A | N | - | N/A | N/A | N/A | N/A | |

* with documentation

## Terms To Know

**dental implant.** Surgical implantation of a device within the mandible or maxilla for dental replacement.

**fixed partial denture.** Prosthetic replacement of one or more missing teeth attached to the abutment teeth or implant replacements.

**retainer.** In dentistry, portion of a fixed partial denture that attaches an artificial tooth to the abutment tooth or implant.

# D6080

**D6080** implant maintenance procedures when prostheses are removed and reinserted, including cleansing of prostheses and abutments

*This procedure includes active debriding of the implant(s) and examination of all aspects of the implant system(s), including the occlusion and stability of the superstructure. The patient is also instructed in thorough daily cleansing of the implant(s). This is not a per implant code, and is indicated for implant supported fixed prostheses.*

## Explanation

Maintenance with plaque control of the abutments and care of the root face is imperative to the longevity of the implant. Regular appointments with the oral hygienist may be mandatory, and the dentist may prescribe a fluoride gel to place in the recess of the denture where it contacts the denture. In the first year, the patient may be assessed every three months. Appointments after the first year should be based on the patient's needs, such as periodontal health of the surrounding teeth and the patient's ability and willingness to participate in effective home care procedures. During each visit, the dental hygienist may assess the client's oral hygiene and make necessary modifications. Home care should be reviewed and reinforced with written instruction.

## Coding Tips

Local anesthesia is generally considered part of restorative procedures.

## Reimbursement Tips

The third-party payer may require an x-ray or x-ray report. Coverage of implant procedures varies by payer and by individual contract. Check with payers for specific coverage guidelines.

## ICD-10-CM Diagnostic Codes

| | |
|---|---|
| K13.24 | Leukokeratosis nicotina palati |
| Z46.3 | Encounter for fitting and adjustment of dental prosthetic device |
| Z48.814 | Encounter for surgical aftercare following surgery on the teeth or oral cavity |

## Relative Value Units/Medicare Edits

| Non-Facility RVU | Work | PE | MP | Total |
|---|---|---|---|---|
| D6080 | 0.75 | 0.66 | 0.15 | 1.56 |
| **Facility RVU** | **Work** | **PE** | **MP** | **Total** |
| D6080 | 0.75 | 0.66 | 0.15 | 1.56 |

| | FUD | Status | MUE | Modifiers | | | | IOM Reference |
|---|---|---|---|---|---|---|---|---|
| D6080 | N/A | I | - | N/A | N/A | N/A | N/A | None |

* with documentation

## Terms To Know

**abutment.** Tooth or implant fixture supporting a prosthesis.

**debridement.** Removal of dead or contaminated tissue and foreign matter from a wound.

**plaque.** Accumulation of a soft sticky substance on the teeth largely composed of bacteria and its byproducts.

**prophylaxis.** Intervention or protective therapy intended to prevent a disease.

# D6081

**D6081** scaling and debridement in the presence of inflammation or mucositis of a single implant, including cleaning of the implant surfaces, without flap entry and closure

*This procedure is not performed in conjunction with D1110, D4910 or D4346.*

## Explanation

The provider removes plaque and calculus from an implant when there inflammation and/or ulceration of the oral mucosa. Depending on the depth of the accretions, it may be necessary for the provider to incise the gingiva, forming a flap in which to reach the post. Debridement of the implant restoration is directed to the three components of the implant: the prosthesis, the abutment, and the implant fixture surface. This may be accomplished using a variety of instruments including plastic scaler and curettes, power instruments, Piezo tips, ultrasonic inserts, and Eva tips.

## Coding Tips

Do not report this service in addition to D1110, D4910, or D4346. Local anesthesia is included in this service. Any evaluation or radiograph is reported separately.

## Documentation Tips

This service should only be reported when the medical documentation indicates the presence of mucositis.

## ICD-10-CM Diagnostic Codes

| | |
|---|---|
| K12.31 | Oral mucositis (ulcerative) due to antineoplastic therapy |
| K12.32 | Oral mucositis (ulcerative) due to other drugs |
| K12.33 | Oral mucositis (ulcerative) due to radiation |
| K12.39 | Other oral mucositis (ulcerative) |
| T85.79XA | Infection and inflammatory reaction due to other internal prosthetic devices, implants and grafts, initial encounter |

## Relative Value Units/Medicare Edits

| Non-Facility RVU | Work | PE | MP | Total |
|---|---|---|---|---|
| D6081 | 1.19 | 1.05 | 0.25 | 2.49 |
| **Facility RVU** | **Work** | **PE** | **MP** | **Total** |
| D6081 | 1.19 | 1.05 | 0.25 | 2.49 |

| | FUD | Status | MUE | Modifiers | | | | IOM Reference |
|---|---|---|---|---|---|---|---|---|
| D6081 | N/A | N | - | N/A | N/A | N/A | N/A | None |

* with documentation

## Terms To Know

**debridement.** Removal of dead or contaminated tissue and foreign matter from a wound.

**implant.** Material or device inserted or placed within the body for therapeutic, reconstructive, or diagnostic purposes.

**scaling.** Removal of plaque, calculus, and stains from teeth.

# D6082-D6084

**D6082** implant supported crown - porcelain fused to predominantly base alloys

*A single metal-ceramic crown restoration that is retained, supported and stabilized by an implant.*

**D6083** implant supported crown - porcelain fused to noble alloys

*A single metal-ceramic crown restoration that is retained, supported and stabilized by an implant.*

**D6084** implant supported crown - porcelain fused to titanium and titanium alloys

*A single metal-ceramic crown restoration that is retained, supported and stabilized by an implant.*

## Explanation

The dentist provides an implant-supported crown that replaces missing teeth of a jaw. Following the development of a dental plan and preparation for the missing tooth, including necessary periodontal work previously performed, the crown is fused to the implant. Code assignment is dependent upon the type of implant. When porcelain is fused to predominately base alloys, report D6082; porcelain to titanium and titanium alloys, report D6083; or porcelain fused to noble alloys, report D6084.

## Coding Tips

Correct code assignment is dependent upon the substances used. Porcelain/ceramic refers to pressed, fired, polished, or milled substances, which predominantly contain inorganic refractory compounds such as porcelains, glasses, ceramics, and glass-ceramics.

## ICD-10-CM Diagnostic Codes

| | |
|---|---|
| K08.411 | Partial loss of teeth due to trauma, class I |
| K08.412 | Partial loss of teeth due to trauma, class II |
| K08.413 | Partial loss of teeth due to trauma, class III |
| K08.414 | Partial loss of teeth due to trauma, class IV |
| K08.421 | Partial loss of teeth due to periodontal diseases, class I |
| K08.422 | Partial loss of teeth due to periodontal diseases, class II |
| K08.423 | Partial loss of teeth due to periodontal diseases, class III |
| K08.424 | Partial loss of teeth due to periodontal diseases, class IV |
| K08.431 | Partial loss of teeth due to caries, class I |
| K08.432 | Partial loss of teeth due to caries, class II |
| K08.433 | Partial loss of teeth due to caries, class III |
| K08.434 | Partial loss of teeth due to caries, class IV |
| K08.491 | Partial loss of teeth due to other specified cause, class I |
| K08.492 | Partial loss of teeth due to other specified cause, class II |
| K08.493 | Partial loss of teeth due to other specified cause, class III |
| K08.494 | Partial loss of teeth due to other specified cause, class IV |

## Relative Value Units/Medicare Edits

| Non-Facility RVU | Work | PE | MP | Total |
|---|---|---|---|---|
| D6082 | 5.26 | 4.64 | 1.08 | 10.98 |
| D6083 | 5.97 | 5.27 | 1.23 | 12.47 |
| D6084 | 5.97 | 5.27 | 1.23 | 12.47 |
| **Facility RVU** | **Work** | **PE** | **MP** | **Total** |
| D6082 | 5.26 | 4.64 | 1.08 | 10.98 |
| D6083 | 5.97 | 5.27 | 1.23 | 12.47 |
| D6084 | 5.97 | 5.27 | 1.23 | 12.47 |

| | FUD | Status | MUE | Modifiers | | | | IOM Reference |
|---|---|---|---|---|---|---|---|---|
| D6082 | N/A | N | - | N/A | N/A | N/A | N/A | None |
| D6083 | N/A | N | - | N/A | N/A | N/A | N/A | |
| D6084 | N/A | N | - | N/A | N/A | N/A | N/A | |

* with documentation

## Terms To Know

**crown.** Dental restoration that completely caps or encircles a tooth or dental implant.

**edentulism.** Partial or complete absence of teeth due to a congenital defect involving the tooth bud or acquired as a result of caries, trauma, extraction, or periodontal disease. ***Synonym(s):*** *adontia, anodontia, anodontism, edentia.*

Dental - Implant Services

# D6085

▲ **D6085** interim implant crown

*Placed when a period of healing is necessary prior to fabrication and placement of the definitive prosthesis.*

## Explanation

A provisional implant crown is placed to allow healing for an extended time prior to final restoration. The temporary crown can be fabricated either intraorally or extraorally at the surgical appointment or for placement at a later date. Temporary abutments are either affixed to the implants intraorally or to a cast made from an implant impression. The temporary crown is positioned and inserted over the abutments either intraorally or on the cast. The provisional resin is allowed to fully set.

## Coding Tips

For a provisional crown prior to completion of a routine restoration not related to implant services, see D2799. For removal of an interim implant crown, see D6198.

## ICD-10-CM Diagnostic Codes

K02.51 Dental caries on pit and fissure surface limited to enamel
K02.52 Dental caries on pit and fissure surface penetrating into dentin
K02.53 Dental caries on pit and fissure surface penetrating into pulp
K02.61 Dental caries on smooth surface limited to enamel
K02.62 Dental caries on smooth surface penetrating into dentin
K02.63 Dental caries on smooth surface penetrating into pulp
K02.7 Dental root caries
K02.9 Dental caries, unspecified
K03.0 Excessive attrition of teeth
K03.1 Abrasion of teeth
K03.2 Erosion of teeth
K03.3 Pathological resorption of teeth
K03.4 Hypercementosis
K03.5 Ankylosis of teeth
K03.6 Deposits [accretions] on teeth
K03.7 Posteruptive color changes of dental hard tissues
K03.81 Cracked tooth
K03.89 Other specified diseases of hard tissues of teeth
K03.9 Disease of hard tissues of teeth, unspecified
K04.01 Reversible pulpitis
K04.02 Irreversible pulpitis
K04.1 Necrosis of pulp
K04.2 Pulp degeneration
K04.3 Abnormal hard tissue formation in pulp
K08.50 Unsatisfactory restoration of tooth, unspecified
K08.51 Open restoration margins of tooth
K08.52 Unrepairable overhanging of dental restorative materials
K08.530 Fractured dental restorative material without loss of material
K08.531 Fractured dental restorative material with loss of material
K08.539 Fractured dental restorative material, unspecified
K08.55 Allergy to existing dental restorative material
K08.56 Poor aesthetic of existing restoration of tooth
K08.59 Other unsatisfactory restoration of tooth
K08.81 Primary occlusal trauma
K08.82 Secondary occlusal trauma
K08.89 Other specified disorders of teeth and supporting structures
K08.9 Disorder of teeth and supporting structures, unspecified

## Relative Value Units/Medicare Edits

| Non-Facility RVU | Work | PE | MP | Total |
|---|---|---|---|---|
| **D6085** | 1.43 | 1.26 | 0.29 | 2.98 |
| **Facility RVU** | **Work** | **PE** | **MP** | **Total** |
| **D6085** | 1.43 | 1.26 | 0.29 | 2.98 |

| | FUD | Status | MUE | Modifiers | | | | IOM Reference |
|---|---|---|---|---|---|---|---|---|
| **D6085** | N/A | N | - | N/A | N/A | N/A | N/A | None |

* with documentation

## Terms To Know

**abutment.** Tooth or implant fixture supporting a prosthesis.

**attrition.** In dentistry, wearing away or erosion of tooth surface from abrasive food or grinding teeth.

**caries.** Localized section of tooth decay that begins on the tooth surface with destruction of the calcified enamel, allowing bacterial destruction to continue and form cavities and may extend to the dentin and pulp.

**extraoral.** Outside of the mouth or oral cavity.

**implant.** Material or device inserted or placed within the body for therapeutic, reconstructive, or diagnostic purposes.

**intraoral.** Within the mouth.

# D6086-D6088

**D6086** implant supported crown - predominantly base alloys

*A single metal crown restoration that is retained, supported and stabilized by an implant.*

**D6087** implant supported crown - noble alloys

*A single metal crown restoration that is retained, supported and stabilized by an implant.*

**D6088** implant supported crown - titanium and titanium alloys

*A single metal crown restoration that is retained, supported and stabilized by an implant.*

## Explanation

The dentist provides an implant supported crown that replaces missing teeth of a jaw. Following the development of a dental plan and preparation for the missing tooth, including necessary periodontal work, previously performed the crown is fused to the implant. Code assignment is dependent upon the type of implant. When porcelain is fused to predominately base alloys, report D6086; porcelain to noble alloys, report D6087; or porcelain fused to titanium and titanium alloys, report D6088.

## Coding Tips

Correct code assignment is dependent upon the substances used. Porcelain/ceramic refers to pressed, fired, polished, or milled substances, which predominantly contain inorganic refractory compounds such as porcelains, glasses, ceramics, and glass-ceramics.

## ICD-10-CM Diagnostic Codes

K08.411 Partial loss of teeth due to trauma, class I
K08.412 Partial loss of teeth due to trauma, class II
K08.413 Partial loss of teeth due to trauma, class III
K08.414 Partial loss of teeth due to trauma, class IV
K08.421 Partial loss of teeth due to periodontal diseases, class I
K08.422 Partial loss of teeth due to periodontal diseases, class II
K08.423 Partial loss of teeth due to periodontal diseases, class III
K08.424 Partial loss of teeth due to periodontal diseases, class IV
K08.431 Partial loss of teeth due to caries, class I
K08.432 Partial loss of teeth due to caries, class II
K08.433 Partial loss of teeth due to caries, class III
K08.434 Partial loss of teeth due to caries, class IV
K08.491 Partial loss of teeth due to other specified cause, class I
K08.492 Partial loss of teeth due to other specified cause, class II
K08.493 Partial loss of teeth due to other specified cause, class III
K08.494 Partial loss of teeth due to other specified cause, class IV

## Relative Value Units/Medicare Edits

| Non-Facility RVU | Work | PE | MP | Total |
|---|---|---|---|---|
| **D6086** | 4.06 | 3.58 | 0.84 | 8.48 |
| **D6087** | 4.78 | 4.22 | 0.98 | 9.98 |
| **D6088** | 4.54 | 4.01 | 0.93 | 9.48 |
| **Facility RVU** | **Work** | **PE** | **MP** | **Total** |
| **D6086** | 4.06 | 3.58 | 0.84 | 8.48 |
| **D6087** | 4.78 | 4.22 | 0.98 | 9.98 |
| **D6088** | 4.54 | 4.01 | 0.93 | 9.48 |

| | FUD | Status | MUE | Modifiers | | | | IOM Reference |
|---|---|---|---|---|---|---|---|---|
| **D6086** | N/A | N | - | N/A | N/A | N/A | N/A | None |
| **D6087** | N/A | N | - | N/A | N/A | N/A | N/A | |
| **D6088** | N/A | N | - | N/A | N/A | N/A | N/A | |

* with documentation

## Terms To Know

**crown.** Dental restoration that completely caps or encircles a tooth or dental implant.

**edentulism.** Partial or complete absence of teeth due to a congenital defect involving the tooth bud or acquired as a result of caries, trauma, extraction, or periodontal disease. ***Synonym(s):*** *adontia, anodontia, anodontism, edentia.*

# D6090

**D6090** repair implant supported prosthesis, by report

*This procedure involves the repair or replacement of any part of the implant supported prosthesis.*

## Explanation

Changes in implant health can indicate an ailing or a failed implant. The ailing implant-supported prosthesis may show radiological bone loss without clinical inflammation, and the implant must be monitored closely to prevent failure and removal of the implant. An ailing implant may be saved through treatments that include surgical intervention and detoxification of the implant surface. Code D6090 requires pertinent documentation to evaluate the medical appropriateness of repair.

## Coding Tips

Local anesthesia is generally considered part of restorative procedures. Pertinent documentation to evaluate medical appropriateness should be incuded when this code is reported. The third-party payer may require an x-ray or x-ray report. Coverage of implant procedures varies by payer and by individual contract. Check with payers for their specific coverage guidelines.

## Reimbursement Tips

The third-party payer may require an x-ray or x-ray report. Coverage of implant procedures varies by payer and by individual contract. Check with payers for specific coverage guidelines.

## ICD-10-CM Diagnostic Codes

Z46.3 Encounter for fitting and adjustment of dental prosthetic device

## Relative Value Units/Medicare Edits

| Non-Facility RVU | Work | PE | MP | Total |
|---|---|---|---|---|
| D6090 | 2.68 | 2.36 | 0.55 | 5.59 |
| **Facility RVU** | **Work** | **PE** | **MP** | **Total** |
| D6090 | 2.68 | 2.36 | 0.55 | 5.59 |

| | FUD | Status | MUE | Modifiers | | | | IOM Reference |
|---|---|---|---|---|---|---|---|---|
| D6090 | N/A | I | - | N/A | N/A | N/A | N/A | None |

* with documentation

## Terms To Know

**dental implant.** Surgical implantation of a device within the mandible or maxilla for dental replacement.

# D6091-D6093

▲ **D6091** replacement of replaceable part of semi-precision or precision attachment of implant/abutment supported prosthesis, per attachment

**D6092** re-cement or re-bond implant/abutment supported crown

**D6093** re-cement or re-bond implant/abutment supported fixed partial denture

## Explanation

The dentist replaces a replaceable component of a fixed partial denture (FPD) in D6091. The dentist recements or rebonds portions of the implant of an abutment-supported crown in D6092 or FPD in D6093. The type of retainer the dentist repairs or replaces depends upon the retention required by the patient, the bridge design, the extent of existing restorations, and the amount of metal display the patient finds tolerable (aesthetics).

## Coding Tips

Local anesthesia is generally considered part of restorative procedures.

## Reimbursement Tips

Coverage of implant procedures varies by payer and by individual contract. Check with payers for specific coverage guidelines. The third-party payer may require an x-ray or x-ray report.

## ICD-10-CM Diagnostic Codes

K08.530 Fractured dental restorative material without loss of material

K08.531 Fractured dental restorative material with loss of material

K08.539 Fractured dental restorative material, unspecified

K08.56 Poor aesthetic of existing restoration of tooth

K08.59 Other unsatisfactory restoration of tooth

Z46.3 Encounter for fitting and adjustment of dental prosthetic device

Z48.814 Encounter for surgical aftercare following surgery on the teeth or oral cavity

## Relative Value Units/Medicare Edits

| Non-Facility RVU | Work | PE | MP | Total |
|---|---|---|---|---|
| D6091 | 2.93 | 2.59 | 0.60 | 6.12 |
| D6092 | 0.62 | 0.55 | 0.13 | 1.30 |
| D6093 | 0.88 | 0.78 | 0.18 | 1.84 |
| **Facility RVU** | **Work** | **PE** | **MP** | **Total** |
| D6091 | 2.93 | 2.59 | 0.60 | 6.12 |
| D6092 | 0.62 | 0.55 | 0.13 | 1.30 |
| D6093 | 0.88 | 0.78 | 0.18 | 1.84 |

| | FUD | Status | MUE | Modifiers | | | | IOM Reference |
|---|---|---|---|---|---|---|---|---|
| D6091 | N/A | N | - | N/A | N/A | N/A | N/A | None |
| D6092 | N/A | N | - | N/A | N/A | N/A | N/A | |
| D6093 | N/A | N | - | N/A | N/A | N/A | N/A | |

* with documentation

# D6094

**D6094** abutment supported crown - titanium and titanium alloys

*A single crown restoration that is retained, supported and stabilized by an abutment on an implant.*

## Explanation

An implant is placed. After adequate healing time, the provider attaches the abutment that includes the titanium or titanium alloy crown. To seat the abutment, the provider inserts a guide pin into the well of the implant. A sulcus reamer is passed over the guide pin and rotated while pressing it toward the alveolar crest to remove all bony interferences. The abutment is placed within the well and rotated to the desired position. The abutment is seated according to the manufacturer's specification.

## Coding Tips

This is an out-of-sequence code and will not display in numeric order in the CDT book. Local anesthesia is generally considered part of restorative procedures.

## Reimbursement Tips

The third-party payer may require an x-ray or x-ray report. Coverage of implant procedures varies by payer and by individual contract. Check with payers for specific coverage guidelines.

## ICD-10-CM Diagnostic Codes

| | |
|---|---|
| K08.411 | Partial loss of teeth due to trauma, class I |
| K08.412 | Partial loss of teeth due to trauma, class II |
| K08.413 | Partial loss of teeth due to trauma, class III |
| K08.414 | Partial loss of teeth due to trauma, class IV |
| K08.421 | Partial loss of teeth due to periodontal diseases, class I |
| K08.422 | Partial loss of teeth due to periodontal diseases, class II |
| K08.423 | Partial loss of teeth due to periodontal diseases, class III |
| K08.424 | Partial loss of teeth due to periodontal diseases, class IV |
| K08.431 | Partial loss of teeth due to caries, class I |
| K08.432 | Partial loss of teeth due to caries, class II |
| K08.433 | Partial loss of teeth due to caries, class III |
| K08.434 | Partial loss of teeth due to caries, class IV |
| K08.491 | Partial loss of teeth due to other specified cause, class I |
| K08.492 | Partial loss of teeth due to other specified cause, class II |
| K08.493 | Partial loss of teeth due to other specified cause, class III |
| K08.494 | Partial loss of teeth due to other specified cause, class IV |

## Relative Value Units/Medicare Edits

| Non-Facility RVU | Work | PE | MP | Total |
|---|---|---|---|---|
| D6094 | 5.77 | 5.09 | 1.19 | 12.05 |
| **Facility RVU** | **Work** | **PE** | **MP** | **Total** |
| D6094 | 5.77 | 5.09 | 1.19 | 12.05 |

| | FUD | Status | MUE | Modifiers | | | | IOM Reference |
|---|---|---|---|---|---|---|---|---|
| D6094 | N/A | N | - | N/A | N/A | N/A | N/A | None |

* with documentation

## Terms To Know

**abutment crown.** Artificial tooth cap for the retention and/or support of a dental prosthesis.

# D6095

**D6095** repair implant abutment, by report

*This procedure involves the repair or replacement of any part of the implant abutment.*

## Explanation

Changes in implant health can indicate an ailing or a failed implant. The ailing implant abutment may show radiological bone loss without clinical inflammation, and the implant must be monitored closely to prevent failure and removal of the implant. An ailing implant may be saved through treatments that include repair or replacement. Code D6095 requires pertinent documentation to evaluate the medical appropriateness of the repair.

## Coding Tips

This is an out-of-sequence code and will not display in numeric order in the CDT manual. For repair of implant-supported prosthesis, see code D6090. Local anesthesia is generally considered part of restorative procedures.

## Reimbursement Tips

Pertinent documentation to evaluate the medical appropriateness should be included when this code is reported. Coverage of implant services varies by payer and by individual contract. Check with payers for specific coverage guidelines.

## ICD-10-CM Diagnostic Codes

| | |
|---|---|
| K08.21 | Minimal atrophy of the mandible |
| K08.22 | Moderate atrophy of the mandible |
| K08.23 | Severe atrophy of the mandible |
| K08.24 | Minimal atrophy of maxilla |
| K08.25 | Moderate atrophy of the maxilla |
| K08.26 | Severe atrophy of the maxilla |
| K08.51 | Open restoration margins of tooth |
| K08.52 | Unrepairable overhanging of dental restorative materials |
| K08.530 | Fractured dental restorative material without loss of material |
| K08.531 | Fractured dental restorative material with loss of material |
| K08.54 | Contour of existing restoration of tooth biologically incompatible with oral health |
| K08.55 | Allergy to existing dental restorative material |
| K08.56 | Poor aesthetic of existing restoration of tooth |
| K08.59 | Other unsatisfactory restoration of tooth |
| Z46.3 | Encounter for fitting and adjustment of dental prosthetic device |
| Z97.2 | Presence of dental prosthetic device (complete) (partial) |

## Relative Value Units/Medicare Edits

| Non-Facility RVU | Work | PE | MP | Total |
|---|---|---|---|---|
| D6095 | 2.89 | 2.55 | 0.60 | 6.04 |
| **Facility RVU** | **Work** | **PE** | **MP** | **Total** |
| D6095 | 2.89 | 2.55 | 0.60 | 6.04 |

| | FUD | Status | MUE | Modifiers | | | | IOM Reference |
|---|---|---|---|---|---|---|---|---|
| D6095 | N/A | I | - | N/A | N/A | N/A | N/A | None |

* with documentation

## Terms To Know

**abutment.** Tooth or implant fixture supporting a prosthesis.

# D6096

**D6096** remove broken implant retaining screw

## Explanation

The provider removes a broken retaining screw that is used to hold a dental implant. There are several methods that can be used. When using an ultrasonic scaler, the provider uses a tissue punch to expose the screw after providing local anesthesia. Using a ¼ round bur in a high-speed hand piece, the provider makes a deep pit across the broken screw fragment. Using an ultrasonic scaler and moving in the anticlockwise direction, the fractured abutment screw is retrieved. If a round bur and hand piece is used, the provider makes contact with the outer edge of the retainer screw and rotates the bur in a rotating clockwise rotation to loosen the remaining fragment. A secondary alternative is to create a horizontal slot in the shank of what remains of the abutment screw and using a small straight blade driver remove the fragment. A third method could be for the provider to use a reverse-tapping rotary instrument to mechanically remove the abutment screw.

## Coding Tips

Local anesthesia is generally considered to be part of removable prosthodontic procedures.

## ICD-10-CM Diagnostic Codes

Z46.3 Encounter for fitting and adjustment of dental prosthetic device
Z97.2 Presence of dental prosthetic device (complete) (partial)

## Relative Value Units/Medicare Edits

| Non-Facility RVU | Work | PE | MP | Total |
|---|---|---|---|---|
| D6096 | 0.00 | 0.00 | 0.00 | 0.00 |
| **Facility RVU** | **Work** | **PE** | **MP** | **Total** |
| D6096 | 0.00 | 0.00 | 0.00 | 0.00 |

| | FUD | Status | MUE | Modifiers | | | | IOM Reference |
|---|---|---|---|---|---|---|---|---|
| D6096 | N/A | N | - | N/A | N/A | N/A | N/A | None |

* with documentation

## Terms To Know

**implant.** Material or device inserted or placed within the body for therapeutic, reconstructive, or diagnostic purposes.

# D6097

**D6097** abutment supported crown - porcelain fused to titanium and titanium alloys

*A single metal-ceramic crown restoration that is retained, supported, and stabilized by an abutment on an implant.*

## Explanation

An implant replaces lost teeth with a nonremovable restoration to help restore function, aesthetics, and speech. Most implant treatment consists of a two-stage procedure. After treatment planning, the bone is surgically exposed and an implant is placed. The implant is left buried in the bone and unloaded, usually for three months in the mandible and six months in the maxilla. After the healing period, the implant is uncovered. The second step of the procedure is necessary to uncover the implant and attach an extension. This small metal post, called an abutment, completes the foundation on which the tooth will be placed. The prosthesis (abutment) is screwed into the implant using a screwdriver and ratchet and fixed to the implant. Before cementing the crown, the screw channel is sealed off with wax or gutta-percha to allow release of the screw if required. A transfer coping at the impression stage is given to the laboratory to assist in the crown manufacture. During this time, a temporary tooth replacement option can be worn over the implant site. Appropriate code selection depends upon the type of crown. Code D6097 represents a porcelain crown fused to titanium and titanium alloys.

## Coding Tips

Local anesthesia is generally considered part of restorative procedures. The third-party payer may require an x-ray or x-ray report.

## ICD-10-CM Diagnostic Codes

K02.51 Dental caries on pit and fissure surface limited to enamel
K02.52 Dental caries on pit and fissure surface penetrating into dentin
K02.53 Dental caries on pit and fissure surface penetrating into pulp
K02.61 Dental caries on smooth surface limited to enamel
K02.62 Dental caries on smooth surface penetrating into dentin
K02.63 Dental caries on smooth surface penetrating into pulp
K02.7 Dental root caries
K03.0 Excessive attrition of teeth
K03.1 Abrasion of teeth
K03.2 Erosion of teeth
K03.3 Pathological resorption of teeth
K03.4 Hypercementosis
K03.5 Ankylosis of teeth
K03.6 Deposits [accretions] on teeth
K03.7 Posteruptive color changes of dental hard tissues
K03.81 Cracked tooth
K03.89 Other specified diseases of hard tissues of teeth
K03.9 Disease of hard tissues of teeth, unspecified
K04.01 Reversible pulpitis
K04.02 Irreversible pulpitis
K04.1 Necrosis of pulp
K04.2 Pulp degeneration
K04.3 Abnormal hard tissue formation in pulp
K08.50 Unsatisfactory restoration of tooth, unspecified
K08.51 Open restoration margins of tooth
K08.52 Unrepairable overhanging of dental restorative materials
K08.530 Fractured dental restorative material without loss of material
K08.531 Fractured dental restorative material with loss of material

K08.539 Fractured dental restorative material, unspecified
K08.55 Allergy to existing dental restorative material
K08.56 Poor aesthetic of existing restoration of tooth
K08.59 Other unsatisfactory restoration of tooth
K08.81 Primary occlusal trauma
K08.82 Secondary occlusal trauma

## Relative Value Units/Medicare Edits

| Non-Facility RVU | Work | PE | MP | Total |
|---|---|---|---|---|
| D6097 | 4.52 | 3.99 | 0.93 | 9.44 |
| Facility RVU | Work | PE | MP | Total |
| D6097 | 4.52 | 3.99 | 0.93 | 9.44 |

| | FUD | Status | MUE | Modifiers | | | | IOM Reference |
|---|---|---|---|---|---|---|---|---|
| D6097 | N/A | N | - | N/A | N/A | N/A | N/A | None |

* with documentation

## Terms To Know

**abutment.** Tooth or implant fixture supporting a prosthesis.

# D6098-D6099

**D6098** implant supported retainer - porcelain fused to predominantly base alloys

*A metal-ceramic retainer for a fixed partial denture that gains retention, support, and stability from an implant.*

**D6099** implant supported retainer for FPD - porcelain fused to noble alloys

*A metal-ceramic retainer for a fixed partial denture that gains retention, support, and stability from an implant.*

## Explanation

A prosthodontic retainer is a part of a fixed partial denture (FPD) that attaches a bridge to an adjacent tooth, an implant abutment, or an implant. The retainer provides support, retention, and stability to the dental prosthesis. The type of retainer the dentist selects depends upon the retention required, the bridge design, the extent of existing restorations, and the amount of metal display the patient finds tolerable (aesthetics). The retainer is designed during the diagnostic wax-up of the bridge being made to replace the lost tooth. Code selection depends on the type of FPD as well as whether the abutment is implant-supported and the alloys used. Report D6098 for porcelain fused to predominantly base alloys; D6099 for porcelain fused to noble alloys.

## Coding Tips

Local anesthesia is generally considered part of restorative procedures. High noble metals include gold, palladium, and platinum and are reported with D6069. Noble metals include 25 percent or less gold plus platinum group and are reported with D6071.

## Reimbursement Tips

The third-party payer may require an x-ray or x-ray report. Coverage of implant procedures varies by payer and by individual contract. Check with payers for specific coverage guidelines.

## ICD-10-CM Diagnostic Codes

K02.51 Dental caries on pit and fissure surface limited to enamel
K02.52 Dental caries on pit and fissure surface penetrating into dentin
K02.53 Dental caries on pit and fissure surface penetrating into pulp
K02.61 Dental caries on smooth surface limited to enamel
K02.62 Dental caries on smooth surface penetrating into dentin
K02.63 Dental caries on smooth surface penetrating into pulp
K02.7 Dental root caries
K03.0 Excessive attrition of teeth
K03.1 Abrasion of teeth
K03.2 Erosion of teeth
K03.3 Pathological resorption of teeth
K03.4 Hypercementosis
K03.5 Ankylosis of teeth
K03.6 Deposits [accretions] on teeth
K03.7 Posteruptive color changes of dental hard tissues
K03.81 Cracked tooth
K03.89 Other specified diseases of hard tissues of teeth
K03.9 Disease of hard tissues of teeth, unspecified
K04.01 Reversible pulpitis
K04.02 Irreversible pulpitis
K04.1 Necrosis of pulp
K04.2 Pulp degeneration
K04.3 Abnormal hard tissue formation in pulp
K08.50 Unsatisfactory restoration of tooth, unspecified

K08.51 Open restoration margins of tooth
K08.52 Unrepairable overhanging of dental restorative materials
K08.530 Fractured dental restorative material without loss of material
K08.531 Fractured dental restorative material with loss of material
K08.539 Fractured dental restorative material, unspecified
K08.55 Allergy to existing dental restorative material
K08.56 Poor aesthetic of existing restoration of tooth
K08.59 Other unsatisfactory restoration of tooth
K08.81 Primary occlusal trauma
K08.82 Secondary occlusal trauma

## Relative Value Units/Medicare Edits

| Non-Facility RVU | Work | PE | MP | Total |
|---|---|---|---|---|
| **D6098** | 0.00 | 0.00 | 0.00 | 0.00 |
| **D6099** | 0.00 | 0.00 | 0.00 | 0.00 |
| **Facility RVU** | **Work** | **PE** | **MP** | **Total** |
| **D6098** | 0.00 | 0.00 | 0.00 | 0.00 |
| **D6099** | 0.00 | 0.00 | 0.00 | 0.00 |

| | FUD | Status | MUE | Modifiers | | | | IOM Reference |
|---|---|---|---|---|---|---|---|---|
| **D6098** | N/A | N | - | N/A | N/A | N/A | N/A | None |
| **D6099** | N/A | N | - | N/A | N/A | N/A | N/A | |

* with documentation

## Terms To Know

**fixed partial denture.** Prosthetic replacement of one or more missing teeth attached to the abutment teeth or implant replacements.

**retainer.** In dentistry, portion of a fixed partial denture that attaches an artificial tooth to the abutment tooth or implant.

# D6100

▲ **D6100** surgical removal of implant body

## Explanation

The provider removes a dental implant. Removal steps vary depending upon the type of implant being removed.

## Coding Tips

This is an out-of-sequence code and will not display in numeric order in the CDT manual. Removal steps vary depending on the type of implant. Determine if another, more specific code may be appropriate before assigning this code.

## Reimbursement Tips

The third-party payer may require an x-ray or x-ray report. Coverage of implant procedures varies by payer and by individual contract. Check with payers for specific coverage guidelines.

## Associated CPT Codes

20670 Removal of implant; superficial (eg, buried wire, pin or rod) (separate procedure)
20680 Removal of implant; deep (eg, buried wire, pin, screw, metal band, nail, rod or plate)

## ICD-10-CM Diagnostic Codes

K08.21 Minimal atrophy of the mandible
K08.22 Moderate atrophy of the mandible
K08.23 Severe atrophy of the mandible
K08.24 Minimal atrophy of maxilla
K08.25 Moderate atrophy of the maxilla
K08.26 Severe atrophy of the maxilla
K08.51 Open restoration margins of tooth
K08.52 Unrepairable overhanging of dental restorative materials
K08.530 Fractured dental restorative material without loss of material
K08.531 Fractured dental restorative material with loss of material
K08.54 Contour of existing restoration of tooth biologically incompatible with oral health
K08.55 Allergy to existing dental restorative material
K08.56 Poor aesthetic of existing restoration of tooth
K08.59 Other unsatisfactory restoration of tooth
M27.63 Post-osseointegration mechanical failure of dental implant
Z46.3 Encounter for fitting and adjustment of dental prosthetic device
Z97.2 Presence of dental prosthetic device (complete) (partial)

## Relative Value Units/Medicare Edits

| Non-Facility RVU | Work | PE | MP | Total |
|---|---|---|---|---|
| **D6100** | 3.08 | 2.72 | 0.63 | 6.43 |
| **Facility RVU** | **Work** | **PE** | **MP** | **Total** |
| **D6100** | 3.08 | 2.72 | 0.63 | 6.43 |

| | FUD | Status | MUE | Modifiers | | | | IOM Reference |
|---|---|---|---|---|---|---|---|---|
| **D6100** | N/A | I | - | N/A | N/A | N/A | N/A | None |

* with documentation

# D6101

**D6101** debridement of a peri-implant defect or defects surrounding a single implant, and surface cleaning of the exposed implant surfaces, including flap entry and closure

## Explanation

The provider removes plaque and calculus from a peri-implant. Depending on the depth of the accretions, it may be necessary for the provider to incise the gingiva, forming a flap in which to reach the post. Debridement of the implant restoration is directed that the three components of the implant: the prosthesis, the abutment, and the implant fixture surface. This may be accomplished using a variety of instruments including plastic scaler and curettes, power instruments, Piezo tips, ultrasonic inserts, and Eva tips.

## Coding Tips

This is an out-of-sequence code and will not display in numeric order in the CDT manual. The creation of the flap and its closure is an integral part of the procedure and should not be reported separately. Local anesthesia is generally considered part of this procedure. Necessary radiographs are included and should not be reported separately.

## Reimbursement Tips

Coverage of implant procedures vary by payer and by individual contract. Check with the payer for specific coverage guidelines.

## ICD-10-CM Diagnostic Codes

M27.59 Other periradicular pathology associated with previous endodontic treatment

## Relative Value Units/Medicare Edits

| Non-Facility RVU | Work | PE | MP | Total |
|---|---|---|---|---|
| D6101 | 1.53 | 1.35 | 0.31 | 3.19 |
| **Facility RVU** | **Work** | **PE** | **MP** | **Total** |
| D6101 | 1.53 | 1.35 | 0.31 | 3.19 |

| | FUD | Status | MUE | Modifiers | | | | IOM Reference |
|---|---|---|---|---|---|---|---|---|
| D6101 | N/A | I | - | N/A | N/A | N/A | N/A | None |

* with documentation

## Terms To Know

**debridement.** Removal of dead or contaminated tissue and foreign matter from a wound.

**implant.** Material or device inserted or placed within the body for therapeutic, reconstructive, or diagnostic purposes.

# D6102

**D6102** debridement and osseous contouring of a peri-implant defect or defects surrounding a single implant and includes surface cleaning of the exposed implant surfaces, including flap entry and closure

## Explanation

The provider removes plaque and calculus from a peri-implant and contours the surrounding bony structure. Depending on the depth of the accretions it may be necessary for the provider to incise the gingiva, forming a flap in which to reach the post. Debridement of the implant restoration is directed at the three components of the implant: the prosthesis, the abutment, and the implant fixture surface. This may be accomplished using a variety of instruments including plastic scaler and curettes, power instruments, Piezo tips, ultrasonic inserts, and Eva tips. The surrounding bony structures are contoured using files and/or power instruments.

## Coding Tips

This is an out-of-sequence code and will not display in numeric order in the CDT manual. The creation of the flap and its closure is an integral part of the procedure and should not be reported separately. Local anesthesia is generally considered part of this procedure. Necessary radiographs are included and should not be reported separately.

## Reimbursement Tips

Coverage of implant procedures vary by payer and by individual contract. Check with the payer for specific coverage guidelines.

## ICD-10-CM Diagnostic Codes

M27.59 Other periradicular pathology associated with previous endodontic treatment

M27.61 Osseointegration failure of dental implant

M27.62 Post-osseointegration biological failure of dental implant

M27.63 Post-osseointegration mechanical failure of dental implant

M27.69 Other endosseous dental implant failure

## Relative Value Units/Medicare Edits

| Non-Facility RVU | Work | PE | MP | Total |
|---|---|---|---|---|
| D6102 | 2.68 | 2.36 | 0.55 | 5.59 |
| **Facility RVU** | **Work** | **PE** | **MP** | **Total** |
| D6102 | 2.68 | 2.36 | 0.55 | 5.59 |

| | FUD | Status | MUE | Modifiers | | | | IOM Reference |
|---|---|---|---|---|---|---|---|---|
| D6102 | N/A | I | - | N/A | N/A | N/A | N/A | None |

* with documentation

## Terms To Know

**debridement.** Removal of dead or contaminated tissue and foreign matter from a wound.

**dental implant.** Surgical implantation of a device within the mandible or maxilla for dental replacement.

**osseous.** Related to, consisting of, or resembling bone.

# D6103-D6104

**D6103** bone graft for repair of peri-implant defect - does not include flap entry and closure

*Placement of a barrier membrane or biologic materials to aid in osseous regeneration, are reported separately.*

**D6104** bone graft at time of implant placement

*Placement of a barrier membrane, or biologic materials to aid in osseous regeneration are reported separately.*

## Explanation

The provider performs a bone graft to repair a defect near an implant to stabilize or increase the level of the bone or to fill structural defects. The area is exposed; the method used is dependent upon the area where the graft will be inserted. The physician dissects tissues away and the site is exposed. The graft is placed on the site and contoured until desired shape is achieved. The graft is secured and the site is closed.

## Coding Tips

These codes are out-of-sequence codes and will not display in numeric order in the CDT book. When flap entry is performed, this may be reported separately (D4240–D4245). When performed, the placement of a barrier membrane or other biologic material to aid in soft and osseous tissue regeneration may be reported separately (D4265–D4267).

## ICD-10-CM Diagnostic Codes

The application of this code is too broad to adequately present ICD-10-CM diagnostic code links here. Refer to your ICD-10-CM book.

## Relative Value Units/Medicare Edits

| Non-Facility RVU | Work | PE | MP | Total |
|---|---|---|---|---|
| D6103 | 1.79 | 1.58 | 0.37 | 3.74 |
| D6104 | 2.41 | 2.13 | 0.50 | 5.04 |
| **Facility RVU** | **Work** | **PE** | **MP** | **Total** |
| D6103 | 1.79 | 1.58 | 0.37 | 3.74 |
| D6104 | 2.41 | 2.13 | 0.50 | 5.04 |

| | FUD | Status | MUE | Modifiers | | | | IOM Reference |
|---|---|---|---|---|---|---|---|---|
| D6103 | N/A | I | - | N/A | N/A | N/A | N/A | None |
| D6104 | N/A | I | - | N/A | N/A | N/A | N/A | |

* with documentation

## Terms To Know

**bone graft.** Bone that is removed from one part of the body and placed into another bone site without direct re-establishment of blood supply.

**implant.** Material or device inserted or placed within the body for therapeutic, reconstructive, or diagnostic purposes.

# D6110-D6111

**D6110** implant /abutment supported removable denture for edentulous arch - maxillary

**D6111** implant /abutment supported removable denture for edentulous arch - mandibular

## Explanation

The dentist provides an implant/abutment supported removable denture for the upper (D6110) or lower jaw (D6111) that is completely toothless. Following the drawing up of a dental plan and preparation for the denture, including placement of the abutments and/or implants (see codes D6010-D6050) previously performed, the patient receives the removable denture. The denture is snapped into place and the fit and comfort of the denture is determined. Minor adjustments may be made if required. The patient is instructed as to the removal and care of the denture.

## Coding Tips

To report implant/abutment-supported removable denture for a partially edentulous arch, see D6112–D6113. To report implant/abutment-supported fixed denture for completely edentulous arch, see D6114–D6115.

## ICD-10-CM Diagnostic Codes

| | |
|---|---|
| K08.111 | Complete loss of teeth due to trauma, class I |
| K08.112 | Complete loss of teeth due to trauma, class II |
| K08.113 | Complete loss of teeth due to trauma, class III |
| K08.114 | Complete loss of teeth due to trauma, class IV |
| K08.121 | Complete loss of teeth due to periodontal diseases, class I |
| K08.122 | Complete loss of teeth due to periodontal diseases, class II |
| K08.123 | Complete loss of teeth due to periodontal diseases, class III |
| K08.124 | Complete loss of teeth due to periodontal diseases, class IV |
| K08.131 | Complete loss of teeth due to caries, class I |
| K08.132 | Complete loss of teeth due to caries, class II |
| K08.133 | Complete loss of teeth due to caries, class III |
| K08.134 | Complete loss of teeth due to caries, class IV |
| K08.191 | Complete loss of teeth due to other specified cause, class I |
| K08.192 | Complete loss of teeth due to other specified cause, class II |
| K08.193 | Complete loss of teeth due to other specified cause, class III |
| K08.194 | Complete loss of teeth due to other specified cause, class IV |

## Relative Value Units/Medicare Edits

| Non-Facility RVU | Work | PE | MP | Total |
|---|---|---|---|---|
| D6110 | 9.01 | 7.95 | 1.85 | 18.81 |
| D6111 | 9.01 | 7.95 | 1.85 | 18.81 |
| **Facility RVU** | **Work** | **PE** | **MP** | **Total** |
| D6110 | 9.01 | 7.95 | 1.85 | 18.81 |
| D6111 | 9.01 | 7.95 | 1.85 | 18.81 |

| | FUD | Status | MUE | Modifiers | | | | IOM Reference |
|---|---|---|---|---|---|---|---|---|
| D6110 | N/A | N | - | N/A | N/A | N/A | N/A | None |
| D6111 | N/A | N | - | N/A | N/A | N/A | N/A | |

* with documentation

## Terms To Know

**abutment.** Tooth or implant fixture supporting a prosthesis.

# D6112-D6113

**D6112** implant /abutment supported removable denture for partially edentulous arch - maxillary

**D6113** implant /abutment supported removable denture for partially edentulous arch - mandibular

## Explanation

The dentist provides an implant/abutment-supported removable denture for the upper (D6112) or lower jaw (D6113) that replaces missing teeth of a jaw that is only partially edentulous. Following the drawing up of a dental plan and preparation for the denture, including necessary periodontal work, root canal treatment, and placement of the abutments and/or implants (see codes D6010-D6050) previously performed, the patient receives the removable denture. The denture is snapped into place and the fit and comfort of the denture is determined. Minor adjustments may be made if required. The patient is instructed as to the removal and care of the denture.

## Coding Tips

To report implant/abutment-supported removable denture for a completely edentulous arch, see D6110–D6111. To report implant/abutment-supported fixed denture for partially edentulous arch, see D6116–D6117.

## ICD-10-CM Diagnostic Codes

| | |
|---|---|
| K08.411 | Partial loss of teeth due to trauma, class I |
| K08.412 | Partial loss of teeth due to trauma, class II |
| K08.413 | Partial loss of teeth due to trauma, class III |
| K08.414 | Partial loss of teeth due to trauma, class IV |
| K08.421 | Partial loss of teeth due to periodontal diseases, class I |
| K08.422 | Partial loss of teeth due to periodontal diseases, class II |
| K08.423 | Partial loss of teeth due to periodontal diseases, class III |
| K08.424 | Partial loss of teeth due to periodontal diseases, class IV |
| K08.431 | Partial loss of teeth due to caries, class I |
| K08.432 | Partial loss of teeth due to caries, class II |
| K08.433 | Partial loss of teeth due to caries, class III |
| K08.434 | Partial loss of teeth due to caries, class IV |
| K08.491 | Partial loss of teeth due to other specified cause, class I |
| K08.492 | Partial loss of teeth due to other specified cause, class II |
| K08.493 | Partial loss of teeth due to other specified cause, class III |
| K08.494 | Partial loss of teeth due to other specified cause, class IV |

## Relative Value Units/Medicare Edits

| Non-Facility RVU | Work | PE | MP | Total |
|---|---|---|---|---|
| D6112 | 8.93 | 7.89 | 1.84 | 18.66 |
| D6113 | 8.93 | 7.89 | 1.84 | 18.66 |
| **Facility RVU** | **Work** | **PE** | **MP** | **Total** |
| D6112 | 8.93 | 7.89 | 1.84 | 18.66 |
| D6113 | 8.93 | 7.89 | 1.84 | 18.66 |

| | FUD | Status | MUE | Modifiers | | | | IOM Reference |
|---|---|---|---|---|---|---|---|---|
| D6112 | N/A | N | - | N/A | N/A | N/A | N/A | None |
| D6113 | N/A | N | - | N/A | N/A | N/A | N/A | |

* with documentation

## Terms To Know

**abutment.** Tooth or implant fixture supporting a prosthesis.

# D6114-D6115

**D6114** implant /abutment supported fixed denture for edentulous arch - maxillary

**D6115** implant /abutment supported fixed denture for edentulous arch - mandibular

## Explanation

The dentist provides an implant/abutment-supported fixed denture for the upper (D6114) or lower jaw (D6115) that is completely toothless. Following the drawing up of a dental plan and preparation for the denture, including the placement of the abutments and/or implants (see codes D6010-D6050) and supporting structures (D6052-D6055) previously performed, the patient receives the fixed denture. The fit and comfort of the denture is determined and minor adjustments may be made if required. The denture is fastened using screws (screw-retained) or clips (bar-retained). The patient is instructed as to the care of the denture.

## Coding Tips

To report implant/abutment-supported removable denture for a completely edentulous arch, see D6110–D6111. To report implant/abutment-supported fixed denture for partially edentulous arch, see D6116–D6117.

## ICD-10-CM Diagnostic Codes

| | |
|---|---|
| K08.111 | Complete loss of teeth due to trauma, class I |
| K08.112 | Complete loss of teeth due to trauma, class II |
| K08.113 | Complete loss of teeth due to trauma, class III |
| K08.114 | Complete loss of teeth due to trauma, class IV |
| K08.121 | Complete loss of teeth due to periodontal diseases, class I |
| K08.122 | Complete loss of teeth due to periodontal diseases, class II |
| K08.123 | Complete loss of teeth due to periodontal diseases, class III |
| K08.124 | Complete loss of teeth due to periodontal diseases, class IV |
| K08.131 | Complete loss of teeth due to caries, class I |
| K08.132 | Complete loss of teeth due to caries, class II |
| K08.133 | Complete loss of teeth due to caries, class III |
| K08.134 | Complete loss of teeth due to caries, class IV |
| K08.191 | Complete loss of teeth due to other specified cause, class I |
| K08.192 | Complete loss of teeth due to other specified cause, class II |
| K08.193 | Complete loss of teeth due to other specified cause, class III |
| K08.194 | Complete loss of teeth due to other specified cause, class IV |

## Relative Value Units/Medicare Edits

| Non-Facility RVU | Work | PE | MP | Total |
|---|---|---|---|---|
| D6114 | 15.67 | 13.83 | 3.23 | 32.73 |
| D6115 | 15.67 | 13.83 | 3.23 | 32.73 |
| **Facility RVU** | **Work** | **PE** | **MP** | **Total** |
| D6114 | 15.67 | 13.83 | 3.23 | 32.73 |
| D6115 | 15.67 | 13.83 | 3.23 | 32.73 |

| | FUD | Status | MUE | Modifiers | | | | IOM Reference |
|---|---|---|---|---|---|---|---|---|
| D6114 | N/A | N | - | N/A | N/A | N/A | N/A | None |
| D6115 | N/A | N | - | N/A | N/A | N/A | N/A | |

* with documentation

## Terms To Know

**abutment.** Tooth or implant fixture supporting a prosthesis.

# D6116-D6117

**D6116** implant /abutment supported fixed denture for partially edentulous arch - maxillary

**D6117** implant /abutment supported fixed denture for partially edentulous arch - mandibular

## Explanation

The dentist provides an implant/abutment-supported fixed denture for the upper (D6116) or lower jaw (D6117) replacing missing teeth from a partially edentulous jaw. Following the drawing up of a dental plan and preparation for the denture, including the placement of the abutments and/or implants (see codes D6010-D6050) and supporting structures (D6052-D6055) previously performed, the patient receives the fixed denture. The fit and comfort of the denture is determined and minor adjustments may be made if required. The denture is fastened using screws (screw-retained) or clips (bar-retained). The patient is instructed as to the care of the denture.

## Coding Tips

To report implant/abutment-supported removable denture for a partially edentulous arch, see D6112–D6113. To report implant/abutment-supported fixed denture for completely edentulous arch, see D6114–D6115.

## ICD-10-CM Diagnostic Codes

K08.411 Partial loss of teeth due to trauma, class I
K08.412 Partial loss of teeth due to trauma, class II
K08.413 Partial loss of teeth due to trauma, class III
K08.414 Partial loss of teeth due to trauma, class IV
K08.421 Partial loss of teeth due to periodontal diseases, class I
K08.422 Partial loss of teeth due to periodontal diseases, class II
K08.423 Partial loss of teeth due to periodontal diseases, class III
K08.424 Partial loss of teeth due to periodontal diseases, class IV
K08.431 Partial loss of teeth due to caries, class I
K08.432 Partial loss of teeth due to caries, class II
K08.433 Partial loss of teeth due to caries, class III
K08.434 Partial loss of teeth due to caries, class IV
K08.491 Partial loss of teeth due to other specified cause, class I
K08.492 Partial loss of teeth due to other specified cause, class II
K08.493 Partial loss of teeth due to other specified cause, class III
K08.494 Partial loss of teeth due to other specified cause, class IV

## Relative Value Units/Medicare Edits

| Non-Facility RVU | Work | PE | MP | Total |
|---|---|---|---|---|
| **D6116** | 12.02 | 10.61 | 2.47 | 25.10 |
| **D6117** | 12.02 | 10.61 | 2.47 | 25.10 |
| **Facility RVU** | **Work** | **PE** | **MP** | **Total** |
| **D6116** | 12.02 | 10.61 | 2.47 | 25.10 |
| **D6117** | 12.02 | 10.61 | 2.47 | 25.10 |

| | FUD | Status | MUE | Modifiers | | | | IOM Reference |
|---|---|---|---|---|---|---|---|---|
| **D6116** | N/A | N | - | N/A | N/A | N/A | N/A | None |
| **D6117** | N/A | N | - | N/A | N/A | N/A | N/A | |

* with documentation

## Terms To Know

**abutment.** Tooth or implant fixture supporting a prosthesis.

# D6118-D6119

**D6118** implant/abutment supported interim fixed denture for edentulous arch - mandibular

*Used when a period of healing is necessary prior to fabrication and placement of a permanent prosthetic.*

**D6119** implant/abutment supported interim fixed denture for edentulous arch - maxillary

*Used when a period of healing is necessary prior to fabrication and placement of a permanent prosthetic.*

## Explanation

The dentist provides an interim implant/abutment supported removable denture for the upper (D6118) or lower jaw (D6619) that is completely toothless during a period of healing and prior to the fabrication and placement of a permanent prosthetic. Following the drawing up of a dental plan and preparation for the denture, including placement of the abutments and/or implants (see codes D6010–D6050), the patient receives the removable denture. The interim denture is snapped into place and the fit and comfort of the denture is determined. Minor adjustments may be made if required.

## Coding Tips

To report the placement of a permanent implant/abutment supported fixed denture for an edentulous arch, see D6116–D6117.

## ICD-10-CM Diagnostic Codes

K08.111 Complete loss of teeth due to trauma, class I
K08.112 Complete loss of teeth due to trauma, class II
K08.113 Complete loss of teeth due to trauma, class III
K08.114 Complete loss of teeth due to trauma, class IV
K08.121 Complete loss of teeth due to periodontal diseases, class I
K08.122 Complete loss of teeth due to periodontal diseases, class II
K08.123 Complete loss of teeth due to periodontal diseases, class III
K08.124 Complete loss of teeth due to periodontal diseases, class IV
K08.131 Complete loss of teeth due to caries, class I
K08.132 Complete loss of teeth due to caries, class II
K08.133 Complete loss of teeth due to caries, class III
K08.134 Complete loss of teeth due to caries, class IV
K08.191 Complete loss of teeth due to other specified cause, class I
K08.192 Complete loss of teeth due to other specified cause, class II
K08.193 Complete loss of teeth due to other specified cause, class III
K08.194 Complete loss of teeth due to other specified cause, class IV

## Relative Value Units/Medicare Edits

| Non-Facility RVU | Work | PE | MP | Total |
|---|---|---|---|---|
| **D6118** | 0.00 | 0.00 | 0.00 | 0.00 |
| **D6119** | 0.00 | 0.00 | 0.00 | 0.00 |
| **Facility RVU** | **Work** | **PE** | **MP** | **Total** |
| **D6118** | 0.00 | 0.00 | 0.00 | 0.00 |
| **D6119** | 0.00 | 0.00 | 0.00 | 0.00 |

| | FUD | Status | MUE | Modifiers | | | | IOM Reference |
|---|---|---|---|---|---|---|---|---|
| **D6118** | N/A | N | - | N/A | N/A | N/A | N/A | None |
| **D6119** | N/A | N | - | N/A | N/A | N/A | N/A | |

* with documentation

# D6120-D6123

**D6120** implant supported retainer - porcelain fused to titanium and titanium alloys

*A metal-ceramic retainer for a fixed partial denture that gains retention, support, and stability from an implant.*

**D6121** implant supported retainer for metal FPD - predominantly base alloys

*A metal retainer for a fixed partial denture that gains retention, support, and stability from an implant.*

**D6122** implant supported retainer for metal FPD - noble alloys

*A metal retainer for a fixed partial denture that gains retention, support, and stability from an implant.*

**D6123** implant supported retainer for metal FPD - titanium and titanium alloys

*A metal retainer for a fixed partial denture that gains retention, support, and stability from an implant.*

## Explanation

The provider creates a retainer for a fixed partial denture (FPD), replacing missing teeth from a partially edentulous jaw. Following the development of a dental plan and preparation of the partial denture, including the previously placed implant(s), the retainer is placed. The retainer is supported, stabilized by the implant. Correct code assignment is dependent upon the materials used. For porcelain fused to titanium and titanium alloy, report D6120; predominately base alloys, report D6121; noble alloys, report D6122; titanium and titanium alloys, see D6123.

## Coding Tips

To report implant- or abutment-supported, removable denture for a partially edentulous arch, see D6112–D6113. To report implant/abutment-supported fixed denture for partially edentulous arch, see D6116–D6117.

## Documentation Tips

Documentation should indicate the location and number of missing teeth.

## Reimbursement Tips

Coverage guidelines vary by payer and by patient contract. Patients are often responsible for copayments or may reach contract limitations. Check with the payer to determine coverage policies and patient responsibility.

## ICD-10-CM Diagnostic Codes

| | |
|---|---|
| K08.411 | Partial loss of teeth due to trauma, class I |
| K08.412 | Partial loss of teeth due to trauma, class II |
| K08.413 | Partial loss of teeth due to trauma, class III |
| K08.414 | Partial loss of teeth due to trauma, class IV |
| K08.421 | Partial loss of teeth due to periodontal diseases, class I |
| K08.422 | Partial loss of teeth due to periodontal diseases, class II |
| K08.423 | Partial loss of teeth due to periodontal diseases, class III |
| K08.424 | Partial loss of teeth due to periodontal diseases, class IV |
| K08.431 | Partial loss of teeth due to caries, class I |
| K08.432 | Partial loss of teeth due to caries, class II |
| K08.433 | Partial loss of teeth due to caries, class III |
| K08.434 | Partial loss of teeth due to caries, class IV |
| K08.491 | Partial loss of teeth due to other specified cause, class I |
| K08.492 | Partial loss of teeth due to other specified cause, class II |
| K08.493 | Partial loss of teeth due to other specified cause, class III |
| K08.494 | Partial loss of teeth due to other specified cause, class IV |

## Relative Value Units/Medicare Edits

| Non-Facility RVU | Work | PE | MP | Total |
|---|---|---|---|---|
| D6120 | 0.00 | 0.00 | 0.00 | 0.00 |
| D6121 | 0.00 | 0.00 | 0.00 | 0.00 |
| D6122 | 0.00 | 0.00 | 0.00 | 0.00 |
| D6123 | 0.00 | 0.00 | 0.00 | 0.00 |
| **Facility RVU** | **Work** | **PE** | **MP** | **Total** |
| D6120 | 0.00 | 0.00 | 0.00 | 0.00 |
| D6121 | 0.00 | 0.00 | 0.00 | 0.00 |
| D6122 | 0.00 | 0.00 | 0.00 | 0.00 |
| D6123 | 0.00 | 0.00 | 0.00 | 0.00 |

| | FUD | Status | MUE | Modifiers | | | | IOM Reference |
|---|---|---|---|---|---|---|---|---|
| D6120 | N/A | N | - | N/A | N/A | N/A | N/A | None |
| D6121 | N/A | N | - | N/A | N/A | N/A | N/A | |
| D6122 | N/A | N | - | N/A | N/A | N/A | N/A | |
| D6123 | N/A | N | - | N/A | N/A | N/A | N/A | |

* with documentation

## Terms To Know

**edentulous.** Loss of all or some of the natural teeth.

**implant.** Material or device inserted or placed within the body for therapeutic, reconstructive, or diagnostic purposes.

**retainer.** In dentistry, portion of a fixed partial denture that attaches an artificial tooth to the abutment tooth or implant.

Dental - Implant Services

# D6190

**D6190** radiographic/surgical implant index, by report

*An appliance, designed to relate osteotomy or fixture position to existing anatomic structures, to be utilized during radiographic exposure for treatment planning and/or during osteotomy creation for fixture installation.*

## Explanation

A device that is used to indicate osteotomy or fixture position to other anatomical structures, which is used during x-ray procedures to determine a treatment plan or is used during osteotomy creation.

## Coding Tips

This is an out-of-sequence code and will not display in numeric order in the CDT manual.

## ICD-10-CM Diagnostic Codes

K08.101 Complete loss of teeth, unspecified cause, class I
K08.102 Complete loss of teeth, unspecified cause, class II
K08.103 Complete loss of teeth, unspecified cause, class III
K08.104 Complete loss of teeth, unspecified cause, class IV
K08.109 Complete loss of teeth, unspecified cause, unspecified class
K08.111 Complete loss of teeth due to trauma, class I
K08.112 Complete loss of teeth due to trauma, class II
K08.113 Complete loss of teeth due to trauma, class III
K08.114 Complete loss of teeth due to trauma, class IV
K08.119 Complete loss of teeth due to trauma, unspecified class
K08.121 Complete loss of teeth due to periodontal diseases, class I
K08.122 Complete loss of teeth due to periodontal diseases, class II
K08.123 Complete loss of teeth due to periodontal diseases, class III
K08.124 Complete loss of teeth due to periodontal diseases, class IV
K08.129 Complete loss of teeth due to periodontal diseases, unspecified class
K08.131 Complete loss of teeth due to caries, class I
K08.132 Complete loss of teeth due to caries, class II
K08.133 Complete loss of teeth due to caries, class III
K08.134 Complete loss of teeth due to caries, class IV
K08.139 Complete loss of teeth due to caries, unspecified class
K08.191 Complete loss of teeth due to other specified cause, class I
K08.192 Complete loss of teeth due to other specified cause, class II
K08.193 Complete loss of teeth due to other specified cause, class III
K08.194 Complete loss of teeth due to other specified cause, class IV
K08.199 Complete loss of teeth due to other specified cause, unspecified class
K08.20 Unspecified atrophy of edentulous alveolar ridge
K08.21 Minimal atrophy of the mandible
K08.22 Moderate atrophy of the mandible
K08.23 Severe atrophy of the mandible
K08.24 Minimal atrophy of maxilla
K08.25 Moderate atrophy of the maxilla
K08.26 Severe atrophy of the maxilla
K08.3 Retained dental root
K08.401 Partial loss of teeth, unspecified cause, class I
K08.402 Partial loss of teeth, unspecified cause, class II
K08.403 Partial loss of teeth, unspecified cause, class III
K08.404 Partial loss of teeth, unspecified cause, class IV
K08.409 Partial loss of teeth, unspecified cause, unspecified class
K08.411 Partial loss of teeth due to trauma, class I
K08.412 Partial loss of teeth due to trauma, class II
K08.413 Partial loss of teeth due to trauma, class III
K08.414 Partial loss of teeth due to trauma, class IV
K08.419 Partial loss of teeth due to trauma, unspecified class
K08.421 Partial loss of teeth due to periodontal diseases, class I
K08.422 Partial loss of teeth due to periodontal diseases, class II
K08.423 Partial loss of teeth due to periodontal diseases, class III
K08.424 Partial loss of teeth due to periodontal diseases, class IV
K08.429 Partial loss of teeth due to periodontal diseases, unspecified class
K08.431 Partial loss of teeth due to caries, class I
K08.432 Partial loss of teeth due to caries, class II
K08.433 Partial loss of teeth due to caries, class III
K08.434 Partial loss of teeth due to caries, class IV
K08.439 Partial loss of teeth due to caries, unspecified class
K08.491 Partial loss of teeth due to other specified cause, class I
K08.492 Partial loss of teeth due to other specified cause, class II
K08.493 Partial loss of teeth due to other specified cause, class III
K08.494 Partial loss of teeth due to other specified cause, class IV
K08.499 Partial loss of teeth due to other specified cause, unspecified class

## Relative Value Units/Medicare Edits

| Non-Facility RVU | Work | PE | MP | Total |
|---|---|---|---|---|
| **D6190** | 1.31 | 1.15 | 0.27 | 2.73 |
| **Facility RVU** | **Work** | **PE** | **MP** | **Total** |
| **D6190** | 1.31 | 1.15 | 0.27 | 2.73 |

| | FUD | Status | MUE | Modifiers | | | | IOM Reference |
|---|---|---|---|---|---|---|---|---|
| **D6190** | N/A | N | - | N/A | N/A | N/A | N/A | None |

* with documentation

## Terms To Know

**denture.** Manmade substitution of natural teeth and neighboring structures.

**edentulous.** Loss of all or some of the natural teeth.

**implant.** Material or device inserted or placed within the body for therapeutic, reconstructive, or diagnostic purposes.

**osseous.** Related to, consisting of, or resembling bone.

# D6191-D6192

**D6191** semi-precision abutment - placement

*This procedure is the initial placement, or replacement, of a semi-precision abutment on the implant body.*

**D6192** semi-precision attachment - placement

*This procedure involves the luting of the initial, or replacement, semi-precision attachment to the removable prosthesis.*

## Explanation

The dental health care provider fabricates a semi-precision abutment or attachment by direct casting of plastiwax or refractory patterns. The semi-precision abutment or attachment is a specially shaped extension of the partial denture that fits into or onto a corresponding receiving area or projection on a natural tooth that has been crowned. The components fit snugly and consist of a semi-rigid metal to other surface interface, which may also be metal or some other resilient material such as nylon. Report D6191 for abutment placement and D6192 for attachment placement.

## Coding Tips

To report a connecting bar, see D6055. To report a prefabricated abutment, see D6056. To report a custom fabricated abutment, see D6057. An interim abutment is reported using D6051.

## ICD-10-CM Diagnostic Codes

| | |
|---|---|
| K08.401 | Partial loss of teeth, unspecified cause, class I |
| K08.402 | Partial loss of teeth, unspecified cause, class II |
| K08.403 | Partial loss of teeth, unspecified cause, class III |
| K08.404 | Partial loss of teeth, unspecified cause, class IV |
| K08.409 | Partial loss of teeth, unspecified cause, unspecified class |
| K08.411 | Partial loss of teeth due to trauma, class I |
| K08.412 | Partial loss of teeth due to trauma, class II |
| K08.413 | Partial loss of teeth due to trauma, class III |
| K08.414 | Partial loss of teeth due to trauma, class IV |
| K08.419 | Partial loss of teeth due to trauma, unspecified class |
| K08.421 | Partial loss of teeth due to periodontal diseases, class I |
| K08.422 | Partial loss of teeth due to periodontal diseases, class II |
| K08.423 | Partial loss of teeth due to periodontal diseases, class III |
| K08.424 | Partial loss of teeth due to periodontal diseases, class IV |
| K08.429 | Partial loss of teeth due to periodontal diseases, unspecified class |
| K08.431 | Partial loss of teeth due to caries, class I |
| K08.432 | Partial loss of teeth due to caries, class II |
| K08.433 | Partial loss of teeth due to caries, class III |
| K08.434 | Partial loss of teeth due to caries, class IV |
| K08.439 | Partial loss of teeth due to caries, unspecified class |
| K08.491 | Partial loss of teeth due to other specified cause, class I |
| K08.492 | Partial loss of teeth due to other specified cause, class II |
| K08.493 | Partial loss of teeth due to other specified cause, class III |
| K08.494 | Partial loss of teeth due to other specified cause, class IV |
| K08.499 | Partial loss of teeth due to other specified cause, unspecified class |

## Relative Value Units/Medicare Edits

| Non-Facility RVU | Work | PE | MP | Total |
|---|---|---|---|---|
| D6191 | | | | |
| D6192 | | | | |
| **Facility RVU** | **Work** | **PE** | **MP** | **Total** |
| D6191 | | | | |
| D6192 | | | | |

| | FUD | Status | MUE | Modifiers | | | | IOM Reference |
|---|---|---|---|---|---|---|---|---|
| D6191 | N/A | | - | N/A | N/A | N/A | N/A | |
| D6192 | N/A | | - | N/A | N/A | N/A | N/A | |

* with documentation

## Terms To Know

**abutment.** Tooth or implant fixture supporting a prosthesis.

**dental attachment.** Two or more components connecting a prosthesis to a tooth, tooth root, or implant, often incorporated into the crown of a tooth.

**implant.** Material or device inserted or placed within the body for therapeutic, reconstructive, or diagnostic purposes.

**prosthesis.** Man-made substitute for a missing body part.

**prosthodontics.** Branch of dentistry that specializes in the replacement of missing or damaged teeth.

# D6194-D6195

**D6194** abutment supported retainer crown for FPD- titanium and titanium alloys

*A retainer for a fixed partial denture that gains retention, support and stability from an abutment on an implant.*

**D6195** abutment supported retainer - porcelain fused to titanium and titanium alloys

*A metal-ceramic retainer for a fixed partial denture that gains retention, support, and stability from an abutment on an implant.*

## Explanation

Individual crowns may serve as retainers on abutment teeth when replacing a missing tooth or teeth. The prostheses may be fabricated from composite or acrylic resin, to resin bonded to metal, complete metal, all-ceramic materials, and metal-ceramic. The decision depends on the materials available, preference, and economics. Code D6194 reports a titanium or titanium alloy retainer crown. Code D6195 reports porcelain fused to titanium and titanium alloys.

## Coding Tips

These codes are out-of-sequence codes and will not display in numeric order in the CDT book. Local anesthesia is generally considered part of restorative procedures.

## Reimbursement Tips

The third-party payer may require an x-ray or x-ray report. Coverage of implant procedures varies by payer and by individual contract. Check with payers for specific coverage guidelines.

## ICD-10-CM Diagnostic Codes

K08.411 Partial loss of teeth due to trauma, class I
K08.412 Partial loss of teeth due to trauma, class II
K08.413 Partial loss of teeth due to trauma, class III
K08.414 Partial loss of teeth due to trauma, class IV
K08.421 Partial loss of teeth due to periodontal diseases, class I
K08.422 Partial loss of teeth due to periodontal diseases, class II
K08.423 Partial loss of teeth due to periodontal diseases, class III
K08.424 Partial loss of teeth due to periodontal diseases, class IV
K08.431 Partial loss of teeth due to caries, class I
K08.432 Partial loss of teeth due to caries, class II
K08.433 Partial loss of teeth due to caries, class III
K08.434 Partial loss of teeth due to caries, class IV
K08.491 Partial loss of teeth due to other specified cause, class I
K08.492 Partial loss of teeth due to other specified cause, class II
K08.493 Partial loss of teeth due to other specified cause, class III
K08.494 Partial loss of teeth due to other specified cause, class IV

## Relative Value Units/Medicare Edits

| Non-Facility RVU | Work | PE | MP | Total |
|---|---|---|---|---|
| **D6194** | 6.18 | 5.45 | 1.27 | 12.90 |
| **D6195** | 5.31 | 4.68 | 1.09 | 11.08 |
| **Facility RVU** | **Work** | **PE** | **MP** | **Total** |
| **D6194** | 6.18 | 5.45 | 1.27 | 12.90 |
| **D6195** | 5.31 | 4.68 | 1.09 | 11.08 |

| | FUD | Status | MUE | Modifiers | | | | IOM Reference |
|---|---|---|---|---|---|---|---|---|
| **D6194** | N/A | N | - | N/A | N/A | N/A | N/A | None |
| **D6195** | N/A | N | - | N/A | N/A | N/A | N/A | |

* with documentation

## Terms To Know

**abutment.** Tooth or implant fixture supporting a prosthesis.

**crown.** Dental restoration that completely caps or encircles a tooth or dental implant.

**retainer.** In dentistry, portion of a fixed partial denture that attaches an artificial tooth to the abutment tooth or implant.

Dental - Implant Services

# D6198

- **D6198** remove interim implant component

  *Removal of implant component (e.g., interim abutment; provisional implant crown) originally placed for a specific clinical purpose and period of time determined by the dentist.*

## Explanation

A temporary abutment is an abutment used for the fabrication of an interim restoration. Temporary abutments are either affixed to the implants intraorally or to a cast made from an implant impression. Temporary abutments are an essential component in restorative dentistry procedures. They allow the tissue around the implant to heal while also providing an attachment point for the crown, bridge, or other dental restoration. Following implant osseointegration with the surrounding bone, the temporary abutment may be removed for a permanent abutment to take its place. A provisional implant crown is placed to allow healing for an extended time prior to final restoration. The temporary crown is positioned and inserted over the abutments either intraorally or on the cast. Code D6198 reports the removal of the interim implant component (e.g., interim abutment, provisional implant crown). Removal of an interim abutment may require incision of the gingival tissue.

## Coding Tips

For initial placement of the interim abutment, see D6051. For initial placement of the interim crown, see D6085. For replacement of an implant/abutment, see D6091. For removal of the surgical implant body, see D6100.

## ICD-10-CM Diagnostic Codes

| | |
|---|---|
| K08.401 | Partial loss of teeth, unspecified cause, class I |
| K08.402 | Partial loss of teeth, unspecified cause, class II |
| K08.403 | Partial loss of teeth, unspecified cause, class III |
| K08.404 | Partial loss of teeth, unspecified cause, class IV |
| K08.409 | Partial loss of teeth, unspecified cause, unspecified class |
| K08.411 | Partial loss of teeth due to trauma, class I |
| K08.412 | Partial loss of teeth due to trauma, class II |
| K08.413 | Partial loss of teeth due to trauma, class III |
| K08.414 | Partial loss of teeth due to trauma, class IV |
| K08.419 | Partial loss of teeth due to trauma, unspecified class |
| K08.421 | Partial loss of teeth due to periodontal diseases, class I |
| K08.422 | Partial loss of teeth due to periodontal diseases, class II |
| K08.423 | Partial loss of teeth due to periodontal diseases, class III |
| K08.424 | Partial loss of teeth due to periodontal diseases, class IV |
| K08.429 | Partial loss of teeth due to periodontal diseases, unspecified class |
| K08.431 | Partial loss of teeth due to caries, class I |
| K08.432 | Partial loss of teeth due to caries, class II |
| K08.433 | Partial loss of teeth due to caries, class III |
| K08.434 | Partial loss of teeth due to caries, class IV |
| K08.439 | Partial loss of teeth due to caries, unspecified class |
| K08.491 | Partial loss of teeth due to other specified cause, class I |
| K08.492 | Partial loss of teeth due to other specified cause, class II |
| K08.493 | Partial loss of teeth due to other specified cause, class III |
| K08.494 | Partial loss of teeth due to other specified cause, class IV |
| K08.499 | Partial loss of teeth due to other specified cause, unspecified class |

## Relative Value Units/Medicare Edits

| Non-Facility RVU | Work | PE | MP | Total |
|---|---|---|---|---|
| D6198 | | | | |

| Facility RVU | Work | PE | MP | Total |
|---|---|---|---|---|
| D6198 | | | | |

| | FUD | Status | MUE | Modifiers | | | | IOM Reference |
|---|---|---|---|---|---|---|---|---|
| D6198 | N/A | | - | N/A | N/A | N/A | N/A | |

* with documentation

## Terms To Know

**abutment.** Tooth or implant fixture supporting a prosthesis.

**abutment crown.** Artificial tooth cap for the retention and/or support of a dental prosthesis.

**crown.** Dental restoration that completely caps or encircles a tooth or dental implant.

# D6205-D6214

**D6205** pontic - indirect resin based composite

*Not to be used as a temporary or provisional prosthesis.*

**D6210** pontic - cast high noble metal
**D6211** pontic - cast predominantly base metal
**D6212** pontic - cast noble metal
**D6214** pontic - titanium and titanium alloys

## Explanation

A pontic is a bridge made to fill an edentulous space in the mouth with substitute or false teeth in between abutments, or caps for anchoring onto the neighboring teeth on either side of the space. This prosthetic is made all in one continuous piece. First the dentist makes an impression of the space and neighboring teeth for the lab. The impression is filled with plaster and a working mold is made. The pontic teeth are designed and then created in wax along with the model of the anchoring caps and the connection of each unit to the other, for a one piece, aesthetically correct bridge. When the wax model is complete, it is set in high-density plaster along with a channel leading to it and the wax is burned out. For cast metal pontics, the three-dimensional model is then filled with molten metal from a little reservoir by being spun on the arm of a centrifuge. If the patient does not prefer the metal appearance, an opaque layer is applied. The dentist then tries in the fixed partial denture pontic piece, checking all fitting points and cements the anchoring caps onto the neighboring teeth. Report D6205 for a pontic cast of a resin-based composite, including fiber-or ceramic-reinforced polymer compounds. Report D6210 for a pontic cast from high noble metal, containing at least 60 percent gold, platinum, or palladium; D6211 for a predominantly base metal, an alloy of less than 25 percent noble metals; D6212 for noble metal of a minimum of 25 percent or greater; and D6214 for titanium and titanium alloys. A prosthetic with one substitute tooth and the neighboring abutments is considered a three-unit pontic.

## Coding Tips

Code D6214 is an out-of-sequence code and will not display in numeric order in the CDT book. To report a provisional pontic, see D2799 (provisional crown) or D6253 (provisional pontic). To report fixed partial dentures (FPD), see D6205-D6252. Local anesthesia is included in these services. Any evaluation, radiograph, core buildup, or post or preparation service is reported separately. Each abutment and each pontic constitute a unit in a prosthesis. High noble metals include gold, palladium, and platinum. The content must be ≥ 60 percent gold plus platinum and a minimum ≥ 40 percent gold. Noble metals include 25 percent or less gold plus platinum group. Predominantly base alloys contain a noble metal content of < 25 percent gold plus platinum group. The metals of the platinum group include platinum, palladium, rhodium, iridium, osmium, and ruthenium.

## Reimbursement Tips

Payers may require documentation including the tooth number and preoperative periapical x-rays showing the entire treatment site.

## ICD-10-CM Diagnostic Codes

| | |
|---|---|
| K08.401 | Partial loss of teeth, unspecified cause, class I |
| K08.402 | Partial loss of teeth, unspecified cause, class II |
| K08.403 | Partial loss of teeth, unspecified cause, class III |
| K08.404 | Partial loss of teeth, unspecified cause, class IV |
| K08.409 | Partial loss of teeth, unspecified cause, unspecified class |
| K08.411 | Partial loss of teeth due to trauma, class I |
| K08.412 | Partial loss of teeth due to trauma, class II |
| K08.413 | Partial loss of teeth due to trauma, class III |
| K08.414 | Partial loss of teeth due to trauma, class IV |
| K08.419 | Partial loss of teeth due to trauma, unspecified class |
| K08.421 | Partial loss of teeth due to periodontal diseases, class I |
| K08.422 | Partial loss of teeth due to periodontal diseases, class II |
| K08.423 | Partial loss of teeth due to periodontal diseases, class III |
| K08.424 | Partial loss of teeth due to periodontal diseases, class IV |
| K08.429 | Partial loss of teeth due to periodontal diseases, unspecified class |
| K08.431 | Partial loss of teeth due to caries, class I |
| K08.432 | Partial loss of teeth due to caries, class II |
| K08.433 | Partial loss of teeth due to caries, class III |
| K08.434 | Partial loss of teeth due to caries, class IV |
| K08.439 | Partial loss of teeth due to caries, unspecified class |
| K08.491 | Partial loss of teeth due to other specified cause, class I |
| K08.492 | Partial loss of teeth due to other specified cause, class II |
| K08.493 | Partial loss of teeth due to other specified cause, class III |
| K08.494 | Partial loss of teeth due to other specified cause, class IV |
| K08.499 | Partial loss of teeth due to other specified cause, unspecified class |

## Relative Value Units/Medicare Edits

| Non-Facility RVU | Work | PE | MP | Total |
|---|---|---|---|---|
| **D6205** | 3.96 | 3.49 | 0.82 | 8.27 |
| **D6210** | 5.87 | 5.18 | 1.21 | 12.26 |
| **D6211** | 5.11 | 4.51 | 1.05 | 10.67 |
| **D6212** | 5.43 | 4.80 | 1.12 | 11.35 |
| **D6214** | 5.52 | 4.87 | 1.14 | 11.53 |
| **Facility RVU** | **Work** | **PE** | **MP** | **Total** |
| **D6205** | 3.96 | 3.49 | 0.82 | 8.27 |
| **D6210** | 5.87 | 5.18 | 1.21 | 12.26 |
| **D6211** | 5.11 | 4.51 | 1.05 | 10.67 |
| **D6212** | 5.43 | 4.80 | 1.12 | 11.35 |
| **D6214** | 5.52 | 4.87 | 1.14 | 11.53 |

| | FUD | Status | MUE | Modifiers | | | | IOM Reference |
|---|---|---|---|---|---|---|---|---|
| **D6205** | N/A | N | - | N/A | N/A | N/A | N/A | None |
| **D6210** | N/A | N | - | N/A | N/A | N/A | N/A | |
| **D6211** | N/A | N | - | N/A | N/A | N/A | N/A | |
| **D6212** | N/A | N | - | N/A | N/A | N/A | N/A | |
| **D6214** | N/A | N | - | N/A | N/A | N/A | N/A | |

* with documentation

## Terms To Know

**abutment crown.** Artificial tooth cap for the retention and/or support of a dental prosthesis.

**coping.** Thin covering that is placed over a tooth before attaching a crown or overdenture.

**dental bridge.** Partial denture anchoring onto adjacent teeth on either side.

**pontic.** Artificial tooth on a bridge.

# D6240-D6243

**D6240** pontic - porcelain fused to high noble metal
**D6241** pontic - porcelain fused to predominantly base metal
**D6242** pontic - porcelain fused to noble metal
**D6243** pontic - porcelain fused to titanium and titanium alloys

## Explanation

A pontic is a bridge made to fill an edentulous space in the mouth with substitute or false teeth in between abutments, or caps for anchoring onto the neighboring teeth on either side of the space. This prosthetic is made all in one continuous piece. First the dentist makes an impression of the space and neighboring teeth for the lab. The impression is filled with plaster and a working mold is made. The pontic teeth are designed and then created in wax along with the model of the anchoring caps and the connection of each unit to the other, for a one piece, aesthetically correct bridge. When the wax model is complete, it is set in high-density plaster along with a channel leading to it and the wax is burned out. For porcelain fused to metal pontics, the three-dimensional model for the metal portion is then filled with molten metal from a little reservoir by being spun on the arm of a centrifuge. The cast metal part is cleaned and prepped for bonding. The porcelain layers are completed on it, contoured, shaped, and checked for stain and color, then sent back to the dentist who tries in the fixed partial denture pontic piece, checking all fitting points, and cements the anchoring caps onto the neighboring teeth. Report D6240 for porcelain fused to high noble metal, D6241 for porcelain fused to predominantly base metal, D6242 for porcelain fused to noble metal and D6243 for porcelain fused to titanium and titanium alloys.

## Coding Tips

Local anesthesia is included in these services. Any evaluation, radiograph, core buildup, or post or preparation service is reported separately. Each abutment and each pontic constitute a unit in a prosthesis. High noble metals include gold, palladium, and platinum. The content must be ≥ 60 percent gold plus platinum and a minimum ≥ 40 percent gold. Noble metals include 25 percent or less gold plus platinum group. Predominantly base alloys contain a noble metal content of < 25 percent gold plus platinum group. The metals of the platinum group include platinum, palladium, rhodium, iridium, osmium, and ruthenium.

## Reimbursement Tips

Payers may require documentation including the tooth number and preoperative periapical x-rays showing the entire treatment site.

## ICD-10-CM Diagnostic Codes

| | |
|---|---|
| K08.401 | Partial loss of teeth, unspecified cause, class I |
| K08.402 | Partial loss of teeth, unspecified cause, class II |
| K08.403 | Partial loss of teeth, unspecified cause, class III |
| K08.404 | Partial loss of teeth, unspecified cause, class IV |
| K08.409 | Partial loss of teeth, unspecified cause, unspecified class |
| K08.411 | Partial loss of teeth due to trauma, class I |
| K08.412 | Partial loss of teeth due to trauma, class II |
| K08.413 | Partial loss of teeth due to trauma, class III |
| K08.414 | Partial loss of teeth due to trauma, class IV |
| K08.419 | Partial loss of teeth due to trauma, unspecified class |
| K08.421 | Partial loss of teeth due to periodontal diseases, class I |
| K08.422 | Partial loss of teeth due to periodontal diseases, class II |
| K08.423 | Partial loss of teeth due to periodontal diseases, class III |
| K08.424 | Partial loss of teeth due to periodontal diseases, class IV |
| K08.429 | Partial loss of teeth due to periodontal diseases, unspecified class |
| K08.431 | Partial loss of teeth due to caries, class I |
| K08.432 | Partial loss of teeth due to caries, class II |
| K08.433 | Partial loss of teeth due to caries, class III |
| K08.434 | Partial loss of teeth due to caries, class IV |
| K08.439 | Partial loss of teeth due to caries, unspecified class |
| K08.491 | Partial loss of teeth due to other specified cause, class I |
| K08.492 | Partial loss of teeth due to other specified cause, class II |
| K08.493 | Partial loss of teeth due to other specified cause, class III |
| K08.494 | Partial loss of teeth due to other specified cause, class IV |
| K08.499 | Partial loss of teeth due to other specified cause, unspecified class |

## Relative Value Units/Medicare Edits

| Non-Facility RVU | Work | PE | MP | Total |
|---|---|---|---|---|
| **D6240** | 5.99 | 5.28 | 1.23 | 12.50 |
| **D6241** | 5.33 | 4.71 | 1.10 | 11.14 |
| **D6242** | 5.71 | 5.04 | 1.18 | 11.93 |
| **D6243** | 4.54 | 4.01 | 0.93 | 9.48 |
| **Facility RVU** | **Work** | **PE** | **MP** | **Total** |
| **D6240** | 5.99 | 5.28 | 1.23 | 12.50 |
| **D6241** | 5.33 | 4.71 | 1.10 | 11.14 |
| **D6242** | 5.71 | 5.04 | 1.18 | 11.93 |
| **D6243** | 4.54 | 4.01 | 0.93 | 9.48 |

| | FUD | Status | MUE | Modifiers | | | | IOM Reference |
|---|---|---|---|---|---|---|---|---|
| **D6240** | N/A | N | - | N/A | N/A | N/A | N/A | None |
| **D6241** | N/A | N | - | N/A | N/A | N/A | N/A | |
| **D6242** | N/A | N | - | N/A | N/A | N/A | N/A | |
| **D6243** | N/A | N | - | N/A | N/A | N/A | N/A | |

* with documentation

## Terms To Know

**abutment crown.** Artificial tooth cap for the retention and/or support of a dental prosthesis.

**coping.** Thin covering that is placed over a tooth before attaching a crown or overdenture.

**dental bridge.** Partial denture anchoring onto adjacent teeth on either side.

**pontic.** Artificial tooth on a bridge.

# D6245

**D6245** pontic - porcelain/ceramic

## Explanation

A pontic is a bridge made to fill an edentulous space in the mouth with substitute or false teeth in between abutments, or caps for anchoring onto the neighboring teeth on either side of the space. This prosthetic is made all in one continuous piece. First the dentist makes an impression of the space and neighboring teeth for the lab. The impression is filled with plaster and a working mold is made. The pontic teeth are designed and then created in wax along with the model of the anchoring caps and the connection of each unit to the other, for a one piece, aesthetically correct bridge. When the wax model is complete, it is set in high-density plaster and the wax burned out. For an all porcelain/ceramic prosthesis, the three-dimensional model in plaster is placed in a pressing furnace with an ingot of porcelain. At the right temperature for the melting ingot, a mechanical arm will press the porcelain into the mold at a controlled speed to fill the model. Other layers of porcelain may be hand applied to finish the piece with correct color and shading. The porcelain pontic is sandblasted for shaping and polishing and returned to the dentist who tries in the fixed partial denture pontic piece, checking all fitting points, and cements the anchoring caps onto the neighboring teeth.

## Coding Tips

Payers may require documentation including the tooth number and preoperative periapical x-rays showing the entire treatment site. Local anesthesia is included in this service. Any evaluation, radiograph, core buildup, or post or preparation service is reported separately. Porcelain/ceramic refers to pressed, fired, polished, or milled substances, which predominantly contain inorganic refractory compounds such as porcelains, glasses, ceramics, and glass-ceramics.

## Documentation Tips

Documentation should indicate the location and number of missing teeth.

## Reimbursement Tips

Payers may require documentation including the tooth number and preoperative periapical x-rays showing the entire treatment site. Coverage guidelines vary by payer and by patient contract. Patients are often responsible for copayments or may reach contract limitations. Check with the payer to determine coverage policies and patient responsibility.

## ICD-10-CM Diagnostic Codes

K08.401 Partial loss of teeth, unspecified cause, class I
K08.402 Partial loss of teeth, unspecified cause, class II
K08.403 Partial loss of teeth, unspecified cause, class III
K08.404 Partial loss of teeth, unspecified cause, class IV
K08.409 Partial loss of teeth, unspecified cause, unspecified class
K08.411 Partial loss of teeth due to trauma, class I
K08.412 Partial loss of teeth due to trauma, class II
K08.413 Partial loss of teeth due to trauma, class III
K08.414 Partial loss of teeth due to trauma, class IV
K08.419 Partial loss of teeth due to trauma, unspecified class
K08.421 Partial loss of teeth due to periodontal diseases, class I
K08.422 Partial loss of teeth due to periodontal diseases, class II
K08.423 Partial loss of teeth due to periodontal diseases, class III
K08.424 Partial loss of teeth due to periodontal diseases, class IV
K08.429 Partial loss of teeth due to periodontal diseases, unspecified class
K08.431 Partial loss of teeth due to caries, class I
K08.432 Partial loss of teeth due to caries, class II
K08.433 Partial loss of teeth due to caries, class III
K08.434 Partial loss of teeth due to caries, class IV
K08.439 Partial loss of teeth due to caries, unspecified class
K08.491 Partial loss of teeth due to other specified cause, class I
K08.492 Partial loss of teeth due to other specified cause, class II
K08.493 Partial loss of teeth due to other specified cause, class III
K08.494 Partial loss of teeth due to other specified cause, class IV
K08.499 Partial loss of teeth due to other specified cause, unspecified class

## Relative Value Units/Medicare Edits

| Non-Facility RVU | Work | PE | MP | Total |
|---|---|---|---|---|
| D6245 | 5.54 | 4.89 | 1.14 | 11.57 |
| Facility RVU | Work | PE | MP | Total |
| D6245 | 5.54 | 4.89 | 1.14 | 11.57 |

| | FUD | Status | MUE | Modifiers | | | | IOM Reference |
|---|---|---|---|---|---|---|---|---|
| D6245 | N/A | N | - | N/A | N/A | N/A | N/A | None |

* with documentation

## Terms To Know

**abutment crown.** Artificial tooth cap for the retention and/or support of a dental prosthesis.

**coping.** Thin covering that is placed over a tooth before attaching a crown or overdenture.

**dental bridge.** Partial denture anchoring onto adjacent teeth on either side.

**pontic.** Artificial tooth on a bridge.

# D6250-D6252

**D6250** pontic - resin with high noble metal
**D6251** pontic - resin with predominantly base metal
**D6252** pontic - resin with noble metal

## Explanation

A pontic is a bridge made to fill an edentulous space in the mouth with substitute or false teeth in between abutments, or caps for anchoring onto the neighboring teeth on either side of the space. This prosthetic is made all in one continuous piece. First the dentist makes an impression of the space and neighboring teeth for the lab. The impression is filled with plaster and a working mold is made. The pontic teeth are designed and then created in wax along with the model of the anchoring caps and the connection of each unit to the other, for a one piece, aesthetically correct bridge. When the wax model is complete, it is set in high-density plaster along with a channel leading to it and the wax is burned out. For resin with metal pontics, the three-dimensional model for the metal portion is then filled with molten metal from a little reservoir by being spun on the arm of a centrifuge. The cast metal part is cleaned and prepped for bonding. The acrylic or resin layers are chosen for coloring; applied, cured, and shaped to complete the piece; then sent back to the dentist who tries in the fixed partial denture pontic piece, checking all fitting points, and cements the anchoring caps onto the neighboring teeth. Report D6250 for resin with high noble metal, D6251 for resin with predominantly base metal, and D6252 for resin with noble metal.

## Coding Tips

Local anesthesia is included in these services. Any evaluation, radiograph, core buildup, or post or preparation service is reported separately. Each abutment and each pontic constitute a unit in a prosthesis. High noble metals include gold, palladium, and platinum. The content must be ≥ 60 percent gold plus platinum and ≥ 40 percent gold. Noble metals include 25 percent or less gold plus platinum group. Predominantly base alloys contain a noble metal content of < 25 percent gold plus platinum group. The metals of the platinum group include platinum, palladium, rhodium, iridium, osmium, and ruthenium. Resin-based composite includes fiber or ceramic reinforced polymer compounds.

## Documentation Tips

Documentation should indicate the location and number of missing teeth.

## Reimbursement Tips

Payers may require documentation including the tooth number and preoperative periapical x-rays showing the entire treatment site. Coverage guidelines vary by payer and by patient contract. Patients are often responsible for copayments or may reach contract limitations. Check with the payer to determine coverage policies and patient responsibility.

## ICD-10-CM Diagnostic Codes

| | |
|---|---|
| K08.411 | Partial loss of teeth due to trauma, class I |
| K08.412 | Partial loss of teeth due to trauma, class II |
| K08.413 | Partial loss of teeth due to trauma, class III |
| K08.414 | Partial loss of teeth due to trauma, class IV |
| K08.421 | Partial loss of teeth due to periodontal diseases, class I |
| K08.422 | Partial loss of teeth due to periodontal diseases, class II |
| K08.423 | Partial loss of teeth due to periodontal diseases, class III |
| K08.424 | Partial loss of teeth due to periodontal diseases, class IV |
| K08.431 | Partial loss of teeth due to caries, class I |
| K08.432 | Partial loss of teeth due to caries, class II |
| K08.433 | Partial loss of teeth due to caries, class III |
| K08.434 | Partial loss of teeth due to caries, class IV |
| K08.491 | Partial loss of teeth due to other specified cause, class I |
| K08.492 | Partial loss of teeth due to other specified cause, class II |
| K08.493 | Partial loss of teeth due to other specified cause, class III |
| K08.494 | Partial loss of teeth due to other specified cause, class IV |

## Relative Value Units/Medicare Edits

| Non-Facility RVU | Work | PE | MP | Total |
|---|---|---|---|---|
| **D6250** | 5.76 | 5.09 | 1.19 | 12.04 |
| **D6251** | 4.95 | 4.37 | 1.02 | 10.34 |
| **D6252** | 5.40 | 4.77 | 1.11 | 11.28 |
| **Facility RVU** | **Work** | **PE** | **MP** | **Total** |
| **D6250** | 5.76 | 5.09 | 1.19 | 12.04 |
| **D6251** | 4.95 | 4.37 | 1.02 | 10.34 |
| **D6252** | 5.40 | 4.77 | 1.11 | 11.28 |

| | FUD | Status | MUE | Modifiers | | | | IOM Reference |
|---|---|---|---|---|---|---|---|---|
| **D6250** | N/A | N | - | N/A | N/A | N/A | N/A | None |
| **D6251** | N/A | N | - | N/A | N/A | N/A | N/A | |
| **D6252** | N/A | N | - | N/A | N/A | N/A | N/A | |

* with documentation

## Terms To Know

**abutment crown.** Artificial tooth cap for the retention and/or support of a dental prosthesis.

**coping.** Thin covering that is placed over a tooth before attaching a crown or overdenture.

**dental bridge.** Partial denture anchoring onto adjacent teeth on either side.

**pontic.** Artificial tooth on a bridge.

# D6253

▲ **D6253** interim pontic - further treatment or completion of diagnosis necessary prior to final impression

*Not to be used as a temporary pontic for a routine prosthetic restoration.*

## Explanation

A pontic is a bridge made to fill an edentulous space in the mouth with substitute or false teeth in between abutments, or caps for anchoring onto the neighboring teeth on either side of the space. This prosthetic is made all in one continuous piece. A provisional pontic (D6253) is made and applied for an intended minimal interim of six months to allow enough time for adequate healing to occur or for the completion of other procedures that require extended periods of time.

## Coding Tips

To report fixed partial dentures, see D6205–D6252. To report a provisional crown, see D2799. Local anesthesia is included in this service. Any evaluation, radiograph, core buildup, or post or preparation service is reported separately. Most third-party payers do not cover interim or temporary pontics. However, long-term (six months or longer) use may be covered on a by-report basis. Check with third-party payers for their specific guidelines.

## Documentation Tips

Documentation should indicate the location and number of missing teeth.

## Reimbursement Tips

Coverage guidelines vary by payer and by patient contract. Patients are often responsible for copayments or they may reach contract limitations. Check with the payer to determine coverage policies and patient responsibility. Tooth numbering may be required by some payers.

## ICD-10-CM Diagnostic Codes

K08.401 Partial loss of teeth, unspecified cause, class I
K08.402 Partial loss of teeth, unspecified cause, class II
K08.403 Partial loss of teeth, unspecified cause, class III
K08.404 Partial loss of teeth, unspecified cause, class IV
K08.409 Partial loss of teeth, unspecified cause, unspecified class
K08.411 Partial loss of teeth due to trauma, class I
K08.412 Partial loss of teeth due to trauma, class II
K08.413 Partial loss of teeth due to trauma, class III
K08.414 Partial loss of teeth due to trauma, class IV
K08.419 Partial loss of teeth due to trauma, unspecified class
K08.421 Partial loss of teeth due to periodontal diseases, class I
K08.422 Partial loss of teeth due to periodontal diseases, class II
K08.423 Partial loss of teeth due to periodontal diseases, class III
K08.424 Partial loss of teeth due to periodontal diseases, class IV
K08.429 Partial loss of teeth due to periodontal diseases, unspecified class
K08.431 Partial loss of teeth due to caries, class I
K08.432 Partial loss of teeth due to caries, class II
K08.433 Partial loss of teeth due to caries, class III
K08.434 Partial loss of teeth due to caries, class IV
K08.439 Partial loss of teeth due to caries, unspecified class
K08.491 Partial loss of teeth due to other specified cause, class I
K08.492 Partial loss of teeth due to other specified cause, class II
K08.493 Partial loss of teeth due to other specified cause, class III
K08.494 Partial loss of teeth due to other specified cause, class IV
K08.499 Partial loss of teeth due to other specified cause, unspecified class

## Relative Value Units/Medicare Edits

| Non-Facility RVU | Work | PE | MP | Total |
|---|---|---|---|---|
| **D6253** | 2.65 | 2.34 | 0.55 | 5.54 |
| **Facility RVU** | **Work** | **PE** | **MP** | **Total** |
| **D6253** | 2.65 | 2.34 | 0.55 | 5.54 |

| | FUD | Status | MUE | Modifiers | | | | IOM Reference |
|---|---|---|---|---|---|---|---|---|
| **D6253** | N/A | N | - | N/A | N/A | N/A | N/A | None |

* with documentation

## Terms To Know

**abutment crown.** Artificial tooth cap for the retention and/or support of a dental prosthesis.

**coping.** Thin covering that is placed over a tooth before attaching a crown or overdenture.

**dental bridge.** Partial denture anchoring onto adjacent teeth on either side.

**pontic.** Artificial tooth on a bridge.

Dental - Fixed Prosthodontics

# D6545-D6549

**D6545** retainer - cast metal for resin bonded fixed prosthesis
**D6548** retainer - porcelain/ceramic for resin bonded fixed prosthesis
**D6549** retainer - for resin bonded fixed prosthesis

## Explanation

The retainer attaches the prosthesis to the abutment tooth, implant abutment or implant, and these three codes report retainers for resin-bonded fixed prostheses. A resin-bonded fixed prosthesis is a tooth-colored restoration; the resin is bonded to the bridge either directly, while in the patient's mouth, or indirectly, in the laboratory. Code D6545 reports a cast-metal retainer, code D6548 reports a porcelain/ceramic retainer, and D6549 reports a resin retainer. The porcelain/ceramic dental materials include porcelain, ceramic, or glasslike fillings and crowns.

## Coding Tips

Use these codes to report the retainer of a Maryland bridge. The pontic is reported separately. Local anesthesia is generally considered part of restorative procedures. Porcelain/ceramic refers to pressed, fired, polished, or milled substances, which predominantly contain inorganic refractory compounds such as porcelains, glasses, ceramics, and glass-ceramics.

## Reimbursement Tips

Payers may require documentation including the tooth number and preoperative periapical x-rays showing the entire treatment site. Most third-party payers define a specified time period during which any rebonding or repair services are included. Check with payers for specific guidelines.

## ICD-10-CM Diagnostic Codes

K08.401 Partial loss of teeth, unspecified cause, class I
K08.402 Partial loss of teeth, unspecified cause, class II
K08.403 Partial loss of teeth, unspecified cause, class III
K08.404 Partial loss of teeth, unspecified cause, class IV
K08.409 Partial loss of teeth, unspecified cause, unspecified class
K08.411 Partial loss of teeth due to trauma, class I
K08.412 Partial loss of teeth due to trauma, class II
K08.413 Partial loss of teeth due to trauma, class III
K08.414 Partial loss of teeth due to trauma, class IV
K08.419 Partial loss of teeth due to trauma, unspecified class
K08.421 Partial loss of teeth due to periodontal diseases, class I
K08.422 Partial loss of teeth due to periodontal diseases, class II
K08.423 Partial loss of teeth due to periodontal diseases, class III
K08.424 Partial loss of teeth due to periodontal diseases, class IV
K08.429 Partial loss of teeth due to periodontal diseases, unspecified class
K08.431 Partial loss of teeth due to caries, class I
K08.432 Partial loss of teeth due to caries, class II
K08.433 Partial loss of teeth due to caries, class III
K08.434 Partial loss of teeth due to caries, class IV
K08.439 Partial loss of teeth due to caries, unspecified class
K08.491 Partial loss of teeth due to other specified cause, class I
K08.492 Partial loss of teeth due to other specified cause, class II
K08.493 Partial loss of teeth due to other specified cause, class III
K08.494 Partial loss of teeth due to other specified cause, class IV
K08.499 Partial loss of teeth due to other specified cause, unspecified class

## Relative Value Units/Medicare Edits

| Non-Facility RVU | Work | PE | MP | Total |
|---|---|---|---|---|
| **D6545** | 2.54 | 2.24 | 0.52 | 5.30 |
| **D6548** | 3.06 | 2.70 | 0.63 | 6.39 |
| **D6549** | 2.27 | 2.00 | 0.47 | 4.74 |
| **Facility RVU** | **Work** | **PE** | **MP** | **Total** |
| **D6545** | 2.54 | 2.24 | 0.52 | 5.30 |
| **D6548** | 3.06 | 2.70 | 0.63 | 6.39 |
| **D6549** | 2.27 | 2.00 | 0.47 | 4.74 |

| | FUD | Status | MUE | Modifiers | | | | IOM Reference |
|---|---|---|---|---|---|---|---|---|
| **D6545** | N/A | N | - | N/A | N/A | N/A | N/A | None |
| **D6548** | N/A | N | - | N/A | N/A | N/A | N/A | |
| **D6549** | N/A | N | - | N/A | N/A | N/A | N/A | |

* with documentation

## Terms To Know

**abutment.** Tooth or implant fixture supporting a prosthesis.

**bridge.** Connection between two parts of an organ or body part.

**implant.** Material or device inserted or placed within the body for therapeutic, reconstructive, or diagnostic purposes.

# D6600-D6601

**D6600** retainer inlay - porcelain/ceramic, two surfaces
**D6601** retainer inlay - porcelain/ceramic, three or more surfaces

## Explanation

An inlay fixed partial denture (IFPD) is used to replace missing teeth in patients refusing implant surgery. It is an alternative to a conventional, metal-ceramic, three-unit bridge. The intracoronal restoration is made outside of the mouth to correspond to the form of the hollow space and cemented into the space by use of adhesive products. Code selection depends on the material used for the inlay. These codes describe porcelain/ceramic inlays; code D6600 reports two inlay surfaces, and code D6601 reports three or more inlay surfaces. The porcelain/ceramic dental materials include porcelain, ceramic, or glasslike fillings and crowns.

## Coding Tips

Local anesthesia is generally considered part of restorative procedures. Inlays using high noble metal are reported with the appropriate code from the D6602–D6603 range. To report inlay with base metal, see D6604–D6605; inlay with noble metal, see D6606–D6607. Report D6624 when the inlay is made of titanium. Porcelain/ceramic refers to pressed, fired, polished, or milled substances, which predominantly contain inorganic refractory compounds such as porcelains, glasses, ceramics, and glass-ceramics.

## Documentation Tips

Documentation should indicate the location and number of missing teeth.

## Reimbursement Tips

Coverage for these procedures varies by payer and by individual contract. Check with payers for specific coverage guidelines.

## ICD-10-CM Diagnostic Codes

K08.401 Partial loss of teeth, unspecified cause, class I
K08.402 Partial loss of teeth, unspecified cause, class II
K08.403 Partial loss of teeth, unspecified cause, class III
K08.404 Partial loss of teeth, unspecified cause, class IV
K08.409 Partial loss of teeth, unspecified cause, unspecified class
K08.411 Partial loss of teeth due to trauma, class I
K08.412 Partial loss of teeth due to trauma, class II
K08.413 Partial loss of teeth due to trauma, class III
K08.414 Partial loss of teeth due to trauma, class IV
K08.419 Partial loss of teeth due to trauma, unspecified class
K08.421 Partial loss of teeth due to periodontal diseases, class I
K08.422 Partial loss of teeth due to periodontal diseases, class II
K08.423 Partial loss of teeth due to periodontal diseases, class III
K08.424 Partial loss of teeth due to periodontal diseases, class IV
K08.429 Partial loss of teeth due to periodontal diseases, unspecified class
K08.431 Partial loss of teeth due to caries, class I
K08.432 Partial loss of teeth due to caries, class II
K08.433 Partial loss of teeth due to caries, class III
K08.434 Partial loss of teeth due to caries, class IV
K08.439 Partial loss of teeth due to caries, unspecified class
K08.491 Partial loss of teeth due to other specified cause, class I
K08.492 Partial loss of teeth due to other specified cause, class II
K08.493 Partial loss of teeth due to other specified cause, class III
K08.494 Partial loss of teeth due to other specified cause, class IV
K08.499 Partial loss of teeth due to other specified cause, unspecified class

## Relative Value Units/Medicare Edits

| Non-Facility RVU | Work | PE | MP | Total |
|---|---|---|---|---|
| D6600 | 4.65 | 4.11 | 0.96 | 9.72 |
| D6601 | 4.92 | 4.34 | 1.01 | 10.27 |
| **Facility RVU** | **Work** | **PE** | **MP** | **Total** |
| D6600 | 4.65 | 4.11 | 0.96 | 9.72 |
| D6601 | 4.92 | 4.34 | 1.01 | 10.27 |

| | FUD | Status | MUE | Modifiers | | | | IOM Reference |
|---|---|---|---|---|---|---|---|---|
| D6600 | N/A | N | - | N/A | N/A | N/A | N/A | None |
| D6601 | N/A | N | - | N/A | N/A | N/A | N/A | |

* with documentation

## Terms To Know

**fixed partial denture.** Prosthetic replacement of one or more missing teeth attached to the abutment teeth or implant replacements.

**inlay.** Restoration made outside of the mouth to fit a prepared cavity and placed on the tooth.

**retainer.** In dentistry, portion of a fixed partial denture that attaches an artificial tooth to the abutment tooth or implant.

# D6602-D6603

**D6602** retainer inlay - cast high noble metal, two surfaces
**D6603** retainer inlay - cast high noble metal, three or more surfaces

## Explanation

An inlay fixed partial denture (IFPD) is used to replace missing teeth in patients refusing implant surgery. It is an alternative to a conventional, metal-ceramic three-unit bridge. The intracoronal restoration is made outside of the mouth to correspond to the form of the hollow space and cemented into the space by use of adhesive products. Code selection depends on the material used for the inlay. These codes report cast high noble metals (gold); code D6602 reports two inlay surfaces; and code D6603 reports three or more inlay surfaces.

## Coding Tips

Local anesthesia is generally considered part of restorative procedures. To report inlay using predominantly base metal, see D6604-D6605; using cast noble metal, see D6606-D6607. Inlays using porcelain or ceramic are reported using D6600-D6601. Report D6624 when the inlay is made of titanium. High noble metals include gold, palladium, and platinum. The content must be ≥ 60 percent gold plus platinum and ≥ 40 percent gold. Noble metals include 25 percent or less gold plus platinum group. Predominantly base alloys contain a noble metal content of < 25 percent gold plus platinum group. The metals of the platinum group include platinum, palladium, rhodium, iridium, osmium, and ruthenium.

## Reimbursement Tips

Coverage for these procedures varies by payer and by individual contract. Check with payers for specific coverage guidelines.

## ICD-10-CM Diagnostic Codes

| | |
|---|---|
| K08.401 | Partial loss of teeth, unspecified cause, class I |
| K08.402 | Partial loss of teeth, unspecified cause, class II |
| K08.403 | Partial loss of teeth, unspecified cause, class III |
| K08.404 | Partial loss of teeth, unspecified cause, class IV |
| K08.409 | Partial loss of teeth, unspecified cause, unspecified class |
| K08.411 | Partial loss of teeth due to trauma, class I |
| K08.412 | Partial loss of teeth due to trauma, class II |
| K08.413 | Partial loss of teeth due to trauma, class III |
| K08.414 | Partial loss of teeth due to trauma, class IV |
| K08.419 | Partial loss of teeth due to trauma, unspecified class |
| K08.421 | Partial loss of teeth due to periodontal diseases, class I |
| K08.422 | Partial loss of teeth due to periodontal diseases, class II |
| K08.423 | Partial loss of teeth due to periodontal diseases, class III |
| K08.424 | Partial loss of teeth due to periodontal diseases, class IV |
| K08.429 | Partial loss of teeth due to periodontal diseases, unspecified class |
| K08.431 | Partial loss of teeth due to caries, class I |
| K08.432 | Partial loss of teeth due to caries, class II |
| K08.433 | Partial loss of teeth due to caries, class III |
| K08.434 | Partial loss of teeth due to caries, class IV |
| K08.439 | Partial loss of teeth due to caries, unspecified class |
| K08.491 | Partial loss of teeth due to other specified cause, class I |
| K08.492 | Partial loss of teeth due to other specified cause, class II |
| K08.493 | Partial loss of teeth due to other specified cause, class III |
| K08.494 | Partial loss of teeth due to other specified cause, class IV |
| K08.499 | Partial loss of teeth due to other specified cause, unspecified class |

## Relative Value Units/Medicare Edits

| Non-Facility RVU | Work | PE | MP | Total |
|---|---|---|---|---|
| **D6602** | 4.93 | 4.35 | 1.01 | 10.29 |
| **D6603** | 5.32 | 4.70 | 1.10 | 11.12 |
| **Facility RVU** | **Work** | **PE** | **MP** | **Total** |
| **D6602** | 4.93 | 4.35 | 1.01 | 10.29 |
| **D6603** | 5.32 | 4.70 | 1.10 | 11.12 |

| | FUD | Status | MUE | Modifiers | | | | IOM Reference |
|---|---|---|---|---|---|---|---|---|
| **D6602** | N/A | N | - | N/A | N/A | N/A | N/A | None |
| **D6603** | N/A | N | - | N/A | N/A | N/A | N/A | |

* with documentation

## Terms To Know

**inlay.** Restoration made outside of the mouth to fit a prepared cavity and placed on the tooth.

**retainer.** In dentistry, portion of a fixed partial denture that attaches an artificial tooth to the abutment tooth or implant.

# D6604-D6605

**D6604** retainer inlay - cast predominantly base metal, two surfaces
**D6605** retainer inlay - cast predominantly base metal, three or more surfaces

## Explanation

An inlay fixed partial denture (IFPD) is used to replace missing teeth in patients refusing implant surgery. It is an alternative to a conventional, metal-ceramic, three-unit bridge. The intracoronal restoration is made outside of the mouth to correspond to the form of the hollow space and cemented into the space by use of adhesive products. Code selection depends on the material used for the inlay. These codes report a predominantly base-metal cast (non-noble metals with a silver appearance); code D6604 reports two inlay surfaces; and code D6605 reports three or more inlay surfaces.

## Coding Tips

For inlays using high noble metals, see D6602–D6603; using noble metals, see D6606–D6607. Porcelain or ceramic inlays are reported using D6600–D6601. Report D6624 when the inlay is made of titanium. High noble metals include gold, palladium, and platinum. The content must be ≥ 60 percent gold plus platinum and ≥ 40 percent gold. Noble metals include 25 percent or less gold plus platinum group. Predominantly base alloys contain a noble metal content of < 25 percent gold plus platinum group. The metals of the platinum group include platinum, palladium, rhodium, iridium, osmium, and ruthenium.

## Reimbursement Tips

Coverage for these procedures varies by payer and by individual contract.

## ICD-10-CM Diagnostic Codes

K08.401 Partial loss of teeth, unspecified cause, class I
K08.402 Partial loss of teeth, unspecified cause, class II
K08.403 Partial loss of teeth, unspecified cause, class III
K08.404 Partial loss of teeth, unspecified cause, class IV
K08.409 Partial loss of teeth, unspecified cause, unspecified class
K08.411 Partial loss of teeth due to trauma, class I
K08.412 Partial loss of teeth due to trauma, class II
K08.413 Partial loss of teeth due to trauma, class III
K08.414 Partial loss of teeth due to trauma, class IV
K08.419 Partial loss of teeth due to trauma, unspecified class
K08.421 Partial loss of teeth due to periodontal diseases, class I
K08.422 Partial loss of teeth due to periodontal diseases, class II
K08.423 Partial loss of teeth due to periodontal diseases, class III
K08.424 Partial loss of teeth due to periodontal diseases, class IV
K08.429 Partial loss of teeth due to periodontal diseases, unspecified class
K08.431 Partial loss of teeth due to caries, class I
K08.432 Partial loss of teeth due to caries, class II
K08.433 Partial loss of teeth due to caries, class III
K08.434 Partial loss of teeth due to caries, class IV
K08.439 Partial loss of teeth due to caries, unspecified class
K08.491 Partial loss of teeth due to other specified cause, class I
K08.492 Partial loss of teeth due to other specified cause, class II
K08.493 Partial loss of teeth due to other specified cause, class III
K08.494 Partial loss of teeth due to other specified cause, class IV
K08.499 Partial loss of teeth due to other specified cause, unspecified class

## Relative Value Units/Medicare Edits

| Non-Facility RVU | Work | PE | MP | Total |
|---|---|---|---|---|
| **D6604** | 4.79 | 4.23 | 0.99 | 10.01 |
| **D6605** | 5.10 | 4.50 | 1.05 | 10.65 |
| **Facility RVU** | **Work** | **PE** | **MP** | **Total** |
| **D6604** | 4.79 | 4.23 | 0.99 | 10.01 |
| **D6605** | 5.10 | 4.50 | 1.05 | 10.65 |

| | FUD | Status | MUE | Modifiers | | | | IOM Reference |
|---|---|---|---|---|---|---|---|---|
| **D6604** | N/A | N | - | N/A | N/A | N/A | N/A | None |
| **D6605** | N/A | N | - | N/A | N/A | N/A | N/A | |

* with documentation

## Terms To Know

**inlay.** Restoration made outside of the mouth to fit a prepared cavity and placed on the tooth.

**retainer.** In dentistry, portion of a fixed partial denture that attaches an artificial tooth to the abutment tooth or implant.

# D6606-D6607

**D6606** retainer inlay - cast noble metal, two surfaces
**D6607** retainer inlay - cast noble metal, three or more surfaces

## Explanation

An inlay fixed partial denture (IFPD) is used to replace missing teeth in patients refusing implant surgery. It is an alternative to a conventional, metal-ceramic three-unit bridge. The intracoronal restoration is made outside of the mouth to correspond to the form of the hollow space and cemented into the space by use of adhesive products. Code selection depends on the material used for the inlay. These codes report a noble metal cast (a gold alloy containing gold, copper and other metals); code D6606 reports two inlay surfaces; and code D6607 reports three or more inlay surfaces.

## Coding Tips

Local anesthesia is generally considered part of restorative procedures. To report inlays using high noble metal, see D6602–D6603; using base metal, see D6604–D6605. Porcelain or ceramic inlays are reported using D6600–D6601. Report D6624 when the inlay is made of titanium. High noble metals include gold, palladium, and platinum. The content must be ≥ 60 percent gold plus platinum and ≥ 40 percent gold. Noble metals include 25 percent or less gold plus platinum group. Predominantly base alloys contain a noble metal content of < 25 percent gold plus platinum group. The metals of the platinum group include platinum, palladium, rhodium, iridium, osmium, and ruthenium.

## Documentation Tips

The following information should be documented on a tooth chart: treatment/location of caries, endodontic procedures, prosthetic services, preventive services, treatment of lesions and dental disease, or other special procedures. A tooth chart may also be used to identify structure and rationale of disease process, and the type of service performed on intraoral structures other than teeth.

## Reimbursement Tips

Coverage guidelines vary by payer and by patient contract. Patients are often responsible for copayments or may reach contract limitations. Check with the payer to determine coverage policies and patient responsibility.

## ICD-10-CM Diagnostic Codes

| | |
|---|---|
| K08.411 | Partial loss of teeth due to trauma, class I |
| K08.412 | Partial loss of teeth due to trauma, class II |
| K08.413 | Partial loss of teeth due to trauma, class III |
| K08.414 | Partial loss of teeth due to trauma, class IV |
| K08.421 | Partial loss of teeth due to periodontal diseases, class I |
| K08.422 | Partial loss of teeth due to periodontal diseases, class II |
| K08.423 | Partial loss of teeth due to periodontal diseases, class III |
| K08.424 | Partial loss of teeth due to periodontal diseases, class IV |
| K08.431 | Partial loss of teeth due to caries, class I |
| K08.432 | Partial loss of teeth due to caries, class II |
| K08.433 | Partial loss of teeth due to caries, class III |
| K08.434 | Partial loss of teeth due to caries, class IV |
| K08.491 | Partial loss of teeth due to other specified cause, class I |
| K08.492 | Partial loss of teeth due to other specified cause, class II |
| K08.493 | Partial loss of teeth due to other specified cause, class III |
| K08.494 | Partial loss of teeth due to other specified cause, class IV |

## Relative Value Units/Medicare Edits

| Non-Facility RVU | Work | PE | MP | Total |
|---|---|---|---|---|
| D6606 | 4.75 | 4.20 | 0.98 | 9.93 |
| D6607 | 5.24 | 4.62 | 1.08 | 10.94 |
| **Facility RVU** | **Work** | **PE** | **MP** | **Total** |
| D6606 | 4.75 | 4.20 | 0.98 | 9.93 |
| D6607 | 5.24 | 4.62 | 1.08 | 10.94 |

| | FUD | Status | MUE | Modifiers | | | | IOM Reference |
|---|---|---|---|---|---|---|---|---|
| D6606 | N/A | N | - | N/A | N/A | N/A | N/A | None |
| D6607 | N/A | N | - | N/A | N/A | N/A | N/A | |

* with documentation

## Terms To Know

**inlay.** Restoration made outside of the mouth to fit a prepared cavity and placed on the tooth.

**retainer.** In dentistry, portion of a fixed partial denture that attaches an artificial tooth to the abutment tooth or implant.

Dental - Fixed Prosthodontics

# D6608-D6609

**D6608** retainer onlay - porcelain/ceramic, two surfaces
**D6609** retainer onlay - porcelain/ceramic, three or more surfaces

## Explanation

An overlay, or overdenture, fastens a denture to the jawbone, and it is secured by precision dental attachments placed in tooth roots or dental implants. Types of overdentures include bar joint dentures and telescopic dentures. The adjacent teeth may be altered with locking devices or connecting bars to ensure the denture fits properly. Bars on the upper arch always require more implants than do bars on the lower arch due to the lesser bone density in the upper jaw. A telescopic denture is often the choice for patients with compromised bone density due to age or poor oral hygiene. The procedure consists of a double crown system, the telescopic, and involves fitting inner crowns, outer crowns, and copings on the remaining natural teeth to create a natural-looking, removable overdenture. Copings consist of either a gold thimble over the tooth or a post-retained dome and are used to protect a weakened tooth from fracture and wear, but they do not prevent caries. Code selection depends on the number of surfaces and the type of material used for the onlay. These codes report porcelain/ceramic onlays; code D6608 reports two cusps; and code D6609 reports three or more cusps. The porcelain/ceramic dental materials include porcelain, ceramic, or glasslike fillings and crowns.

## Coding Tips

Local anesthesia is generally considered part of restorative procedures.To report onlay using high noble metal, see D6610–D6611; using base metal, see D6612–D6613, noble metal, see D6614–D6615. A titanium onlay is reported using D6634. Porcelain/ceramic refers to pressed, fired, polished, or milled substances, which predominantly contain inorganic refractory compounds such as porcelains, glasses, ceramics, and glass-ceramics.

## Documentation Tips

The following information should be documented on a tooth chart: treatment/location of caries, endodontic procedures, prosthetic services, preventive services, treatment of lesions and dental disease, or other special procedures. A tooth chart may also be used to identify structure and rationale of disease process, and the type of service performed on intraoral structures other than teeth.

## Reimbursement Tips

Payers may require documentation including the tooth number and preoperative periapical x-rays showing the entire treatment site. Coverage for these procedures varies by payer and by individual contract. Check with payers for specific coverage guidelines.

## ICD-10-CM Diagnostic Codes

K08.401 Partial loss of teeth, unspecified cause, class I
K08.402 Partial loss of teeth, unspecified cause, class II
K08.403 Partial loss of teeth, unspecified cause, class III
K08.404 Partial loss of teeth, unspecified cause, class IV
K08.409 Partial loss of teeth, unspecified cause, unspecified class
K08.411 Partial loss of teeth due to trauma, class I
K08.412 Partial loss of teeth due to trauma, class II
K08.413 Partial loss of teeth due to trauma, class III
K08.414 Partial loss of teeth due to trauma, class IV
K08.419 Partial loss of teeth due to trauma, unspecified class
K08.421 Partial loss of teeth due to periodontal diseases, class I
K08.422 Partial loss of teeth due to periodontal diseases, class II
K08.423 Partial loss of teeth due to periodontal diseases, class III
K08.424 Partial loss of teeth due to periodontal diseases, class IV
K08.429 Partial loss of teeth due to periodontal diseases, unspecified class
K08.431 Partial loss of teeth due to caries, class I
K08.432 Partial loss of teeth due to caries, class II
K08.433 Partial loss of teeth due to caries, class III
K08.434 Partial loss of teeth due to caries, class IV
K08.439 Partial loss of teeth due to caries, unspecified class
K08.491 Partial loss of teeth due to other specified cause, class I
K08.492 Partial loss of teeth due to other specified cause, class II
K08.493 Partial loss of teeth due to other specified cause, class III
K08.494 Partial loss of teeth due to other specified cause, class IV
K08.499 Partial loss of teeth due to other specified cause, unspecified class

## Relative Value Units/Medicare Edits

| Non-Facility RVU | Work | PE | MP | Total |
|---|---|---|---|---|
| **D6608** | 5.06 | 4.46 | 1.04 | 10.56 |
| **D6609** | 5.31 | 4.69 | 1.09 | 11.09 |
| **Facility RVU** | **Work** | **PE** | **MP** | **Total** |
| **D6608** | 5.06 | 4.46 | 1.04 | 10.56 |
| **D6609** | 5.31 | 4.69 | 1.09 | 11.09 |

| | FUD | Status | MUE | Modifiers | | | | IOM Reference |
|---|---|---|---|---|---|---|---|---|
| **D6608** | N/A | N | - | N/A | N/A | N/A | N/A | None |
| **D6609** | N/A | N | - | N/A | N/A | N/A | N/A | |

* with documentation

## Terms To Know

**onlay.** In dentistry, restoration made outside of the mouth that is cemented over a cusp or cusps of the tooth.

**retainer.** In dentistry, portion of a fixed partial denture that attaches an artificial tooth to the abutment tooth or implant.

Dental - Fixed Prosthodontics

# D6610-D6611

**D6610** retainer onlay - cast high noble metal, two surfaces
**D6611** retainer onlay - cast high noble metal, three or more surfaces

## Explanation

An overlay, or overdenture, fastens a denture to the jawbone, and it is secured by precision dental attachments placed in tooth roots or dental implants. Types of overdentures include bar joint dentures and telescopic dentures. The adjacent teeth may be altered with locking devices or connecting bars to ensure the denture fits properly. Bars on the upper arch always require more implants than do bars on the lower arch due to the lesser bone density in the upper jaw. A telescopic denture is often the choice for patients with compromised bone density due to age or poor oral hygiene. The procedure consists of a double-crown system, the telescopic, and involves fitting inner crowns, outer crowns and copings on the remaining natural teeth to create a natural-looking, removable overdenture. Copings consist of either a gold thimble over the tooth or a post-retained dome and are used to protect a weakened tooth from fracture and wear, but they do not prevent caries. Code selection depends on the number of cusp surfaces and the type of material used for the onlay. These codes report cast high noble metal (gold); code D6610 reports two cusps; and code D6611 reports three or more cusps.

## Coding Tips

Local anesthesia is generally considered part of restorative procedures. To report onlay using noble metal, see D6614-D6615; using base metal, see D6612-D6613. A titanium onlay is reported using D6634. Onlays made or porcelain or ceramic are reported using D6608-D6609. High noble metals include gold, palladium, and platinum. The content must be ≥ 60 percent gold plus platinum and ≥ 40 percent gold. Noble metals include 25 percent or less gold plus platinum group. Predominantly base alloys contain a noble metal content of < 25 percent gold plus platinum group. The metals of the platinum group include platinum, palladium, rhodium, iridium, osmium and ruthenium.

## Documentation Tips

Documentation should indicate the location and number of missing teeth.

## Reimbursement Tips

Payers may require documentation including the tooth number and preoperative periapical x-rays showing the entire treatment site. Coverage guidelines vary by payer and by patient contract. Patients are often responsible for copayments or may reach contract limitations. Check with the payer to determine coverage policies and patient responsibility.

## ICD-10-CM Diagnostic Codes

K08.401 Partial loss of teeth, unspecified cause, class I
K08.402 Partial loss of teeth, unspecified cause, class II
K08.403 Partial loss of teeth, unspecified cause, class III
K08.404 Partial loss of teeth, unspecified cause, class IV
K08.409 Partial loss of teeth, unspecified cause, unspecified class
K08.411 Partial loss of teeth due to trauma, class I
K08.412 Partial loss of teeth due to trauma, class II
K08.413 Partial loss of teeth due to trauma, class III
K08.414 Partial loss of teeth due to trauma, class IV
K08.419 Partial loss of teeth due to trauma, unspecified class
K08.421 Partial loss of teeth due to periodontal diseases, class I
K08.422 Partial loss of teeth due to periodontal diseases, class II
K08.423 Partial loss of teeth due to periodontal diseases, class III
K08.424 Partial loss of teeth due to periodontal diseases, class IV
K08.429 Partial loss of teeth due to periodontal diseases, unspecified class
K08.431 Partial loss of teeth due to caries, class I
K08.432 Partial loss of teeth due to caries, class II
K08.433 Partial loss of teeth due to caries, class III
K08.434 Partial loss of teeth due to caries, class IV
K08.439 Partial loss of teeth due to caries, unspecified class
K08.491 Partial loss of teeth due to other specified cause, class I
K08.492 Partial loss of teeth due to other specified cause, class II
K08.493 Partial loss of teeth due to other specified cause, class III
K08.494 Partial loss of teeth due to other specified cause, class IV
K08.499 Partial loss of teeth due to other specified cause, unspecified class

## Relative Value Units/Medicare Edits

| Non-Facility RVU | Work | PE | MP | Total |
|---|---|---|---|---|
| **D6610** | 5.32 | 4.70 | 1.10 | 11.12 |
| **D6611** | 5.77 | 5.09 | 1.19 | 12.05 |
| **Facility RVU** | **Work** | **PE** | **MP** | **Total** |
| **D6610** | 5.32 | 4.70 | 1.10 | 11.12 |
| **D6611** | 5.77 | 5.09 | 1.19 | 12.05 |

| | FUD | Status | MUE | Modifiers | | | | IOM Reference |
|---|---|---|---|---|---|---|---|---|
| **D6610** | N/A | N | - | N/A | N/A | N/A | N/A | None |
| **D6611** | N/A | N | - | N/A | N/A | N/A | N/A | |

* with documentation

## Terms To Know

**onlay.** In dentistry, restoration made outside of the mouth that is cemented over a cusp or cusps of the tooth.

**retainer.** In dentistry, portion of a fixed partial denture that attaches an artificial tooth to the abutment tooth or implant.

# D6612-D6613

**D6612** retainer onlay - cast predominantly base metal, two surfaces
**D6613** retainer onlay - cast predominantly base metal, three or more surfaces

## Explanation

An overlay, or overdenture, fastens a denture to the jawbone, and it is secured by precision dental attachments placed in tooth roots or dental implants. Types of overdentures include bar joint dentures and telescopic dentures. The adjacent teeth may be altered with locking devices or connecting bars to ensure the denture fits properly. Bars on the upper arch always require more implants than do bars on the lower arch due to the lesser bone density in the upper jaw. A telescopic denture is often the choice for patients with compromised bone density due to age or poor oral hygiene. The procedure consists of a double-crown system, the telescopic, and involves fitting inner crowns, outer crowns, and copings on the remaining natural teeth to create a natural-looking, removable overdenture. Copings consist of either a gold thimble over the tooth or a post-retained dome and are used to protect a weakened tooth from fracture and wear, but they do not prevent caries. Code selection depends on the number of cusp surfaces and the type of material used for the onlay. These codes report a cast of predominantly base metal (non-noble metals with a silver appearance); code D6612 reports two surfaces; and code D6613 reports three or more cusps.

## Coding Tips

Local anesthesia is generally considered part of restorative procedures. To report onlays using high noble metal, see D6610–D6611; noble metal, see D6614–D6615. A titanium onlay is reported using D6634. Onlays made of porcelain or ceramic are reported using D6608–D6609. High noble metals include gold, palladium, and platinum. The content must be ≥ 60 percent gold plus platinum and ≥ 40 percent gold. Noble metals include 25 percent or less gold plus platinum group. Predominantly base alloys contain a noble metal content of < 25 percent gold plus platinum group. The metals of the platinum group include platinum, palladium, rhodium, iridium, osmium, and ruthenium.

## Documentation Tips

Documentation should indicate the location and number of missing teeth.

## Reimbursement Tips

Payers may require documentation including the tooth number and preoperative periapical x-rays showing the entire treatment site. Coverage guidelines vary by payer and by patient contract. Patients are often responsible for copayments or may reach contract limitations. Check with the payer to determine coverage policies and patient responsibility.

## ICD-10-CM Diagnostic Codes

K08.401 Partial loss of teeth, unspecified cause, class I
K08.402 Partial loss of teeth, unspecified cause, class II
K08.403 Partial loss of teeth, unspecified cause, class III
K08.404 Partial loss of teeth, unspecified cause, class IV
K08.409 Partial loss of teeth, unspecified cause, unspecified class
K08.411 Partial loss of teeth due to trauma, class I
K08.412 Partial loss of teeth due to trauma, class II
K08.413 Partial loss of teeth due to trauma, class III
K08.414 Partial loss of teeth due to trauma, class IV
K08.419 Partial loss of teeth due to trauma, unspecified class
K08.421 Partial loss of teeth due to periodontal diseases, class I
K08.422 Partial loss of teeth due to periodontal diseases, class II
K08.423 Partial loss of teeth due to periodontal diseases, class III
K08.424 Partial loss of teeth due to periodontal diseases, class IV
K08.429 Partial loss of teeth due to periodontal diseases, unspecified class
K08.431 Partial loss of teeth due to caries, class I
K08.432 Partial loss of teeth due to caries, class II
K08.433 Partial loss of teeth due to caries, class III
K08.434 Partial loss of teeth due to caries, class IV
K08.439 Partial loss of teeth due to caries, unspecified class
K08.491 Partial loss of teeth due to other specified cause, class I
K08.492 Partial loss of teeth due to other specified cause, class II
K08.493 Partial loss of teeth due to other specified cause, class III
K08.494 Partial loss of teeth due to other specified cause, class IV
K08.499 Partial loss of teeth due to other specified cause, unspecified class

## Relative Value Units/Medicare Edits

| Non-Facility RVU | Work | PE | MP | Total |
|---|---|---|---|---|
| **D6612** | 5.23 | 4.61 | 1.08 | 10.92 |
| **D6613** | 5.53 | 4.88 | 1.14 | 11.55 |
| **Facility RVU** | **Work** | **PE** | **MP** | **Total** |
| **D6612** | 5.23 | 4.61 | 1.08 | 10.92 |
| **D6613** | 5.53 | 4.88 | 1.14 | 11.55 |

| | FUD | Status | MUE | Modifiers | | | | IOM Reference |
|---|---|---|---|---|---|---|---|---|
| **D6612** | N/A | N | - | N/A | N/A | N/A | N/A | None |
| **D6613** | N/A | N | - | N/A | N/A | N/A | N/A | |

* with documentation

## Terms To Know

**onlay.** In dentistry, restoration made outside of the mouth that is cemented over a cusp or cusps of the tooth.

**retainer.** In dentistry, portion of a fixed partial denture that attaches an artificial tooth to the abutment tooth or implant.

Dental - Fixed Prosthodontics

# D6614-D6615

**D6614** retainer onlay - cast noble metal, two surfaces
**D6615** retainer onlay - cast noble metal, three or more surfaces

## Explanation

An overlay, or overdenture, fastens a denture to the jawbone, and it is secured by precision dental attachments placed in tooth roots or dental implants. Types of overdentures include bar joint dentures and telescopic dentures. The adjacent teeth may be altered with locking devices or connecting bars to ensure the denture fits properly. Bars on the upper arch always require more implants than do bars on the lower arch due to the lesser bone density in the upper jaw. A telescopic denture is often the choice for patients with compromised bone density due to age or poor oral hygiene. The procedure consists of a double-crown system, the telescopic, and involves fitting inner crowns, outer crowns, and copings on the remaining natural teeth to create a natural-looking, removable overdenture. Copings consist of either a gold thimble over the tooth or a post-retained dome and are used to protect a weakened tooth from fracture and wear, but they do not prevent caries. Code selection depends on the number of cusp surfaces and the type of material used for the onlay. These codes report a noble metal cast (a gold alloy containing gold, copper and other metals); code D6614 reports two cusps; and code D6615 reports three or more cusps.

## Coding Tips

Local anesthesia is generally considered part of restorative procedures. Porcelain or ceramic onlays are reported using D6608-D6609. Onlays fabricated with titanium are reported using D6634. High noble metals include gold, palladium, and platinum. The content must be ≥ 60 percent gold plus platinum and ≥ 40 percent gold. Noble metals include 25 percent or less gold plus platinum group. Predominantly base alloys contain a noble metal content of < 25 percent gold plus platinum group. The metals of the platinum group include platinum, palladium, rhodium, iridium, osmium, and ruthenium.

## Documentation Tips

The following information should be documented on a tooth chart: treatment/location of caries, endodontic procedures, prosthetic services, preventive services, treatment of lesions and dental disease, or other special procedures. A tooth chart may also be used to identify structure and rationale of disease process, and the type of service performed on intraoral structures other than teeth.

## Reimbursement Tips

Payers may require documentation including the tooth number and preoperative periapical x-rays showing the entire treatment site.

## ICD-10-CM Diagnostic Codes

K08.401 Partial loss of teeth, unspecified cause, class I
K08.402 Partial loss of teeth, unspecified cause, class II
K08.403 Partial loss of teeth, unspecified cause, class III
K08.404 Partial loss of teeth, unspecified cause, class IV
K08.409 Partial loss of teeth, unspecified cause, unspecified class
K08.411 Partial loss of teeth due to trauma, class I
K08.412 Partial loss of teeth due to trauma, class II
K08.413 Partial loss of teeth due to trauma, class III
K08.414 Partial loss of teeth due to trauma, class IV
K08.419 Partial loss of teeth due to trauma, unspecified class
K08.421 Partial loss of teeth due to periodontal diseases, class I
K08.422 Partial loss of teeth due to periodontal diseases, class II
K08.423 Partial loss of teeth due to periodontal diseases, class III
K08.424 Partial loss of teeth due to periodontal diseases, class IV
K08.429 Partial loss of teeth due to periodontal diseases, unspecified class
K08.431 Partial loss of teeth due to caries, class I
K08.432 Partial loss of teeth due to caries, class II
K08.433 Partial loss of teeth due to caries, class III
K08.434 Partial loss of teeth due to caries, class IV
K08.439 Partial loss of teeth due to caries, unspecified class
K08.491 Partial loss of teeth due to other specified cause, class I
K08.492 Partial loss of teeth due to other specified cause, class II
K08.493 Partial loss of teeth due to other specified cause, class III
K08.494 Partial loss of teeth due to other specified cause, class IV
K08.499 Partial loss of teeth due to other specified cause, unspecified class

## Relative Value Units/Medicare Edits

| Non-Facility RVU | Work | PE | MP | Total |
|---|---|---|---|---|
| **D6614** | 5.20 | 4.59 | 1.07 | 10.86 |
| **D6615** | 5.45 | 4.81 | 1.12 | 11.38 |
| **Facility RVU** | **Work** | **PE** | **MP** | **Total** |
| **D6614** | 5.20 | 4.59 | 1.07 | 10.86 |
| **D6615** | 5.45 | 4.81 | 1.12 | 11.38 |

| | FUD | Status | MUE | Modifiers | | | | IOM Reference |
|---|---|---|---|---|---|---|---|---|
| **D6614** | N/A | N | - | N/A | N/A | N/A | N/A | None |
| **D6615** | N/A | N | - | N/A | N/A | N/A | N/A | |

* with documentation

## Terms To Know

**onlay.** In dentistry, restoration made outside of the mouth that is cemented over a cusp or cusps of the tooth.

**retainer.** In dentistry, portion of a fixed partial denture that attaches an artificial tooth to the abutment tooth or implant.

# D6624

**D6624** retainer inlay - titanium

## Explanation

An inlay fixed partial denture (IFPD) is used to replace missing teeth in patients refusing implant surgery. It is an alternative to a conventional, metal-ceramic three-unit bridge. The intracoronal restoration is made outside of the mouth to correspond to the form of the hollow space, and cemented into the space by use of adhesive products. This code reports a titanium inlay and it is reported once for each inlay.

## Coding Tips

This is an out of sequence code and will not display in numeric order in the CDT manual. Local anesthesia is generally considered part of restorative procedures. For high noble metal inlays, see D6610–D6611; for cast, see D6612–D6613. Cast noble metal onlays are reported with D6614–D6615. Onlays made of porcelain or ceramic are reported with D6608--D6609.

## Documentation Tips

The following information should be documented on a tooth chart: treatment/location of caries, endodontic procedures, prosthetic services, preventive services, treatment of lesions and dental disease, or other special procedures. A tooth chart may also be used to identify structure and rationale of disease process, and the type of service performed on intraoral structures other than teeth.

## Reimbursement Tips

Coverage guidelines vary by payer and by patient contract. Patients are often responsible for copayments or they may reach contract limitations. Check with the payer to determine coverage policies and patient responsibility.

## ICD-10-CM Diagnostic Codes

| | |
|---|---|
| K08.401 | Partial loss of teeth, unspecified cause, class I |
| K08.411 | Partial loss of teeth due to trauma, class I |
| K08.412 | Partial loss of teeth due to trauma, class II |
| K08.413 | Partial loss of teeth due to trauma, class III |
| K08.414 | Partial loss of teeth due to trauma, class IV |
| K08.421 | Partial loss of teeth due to periodontal diseases, class I |
| K08.422 | Partial loss of teeth due to periodontal diseases, class II |
| K08.423 | Partial loss of teeth due to periodontal diseases, class III |
| K08.424 | Partial loss of teeth due to periodontal diseases, class IV |
| K08.431 | Partial loss of teeth due to caries, class I |
| K08.432 | Partial loss of teeth due to caries, class II |
| K08.433 | Partial loss of teeth due to caries, class III |
| K08.434 | Partial loss of teeth due to caries, class IV |
| K08.491 | Partial loss of teeth due to other specified cause, class I |
| K08.492 | Partial loss of teeth due to other specified cause, class II |
| K08.493 | Partial loss of teeth due to other specified cause, class III |
| K08.494 | Partial loss of teeth due to other specified cause, class IV |

## Relative Value Units/Medicare Edits

| Non-Facility RVU | Work | PE | MP | Total |
|---|---|---|---|---|
| **D6624** | 5.03 | 4.44 | 1.04 | 10.51 |
| **Facility RVU** | **Work** | **PE** | **MP** | **Total** |
| **D6624** | 5.03 | 4.44 | 1.04 | 10.51 |

| | FUD | Status | MUE | Modifiers | | | | IOM Reference |
|---|---|---|---|---|---|---|---|---|
| **D6624** | N/A | N | - | N/A | N/A | N/A | N/A | None |

* with documentation

## Terms To Know

**inlay.** Restoration made outside of the mouth to fit a prepared cavity and placed on the tooth.

**retainer.** In dentistry, portion of a fixed partial denture that attaches an artificial tooth to the abutment tooth or implant.

Dental - Fixed Prosthodontics

# D6634

**D6634** retainer onlay - titanium

## Explanation

An overlay, or overdenture, fastens a denture to the jawbone, and it is secured by precision dental attachments placed in tooth roots or dental implants. Types of overdentures include bar joint dentures and telescopic dentures. The adjacent teeth may be altered with locking devices or connecting bars to ensure the denture fits properly. Bars on the upper arch always require more implants than do bars on the lower arch due to the lesser bone density in the upper jaw. A telescopic denture is often the choice for patients with compromised bone density due to age or poor oral hygiene. The procedure consists of a double-crown system, the telescopic, and involves fitting inner crowns, outer crowns, and copings on the remaining natural teeth to create a natural-looking, removable overdenture. The outer crowns of the restoration may be placed with a temporary type of adhesive so that they can be removed for inspection or repair. Copings consist of either a gold thimble over the tooth or a post-retained dome and are used to protect a weakened tooth from fracture and wear, but they do not prevent caries. This code reports a titanium onlay and it is reported once for each onlay.

## Coding Tips

Local anesthesia is generally considered part of restorative procedures. To report onlays fabricated with high noble metal, see D6610-D6611; noble metal, see D6614-D6615. Onlays that are constructed using base metal are reported using D6612-D6613. Porcelain or ceramic onlays are coded using the appropriate code from the D6608-D6609 range.

## Documentation Tips

The following information should be documented on a tooth chart: treatment/location of caries, endodontic procedures, prosthetic services, preventive services, treatment of lesions and dental disease, or other special procedures. A tooth chart may also be used to identify structure and rationale of disease process, and the type of service performed on intraoral structures other than teeth.

## Reimbursement Tips

Payers may require documentation including the tooth number and preoperative periapical x-rays showing the entire treatment site.

## ICD-10-CM Diagnostic Codes

| | |
|---|---|
| K08.401 | Partial loss of teeth, unspecified cause, class I |
| K08.402 | Partial loss of teeth, unspecified cause, class II |
| K08.403 | Partial loss of teeth, unspecified cause, class III |
| K08.404 | Partial loss of teeth, unspecified cause, class IV |
| K08.409 | Partial loss of teeth, unspecified cause, unspecified class |
| K08.411 | Partial loss of teeth due to trauma, class I |
| K08.412 | Partial loss of teeth due to trauma, class II |
| K08.413 | Partial loss of teeth due to trauma, class III |
| K08.414 | Partial loss of teeth due to trauma, class IV |
| K08.419 | Partial loss of teeth due to trauma, unspecified class |
| K08.421 | Partial loss of teeth due to periodontal diseases, class I |
| K08.422 | Partial loss of teeth due to periodontal diseases, class II |
| K08.423 | Partial loss of teeth due to periodontal diseases, class III |
| K08.424 | Partial loss of teeth due to periodontal diseases, class IV |
| K08.429 | Partial loss of teeth due to periodontal diseases, unspecified class |
| K08.431 | Partial loss of teeth due to caries, class I |
| K08.432 | Partial loss of teeth due to caries, class II |
| K08.433 | Partial loss of teeth due to caries, class III |
| K08.434 | Partial loss of teeth due to caries, class IV |
| K08.439 | Partial loss of teeth due to caries, unspecified class |
| K08.491 | Partial loss of teeth due to other specified cause, class I |
| K08.492 | Partial loss of teeth due to other specified cause, class II |
| K08.493 | Partial loss of teeth due to other specified cause, class III |
| K08.494 | Partial loss of teeth due to other specified cause, class IV |
| K08.499 | Partial loss of teeth due to other specified cause, unspecified class |

## Relative Value Units/Medicare Edits

| Non-Facility RVU | Work | PE | MP | Total |
|---|---|---|---|---|
| **D6634** | 5.26 | 4.64 | 1.08 | 10.98 |
| **Facility RVU** | **Work** | **PE** | **MP** | **Total** |
| **D6634** | 5.26 | 4.64 | 1.08 | 10.98 |

| | FUD | Status | MUE | Modifiers | | | | IOM Reference |
|---|---|---|---|---|---|---|---|---|
| **D6634** | N/A | N | - | N/A | N/A | N/A | N/A | None |

* with documentation

## Terms To Know

**onlay.** In dentistry, restoration made outside of the mouth that is cemented over a cusp or cusps of the tooth.

**retainer.** In dentistry, portion of a fixed partial denture that attaches an artificial tooth to the abutment tooth or implant.

# D6710-D6722

**D6710** retainer crown - indirect resin based composite

*Not to be used as a temporary or provisional prosthesis.*

**D6720** retainer crown - resin with high noble metal

**D6721** retainer crown - resin with predominantly base metal

**D6722** retainer crown - resin with noble metal

## Explanation

A fixed partial denture retainer crown is made for a tooth that needs to be the connecting or anchoring tooth for the retainer but may be decayed or damaged enough to require restoration. The crown is made to accommodate the attachment of the retainer from impressions taken of the tooth's anatomy and the tooth with the retainer (see previous restorative crown codes D2710-D2722 for the method). Report D6710 when tooth-colored resin composite is bonded to the crown. Report D6720 for resin with high noble metal; D6721 for resin with predominantly base metal; and D6722 for resin with noble metal.

## Coding Tips

Local anesthesia is included in these services. Any evaluation or radiograph, core buildup, or post or preparation service is reported separately. For individual restorations, see D2710–D2799.Prefabricated crowns are reported using the appropriate code from the D2930–D2934 range; for abutment supported, see D6058–D6064 or D6094. Implant supported crowns are reported with a code from the D6065–D6067 range. Code D6710 should not be used to report a temporary or provisional prosthesis, see D6793. For crowns used as a fixed partial denture retainer fabricated using porcelain or ceramic, see codes D6740–D6752; for 3/4 cast metals or porcelain/ceramics, see D6780–D6783. Full crowns used for partial denture retainers are reported with the appropriate code in the D6790–D6792 range. A titanium fixed partial denture retainer crown is reported with D6794. High noble metals include gold, palladium, and platinum. The content must be ≥ 60 percent gold plus platinum and ≥ 40 percent gold. Noble metals include 25 percent or less gold plus platinum group. Predominantly base alloys contain a noble metal content of < 25 percent gold plus platinum group. The metals of the platinum group include platinum, palladium, rhodium, iridium, osmium, and ruthenium. Resin-based composite includes fiber or ceramic reinforced polymer compounds.

## Documentation Tips

Documentation should indicate the location and number of missing teeth.

## Reimbursement Tips

Payers may require documentation including the tooth number and preoperative periapical x-rays showing the entire treatment site for codes D6720-D6722.

## ICD-10-CM Diagnostic Codes

| | |
|---|---|
| K02.51 | Dental caries on pit and fissure surface limited to enamel |
| K02.52 | Dental caries on pit and fissure surface penetrating into dentin |
| K02.53 | Dental caries on pit and fissure surface penetrating into pulp |
| K02.61 | Dental caries on smooth surface limited to enamel |
| K02.62 | Dental caries on smooth surface penetrating into dentin |
| K02.63 | Dental caries on smooth surface penetrating into pulp |
| K02.7 | Dental root caries |
| K03.0 | Excessive attrition of teeth |
| K03.1 | Abrasion of teeth |
| K03.2 | Erosion of teeth |
| K03.3 | Pathological resorption of teeth |
| K03.4 | Hypercementosis |
| K03.5 | Ankylosis of teeth |
| K03.6 | Deposits [accretions] on teeth |
| K03.7 | Posteruptive color changes of dental hard tissues |
| K03.81 | Cracked tooth |
| K03.89 | Other specified diseases of hard tissues of teeth |

## Relative Value Units/Medicare Edits

| Non-Facility RVU | Work | PE | MP | Total |
|---|---|---|---|---|
| **D6710** | 5.22 | 4.61 | 1.08 | 10.91 |
| **D6720** | 6.29 | 5.55 | 1.30 | 13.14 |
| **D6721** | 5.64 | 4.98 | 1.16 | 11.78 |
| **D6722** | 5.88 | 5.19 | 1.21 | 12.28 |
| **Facility RVU** | **Work** | **PE** | **MP** | **Total** |
| **D6710** | 5.22 | 4.61 | 1.08 | 10.91 |
| **D6720** | 6.29 | 5.55 | 1.30 | 13.14 |
| **D6721** | 5.64 | 4.98 | 1.16 | 11.78 |
| **D6722** | 5.88 | 5.19 | 1.21 | 12.28 |

| | FUD | Status | MUE | Modifiers | | | | IOM Reference |
|---|---|---|---|---|---|---|---|---|
| **D6710** | N/A | N | - | N/A | N/A | N/A | N/A | None |
| **D6720** | N/A | N | - | N/A | N/A | N/A | N/A | |
| **D6721** | N/A | N | - | N/A | N/A | N/A | N/A | |
| **D6722** | N/A | N | - | N/A | N/A | N/A | N/A | |

* with documentation

## Terms To Know

**abutment crown.** Artificial tooth cap for the retention and/or support of a dental prosthesis.

**artificial crown.** In dentistry, a ceramic or metal restoration made to cover or replace a major part of the top of a tooth.

**composite.** In dentistry, synthetic material such as acrylic resin and quartz particles used in tooth restoration.

**coping.** Thin covering that is placed over a tooth before attaching a crown or overdenture.

**denture.** Manmade substitution of natural teeth and neighboring structures.

**moulage.** Model of an anatomical structure formed via a negative impression in wax or plaster.

# D6740-D6753

**D6740** retainer crown - porcelain/ceramic
**D6750** retainer crown - porcelain fused to high noble metal
**D6751** retainer crown - porcelain fused to predominantly base metal
**D6752** retainer crown - porcelain fused to noble metal
**D6753** retainer crown - porcelain fused to titanium and titanium alloys

## Explanation

A fixed partial denture retainer crown is made for a tooth that needs to be the connecting or anchoring tooth for the retainer but may be decayed or damaged enough to require restoration. The crown is made to accommodate the attachment of the retainer from impressions taken of the tooth's anatomy and the tooth with the retainer (see previous restorative crown codes D2740–D2752 for the method). Report D6740 for an all porcelain/ceramic substrate crown; D6750 for porcelain fused to high noble metal, D6751 for porcelain fused to predominantly base metal, D6752 for porcelain fused to noble metal, and D6753 for porcelain fused to titanium and titanium alloys.

## Coding Tips

Local anesthesia is included in these services. Any evaluation or radiograph, core buildup, or post or preparation service is reported separately. For individual restorations, see D2710-D2799. Prefabricated crowns are reported using the appropriate code from the D2930-D2934 range; for abutment supported, see D6058-D6064 or D6094. Implant supported crowns are reported with a code from the D6065-D6067 range. Code D6710 should not be used to report a temporary or provisional prosthesis; see D6793. For crowns used as a fixed partial denture retainer fabricated using porcelain or ceramic, see codes D6740-D6752; for 3/4 cast metals or porcelain/ceramics, see D6780-D6784. Full crowns used for partial denture retainers are reported with the appropriate code in the D6790-D6792 range. A titanium fixed partial denture retainer crown is reported with D6794. High noble metals include gold, palladium, and platinum. The content must be ≥ 60 percent gold plus platinum and a minimum of ≥ 40 percent gold. Noble metals include 25 percent or less gold plus platinum group. Predominantly base alloys contain a noble metal content of < 25 percent gold plus platinum group. The metals of the platinum group include platinum, palladium, rhodium, iridium, osmium, and ruthenium. Resin-based composite includes fiber or ceramic reinforced polymer compounds.

## Documentation Tips

Documentation should indicate the location and number of missing teeth.

## Reimbursement Tips

Payers may require documentation including the tooth number and preoperative periapical x-rays showing the entire treatment site. Any evaluation or radiograph, core buildup, or post or preparation service is reported separately.

## ICD-10-CM Diagnostic Codes

| | |
|---|---|
| K02.3 | Arrested dental caries |
| K02.51 | Dental caries on pit and fissure surface limited to enamel |
| K02.52 | Dental caries on pit and fissure surface penetrating into dentin |
| K02.53 | Dental caries on pit and fissure surface penetrating into pulp |
| K02.61 | Dental caries on smooth surface limited to enamel |
| K02.62 | Dental caries on smooth surface penetrating into dentin |
| K02.63 | Dental caries on smooth surface penetrating into pulp |
| K02.7 | Dental root caries |
| K03.0 | Excessive attrition of teeth |
| K03.1 | Abrasion of teeth |
| K03.2 | Erosion of teeth |
| K03.3 | Pathological resorption of teeth |
| K03.4 | Hypercementosis |
| K03.5 | Ankylosis of teeth |
| K03.6 | Deposits [accretions] on teeth |
| K03.7 | Posteruptive color changes of dental hard tissues |
| K03.81 | Cracked tooth |
| K03.89 | Other specified diseases of hard tissues of teeth |

## Relative Value Units/Medicare Edits

| Non-Facility RVU | Work | PE | MP | Total |
|---|---|---|---|---|
| **D6740** | 6.20 | 5.47 | 1.28 | 12.95 |
| **D6750** | 6.74 | 5.95 | 1.39 | 14.08 |
| **D6751** | 5.76 | 5.08 | 1.19 | 12.03 |
| **D6752** | 6.20 | 5.47 | 1.28 | 12.95 |
| **D6753** | 4.54 | 4.01 | 0.93 | 9.48 |
| **Facility RVU** | **Work** | **PE** | **MP** | **Total** |
| **D6740** | 6.20 | 5.47 | 1.28 | 12.95 |
| **D6750** | 6.74 | 5.95 | 1.39 | 14.08 |
| **D6751** | 5.76 | 5.08 | 1.19 | 12.03 |
| **D6752** | 6.20 | 5.47 | 1.28 | 12.95 |
| **D6753** | 4.54 | 4.01 | 0.93 | 9.48 |

| | FUD | Status | MUE | Modifiers | | | | IOM Reference |
|---|---|---|---|---|---|---|---|---|
| **D6740** | N/A | N | - | N/A | N/A | N/A | N/A | None |
| **D6750** | N/A | N | - | N/A | N/A | N/A | N/A | |
| **D6751** | N/A | N | - | N/A | N/A | N/A | N/A | |
| **D6752** | N/A | N | - | N/A | N/A | N/A | N/A | |
| **D6753** | N/A | N | - | N/A | N/A | N/A | N/A | |

* with documentation

## Terms To Know

**abutment crown.** Artificial tooth cap for the retention and/or support of a dental prosthesis.

**artificial crown.** In dentistry, a ceramic or metal restoration made to cover or replace a major part of the top of a tooth.

**composite.** In dentistry, synthetic material such as acrylic resin and quartz particles used in tooth restoration.

**coping.** Thin covering that is placed over a tooth before attaching a crown or overdenture.

**denture.** Manmade substitution of natural teeth and neighboring structures.

**moulage.** Model of an anatomical structure formed via a negative impression in wax or plaster.

# D6780-D6784

**D6780** retainer crown - 3/4 cast high noble metal
**D6781** retainer crown - 3/4 cast predominantly base metal
**D6782** retainer crown - 3/4 cast noble metal
**D6783** retainer crown - 3/4 porcelain/ceramic
**D6784** retainer crown 3/4 - titanium and titanium alloys

## Explanation

A fixed partial denture retainer crown is made for a tooth that needs to be the connecting or anchoring tooth for the retainer but may be decayed or damaged enough to require restoration. The crown is made to accommodate the attachment of the retainer from impressions taken of the tooth's anatomy and the tooth with the retainer (see previous restorative crown codes D2780–D2783 for the method). Report D6780 for a cast high noble metal crown, D6781 for cast predominantly base metal, D6782 for cast noble metal, D6783 for a cast porcelain crown and D6784 for titanium and titanium alloys.

## Coding Tips

Local anesthesia is included in these services. Any evaluation or radiograph, core buildup, or post or preparation service is reported separately. For individual restorations, see D2710-D2799. Prefabricated crowns are reported using the appropriate code from the D2930-D2934 range; for abutment supported, see D6058-D6064 or D6094. Implant supported crowns are reported with a code from the D6065-D6067 range. Code D6710 should not be used to report a temporary or provisional prosthesis; see D6793. For crowns used as a fixed partial denture retainer fabricated using porcelain or ceramic, see codes D6740-D6752; for crowns used as a fixed partial denture retainer fabricated using resin-based materials, see D6710-D6722. Full crowns used for partial denture retainers are reported with the appropriate code in the D6790-D6792 range. A titanium fixed partial denture retainer crown is reported with D6794. High noble metals include gold, palladium, and platinum. The content must be ≥ 60 percent gold plus platinum and a minimum of ≥ 40 percent gold. Noble metals include 25 percent or less gold plus platinum group. Predominantly base alloys contain a noble metal content of < 25 percent gold plus platinum group. The metals of the platinum group include platinum, palladium, rhodium, iridium, osmium, and ruthenium. Porcelain/ceramic refers to pressed, fired, polished, or milled substances, which predominantly contain inorganic refractory compounds such as porcelains, glasses, ceramics, and glass-ceramics.

## Documentation Tips

Documentation should indicate the location and number of missing teeth.

## Reimbursement Tips

Payers may require documentation including the tooth number and preoperative periapical x-rays showing the entire treatment site.

## ICD-10-CM Diagnostic Codes

| | |
|---|---|
| K02.3 | Arrested dental caries |
| K02.51 | Dental caries on pit and fissure surface limited to enamel |
| K02.52 | Dental caries on pit and fissure surface penetrating into dentin |
| K02.53 | Dental caries on pit and fissure surface penetrating into pulp |
| K02.61 | Dental caries on smooth surface limited to enamel |
| K02.62 | Dental caries on smooth surface penetrating into dentin |
| K02.63 | Dental caries on smooth surface penetrating into pulp |
| K02.7 | Dental root caries |
| K03.0 | Excessive attrition of teeth |
| K03.1 | Abrasion of teeth |
| K03.2 | Erosion of teeth |
| K03.3 | Pathological resorption of teeth |
| K03.4 | Hypercementosis |
| K03.5 | Ankylosis of teeth |
| K03.6 | Deposits [accretions] on teeth |
| K03.7 | Posteruptive color changes of dental hard tissues |
| K03.81 | Cracked tooth |
| K03.89 | Other specified diseases of hard tissues of teeth |

## Relative Value Units/Medicare Edits

| Non-Facility RVU | Work | PE | MP | Total |
|---|---|---|---|---|
| **D6780** | 6.05 | 5.34 | 1.25 | 12.64 |
| **D6781** | 5.77 | 5.09 | 1.19 | 12.05 |
| **D6782** | 5.46 | 4.82 | 1.12 | 11.40 |
| **D6783** | 5.92 | 5.22 | 1.22 | 12.36 |
| **D6784** | 3.75 | 3.31 | 0.77 | 7.83 |
| **Facility RVU** | **Work** | **PE** | **MP** | **Total** |
| **D6780** | 6.05 | 5.34 | 1.25 | 12.64 |
| **D6781** | 5.77 | 5.09 | 1.19 | 12.05 |
| **D6782** | 5.46 | 4.82 | 1.12 | 11.40 |
| **D6783** | 5.92 | 5.22 | 1.22 | 12.36 |
| **D6784** | 3.75 | 3.31 | 0.77 | 7.83 |

| | FUD | Status | MUE | Modifiers | | | | IOM Reference |
|---|---|---|---|---|---|---|---|---|
| **D6780** | N/A | N | - | N/A | N/A | N/A | N/A | None |
| **D6781** | N/A | N | - | N/A | N/A | N/A | N/A | |
| **D6782** | N/A | N | - | N/A | N/A | N/A | N/A | |
| **D6783** | N/A | N | - | N/A | N/A | N/A | N/A | |
| **D6784** | N/A | N | - | N/A | N/A | N/A | N/A | |

* with documentation

## Terms To Know

**abutment crown.** Artificial tooth cap for the retention and/or support of a dental prosthesis.

**artificial crown.** In dentistry, a ceramic or metal restoration made to cover or replace a major part of the top of a tooth.

**composite.** In dentistry, synthetic material such as acrylic resin and quartz particles used in tooth restoration.

**coping.** Thin covering that is placed over a tooth before attaching a crown or overdenture.

**denture.** Manmade substitution of natural teeth and neighboring structures.

**moulage.** Model of an anatomical structure formed via a negative impression in wax or plaster.

# D6790-D6792

**D6790** retainer crown - full cast high noble metal
**D6791** retainer crown - full cast predominantly base metal
**D6792** retainer crown - full cast noble metal

## Explanation

A fixed partial denture retainer crown is made for a tooth that needs to be the connecting or anchoring tooth for the retainer but may be decayed or damaged enough to require restoration. The crown is made to accommodate the attachment of the retainer from impressions taken of the tooth's anatomy and the tooth with the retainer (see previous restorative crown codes D2790-D2792 for the method). Report D6790 for a full cast high noble metal crown, D6791 for full cast of predominantly base metal, and D6792 for full cast noble metal.

## Coding Tips

Local anesthesia is included in these services. Any evaluation or radiograph, core buildup, or post or preparation service is reported separately. For individual restorations, see D2710–D2799. Prefabricated crowns are reported using the appropriate code from the D2930–D2934 range; for abutment supported, see D6058–D6064 or D6094. Implant supported crowns are reported with a code from the D6065–D6067 range. Code D6710 should not be used to report a temporary or provisional prosthesis, see D6793. For crowns used as a fixed partial denture retainer fabricated using porcelain or ceramic, see codes D6740–D6752; for 3/4 cast metals or porcelain/ceramics, see D6780–D6783. For crowns used as a fixed partial denture retainer fabricated using resin based materials, see D6710–D6722. A titanium fixed partial denture retainer crown is reported with D6794. High noble metals include gold, palladium, and platinum. The content must be ≥ 60 percent gold plus platinum and ≥ 40 percent gold. Noble metals include 25 percent or less gold plus platinum group. Predominantly base alloys contain a noble metal content of < 25 percent gold plus platinum group. The metals of the platinum group include platinum, palladium, rhodium, iridium, osmium, and ruthenium.

## Documentation Tips

The following information should be documented on a tooth chart: treatment/location of caries, endodontic procedures, prosthetic services, preventive services, treatment of lesions and dental disease, or other special procedures. A tooth chart may also be used to identify structure and rationale of disease process, and the type of service performed on intraoral structures other than teeth.

## Reimbursement Tips

Payers may require documentation including the tooth number and preoperative periapical x-rays showing the entire treatment site.

## ICD-10-CM Diagnostic Codes

| | |
|---|---|
| K02.51 | Dental caries on pit and fissure surface limited to enamel |
| K02.52 | Dental caries on pit and fissure surface penetrating into dentin |
| K02.53 | Dental caries on pit and fissure surface penetrating into pulp |
| K02.61 | Dental caries on smooth surface limited to enamel |
| K02.62 | Dental caries on smooth surface penetrating into dentin |
| K02.63 | Dental caries on smooth surface penetrating into pulp |
| K02.7 | Dental root caries |
| K03.0 | Excessive attrition of teeth |
| K03.1 | Abrasion of teeth |
| K03.2 | Erosion of teeth |
| K03.3 | Pathological resorption of teeth |
| K03.4 | Hypercementosis |
| K03.5 | Ankylosis of teeth |
| K03.6 | Deposits [accretions] on teeth |
| K03.7 | Posteruptive color changes of dental hard tissues |
| K03.81 | Cracked tooth |
| K03.89 | Other specified diseases of hard tissues of teeth |

## Relative Value Units/Medicare Edits

| Non-Facility RVU | Work | PE | MP | Total |
|---|---|---|---|---|
| **D6790** | 6.16 | 5.43 | 1.27 | 12.86 |
| **D6791** | 5.51 | 4.86 | 1.13 | 11.50 |
| **D6792** | 5.91 | 5.22 | 1.22 | 12.35 |
| **Facility RVU** | **Work** | **PE** | **MP** | **Total** |
| **D6790** | 6.16 | 5.43 | 1.27 | 12.86 |
| **D6791** | 5.51 | 4.86 | 1.13 | 11.50 |
| **D6792** | 5.91 | 5.22 | 1.22 | 12.35 |

| | FUD | Status | MUE | Modifiers | | | | IOM Reference |
|---|---|---|---|---|---|---|---|---|
| **D6790** | N/A | N | - | N/A | N/A | N/A | N/A | None |
| **D6791** | N/A | N | - | N/A | N/A | N/A | N/A | |
| **D6792** | N/A | N | - | N/A | N/A | N/A | N/A | |

* with documentation

## Terms To Know

**abutment crown.** Artificial tooth cap for the retention and/or support of a dental prosthesis.

**artificial crown.** In dentistry, a ceramic or metal restoration made to cover or replace a major part of the top of a tooth.

**composite.** In dentistry, synthetic material such as acrylic resin and quartz particles used in tooth restoration.

**coping.** Thin covering that is placed over a tooth before attaching a crown or overdenture.

**denture.** Manmade substitution of natural teeth and neighboring structures.

**moulage.** Model of an anatomical structure formed via a negative impression in wax or plaster.

# D6793

▲ **D6793** interim retainer crown - further treatment or completion of diagnosis necessary prior to final impression

*Not to be used as a temporary retainer crown for a routine prosthetic restoration.*

## Explanation

A fixed partial denture retainer crown is made for a tooth that needs to be the connecting or anchoring tooth for the retainer but may be decayed or damaged enough to require restoration. The crown is made to accommodate the attachment of the retainer from impressions taken of the tooth's anatomy and the tooth with the retainer (see previous restorative crown codes D2790–D2792 for the method). Use code D6793 to report a provisional retainer crown.

## Coding Tips

Code D6793 is an out-of-sequence code and will not display in numeric order in the CDT manual. It should be reported when the retainer crown will be used for at least six months during the restorative treatment. This code should not be used to report a temporary retainer crown for routine prosthetic fixed partial denture restoration. To report a provisional crown, see D2799. Local anesthesia is included in this service. Any evaluation or radiograph, core buildup, or post or preparation service is reported separately. Most third-party payers do not cover interim or temporary services. However, long-term (six months or longer) use may be covered on a by-report basis. Check with third-party payers for their specific guidelines.

## Documentation Tips

The following information should be documented on a tooth chart: treatment/location of caries, endodontic procedures, prosthetic services, preventive services, treatment of lesions and dental disease, or other special procedures. A tooth chart may also be used to identify structure and rationale of disease process, and the type of service performed on intraoral structures other than teeth.

## Reimbursement Tips

Coverage guidelines vary by payer and by patient contract. Patients are often responsible for copayments or they may reach contract limitations. Check with the payer to determine coverage policies and patient responsibility.
Check with the payer to determine coverage policies and patient responsibility.

## ICD-10-CM Diagnostic Codes

| | |
|---|---|
| K02.3 | Arrested dental caries |
| K02.51 | Dental caries on pit and fissure surface limited to enamel |
| K02.52 | Dental caries on pit and fissure surface penetrating into dentin |
| K02.53 | Dental caries on pit and fissure surface penetrating into pulp |
| K02.61 | Dental caries on smooth surface limited to enamel |
| K02.62 | Dental caries on smooth surface penetrating into dentin |
| K02.63 | Dental caries on smooth surface penetrating into pulp |
| K02.7 | Dental root caries |
| K03.0 | Excessive attrition of teeth |
| K03.1 | Abrasion of teeth |
| K03.2 | Erosion of teeth |
| K03.3 | Pathological resorption of teeth |
| K03.4 | Hypercementosis |
| K03.5 | Ankylosis of teeth |
| K03.6 | Deposits [accretions] on teeth |
| K03.7 | Posteruptive color changes of dental hard tissues |
| K03.81 | Cracked tooth |
| K03.89 | Other specified diseases of hard tissues of teeth |

## Relative Value Units/Medicare Edits

| Non-Facility RVU | Work | PE | MP | Total |
|---|---|---|---|---|
| **D6793** | 2.67 | 2.35 | 0.55 | 5.57 |
| **Facility RVU** | **Work** | **PE** | **MP** | **Total** |
| **D6793** | 2.67 | 2.35 | 0.55 | 5.57 |

| | FUD | Status | MUE | Modifiers | | | | IOM Reference |
|---|---|---|---|---|---|---|---|---|
| **D6793** | N/A | N | - | N/A | N/A | N/A | N/A | None |

* with documentation

## Terms To Know

**abutment crown.** Artificial tooth cap for the retention and/or support of a dental prosthesis.

**artificial crown.** In dentistry, a ceramic or metal restoration made to cover or replace a major part of the top of a tooth.

**composite.** In dentistry, synthetic material such as acrylic resin and quartz particles used in tooth restoration.

**coping.** Thin covering that is placed over a tooth before attaching a crown or overdenture.

**denture.** Manmade substitution of natural teeth and neighboring structures.

**moulage.** Model of an anatomical structure formed via a negative impression in wax or plaster.

Dental - Fixed Prosthodontics

# D6794

**D6794** retainer crown - titanium and titanium alloys

## Explanation

A fixed, partial denture retainer crown is made for a connecting or anchoring tooth that is decayed or damaged. The crown is made to accommodate the attachment of the retainer from impressions taken of the tooth's anatomy. The dentist takes an upper and lower bite impression of the section of the mouth containing the tooth to be crowned and sends it to the lab. Plaster is poured into the impression mold with pins placed for later removal, connected to an articulator with more plaster, and then the poured model is removed. The prepped tooth is isolated. The margins are trimmed and marked. A spacer substance is painted on to represent the exact allowance needed for cementing the crown onto the tooth. A wax layer model, or coping, is made for the support layer of the crown and encased with a channel in high-density plaster. The wax is burned out. The coping model is filled with molten metal, spun on the arm of a centrifuge. If the crown is not made with a metal support, other pressing methods are used to cast the model. The metal support coping is tested on the tooth model, cleaned, and prepped for bonding so the resin layers of the crown may be completed over the metal coping support. The crown is contoured, shaped, checked for stain, color, and all contacts and sent back to the dentist who tries the crown on the patient, checking all contact points, margins, and coloring. When the patient is satisfied with the crown, the dentist cements it onto the tooth. Report D6794 for a titanium or titanium alloy crown.

## Coding Tips

This is an out-of-sequence code and will not display in numeric order in the CDT book. Local anesthesia is included in these services. Any evaluation or radiograph, core buildup, or post or preparation service is reported separately. Payers may require documentation including the tooth number, surface(s), and preoperative periapical x-ray. For individual restorations, see D2710–D2799. Prefabricated crowns are reported using the appropriate code from the D2930–D2934 range; for abutment supported, see D6058–D6064 or D6094. Implant supported crowns are reported with a code from the D6065–D6067 range. Code D6710 should not be used to report a temporary or provisional prosthesis, see D6793. For crowns used as a fixed partial denture retainer fabricated using porcelain or ceramic, see codes D6740–D6752; for 3/4 cast metals or porcelain/ceramics, see D6780–D6783. Full crowns used for partial denture retainers are reported with the appropriate code in the D6790–D6792 range.

## Documentation Tips

The following information should be documented on a tooth chart: treatment/location of caries, endodontic procedures, prosthetic services, preventive services, treatment of lesions and dental disease, or other special procedures. A tooth chart may also be used to identify structure and rationale of disease process, and the type of service performed on intraoral structures other than teeth.

## Reimbursement Tips

Coverage guidelines vary by payer and by patient contract. Patients are often responsible for copayments or they may reach contract limitations. Check with the payer to determine coverage policies and patient responsibility.

## ICD-10-CM Diagnostic Codes

| | |
|---|---|
| K02.3 | Arrested dental caries |
| K02.51 | Dental caries on pit and fissure surface limited to enamel |
| K02.52 | Dental caries on pit and fissure surface penetrating into dentin |
| K02.53 | Dental caries on pit and fissure surface penetrating into pulp |
| K02.61 | Dental caries on smooth surface limited to enamel |
| K02.62 | Dental caries on smooth surface penetrating into dentin |
| K02.63 | Dental caries on smooth surface penetrating into pulp |
| K02.7 | Dental root caries |
| K02.9 | Dental caries, unspecified |
| K03.0 | Excessive attrition of teeth |
| K03.1 | Abrasion of teeth |
| K03.2 | Erosion of teeth |
| K03.3 | Pathological resorption of teeth |
| K03.4 | Hypercementosis |
| K03.5 | Ankylosis of teeth |
| K03.6 | Deposits [accretions] on teeth |
| K03.7 | Posteruptive color changes of dental hard tissues |
| K03.81 | Cracked tooth |
| K03.89 | Other specified diseases of hard tissues of teeth |
| K03.9 | Disease of hard tissues of teeth, unspecified |

## Relative Value Units/Medicare Edits

| Non-Facility RVU | Work | PE | MP | Total |
|---|---|---|---|---|
| **D6794** | 5.65 | 4.98 | 1.16 | 11.79 |
| **Facility RVU** | **Work** | **PE** | **MP** | **Total** |
| **D6794** | 5.65 | 4.98 | 1.16 | 11.79 |

| | FUD | Status | MUE | Modifiers | | | | IOM Reference |
|---|---|---|---|---|---|---|---|---|
| **D6794** | N/A | N | - | N/A | N/A | N/A | N/A | None |

* with documentation

## Terms To Know

**abutment crown.** Artificial tooth cap for the retention and/or support of a dental prosthesis.

**artificial crown.** In dentistry, a ceramic or metal restoration made to cover or replace a major part of the top of a tooth.

**denture.** Manmade substitution of natural teeth and neighboring structures.

# D6920

**D6920** connector bar

*A device attached to fixed partial denture retainer or coping which serves to stabilize and anchor a removable overdenture prosthesis.*

## Explanation

A connector bar can be classified as either minor or major. The minor connector joins the smaller dental components, such as clasps, to the major connector, which unifies the structure of the fixed partial denture and spreads the loading between the abutment teeth. The connectors contribute to the support and bracing of the denture and provide indirect retention by, for example, in the upper jaw covering the palatal mucosa. The design of the connector differs for the upper jaw compared with that for the lower jaw.

## Coding Tips

To report the fixed partial denture, see D5211–D5283. To report overdenture, see D5863–D5866. Local anesthesia is generally considered part of restorative procedures.

## Documentation Tips

Dentists should be certain that sufficient documentation is provided in the dental records to accurately verify and describe the services rendered. Additionally, records should be legible and signed with the appropriate name and title of the provider of the service.

## Reimbursement Tips

Coverage for these procedures varies by payer and by individual contract. Check with payers for specific coverage guidelines.

## ICD-10-CM Diagnostic Codes

| | |
|---|---|
| Z46.3 | Encounter for fitting and adjustment of dental prosthetic device |

## Relative Value Units/Medicare Edits

| Non-Facility RVU | Work | PE | MP | Total |
|---|---|---|---|---|
| D6920 | 2.07 | 1.83 | 0.43 | 4.33 |
| Facility RVU | Work | PE | MP | Total |
| D6920 | 2.07 | 1.83 | 0.43 | 4.33 |

| | FUD | Status | MUE | Modifiers | | | | IOM Reference |
|---|---|---|---|---|---|---|---|---|
| D6920 | N/A | R | - | N/A | N/A | N/A | 80* | 100-02,1,70; 100-04,4,20.5 |

* with documentation

## Terms To Know

**denture.** Manmade substitution of natural teeth and neighboring structures.

# D6930

**D6930** re-cement or re-bond fixed partial denture

## Explanation

The dentist recements the final prosthesis onto fixed abutments. This may be done in cases of allergies to the existing adhesive and to repair or replace damaged prosthesis adhesive.

## Coding Tips

Local anesthesia is generally considered part of restorative procedures. Payers may require the provider to indicate the tooth number of each tooth included in the bridge.

## Documentation Tips

Dentists should be certain that sufficient documentation is provided in the dental records to accurately verify and describe the services rendered. Additionally, records should be legible and signed with the appropriate name and title of the provider of the service.

## Reimbursement Tips

Coverage guidelines vary by payer and by patient contract. Patients are often responsible for copayments or they may reach contract limitations. Check with the payer to determine coverage policies and patient responsibility.

## ICD-10-CM Diagnostic Codes

| | |
|---|---|
| Z46.3 | Encounter for fitting and adjustment of dental prosthetic device |
| Z97.2 | Presence of dental prosthetic device (complete) (partial) |

## Relative Value Units/Medicare Edits

| Non-Facility RVU | Work | PE | MP | Total |
|---|---|---|---|---|
| D6930 | 0.72 | 0.64 | 0.15 | 1.51 |
| Facility RVU | Work | PE | MP | Total |
| D6930 | 0.72 | 0.64 | 0.15 | 1.51 |

| | FUD | Status | MUE | Modifiers | | | | IOM Reference |
|---|---|---|---|---|---|---|---|---|
| D6930 | N/A | N | - | N/A | N/A | N/A | N/A | None |

* with documentation

## Terms To Know

**abutment.** Tooth or implant fixture supporting a prosthesis.

**denture.** Manmade substitution of natural teeth and neighboring structures.

**denture base.** Portion of the artificial substitute for natural teeth that makes contact with the soft tissue of the mouth and serves as the anchor for the artificial teeth.

**fixed.** Not able to be removed easily.

**moulage.** Model of an anatomical structure formed via a negative impression in wax or plaster.

**oral soft tissue.** Subcutaneous fat layers beneath oral mucosa or gingiva; excludes bone and teeth.

**palatal.** Pertaining to the palate or an area toward the palate.

# D6940

**D6940** stress breaker

*A non-rigid connector.*

## Explanation

A stress breaker for a fixed partial denture is designed to relieve the abutment teeth and their supporting tissues from harmful stresses that can cause excessive wear. The stress breaker is often attached to the root using a precision attachment such as a magnet.

## Coding Tips

To report a connector bar, see D6920. To report a precision attachment, see D6950. Local anesthesia is generally considered part of this service. Coverage for these procedures varies by payer and by individual contract.

## Documentation Tips

Dentists should be certain that sufficient documentation is provided in the dental records to accurately verify and describe the services rendered. Additionally, records should be legible and signed with the appropriate name and title of the provider of the service.

## Reimbursement Tips

Payers may require documentation including the tooth number and preoperative periapical x-rays showing the entire treatment site. Coverage guidelines vary by payer and by patient contract. Patients are often responsible for copayments or may reach contract limitations. Check with the payer to determine coverage policies and patient responsibility.

## ICD-10-CM Diagnostic Codes

| | |
|---|---|
| K03.0 | Excessive attrition of teeth |
| K03.1 | Abrasion of teeth |
| K03.2 | Erosion of teeth |

## Relative Value Units/Medicare Edits

| Non-Facility RVU | Work | PE | MP | Total |
|---|---|---|---|---|
| D6940 | 1.68 | 1.48 | 0.35 | 3.51 |
| **Facility RVU** | **Work** | **PE** | **MP** | **Total** |
| D6940 | 1.68 | 1.48 | 0.35 | 3.51 |

| | FUD | Status | MUE | Modifiers | | | | IOM Reference |
|---|---|---|---|---|---|---|---|---|
| D6940 | N/A | N | - | N/A | N/A | N/A | N/A | None |

* with documentation

## Terms To Know

**abutment.** Tooth or implant fixture supporting a prosthesis.

# D6950

▲ **D6950** precision attachment

*A pair of components constitutes one precision attachment that is separate from the prosthesis.*

## Explanation

Precision attachments are used to aid retention from the root for the fixed partial denture. There are several types, including studs, bars, magnets, and balls. Studs are placed in the root face, and the attachment (a clip) is retained in the denture. Bars are placed in the root face, also, but using a post system to hold the denture in place. The bar pattern is cut to follow the arch, and the bar's gingival skirt is shaped to fit the contour of the soft tissue. Magnets are positioned in the mouth and retained in the dentures using a self-care acrylic. Ball attachments permit the use of virtually any tooth to aid in the retention of the denture. The ball is attached below the gingiva to reduce stress on weak abutments.

## Coding Tips

Local anesthesia is generally considered part of this service.

## Reimbursement Tips

Coverage for these procedures varies by payer and by individual contract. Payers may require documentation including the tooth number, surface(s), and preoperative periapical x-ray. Check with payers for specific coverage guidelines.

## ICD-10-CM Diagnostic Codes

| | |
|---|---|
| K08.411 | Partial loss of teeth due to trauma, class I |
| K08.412 | Partial loss of teeth due to trauma, class II |
| K08.413 | Partial loss of teeth due to trauma, class III |
| K08.414 | Partial loss of teeth due to trauma, class IV |
| K08.421 | Partial loss of teeth due to periodontal diseases, class I |
| K08.422 | Partial loss of teeth due to periodontal diseases, class II |
| K08.423 | Partial loss of teeth due to periodontal diseases, class III |
| K08.424 | Partial loss of teeth due to periodontal diseases, class IV |
| K08.431 | Partial loss of teeth due to caries, class I |
| K08.432 | Partial loss of teeth due to caries, class II |
| K08.433 | Partial loss of teeth due to caries, class III |
| K08.434 | Partial loss of teeth due to caries, class IV |
| K08.491 | Partial loss of teeth due to other specified cause, class I |
| K08.492 | Partial loss of teeth due to other specified cause, class II |
| K08.493 | Partial loss of teeth due to other specified cause, class III |
| K08.494 | Partial loss of teeth due to other specified cause, class IV |

## Relative Value Units/Medicare Edits

| Non-Facility RVU | Work | PE | MP | Total |
|---|---|---|---|---|
| D6950 | 3.10 | 2.74 | 0.64 | 6.48 |
| **Facility RVU** | **Work** | **PE** | **MP** | **Total** |
| D6950 | 3.10 | 2.74 | 0.64 | 6.48 |

| | FUD | Status | MUE | Modifiers | | | | IOM Reference |
|---|---|---|---|---|---|---|---|---|
| D6950 | N/A | N | - | N/A | N/A | N/A | N/A | None |

* with documentation

# D6980

**D6980** fixed partial denture repair necessitated by restorative material failure

## Explanation

This code describes the repair of a fixed partial denture, due to restorative material failure. Pertinent documentation to evaluate the medical appropriateness should be included when reporting this code for reimbursement.

## Coding Tips

Local anesthesia is generally considered part of restorative procedures.

## Documentation Tips

The following information should be documented on a tooth chart: treatment/location of caries, endodontic procedures, prosthetic services, preventive services, treatment of lesions and dental disease, or other special procedures. A tooth chart may also be used to identify structure and rationale of disease process, and the type of service performed on intraoral structures other than teeth.

## Reimbursement Tips

Payers allowance for repair of a fixed bridge may be limited to one half of the allowance for the replacement cost of the appliance. Pertinent documentation to evaluate medical appropriateness, the extent, and the duration of the treatment or repair should be provided with the claim. Payers may require documentation including the tooth number, surface(s), and preoperative periapical x-ray. Payment is usually determined after the report is received.

## ICD-10-CM Diagnostic Codes

Z97.2 Presence of dental prosthetic device (complete) (partial)

## Relative Value Units/Medicare Edits

| Non-Facility RVU | Work | PE | MP | Total |
|---|---|---|---|---|
| D6980 | 1.24 | 1.09 | 0.26 | 2.59 |
| **Facility RVU** | **Work** | **PE** | **MP** | **Total** |
| D6980 | 1.24 | 1.09 | 0.26 | 2.59 |

| | FUD | Status | MUE | Modifiers | | | | IOM Reference |
|---|---|---|---|---|---|---|---|---|
| D6980 | N/A | N | - | N/A | N/A | N/A | N/A | None |

* with documentation

## Terms To Know

**partial dentures.** In dentistry, artificial teeth composed of a framework with plastic teeth and gum area replacing part but not all of the natural teeth. The framework can either be formed from an acrylic resin base, cast metal or may be made more flexible using thermoplastics.

# D6985

**D6985** pediatric partial denture, fixed

*This prosthesis is used primarily for aesthetic purposes.*

## Explanation

The pediatric fixed partial denture may be constructed to replace teeth lost due to trauma or disease. Several appointments with a dentist are required to develop a working model of the denture, and follow-up visits may be more frequent than with adults for oral hygiene purposes and to track changing conditions in the mouth of the pediatric patient.

## Coding Tips

The ADA considers a patient to be an adult at age 12 for any service except orthodontics or sealants. This procedure is primarily used for cosmetic purposes and, therefore, may not be reimbursable by the third-party payer.

## Reimbursement Tips

This procedure is primarily used for cosmetic purposes and, therefore, may not be reimbursable by the third-party payer.

## ICD-10-CM Diagnostic Codes

K00.0 Anodontia
K00.6 Disturbances in tooth eruption
K00.8 Other disorders of tooth development
K00.9 Disorder of tooth development, unspecified
K01.0 Embedded teeth
K08.401 Partial loss of teeth, unspecified cause, class I
K08.402 Partial loss of teeth, unspecified cause, class II
K08.403 Partial loss of teeth, unspecified cause, class III
K08.404 Partial loss of teeth, unspecified cause, class IV
K08.409 Partial loss of teeth, unspecified cause, unspecified class
K08.411 Partial loss of teeth due to trauma, class I
K08.412 Partial loss of teeth due to trauma, class II
K08.413 Partial loss of teeth due to trauma, class III
K08.414 Partial loss of teeth due to trauma, class IV
K08.419 Partial loss of teeth due to trauma, unspecified class
K08.421 Partial loss of teeth due to periodontal diseases, class I
K08.422 Partial loss of teeth due to periodontal diseases, class II
K08.423 Partial loss of teeth due to periodontal diseases, class III
K08.424 Partial loss of teeth due to periodontal diseases, class IV
K08.429 Partial loss of teeth due to periodontal diseases, unspecified class
K08.431 Partial loss of teeth due to caries, class I
K08.432 Partial loss of teeth due to caries, class II
K08.433 Partial loss of teeth due to caries, class III
K08.434 Partial loss of teeth due to caries, class IV
K08.439 Partial loss of teeth due to caries, unspecified class
K08.491 Partial loss of teeth due to other specified cause, class I
K08.492 Partial loss of teeth due to other specified cause, class II
K08.493 Partial loss of teeth due to other specified cause, class III
K08.494 Partial loss of teeth due to other specified cause, class IV
K08.499 Partial loss of teeth due to other specified cause, unspecified class

## Relative Value Units/Medicare Edits

| Non-Facility RVU | Work | PE | MP | Total |
|---|---|---|---|---|
| D6985 | 3.24 | 2.86 | 0.67 | 6.77 |
| **Facility RVU** | **Work** | **PE** | **MP** | **Total** |
| D6985 | 3.24 | 2.86 | 0.67 | 6.77 |

| | FUD | Status | MUE | Modifiers | | | | IOM Reference |
|---|---|---|---|---|---|---|---|---|
| D6985 | N/A | N | - | N/A | N/A | N/A | N/A | None |

* with documentation

## Terms To Know

**fixed.** Not able to be removed easily.

**partial dentures.** In dentistry, artificial teeth composed of a framework with plastic teeth and gum area replacing part but not all of the natural teeth. The framework can either be formed from an acrylic resin base, cast metal or may be made more flexible using thermoplastics.

**pediatric patient.** Patient usually younger than 14 years of age.

Dental - Fixed Prosthodontics

# D7111

**D7111** extraction, coronal remnants - primary tooth

*Removal of soft tissue-retained coronal remnants.*

## Explanation

The dentist removes coronal remnants of a primary (deciduous) tooth that have been retained in the oral soft tissue. Local anesthesia is given and the tooth remnants are grasped with hand instruments and removed. If the remnants have become embedded, small incisions may be necessary to locate and remove them. This includes the local anesthesia, the routine postoperative care, and any suturing for closure that may be needed.

## Coding Tips

To report the surgical removal of an erupted tooth, see D7210. To report the removal of an impacted tooth, see D7220–D7250. The removal of an erupted tooth or exposed root is reported using D7140. Local anesthesia is included in this service. Suturing, if needed, is included in this service. Any evaluation or radiograph is reported separately. Pathology exam of tissue with interpretation is reported separately. Conscious sedation or general anesthesia if required for the procedure is reported separately. Routine postoperative care is included in this service.

## Reimbursement Tips

Coverage guidelines vary by payer and by patient contract. Patients are often responsible for copayments or they may reach contract limitations. Check with the payer to determine coverage policies and patient responsibility.

## ICD-10-CM Diagnostic Codes

K08.3 Retained dental root

## Relative Value Units/Medicare Edits

| Non-Facility RVU | Work | PE | MP | Total |
|---|---|---|---|---|
| D7111 | 0.66 | 0.58 | 0.14 | 1.38 |
| **Facility RVU** | **Work** | **PE** | **MP** | **Total** |
| D7111 | 0.66 | 0.58 | 0.14 | 1.38 |

| | FUD | Status | MUE | Modifiers | | | | IOM Reference |
|---|---|---|---|---|---|---|---|---|
| D7111 | N/A | R | - | N/A | N/A | N/A | N/A | 100-04,4,20.5 |

* with documentation

## Terms To Know

**coronal.** Relating to the top of a tooth or the crown of the head.

# D7140

**D7140** extraction, erupted tooth or exposed root (elevation and/or forceps removal)

*Includes removal of tooth structure, minor smoothing of socket bone, and closure, as necessary.*

## Explanation

An erupted tooth or exposed root is extracted by elevation and/or forceps method. This is considered a nonsurgical extraction. After local anesthesia is given and the patient is properly positioned, the socket is dilated by using the elevator between the tooth and the socket wall bone or the forceps blades are driven into the socket, applied to different aspects of the tooth, and pushed along the tooth root or into the bifurcation. The tooth is gripped in the forceps and removed by vertical force. The motion required for extracting the tooth, such as rotation, rocking, or buccal movement is dependent upon the tooth's anatomy. Exposed roots close to the alveolar margin are removed in a similar way, introducing an elevator between bone and the root and directing the root into its removal path or engaging the exposed root with forceps blades. This includes the local anesthesia, routine postoperative care, and any suturing for closure that may be needed.

## Coding Tips

To report the removal of an erupted tooth requiring the removal of bone and/or sectioning of tooth, see D7210. To report the removal of an impacted tooth, see D7220–D7250. The removal of coronal remnants of a deciduous tooth is reported using D7111. Local anesthesia is included in this service. Suturing, if needed, is included in this service. Any evaluation or radiograph is reported separately. Pathology exam of tissue with interpretation is reported separately. Conscious sedation or general anesthesia, if required, for the procedure is reported separately. Routine postoperative care is included in this service.

## Reimbursement Tips

Coverage guidelines vary by payer and by patient contract. Patients are often responsible for copayments or they may reach contract limitations. Check with the payer to determine coverage policies and patient responsibility.

## ICD-10-CM Diagnostic Codes

K02.51 Dental caries on pit and fissure surface limited to enamel
K02.52 Dental caries on pit and fissure surface penetrating into dentin
K02.53 Dental caries on pit and fissure surface penetrating into pulp
K02.61 Dental caries on smooth surface limited to enamel
K02.62 Dental caries on smooth surface penetrating into dentin
K02.63 Dental caries on smooth surface penetrating into pulp
K03.81 Cracked tooth
K05.211 Aggressive periodontitis, localized, slight
K05.212 Aggressive periodontitis, localized, moderate
K05.213 Aggressive periodontitis, localized, severe
K05.219 Aggressive periodontitis, localized, unspecified severity
K05.221 Aggressive periodontitis, generalized, slight
K05.222 Aggressive periodontitis, generalized, moderate
K05.223 Aggressive periodontitis, generalized, severe
K05.229 Aggressive periodontitis, generalized, unspecified severity
K05.30 Chronic periodontitis, unspecified
K05.311 Chronic periodontitis, localized, slight
K05.312 Chronic periodontitis, localized, moderate
K05.313 Chronic periodontitis, localized, severe
K05.319 Chronic periodontitis, localized, unspecified severity

| | |
|---|---|
| K05.321 | Chronic periodontitis, generalized, slight |
| K05.322 | Chronic periodontitis, generalized, moderate |
| K05.323 | Chronic periodontitis, generalized, severe |
| K05.329 | Chronic periodontitis, generalized, unspecified severity |
| K05.4 | Periodontosis |
| K05.5 | Other periodontal diseases |
| S02.5XXA | Fracture of tooth (traumatic), initial encounter for closed fracture |
| S02.5XXB | Fracture of tooth (traumatic), initial encounter for open fracture |

## Relative Value Units/Medicare Edits

| Non-Facility RVU | Work | PE | MP | Total |
|---|---|---|---|---|
| D7140 | 0.82 | 0.72 | 0.17 | 1.71 |
| Facility RVU | Work | PE | MP | Total |
| D7140 | 0.82 | 0.72 | 0.17 | 1.71 |

| | FUD | Status | MUE | Modifiers | | | | IOM Reference |
|---|---|---|---|---|---|---|---|---|
| D7140 | N/A | R | - | N/A | N/A | N/A | N/A | 100-02,1,70; 100-04,4,20.5 |

* with documentation

## Terms To Know

**buccal.** Relating to or toward the cheek.

**deciduous tooth.** Any of 20 teeth that usually erupt between the ages of 6 and 24 months and are later shed as the permanent, adult teeth displace them.

**erupted tooth.** Tooth that protrudes through the gingival soft tissues.

**extraction.** Removal of a tooth and tooth fragments from the alveolus.

**forceps.** Tool used for grasping or compressing tissue.

**furcation.** In dentistry, the area where roots separate in a multirooted tooth.

**local anesthesia.** Induced loss of feeling or sensation restricted to a certain area of the body, including topical, local tissue infiltration, field block, or nerve block methods.

**moderate sedation.** Medically controlled state of depressed consciousness, with or without analgesia, while maintaining the patient's airway, protective reflexes, and ability to respond to stimulation or verbal commands.

# D7210

**D7210** extraction, erupted tooth requiring removal of bone and/or sectioning of tooth, and including elevation of mucoperiosteal flap if indicated

*Includes related cutting of gingiva and bone, removal of tooth structure, minor smoothing of socket bone and closure.*

## Explanation

An erupted tooth is removed requiring removal of bone and/or sectioning of the tooth. It may also be necessary to elevate a mucoperiosteal flap. Surgical extraction is done when the root cannot be delivered. Any obstructions in the tooth's pathway for removal are identified and removed or another pathway for removal is created by sectioning the tooth. The root is exposed next by removing the minimum amount of bone for the maximum diameter of root and an elevator or surgical bur is placed between bone and tooth, applied to the root surface, and directed along the root to its natural withdrawal pathway. When necessary a flap is made along the gingival margin or ridge crest. The flap may be envelope, two or three sided, dependent upon the best way to achieve access. Relieving incisions on the side of the flap may also be used. After removal, the area is debrided and the created wound is closed.

## Coding Tips

To report the removal of an erupted tooth or exposed root by elevation and or forceps, see D7140. For the removal of an impacted tooth covered by soft tissue and requiring mucoperiosteal flap elevation, see D7220–D7250. Local anesthesia is included in this service. Suturing, if needed, is included in this service. Any evaluation or radiograph is reported separately. Pathology exam of tissue with interpretation is reported separately. If conscious sedation or general anesthesia is required for the procedure, it is reported separately. Routine postoperative care is included in this service.

## Documentation Tips

The following information should be documented on a tooth chart: treatment/location of caries, endodontic procedures, prosthetic services, preventive services, treatment of lesions and dental disease, or other special procedures. A tooth chart may also be used to identify structure and rationale of disease process, and the type of service performed on intraoral structures other than teeth.

## Reimbursement Tips

Coverage guidelines vary by payer and by patient contract. Patients are often responsible for copayments or they may reach contract limitations. Check with the payer to determine coverage policies and patient responsibility.

## ICD-10-CM Diagnostic Codes

| | |
|---|---|
| K02.51 | Dental caries on pit and fissure surface limited to enamel |
| K02.52 | Dental caries on pit and fissure surface penetrating into dentin |
| K02.53 | Dental caries on pit and fissure surface penetrating into pulp |
| K02.61 | Dental caries on smooth surface limited to enamel |
| K02.62 | Dental caries on smooth surface penetrating into dentin |
| K02.63 | Dental caries on smooth surface penetrating into pulp |
| K02.7 | Dental root caries |
| K03.0 | Excessive attrition of teeth |
| K03.1 | Abrasion of teeth |
| K03.2 | Erosion of teeth |
| K03.81 | Cracked tooth |
| K04.6 | Periapical abscess with sinus |
| K04.7 | Periapical abscess without sinus |
| K04.8 | Radicular cyst |

| | |
|---|---|
| K04.90 | Unspecified diseases of pulp and periapical tissues |
| K04.99 | Other diseases of pulp and periapical tissues |
| K05.00 | Acute gingivitis, plaque induced |
| K05.01 | Acute gingivitis, non-plaque induced |
| K05.10 | Chronic gingivitis, plaque induced |
| K05.11 | Chronic gingivitis, non-plaque induced |
| K05.20 | Aggressive periodontitis, unspecified |
| K05.30 | Chronic periodontitis, unspecified |
| K05.4 | Periodontosis |
| M27.1 | Giant cell granuloma, central |
| M27.2 | Inflammatory conditions of jaws |
| M27.3 | Alveolitis of jaws |
| M27.8 | Other specified diseases of jaws |
| M27.9 | Disease of jaws, unspecified |
| S02.5XXA | Fracture of tooth (traumatic), initial encounter for closed fracture |
| S02.5XXB | Fracture of tooth (traumatic), initial encounter for open fracture |

## Relative Value Units/Medicare Edits

| Non-Facility RVU | Work | PE | MP | Total |
|---|---|---|---|---|
| D7210 | 1.46 | 1.29 | 0.30 | 3.05 |
| **Facility RVU** | **Work** | **PE** | **MP** | **Total** |
| D7210 | 1.46 | 1.29 | 0.30 | 3.05 |

| | FUD | Status | MUE | Modifiers | | | | IOM Reference |
|---|---|---|---|---|---|---|---|---|
| D7210 | N/A | R | - | N/A | N/A | N/A | 80* | 100-02,1,70; 100-04,4,20.5 |

* with documentation

## Terms To Know

**buccal.** Relating to or toward the cheek.

**erupted tooth.** Tooth that protrudes through the gingival soft tissues.

**extraction.** Removal of a tooth and tooth fragments from the alveolus.

**forceps.** Tool used for grasping or compressing tissue.

**operculum.** Flap of tissue over a tooth that is either unerupted or only partially erupted.

**oral soft tissue.** Subcutaneous fat layers beneath oral mucosa or gingiva; excludes bone and teeth.

# D7220-D7250



**D7220** removal of impacted tooth - soft tissue

*Occlusal surface of tooth covered by soft tissue; requires mucoperiosteal flap elevation.*

**D7230** removal of impacted tooth - partially bony

*Part of crown covered by bone; requires mucoperiosteal flap elevation and bone removal.*

**D7240** removal of impacted tooth - completely bony

*Most or all of crown covered by bone; requires mucoperiosteal flap elevation and bone removal.*

**D7241** removal of impacted tooth - completely bony, with unusual surgical complications

*Most or all of crown covered by bone; unusually difficult or complicated due to factors such as nerve dissection required, separate closure of maxillary sinus required or aberrant tooth position.*

**D7250** removal of residual tooth roots (cutting procedure)

*Includes cutting of soft tissue and bone, removal of tooth structure, and closure.*

## Explanation

An impacted tooth is removed by extraction. For the average third molar impaction, an adequate flap is first made for access with a reverse bevel incision around the second molar, keeping to the crest of the ridge, and down into the buccal sulcus. The incision is extended to bone to reflect the tissue and retract it. The bone overlying the impacted tooth is carefully trephined with a drill while being irrigated and lifted off. This creates space needed for applying an elevator or bur and for tooth removal, especially if the tooth requires splitting to be removed in portions. With chisels or a bur, the pathway for withdrawal is cleared. The tooth may be split with a chisel or sectioned with the bur before removal. Elevators are placed and the tooth or fragments are delivered out with applied force. The socket is debrided and hemostasis is achieved with pressure. The flap is returned and the wound is closed. Report D7220 if the tooth surface is covered in soft tissue only and requires the flap elevation for removal. Report D7230 if the crown is partially covered by bone and D7240 if most of the crown is covered by bone. Report D7241 for removing a tooth completely impacted in bone that presents added difficulties or complications such as an aberrant tooth position, a nerve dissection, or separate closure of a sinus tract. Report D7250 for a similar procedure with cutting of soft tissue and bone to remove residual tooth roots, followed by closure.

## Coding Tips

Correct code assignment is dependent upon to what degree, if any, the crown is covered by bone. To report the removal of an erupted tooth or exposed root by elevation and or forceps, see D7140. For the extraction of an erupted tooth that requires the cutting of gingiva, bone, and tooth structures with minor smoothing of socket bone with closure, report D7210. Local anesthesia is included in these services. Suturing, if needed, is included in these services. Any evaluation or radiograph is reported separately. Pathology exam of tissue with interpretation is reported separately. If conscious sedation or general anesthesia is required for the procedure, it is reported separately. Routine postoperative care is included in these services. When reporting a code from the D7220–D7250 range, please note that some payers may require that x-rays and/or x-ray reports be submitted with the claim.

## Documentation Tips

Dentists should be certain that sufficient documentation is provided in the dental records to accurately verify and describe the services rendered. Additionally, records should be legible and signed with the appropriate name and title of the provider of the service.

## Reimbursement Tips

Coverage guidelines vary by payer and by patient contract. Patients are often responsible for copayments or they may reach contract limitations. Check with the payer to determine coverage policies and patient responsibility.

## ICD-10-CM Diagnostic Codes

K00.6 Disturbances in tooth eruption
K01.0 Embedded teeth
K01.1 Impacted teeth

## Relative Value Units/Medicare Edits

| Non-Facility RVU | Work | PE | MP | Total |
|---|---|---|---|---|
| D7220 | 1.79 | 1.58 | 0.37 | 3.74 |
| D7230 | 2.37 | 2.09 | 0.49 | 4.95 |
| D7240 | 2.79 | 2.46 | 0.57 | 5.82 |
| D7241 | 3.61 | 3.19 | 0.74 | 7.54 |
| D7250 | 1.52 | 1.34 | 0.31 | 3.17 |
| **Facility RVU** | **Work** | **PE** | **MP** | **Total** |
| D7220 | 1.79 | 1.58 | 0.37 | 3.74 |
| D7230 | 2.37 | 2.09 | 0.49 | 4.95 |
| D7240 | 2.79 | 2.46 | 0.57 | 5.82 |
| D7241 | 3.61 | 3.19 | 0.74 | 7.54 |
| D7250 | 1.52 | 1.34 | 0.31 | 3.17 |

| | FUD | Status | MUE | Modifiers | | | | IOM Reference |
|---|---|---|---|---|---|---|---|---|
| D7220 | N/A | R | - | N/A | N/A | N/A | 80* | 100-02,1,70; 100-04,4,20.5 |
| D7230 | N/A | R | - | N/A | N/A | N/A | 80* | |
| D7240 | N/A | R | - | N/A | N/A | N/A | 80* | |
| D7241 | N/A | R | - | N/A | N/A | N/A | 80* | |
| D7250 | N/A | R | - | N/A | N/A | N/A | 80* | |

* with documentation

## Terms To Know

**impacted tooth.** Tooth that is partially or totally unerupted that is unlikely to completely erupt because of its position to adjoining structures.

**residual root.** Remaining root portion after loss of 75 percent or more of the tooth crown.

# D7251

**D7251** coronectomy - intentional partial tooth removal

*Intentional partial tooth removal is performed when a neurovascular complication is likely if the entire impacted tooth is removed.*

## Explanation

A coronectomy is the removal of the clinical crown (exposed portion of the tooth). This procedure is often performed when extraction of lower third molars would result in damage to the inferior alveolar nerve (IAN). After local anesthesia and the patient is properly positioned, a conventional buccal flap incision is made, elevated, and retained with a Minnesota retractor. A lingual flap is raised and lingual tissue retracted after which the lingual nerve is protected using appropriate techniques. The clinical crown is transected and removed with tissue forceps. Following removal of the crown the root fragments are reduced to at least 3 mm below the crest of the lingual and buccal plates. After periosteal release, a watertight primary closure of the socket is performed.

## Coding Tips

To report the extraction of an erupted tooth or exposed root, see D7140. To report the extraction of a tooth or tooth section requiring elevation of mucoperiosteal flap, see D7210. Removal of an impacted tooth is reported with the appropriate code from the D7220–D7250 range.

## ICD-10-CM Diagnostic Codes

K02.51 Dental caries on pit and fissure surface limited to enamel
K02.52 Dental caries on pit and fissure surface penetrating into dentin
K02.53 Dental caries on pit and fissure surface penetrating into pulp
K02.61 Dental caries on smooth surface limited to enamel
K02.62 Dental caries on smooth surface penetrating into dentin
K02.63 Dental caries on smooth surface penetrating into pulp
K02.7 Dental root caries
K03.0 Excessive attrition of teeth
K03.1 Abrasion of teeth
K03.2 Erosion of teeth

## Relative Value Units/Medicare Edits

| Non-Facility RVU | Work | PE | MP | Total |
|---|---|---|---|---|
| D7251 | 3.16 | 2.79 | 0.65 | 6.60 |
| **Facility RVU** | **Work** | **PE** | **MP** | **Total** |
| D7251 | 3.16 | 2.79 | 0.65 | 6.60 |

| | FUD | Status | MUE | Modifiers | | | | IOM Reference |
|---|---|---|---|---|---|---|---|---|
| D7251 | N/A | I | - | N/A | N/A | N/A | N/A | None |

* with documentation

## Terms To Know

**clinical crown.** Part of the tooth that is not covered by any supporting structures such as the gums.

# D7270

**D7270** tooth reimplantation and/or stabilization of accidentally evulsed or displaced tooth

*Includes splinting and/or stabilization.*

## Explanation

A tooth that has been traumatically evulsed or displaced is reimplanted and stabilized with splinting. Dirt is carefully cleaned from the tooth without damaging the cementum. The length is usually recorded. The blood clot that has formed in the socket may be removed by gentle irrigation, if the patient is amenable to the additional procedure without loss of cooperation. There is still debate as to whether the presence of a blood clot between the root surface and the socket wall encourages root resorption or not. The tooth is then pushed firmly up into the socket. The tooth is splinted for seven to 10 days, usually with a practical splint made from a piece of stainless steel wire that is held onto the replanted tooth and its neighbors with acid-etch composite. Antibiotics are also normally prescribed for the immediate period after the reimplantation.

## Coding Tips

Any radiograph is reported separately.

## Reimbursement Tips

Third-party payers may require clinical documentation and/or x-rays before making payment determination. Check with payers to determine their specific requirements.

## ICD-10-CM Diagnostic Codes

| | |
|---|---|
| K08.111 | Complete loss of teeth due to trauma, class I |
| K08.112 | Complete loss of teeth due to trauma, class II |
| K08.113 | Complete loss of teeth due to trauma, class III |
| K08.114 | Complete loss of teeth due to trauma, class IV |
| K08.411 | Partial loss of teeth due to trauma, class I |
| K08.412 | Partial loss of teeth due to trauma, class II |
| K08.413 | Partial loss of teeth due to trauma, class III |
| K08.414 | Partial loss of teeth due to trauma, class IV |

## Relative Value Units/Medicare Edits

| Non-Facility RVU | Work | PE | MP | Total |
|---|---|---|---|---|
| D7270 | 2.78 | 2.45 | 0.57 | 5.80 |
| **Facility RVU** | **Work** | **PE** | **MP** | **Total** |
| D7270 | 2.78 | 2.45 | 0.57 | 5.80 |

| | FUD | Status | MUE | Modifiers | | | | IOM Reference |
|---|---|---|---|---|---|---|---|---|
| D7270 | N/A | N | - | N/A | N/A | N/A | N/A | None |

* with documentation

# D7272

**D7272** tooth transplantation (includes reimplantation from one site to another and splinting and/or stabilization)

## Explanation

A tooth is repositioned by transplanting it from one site to another and stabilizing it. This is normally done only when exposure and subsequent orthodontic movement were rejected. The maxillary canine is most commonly transplanted. First, the available space must be assessed to determine if the retrieved tooth can be accommodated. The tooth is exposed by creating and elevating a flap in the palate or buccal region as appropriate for access. The tooth is extracted only when it may be accomplished atraumatically and a new socket is created using a bur. The retrieved tooth is reimplanted without force up into the new socket space and the flap is closed with sutures. Some form of a splint that is not cemented is placed for seven to 10 days and the tooth is followed for early detection of root resorption.

## Coding Tips

Any radiograph is reported separately.

## Documentation Tips

The following information should be documented on a tooth chart: treatment/location of caries, endodontic procedures, prosthetic services, preventive services, treatment of lesions and dental disease, or other special procedures. A tooth chart may also be used to identify structure and rationale of disease process, and the type of service performed on intraoral structures other than teeth.

## ICD-10-CM Diagnostic Codes

| | |
|---|---|
| K00.6 | Disturbances in tooth eruption |
| K01.0 | Embedded teeth |
| K01.1 | Impacted teeth |
| K08.411 | Partial loss of teeth due to trauma, class I |
| K08.412 | Partial loss of teeth due to trauma, class II |
| K08.413 | Partial loss of teeth due to trauma, class III |
| K08.414 | Partial loss of teeth due to trauma, class IV |
| M26.31 | Crowding of fully erupted teeth |
| M26.32 | Excessive spacing of fully erupted teeth |
| M26.33 | Horizontal displacement of fully erupted tooth or teeth |
| M26.34 | Vertical displacement of fully erupted tooth or teeth |
| M26.35 | Rotation of fully erupted tooth or teeth |
| M26.51 | Abnormal jaw closure |
| S02.5XXA | Fracture of tooth (traumatic), initial encounter for closed fracture |
| S02.5XXB | Fracture of tooth (traumatic), initial encounter for open fracture |
| S03.2XXA | Dislocation of tooth, initial encounter |

## Relative Value Units/Medicare Edits

| Non-Facility RVU | Work | PE | MP | Total |
|---|---|---|---|---|
| D7272 | 3.75 | 3.31 | 0.77 | 7.83 |
| **Facility RVU** | **Work** | **PE** | **MP** | **Total** |
| D7272 | 3.75 | 3.31 | 0.77 | 7.83 |

| | FUD | Status | MUE | Modifiers | | | | IOM Reference |
|---|---|---|---|---|---|---|---|---|
| D7272 | N/A | N | - | N/A | N/A | N/A | N/A | None |

* with documentation

# D7280

**D7280** exposure of an unerupted tooth

*An incision is made and the tissue is reflected and bone removed as necessary to expose the crown of an impacted tooth not intended to be extracted.*

## Explanation

An unerupted tooth is accessed to aid in eruption, usually as preliminary orthodontic treatment help for unerupted canines and incisors when the apices are in good position for eruption. The tooth is exposed by creating a palatal or buccal flap and reflecting or excising some of the mucoperiosteum. Any sacrificable, impeding bone is removed with a chisel and the greatest diameter of crown is exposed. A bracket may be bonded at this time. The wound is packed with appropriate dressing and the flap is repositioned and sutured.

## Coding Tips

For the removal of an impacted tooth, see D7220–D7250. Any radiograph is reported separately.

## Reimbursement Tips

Coverage for these procedures varies by payer and by individual contract. Check with payers for specific coverage guidelines.

## ICD-10-CM Diagnostic Codes

| | |
|---|---|
| K00.2 | Abnormalities of size and form of teeth |
| K00.6 | Disturbances in tooth eruption |
| K01.0 | Embedded teeth |

## Relative Value Units/Medicare Edits

| Non-Facility RVU | Work | PE | MP | Total |
|---|---|---|---|---|
| D7280 | 2.51 | 2.22 | 0.52 | 5.25 |
| **Facility RVU** | **Work** | **PE** | **MP** | **Total** |
| D7280 | 2.51 | 2.22 | 0.52 | 5.25 |

| | FUD | Status | MUE | Modifiers | | | | IOM Reference |
|---|---|---|---|---|---|---|---|---|
| D7280 | N/A | N | - | N/A | N/A | N/A | N/A | None |

* with documentation

## Terms To Know

**apex.** Highest point of a root end of a tooth, or the end of any organ.

**buccal.** Relating to or toward the cheek.

**erupted tooth.** Tooth that protrudes through the gingival soft tissues.

**palatal.** Pertaining to the palate or an area toward the palate.

# D7282

**D7282** mobilization of erupted or malpositioned tooth to aid eruption

*To move/luxate teeth to eliminate ankylosis; not in conjunction with an extraction.*

## Explanation

An erupted or malpositioned tooth is mobilized to eliminate ankylosis, but not in conjunction with any extraction. Ankylosis is a fusion of the root cementum and the alveolar bone with obliteration of the periodontal ligament. This occurs in conjunction with external root resorption and gradual replacement of the root with bone. Ankylosis is a problem in replanted/transplanted teeth and with periapical/periodontal inflammatory disease, especially in younger patients whose alveolar growth has not all taken place. The alveolar process is that part of the jaw bones that supports and forms the tooth sockets. When ankylosis occurs, especially in young people, it creates a discrepancy in the contour of the alveolar bone as the other teeth continue to erupt and alveolar growth continues. The tooth to be mobilized is first accessed and exposed if not enough of the tooth is exposed to facilitate use of the elevator, which is used to luxate teeth. The elevator is a lever with a fulcrum, placed to engage the tooth and the interseptal bone. The operator applies force to the fulcrum point and mobilizes the tooth in its socket, disengaging the root from the bony wall and helping promote the growth of fibroblasts for periodontal ligament regeneration. The mobilized tooth may be stabilized for a few days.

## Coding Tips

Any radiograph is reported separately. Payers may consider this procedure to be part of a more complex procedure and separately reimbursable.

## Documentation Tips

The following information can be documented on a tooth chart: treatment/location of caries, endodontic procedures, prosthetic services, preventive services, treatment of lesions and dental disease, or other special procedures. A tooth chart may also be used to identify structure and rational or disease process and the type of service performed on intra-oral structure other than teeth. The documentation must be authenticated by the provider rendering the service.

## Reimbursement Tips

Coverage guidelines vary by payer and by patient contract. Patients are often responsible for copayments or may reach contract limitations. Check with the payer to determine coverage policies and patient responsibility.

## ICD-10-CM Diagnostic Codes

| | |
|---|---|
| K00.2 | Abnormalities of size and form of teeth |
| K00.6 | Disturbances in tooth eruption |
| K01.0 | Embedded teeth |
| M26.31 | Crowding of fully erupted teeth |
| M26.32 | Excessive spacing of fully erupted teeth |
| M26.33 | Horizontal displacement of fully erupted tooth or teeth |
| M26.34 | Vertical displacement of fully erupted tooth or teeth |
| M26.35 | Rotation of fully erupted tooth or teeth |
| M26.36 | Insufficient interocclusal distance of fully erupted teeth (ridge) |
| M26.37 | Excessive interocclusal distance of fully erupted teeth |
| M26.39 | Other anomalies of tooth position of fully erupted tooth or teeth |

## Relative Value Units/Medicare Edits

| Non-Facility RVU | Work | PE | MP | Total |
|---|---|---|---|---|
| D7282 | 1.73 | 1.53 | 0.36 | 3.62 |
| Facility RVU | Work | PE | MP | Total |
| D7282 | 1.73 | 1.53 | 0.36 | 3.62 |

| | FUD | Status | MUE | Modifiers | | | | IOM Reference |
|---|---|---|---|---|---|---|---|---|
| D7282 | N/A | N | - | N/A | N/A | N/A | N/A | None |

* with documentation

## Terms To Know

**alveolar process.** Bony part of the maxilla or mandible that supports the tooth roots and into which the teeth are implanted.

**ankylosis.** Abnormal union or fusion of bones in a joint, which is normally moveable.

**apex.** Highest point of a root end of a tooth, or the end of any organ.

**buccal.** Relating to or toward the cheek.

**erupted tooth.** Tooth that protrudes through the gingival soft tissues.

**palatal.** Pertaining to the palate or an area toward the palate.

**periodontal.** Relating to the tissues that support and surround the teeth.

# D7283

**D7283** placement of device to facilitate eruption of impacted tooth

*Placement of an attachment on an unerupted tooth, after its exposure, to aid in its eruption. Report the surgical exposure separately using D7280.*

## Explanation

Dense overlying bone, adjacent teeth, or excessive soft tissue may prevent a tooth from erupting within the expected time; the impacted tooth will remain with the patient for a lifetime unless surgically removed. To remove the tooth, the dentist may need to use orthodontic devices to manipulate the impacted tooth into position to facilitate eruption. To do so, the dentist creates a four-corner flap around the tooth, and the overlying bone is removed. The area is debrided, and a bracket is luted (sealed) to the tooth's surface. The bracket is attached by wire to the device, and the tooth is pulled into position for removal. The method of removal from here depends on whether the tooth is positioned toward the lips, toward the palate, or in the middle of the alveolar process. Any of the methods may require several incisions into the gingiva to prevent displacement of the orthodontic device.

## Coding Tips

To report the extraction of an impacted tooth, see D7220-D7250. When it is necessary to perform a surgical access to the tooth's crown, code D7280 may be reported separately.

## Documentation Tips

Treatment plan documentation should reflect any treatment failure, change in diagnosis, and/or a change in treatment plan. There should also be evidence of any initiation or reinstatement of a drug regime, which requires close and continuous skilled medical observation.

## Reimbursement Tips

This procedure may require preauthorization by the payer. Payers may require documentation on the claim form indicating the tooth on which the procedure was performed. Additionally, some payers may allow this procedure for only certain teeth. Check with payers for their specific guidelines. Local anesthesia is generally considered part of this procedure. Medically necessary orthodontia services are mandated under the Affordable Care Act (ACA) for those patients who have a severe handicapping malocclusion related to a medical condition. Medical record documentation must support the severity of the malocclusion and the medical condition. Some payers may require a standardized assessment, such as the Salzmann Evaluation Index be completed and that a specific score (for example 42 or higher) be documented.

## ICD-10-CM Diagnostic Codes

K00.6 Disturbances in tooth eruption
K01.1 Impacted teeth

## Relative Value Units/Medicare Edits

| Non-Facility RVU | Work | PE | MP | Total |
|---|---|---|---|---|
| D7283 | 1.63 | 1.44 | 0.34 | 3.41 |
| Facility RVU | Work | PE | MP | Total |
| D7283 | 1.63 | 1.44 | 0.34 | 3.41 |

| | FUD | Status | MUE | Modifiers | | | | IOM Reference |
|---|---|---|---|---|---|---|---|---|
| D7283 | N/A | R | - | N/A | N/A | N/A | N/A | None |

* with documentation

Dental - Oral and Maxillofacial Surgery

# D7285-D7286

**D7285** incisional biopsy of oral tissue-hard (bone, tooth)

*For partial removal of specimen only. This procedure involves biopsy of osseous lesions and is not used for apicoectomy/periradicular surgery. This procedure does not entail an excision.*

**D7286** incisional biopsy of oral tissue-soft

*For partial removal of an architecturally intact specimen only. This procedure is not used at the same time as codes for apicoectomy/periradicular curettage. This procedure does not entail an excision.*

## Explanation

A biopsy is taken of oral tissue. These codes are for the specimen removal only. Report D7285 for a biopsy sample taken from hard tissue (bone or tooth), such as from an osseous lesion. Report D7286 for a biopsy sample taken from soft tissue, which is all others. Do not use these codes for apicoectomy or periradicular surgery performed at the same time, or for the pathology procedures.

## Coding Tips

Check with the specific payer to determine coverage. To report amputation of apex of tooth (apicoectomy) or periradicular surgery, see D3410–D3426. Any evaluation or radiograph is reported separately. For pathology exam of tissue with interpretation and written report, see D0472, D0473, or D0474. Some payers may require that the pathology report be attached to the claim.

## Reimbursement Tips

This procedure may be covered by medical insurance. When covered by the patient's medical insurance, the payer may require that the appropriate CPT code be reported on the CMS-1500 claim form.

## Associated CPT Codes

| | |
|---|---|
| 20220 | Biopsy, bone, trocar, or needle; superficial (eg, ilium, sternum, spinous process, ribs) |
| 20240 | Biopsy, bone, open; superficial (eg, sternum, spinous process, rib, patella, olecranon process, calcaneus, tarsal, metatarsal, carpal, metacarpal, phalanx) |
| 40808 | Biopsy, vestibule of mouth |
| 41100 | Biopsy of tongue; anterior two-thirds |
| 41105 | Biopsy of tongue; posterior one-third |
| 41108 | Biopsy of floor of mouth |
| 42100 | Biopsy of palate, uvula |
| 42400 | Biopsy of salivary gland; needle |
| 42405 | Biopsy of salivary gland; incisional |
| 42800 | Biopsy; oropharynx |

## ICD-10-CM Diagnostic Codes

The application of this code is too broad to adequately present ICD-10-CM diagnostic code links here. Refer to your ICD-10-CM book.

## Relative Value Units/Medicare Edits

| Non-Facility RVU | Work | PE | MP | Total |
|---|---|---|---|---|
| D7285 | 4.28 | 3.77 | 0.88 | 8.93 |
| D7286 | 2.03 | 1.79 | 0.42 | 4.24 |
| **Facility RVU** | **Work** | **PE** | **MP** | **Total** |
| D7285 | 4.28 | 3.77 | 0.88 | 8.93 |
| D7286 | 2.03 | 1.79 | 0.42 | 4.24 |

| | FUD | Status | MUE | Modifiers | | | | IOM Reference |
|---|---|---|---|---|---|---|---|---|
| D7285 | N/A | I | - | N/A | N/A | N/A | N/A | None |
| D7286 | N/A | I | - | N/A | N/A | N/A | N/A | |

* with documentation

## Terms To Know

**biopsy.** Tissue or fluid removed for diagnostic purposes through analysis of the cells in the biopsy material.

**buccal mucosa.** Tissue from the mucous membrane on the inside of the cheek.

**mucosa.** Moist tissue lining the mouth (buccal mucosa), stomach (gastric mucosa), intestines, and respiratory tract.

**oral soft tissue.** Subcutaneous fat layers beneath oral mucosa or gingiva; excludes bone and teeth.

# D7287

**D7287** exfoliative cytological sample collection

*For collection of non-transepithelial cytology sample via mild scraping of the oral mucosa.*

## Explanation

A sample of cells is taken from the patient's mouth for cytology tests by mildly scraping the oral mucosa. Report this code for the sample collection only, not for the pathology examination.

## Coding Tips

Any evaluation or radiograph is reported separately. For pathology exam of tissue with interpretation and written report, see D0480. Coverage for these procedures varies by payer and by individual contract. Check with payers for their specific coverage guidelines. Additionally, third-party payers may require clinical documentation and/or x-rays before making payment determination.

## Documentation Tips

The following information should be documented on a tooth chart: treatment/location of caries, endodontic procedures, prosthetic services, preventive services, treatment of lesions and dental disease, or other special procedures. A tooth chart may also be used to identify structure and rationale of disease process, and the type of service performed on intraoral structures other than teeth.

## Reimbursement Tips

Coverage for these procedures varies by payer and by individual contract. Check with payers for their specific coverage guidelines. Additionally, third-party payers may require clinical documentation and/or x-rays before making payment determination.

## ICD-10-CM Diagnostic Codes

The application of this code is too broad to adequately present ICD-10-CM diagnostic code links here. Refer to your ICD-10-CM book.

## Relative Value Units/Medicare Edits

| Non-Facility RVU | Work | PE | MP | Total |
|---|---|---|---|---|
| D7287 | 0.88 | 0.77 | 0.18 | 1.83 |
| Facility RVU | Work | PE | MP | Total |
| D7287 | 0.88 | 0.77 | 0.18 | 1.83 |

| | FUD | Status | MUE | Modifiers | | | | IOM Reference |
|---|---|---|---|---|---|---|---|---|
| D7287 | N/A | I | - | N/A | N/A | N/A | N/A | None |

* with documentation

## Terms To Know

**cytology.** Examination of cells for pathology, physiology, and chemistry content.

**leukoplakia.** Thickened white patches or lesions appearing on a mucous membrane, such as oral mucosa or tongue.

**mucosa.** Moist tissue lining the mouth (buccal mucosa), stomach (gastric mucosa), intestines, and respiratory tract.

**pathology.** Medical science, and specialty practice, regarding all aspects of disease, with special reference to the essential nature, causes, and development of abnormal conditions, as well as the structural and functional changes that result from the disease processes.

# D7288

**D7288** brush biopsy - transepithelial sample collection

*For collection of oral disaggregated transepithelial cells via rotational brushing of the oral mucosa.*

## Explanation

The dentist performs a biopsy on a lesion in the vestibule of the mouth. The vestibule consists of the mucosal and submucosal tissue of the lips and cheeks within the oral cavity, not including the dentoalveolar structures. The dentist rubs a brush biopsy forceps along the area of the biopsy to obtain epithelial cells.

## Coding Tips

For biopsy of soft tissue of the oral cavity, see D7286. Documentation will indicate cell sampling of disaggregate transepithelial cells obtained using a rotational brushing.

## Documentation Tips

Dentists should be certain that sufficient documentation is provided in the dental records to accurately verify and describe the services rendered. Additionally, records should be legible and signed with the appropriate name and title of the provider of the service.

## Reimbursement Tips

Coverage for these procedures varies by payer and by individual contract. Check with payers for specific coverage guidelines.

## ICD-10-CM Diagnostic Codes

The application of this code is too broad to adequately present ICD-10-CM diagnostic code links here. Refer to your ICD-10-CM book.

## Relative Value Units/Medicare Edits

| Non-Facility RVU | Work | PE | MP | Total |
|---|---|---|---|---|
| D7288 | 0.91 | 0.80 | 0.19 | 1.90 |
| Facility RVU | Work | PE | MP | Total |
| D7288 | 0.91 | 0.80 | 0.19 | 1.90 |

| | FUD | Status | MUE | Modifiers | | | | IOM Reference |
|---|---|---|---|---|---|---|---|---|
| D7288 | N/A | R | - | N/A | N/A | N/A | N/A | None |

* with documentation

## Terms To Know

**biopsy.** Tissue or fluid removed for diagnostic purposes through analysis of the cells in the biopsy material.

**buccal mucosa.** Tissue from the mucous membrane on the inside of the cheek.

**mucosa.** Moist tissue lining the mouth (buccal mucosa), stomach (gastric mucosa), intestines, and respiratory tract.

**oral soft tissue.** Subcutaneous fat layers beneath oral mucosa or gingiva; excludes bone and teeth.

Dental - Oral and Maxillofacial Surgery

# D7290

**D7290** surgical repositioning of teeth

*Grafting procedure(s) is/are additional.*

## Explanation

A dentist may manipulate a tooth into its proper position using orthodontic appliances. In this procedure, the dentist creates a four-corner flap around the tooth to be repositioned, and the overlying bone tissue is removed. The area is debrided and, once the tooth is prepared by usual standard procedures that include application of primer, a bracket is luted (sealed) to the tooth's surface. The bracket is attached by wire to the orthodontic appliance (such as a gold chain), and the tooth is pulled into place. The soft tissue surrounding the tooth is sutured to provide the maximum coverage of the exposed tissue. A bur may be necessary to remove any overlying bone.

## Coding Tips

Local anesthesia is generally considered part of restorative procedures. Some payers may require that x-rays and/or x-ray reports be submitted with the claim.

## Documentation Tips

Some payers may require that x-rays and/or x-ray reports be submitted with the claim.

## Reimbursement Tips

Coverage may be available through the patient's medical insurance for this service requiring that the service be reported with the appropriate CPT code on a CMS-1500 claim form.

## ICD-10-CM Diagnostic Codes

| | |
|---|---|
| K00.6 | Disturbances in tooth eruption |
| K08.421 | Partial loss of teeth due to periodontal diseases, class I |
| K08.422 | Partial loss of teeth due to periodontal diseases, class II |
| K08.423 | Partial loss of teeth due to periodontal diseases, class III |
| K08.424 | Partial loss of teeth due to periodontal diseases, class IV |
| K08.431 | Partial loss of teeth due to caries, class I |
| K08.432 | Partial loss of teeth due to caries, class II |
| K08.433 | Partial loss of teeth due to caries, class III |
| K08.434 | Partial loss of teeth due to caries, class IV |
| M26.31 | Crowding of fully erupted teeth |
| M26.32 | Excessive spacing of fully erupted teeth |
| M26.33 | Horizontal displacement of fully erupted tooth or teeth |
| M26.34 | Vertical displacement of fully erupted tooth or teeth |
| M26.35 | Rotation of fully erupted tooth or teeth |
| M26.36 | Insufficient interocclusal distance of fully erupted teeth (ridge) |
| M26.37 | Excessive interocclusal distance of fully erupted teeth |

## Relative Value Units/Medicare Edits

| Non-Facility RVU | Work | PE | MP | Total |
|---|---|---|---|---|
| **D7290** | 2.30 | 2.03 | 0.47 | 4.80 |
| **Facility RVU** | **Work** | **PE** | **MP** | **Total** |
| **D7290** | 2.30 | 2.03 | 0.47 | 4.80 |

| | FUD | Status | MUE | Modifiers | | | | IOM Reference |
|---|---|---|---|---|---|---|---|---|
| **D7290** | N/A | N | - | N/A | N/A | N/A | N/A | None |

* with documentation

## Terms To Know

**debride.** To remove all foreign objects and devitalized or infected tissue from a burn or wound to prevent infection and promote healing.

**reposition.** Placement of an organ or structure into another position or return of an organ or structure to its original position.

# D7291

**D7291** transseptal fiberotomy/supra crestal fiberotomy, by report

*The supraosseous connective tissue attachment is surgically severed around the involved teeth. Where there are adjacent teeth, the transseptal fiberotomy of a single tooth will involve a minimum of three teeth. Since the incisions are within the gingival sulcus and tissue and the root surface is not instrumented, this procedure heals by the reunion of connective tissue with the root surface on which viable periodontal tissue is present (reattachment).*

## Explanation

A fiberotomy is a procedure designed to sever the connective tissue around the tooth to reduce the tooth's tendency to relapse into a rotation corrected by dental braces or other treatments. The connective tissue attachment is surgically severed around the involved teeth. Incisions are made within the gingival sulcus and tissue without root surface disruption. The transseptal fiberotomy of a single tooth may require a minimum of three teeth. Pertinent documentation to evaluate medical appropriateness should be included when reporting this code for reimbursement.

## Coding Tips

Local anesthesia is generally considered part of this service. A supra-crestal fiberotomy is appropriately reported with this code.

## Reimbursement Tips

Coverage for these procedures varies by payer and by individual contract. Check with payers for their specific coverage guidelines. Medically necessary orthodontia services are mandated under the Affordable Care Act (ACA) for those patients who have a severe handicapping malocclusion related to a medical condition. Medical record documentation must support the severity of the malocclusion and the medical condition. Some payers may require a standardized assessment, such as the Salzmann Evaluation Index be completed and that a specific score (for example 42 or higher) be documented.

## ICD-10-CM Diagnostic Codes

| | |
|---|---|
| M26.31 | Crowding of fully erupted teeth |
| M26.32 | Excessive spacing of fully erupted teeth |
| M26.33 | Horizontal displacement of fully erupted tooth or teeth |
| M26.34 | Vertical displacement of fully erupted tooth or teeth |
| M26.35 | Rotation of fully erupted tooth or teeth |
| M26.36 | Insufficient interocclusal distance of fully erupted teeth (ridge) |
| M26.37 | Excessive interocclusal distance of fully erupted teeth |

## Relative Value Units/Medicare Edits

| Non-Facility RVU | Work | PE | MP | Total |
|---|---|---|---|---|
| D7291 | 1.42 | 1.25 | 0.29 | 2.96 |
| **Facility RVU** | **Work** | **PE** | **MP** | **Total** |
| D7291 | 1.42 | 1.25 | 0.29 | 2.96 |

| | FUD | Status | MUE | Modifiers | | | | IOM Reference |
|---|---|---|---|---|---|---|---|---|
| D7291 | N/A | R | - | N/A | N/A | N/A | 80* | 100-02,1,70; 100-04,4,20.5 |

* with documentation

# D7292-D7294

▲ **D7292** placement of temporary anchorage device [screw retained plate] requiring flap

▲ **D7293** placement of temporary anchorage device requiring flap

▲ **D7294** placement of temporary anchorage device without flap

## Explanation

In D7292, the doctor makes an incision in the mouth and exposes the bone. A bone plate is bent to lie passively on the bone such that the end of the plate that is planned for attachment of orthodontic appliances is in the correct position. Screws are then placed to secure the plate to the bone. The wound is closed. In D7293 and D7294, the physician makes a small skin incision and places the temporary anchorage device. Report D7293 if the procedure requires a surgical flap for closure. Report D7294 if the procedure does not require a surgical flap.

## Coding Tips

Removal of the anchorage device is included and would not be coded separately.

## Reimbursement Tips

Coverage may be available through the patient's medical insurance for this service. Check with third-party payers for specific coverage information. Services submitted to the medical coverage will require that the service be reported with the appropriate CPT code on a CMS-1500 claim form.

## Associated CPT Codes

| | |
|---|---|
| 20650 | Insertion of wire or pin with application of skeletal traction, including removal (separate procedure) |

## ICD-10-CM Diagnostic Codes

| | |
|---|---|
| S02.80XA | Fracture of other specified skull and facial bones, unspecified side, initial encounter for closed fracture |
| S02.80XB | Fracture of other specified skull and facial bones, unspecified side, initial encounter for open fracture |
| S02.80XD | Fracture of other specified skull and facial bones, unspecified side, subsequent encounter for fracture with routine healing |
| S02.80XG | Fracture of other specified skull and facial bones, unspecified side, subsequent encounter for fracture with delayed healing |
| S02.80XK | Fracture of other specified skull and facial bones, unspecified side, subsequent encounter for fracture with nonunion |
| S02.80XS | Fracture of other specified skull and facial bones, unspecified side, sequela |
| S02.81XA | Fracture of other specified skull and facial bones, right side, initial encounter for closed fracture ☑ |
| S02.81XB | Fracture of other specified skull and facial bones, right side, initial encounter for open fracture ☑ |
| S02.81XD | Fracture of other specified skull and facial bones, right side, subsequent encounter for fracture with routine healing ☑ |
| S02.81XG | Fracture of other specified skull and facial bones, right side, subsequent encounter for fracture with delayed healing ☑ |
| S02.81XK | Fracture of other specified skull and facial bones, right side, subsequent encounter for fracture with nonunion ☑ |
| S02.81XS | Fracture of other specified skull and facial bones, right side, sequela ☑ |
| S02.82XS | Fracture of other specified skull and facial bones, left side, sequela ☑ |
| S03.00XA | Dislocation of jaw, unspecified side, initial encounter |
| S03.00XD | Dislocation of jaw, unspecified side, subsequent encounter |

S03.00XS Dislocation of jaw, unspecified side, sequela
S03.01XA Dislocation of jaw, right side, initial encounter ☑
S03.01XD Dislocation of jaw, right side, subsequent encounter ☑
S03.01XS Dislocation of jaw, right side, sequela ☑
S03.02XA Dislocation of jaw, left side, initial encounter ☑
S03.02XD Dislocation of jaw, left side, subsequent encounter ☑
S03.02XS Dislocation of jaw, left side, sequela ☑
S03.03XA Dislocation of jaw, bilateral, initial encounter ☑
S03.03XD Dislocation of jaw, bilateral, subsequent encounter ☑
S03.03XS Dislocation of jaw, bilateral, sequela ☑

## Relative Value Units/Medicare Edits

| Non-Facility RVU | Work | PE | MP | Total |
|---|---|---|---|---|
| **D7292** | 6.44 | 5.69 | 1.33 | 13.46 |
| **D7293** | 4.45 | 3.93 | 0.92 | 9.30 |
| **D7294** | 3.45 | 3.04 | 0.71 | 7.20 |
| **Facility RVU** | **Work** | **PE** | **MP** | **Total** |
| **D7292** | 6.44 | 5.69 | 1.33 | 13.46 |
| **D7293** | 4.45 | 3.93 | 0.92 | 9.30 |
| **D7294** | 3.45 | 3.04 | 0.71 | 7.20 |

| | FUD | Status | MUE | Modifiers | | | | IOM Reference |
|---|---|---|---|---|---|---|---|---|
| **D7292** | N/A | N | - | N/A | N/A | N/A | N/A | None |
| **D7293** | N/A | N | - | N/A | N/A | N/A | N/A | |
| **D7294** | N/A | N | - | N/A | N/A | N/A | N/A | |

* with documentation

# D7296-D7297

**D7296** corticotomy - one to three teeth or tooth spaces, per quadrant

*This procedure involves creating multiple cuts, perforations, or removal of cortical, alveolar or basal bone of the jaw for the purpose of facilitating orthodontic repositioning of the dentition. This procedure includes flap entry and closure. Graft material and membrane, if used, should be reported separately.*

**D7297** corticotomy - four or more teeth or tooth spaces, per quadrant

*This procedure involves creating multiple cuts, perforations, or removal of cortical, alveolar or basal bone of the jaw for the purpose of facilitating orthodontic repositioning of the dentition. This procedure includes flap entry and closure. Graft material and membrane, if used, should be reported separately.*

## Explanation

Corticotomy-assisted orthodontics uses surgical intervention along with conventional orthodontics to correct bite and tooth spacing. This surgically assisted approach improves tooth movement particularly for molar intrusion, space closure, de-crowding and open bite management. Corticotomy-assisted orthodontics also decrease the time needed under conventional orthodontics. After the administration of local anesthesia, the provider makes a crevicular incision buccally and lingually extending at least two to three teeth past the area to be treated. The full thickness flap is reflected on both buccal and lingual aspects beyond the apices of the teeth. Vertical corticotomy cuts are made between the roots using a diamond round bur (size 2) stopping just short of the alveolar crest (about 3mm) on both the buccal and lingual sides. Report D7296 when one to three teeth or tooth spaces per quadrant are treated. Report D7297 when four or more teeth or tooth spaces are treated.

## Coding Tips

Local anesthesia is generally considered to be part of these procedures. Report the appropriate code for each quadrant treated. Correct code selection is dependent upon the number of teeth or tooth spaces treated with that quadrant.

## ICD-10-CM Diagnostic Codes

K00.5 Hereditary disturbances in tooth structure, not elsewhere classified
K08.401 Partial loss of teeth, unspecified cause, class I
K08.402 Partial loss of teeth, unspecified cause, class II
K08.403 Partial loss of teeth, unspecified cause, class III
K08.404 Partial loss of teeth, unspecified cause, class IV
K08.411 Partial loss of teeth due to trauma, class I
K08.412 Partial loss of teeth due to trauma, class II
K08.413 Partial loss of teeth due to trauma, class III
K08.414 Partial loss of teeth due to trauma, class IV
K08.421 Partial loss of teeth due to periodontal diseases, class I
K08.422 Partial loss of teeth due to periodontal diseases, class II
K08.423 Partial loss of teeth due to periodontal diseases, class III
K08.424 Partial loss of teeth due to periodontal diseases, class IV
K08.431 Partial loss of teeth due to caries, class I
K08.432 Partial loss of teeth due to caries, class II
K08.433 Partial loss of teeth due to caries, class III
K08.434 Partial loss of teeth due to caries, class IV
M26.211 Malocclusion, Angle's class I
M26.212 Malocclusion, Angle's class II
M26.213 Malocclusion, Angle's class III
M26.31 Crowding of fully erupted teeth
M26.32 Excessive spacing of fully erupted teeth

M26.33 Horizontal displacement of fully erupted tooth or teeth
M26.34 Vertical displacement of fully erupted tooth or teeth
M26.35 Rotation of fully erupted tooth or teeth
M26.36 Insufficient interocclusal distance of fully erupted teeth (ridge)
M26.37 Excessive interocclusal distance of fully erupted teeth

## Relative Value Units/Medicare Edits

| Non-Facility RVU | Work | PE | MP | Total |
|---|---|---|---|---|
| **D7296** | 0.00 | 0.00 | 0.00 | 0.00 |
| **D7297** | 0.00 | 0.00 | 0.00 | 0.00 |
| **Facility RVU** | **Work** | **PE** | **MP** | **Total** |
| **D7296** | 0.00 | 0.00 | 0.00 | 0.00 |
| **D7297** | 0.00 | 0.00 | 0.00 | 0.00 |

| | FUD | Status | MUE | Modifiers | | | | IOM Reference |
|---|---|---|---|---|---|---|---|---|
| **D7296** | N/A | N | - | N/A | N/A | N/A | N/A | None |
| **D7297** | N/A | N | - | N/A | N/A | N/A | N/A | |

* with documentation

## Terms To Know

**malocclusion.** Condition in which the teeth are misaligned. Underlying causes may include accessory, impacted, or missing teeth; dentofacial abnormalities; thumb sucking; or sleeping positions.

# D7298-D7300

- **D7298** removal of temporary anchorage device [screw retained plate], requiring flap
- **D7299** removal of temporary anchorage device, requiring flap
- **D7300** removal of temporary anchorage device without flap

## Explanation

In D7298, the doctor makes a flap incision in the mouth exposing the previously place bone plate, the screws are removed and the plate is removed from the bone. The surgical area is cleaned, the flap is reapproximated and sutured into place. In D7299, a surgical flap incision is made, and the temporary anchorage device is located and removed. The surgical area is cleaned, the flap is reapproximated and sutured into place. In D7300, an incision is made exposing the temporary anchorage device. The device is removed, and the incision is sutured.

## Coding Tips

For placement of a temporary anchorage device, see D7292-D7294.

## Reimbursement Tips

Coverage may be available through the patient's medical insurance for this service. Check with third-party payers for specific coverage information. Services submitted to medical coverage require that the service be reported with the appropriate CPT code on a CMS-1500 claim form.

## Associated CPT Codes

20670 Removal of implant; superficial (eg, buried wire, pin or rod) (separate procedure)
20680 Removal of implant; deep (eg, buried wire, pin, screw, metal band, nail, rod or plate)

## ICD-10-CM Diagnostic Codes

S02.80XA Fracture of other specified skull and facial bones, unspecified side, initial encounter for closed fracture
S02.80XB Fracture of other specified skull and facial bones, unspecified side, initial encounter for open fracture
S02.80XD Fracture of other specified skull and facial bones, unspecified side, subsequent encounter for fracture with routine healing
S02.80XG Fracture of other specified skull and facial bones, unspecified side, subsequent encounter for fracture with delayed healing
S02.80XK Fracture of other specified skull and facial bones, unspecified side, subsequent encounter for fracture with nonunion
S02.80XS Fracture of other specified skull and facial bones, unspecified side, sequela
S02.81XA Fracture of other specified skull and facial bones, right side, initial encounter for closed fracture ☑
S02.81XB Fracture of other specified skull and facial bones, right side, initial encounter for open fracture ☑
S02.81XD Fracture of other specified skull and facial bones, right side, subsequent encounter for fracture with routine healing ☑
S02.81XG Fracture of other specified skull and facial bones, right side, subsequent encounter for fracture with delayed healing ☑
S02.81XK Fracture of other specified skull and facial bones, right side, subsequent encounter for fracture with nonunion ☑
S02.81XS Fracture of other specified skull and facial bones, right side, sequela ☑
S02.82XA Fracture of other specified skull and facial bones, left side, initial encounter for closed fracture ☑

| | |
|---|---|
| S02.82XS | Fracture of other specified skull and facial bones, left side, sequela ☑ |
| S03.00XA | Dislocation of jaw, unspecified side, initial encounter |
| S03.00XD | Dislocation of jaw, unspecified side, subsequent encounter |
| S03.00XS | Dislocation of jaw, unspecified side, sequela |
| S03.01XA | Dislocation of jaw, right side, initial encounter ☑ |
| S03.01XD | Dislocation of jaw, right side, subsequent encounter ☑ |
| S03.01XS | Dislocation of jaw, right side, sequela ☑ |
| S03.02XA | Dislocation of jaw, left side, initial encounter ☑ |
| S03.02XD | Dislocation of jaw, left side, subsequent encounter ☑ |
| S03.02XS | Dislocation of jaw, left side, sequela ☑ |
| S03.03XA | Dislocation of jaw, bilateral, initial encounter ☑ |
| S03.03XD | Dislocation of jaw, bilateral, subsequent encounter ☑ |
| S03.03XS | Dislocation of jaw, bilateral, sequela ☑ |

## Relative Value Units/Medicare Edits

| Non-Facility RVU | Work | PE | MP | Total |
|---|---|---|---|---|
| **D7298** | | | | |
| **D7299** | | | | |
| **D7300** | | | | |
| **Facility RVU** | **Work** | **PE** | **MP** | **Total** |
| **D7298** | | | | |
| **D7299** | | | | |
| **D7300** | | | | |

| | FUD | Status | MUE | Modifiers | | | | IOM Reference |
|---|---|---|---|---|---|---|---|---|
| **D7298** | N/A | | - | N/A | N/A | N/A | N/A | |
| **D7299** | N/A | | - | N/A | N/A | N/A | N/A | |
| **D7300** | N/A | | - | N/A | N/A | N/A | N/A | |

* with documentation

## Terms To Know

**flap.** Mass of flesh and skin partially excised from its location but retaining its blood supply that is moved to another site to repair adjacent or distant defects.

**nonunion.** Failure of two ends of a fracture to mend or completely heal.

**sequela.** Abnormality, dysfunction, or other residual condition produced after the acute phase of an illness, injury, or disease is over. There is no time limit as to when sequelae can appear. It may be apparent early, as with a stroke, or it can occur years later, as in arthritis following an injury.

# D7310-D7311

**D7310** alveoloplasty in conjunction with extractions - four or more teeth or tooth spaces, per quadrant

*The alveoloplasty is distinct (separate procedure) from extractions. Usually in preparation for a prosthesis or other treatments such as radiation therapy and transplant surgery.*

**D7311** alveoloplasty in conjunction with extractions - one to three teeth or tooth spaces, per quadrant

*The alveoloplasty is distinct (separate procedure) from extractions. Usually in preparation for a prosthesis or other treatments such as radiation therapy and transplant surgery.*

## Explanation

The contours of the alveolus are altered by selectively performing alveoloplasty to remove sharp areas or undercuts of alveolar bone. The dentist makes incisions in the mucosa overlying the alveolus, exposing the alveolar bone. Drills, osteotomes, or files are used to contour the bone. The mucosa is sutured in place over the contoured bone or a flap graft may be used for closure. Report D7310 for alveoloplasty performed in conjunction with tooth extractions concurrently done involving four or more teeth or tooth spaces per quadrant. Report D7311 for one to three teeth or tooth spaces per quadrant. This is usually in preparation for a prosthesis. Report D7320 for alveoloplasty done per quadrant, not in conjunction with any tooth extractions, such as in an edentulous area.

## Coding Tips

Any evaluation or radiograph is reported separately. Payers often consider procedures D7310 and D7311 to be part of extractions (procedures D7210–D7250) and, therefore, not separately reimbursable when performed in conjunction with the extraction. When not performed at the same time as an extraction, see code D7321.

## Documentation Tips

Payers may require documentation on the claim form indicating the quadrant on which the procedure was performed. The third-party payer may require a preprocedure x-ray or x-ray report before processing the claim.

## Reimbursement Tips

When selecting the procedure or service that accurately identifies the service performed, dentists must use the most accurate code. If the CDT code more accurately identifies the service, this should be used rather than the CPT codes. Third-party payers may consider these procedures to include any associated frenectomy.

## Associated CPT Codes

| | |
|---|---|
| 41874 | Alveoloplasty, each quadrant (specify) |

## ICD-10-CM Diagnostic Codes

| | |
|---|---|
| K02.53 | Dental caries on pit and fissure surface penetrating into pulp |
| K02.61 | Dental caries on smooth surface limited to enamel |
| K02.62 | Dental caries on smooth surface penetrating into dentin |
| K02.63 | Dental caries on smooth surface penetrating into pulp |
| K02.7 | Dental root caries |
| K03.0 | Excessive attrition of teeth |
| K03.1 | Abrasion of teeth |
| K03.2 | Erosion of teeth |
| K03.3 | Pathological resorption of teeth |
| K03.81 | Cracked tooth |

| | |
|---|---|
| K04.01 | Reversible pulpitis |
| K04.02 | Irreversible pulpitis |
| K04.1 | Necrosis of pulp |
| K04.2 | Pulp degeneration |
| K04.3 | Abnormal hard tissue formation in pulp |
| K04.4 | Acute apical periodontitis of pulpal origin |
| K04.5 | Chronic apical periodontitis |
| K04.6 | Periapical abscess with sinus |
| K04.7 | Periapical abscess without sinus |
| K04.8 | Radicular cyst |
| M26.31 | Crowding of fully erupted teeth |
| M26.32 | Excessive spacing of fully erupted teeth |
| M26.33 | Horizontal displacement of fully erupted tooth or teeth |
| M26.34 | Vertical displacement of fully erupted tooth or teeth |
| M26.35 | Rotation of fully erupted tooth or teeth |
| M26.36 | Insufficient interocclusal distance of fully erupted teeth (ridge) |
| M26.37 | Excessive interocclusal distance of fully erupted teeth |

## Relative Value Units/Medicare Edits

| Non-Facility RVU | Work | PE | MP | Total |
|---|---|---|---|---|
| D7310 | 1.52 | 1.34 | 0.31 | 3.17 |
| D7311 | 1.51 | 1.33 | 0.31 | 3.15 |
| Facility RVU | Work | PE | MP | Total |
| D7310 | 1.52 | 1.34 | 0.31 | 3.17 |
| D7311 | 1.51 | 1.33 | 0.31 | 3.15 |

| | FUD | Status | MUE | Modifiers | | | | IOM Reference |
|---|---|---|---|---|---|---|---|---|
| D7310 | N/A | I | - | N/A | N/A | N/A | N/A | None |
| D7311 | N/A | N | - | N/A | N/A | N/A | N/A | |

* with documentation

## Terms To Know

**alveoloplasty.** Surgical recontouring of the bone to which a tooth is attached, usually performed prior to the fitting of prosthesis.

**extraction.** Removal of a tooth and tooth fragments from the alveolus.

**mucosa.** Moist tissue lining the mouth (buccal mucosa), stomach (gastric mucosa), intestines, and respiratory tract.

**osteotome.** Tool used for cutting bone.

# D7320-D7321



**D7320** alveoloplasty not in conjunction with extractions - four or more teeth or tooth spaces, per quadrant

*No extractions performed in an edentulous area. See D7310 if teeth are being extracted concurrently with the alveoloplasty. Usually in preparation for a prosthesis or other treatments such as radiation therapy and transplant surgery.*

**D7321** alveoloplasty not in conjunction with extractions - one to three teeth or tooth spaces, per quadrant

*No extractions performed in an edentulous area. ee D7311 if teeth are being extracted concurrently with the alveoloplasty. Usually in preparation for a prosthesis or other treatments such as radiation therapy and transplant surgery.*

## Explanation

The dentist alters the contours of the alveolus by selectively performing alveoloplasty to remove sharp areas or undercuts of alveolar bone. The dentist makes incisions in the mucosa overlying the alveolus, exposing the alveolar bone. Drills, osteotomes, or files are used to contour the bone. The mucosa is sutured in place over the contoured bone.

## Coding Tips

The third-party payer may require a pre-procedure x-ray or x-ray report before processing the claim. Payers may require documentation on the claim form indicating the quadrant on which the procedure was performed. Local anesthesia is generally considered part of this service. For alveoloplasty performed in conjunction with extractions, see codes D7310-D7311.

## Documentation Tips

Dentists should be certain that sufficient documentation is provided in the dental records to accurately verify and describe the services rendered. Additionally, records should be legible and signed with the appropriate name and title of the provider of the service.

## Reimbursement Tips

When selecting the procedure or service that accurately identifies the service performed, dentists must use the most accurate code. If the CDT code more accurately identifies the service, this should be used rather than the CPT codes. This procedure may be covered by the patient's medical insurance. When covered by medical insurance, the payer may require that the appropriate CPT code be reported on the CMS-1500 claim form.

## Associated CPT Codes

| | |
|---|---|
| 41874 | Alveoloplasty, each quadrant (specify) |

## ICD-10-CM Diagnostic Codes

| | |
|---|---|
| K02.53 | Dental caries on pit and fissure surface penetrating into pulp |
| K02.61 | Dental caries on smooth surface limited to enamel |
| K02.62 | Dental caries on smooth surface penetrating into dentin |
| K02.63 | Dental caries on smooth surface penetrating into pulp |
| K02.7 | Dental root caries |
| K03.0 | Excessive attrition of teeth |
| K03.1 | Abrasion of teeth |
| K03.2 | Erosion of teeth |
| K03.3 | Pathological resorption of teeth |
| K03.81 | Cracked tooth |
| K04.01 | Reversible pulpitis |
| K04.02 | Irreversible pulpitis |
| K04.1 | Necrosis of pulp |
| K04.2 | Pulp degeneration |

K04.3 Abnormal hard tissue formation in pulp
K04.4 Acute apical periodontitis of pulpal origin
K04.5 Chronic apical periodontitis
K04.6 Periapical abscess with sinus
K04.7 Periapical abscess without sinus
K04.8 Radicular cyst
M26.31 Crowding of fully erupted teeth
M26.32 Excessive spacing of fully erupted teeth
M26.33 Horizontal displacement of fully erupted tooth or teeth
M26.34 Vertical displacement of fully erupted tooth or teeth
M26.35 Rotation of fully erupted tooth or teeth
M26.36 Insufficient interocclusal distance of fully erupted teeth (ridge)
M26.37 Excessive interocclusal distance of fully erupted teeth

## Relative Value Units/Medicare Edits

| Non-Facility RVU | Work | PE | MP | Total |
|---|---|---|---|---|
| D7320 | 2.30 | 2.03 | 0.47 | 4.80 |
| D7321 | 2.30 | 2.03 | 0.47 | 4.80 |
| **Facility RVU** | **Work** | **PE** | **MP** | **Total** |
| D7320 | 2.30 | 2.03 | 0.47 | 4.80 |
| D7321 | 2.30 | 2.03 | 0.47 | 4.80 |

| | FUD | Status | MUE | Modifiers | | | | IOM Reference |
|---|---|---|---|---|---|---|---|---|
| D7320 | N/A | I | - | N/A | N/A | N/A | N/A | None |
| D7321 | N/A | R | - | N/A | N/A | N/A | N/A | |

* with documentation

# D7340-D7350

**D7340** vestibuloplasty - ridge extension (secondary epithelialization)
**D7350** vestibuloplasty - ridge extension (including soft tissue grafts, muscle reattachment, revision of soft tissue attachment and management of hypertrophied and hyperplastic tissue)

## Explanation

The surgeon performs a vestibuloplasty and deepens the vestibule of the mouth by any series of surgical procedures for the purpose of increasing the height of the alveolar ridge, allowing a complete denture to be worn. The vestibule refers to the mucosal and submucosal tissue of the inner lips and cheeks, the part of the oral cavity outside of the dentoalveolar structures. This procedure may be performed in several ways. Generally, the surgeon may rearrange the patient's own tissue or the submucosal tissue may be dissected and freed from the bone. The mucosa is moved deeper into the vestibule. For code D7350, soft tissues are also grafted into the mouth.

## Coding Tips

Local anesthesia is generally considered part of these procedures.

## Reimbursement Tips

When selecting the procedure or service that accurately identifies the service performed, dentists must use the most accurate code. If the CDT code more accurately identifies the service, this should be used rather than the CPT codes. Some third-party payers may require that these services be reported using the CMS-1500 claim form and the appropriate CPT codes.

## Associated CPT Codes

40840 Vestibuloplasty; anterior
40842 Vestibuloplasty; posterior, unilateral
40843 Vestibuloplasty; posterior, bilateral
40844 Vestibuloplasty; entire arch
40845 Vestibuloplasty; complex (including ridge extension, muscle repositioning)

## ICD-10-CM Diagnostic Codes

K04.01 Reversible pulpitis
K04.02 Irreversible pulpitis
K04.1 Necrosis of pulp
K04.2 Pulp degeneration
K04.3 Abnormal hard tissue formation in pulp
K04.4 Acute apical periodontitis of pulpal origin
K04.5 Chronic apical periodontitis
K04.6 Periapical abscess with sinus
K04.7 Periapical abscess without sinus
K04.8 Radicular cyst
K08.111 Complete loss of teeth due to trauma, class I
K08.112 Complete loss of teeth due to trauma, class II
K08.113 Complete loss of teeth due to trauma, class III
K08.114 Complete loss of teeth due to trauma, class IV
K08.121 Complete loss of teeth due to periodontal diseases, class I
K08.122 Complete loss of teeth due to periodontal diseases, class II
K08.123 Complete loss of teeth due to periodontal diseases, class III
K08.124 Complete loss of teeth due to periodontal diseases, class IV
K08.131 Complete loss of teeth due to caries, class I
K08.132 Complete loss of teeth due to caries, class II
K08.133 Complete loss of teeth due to caries, class III
K08.134 Complete loss of teeth due to caries, class IV

## Relative Value Units/Medicare Edits

| Non-Facility RVU | Work | PE | MP | Total |
|---|---|---|---|---|
| **D7340** | 8.60 | 7.59 | 1.77 | 17.96 |
| **D7350** | 24.26 | 21.41 | 5.00 | 50.67 |
| **Facility RVU** | **Work** | **PE** | **MP** | **Total** |
| **D7340** | 8.60 | 7.59 | 1.77 | 17.96 |
| **D7350** | 24.26 | 21.41 | 5.00 | 50.67 |

| | FUD | Status | MUE | Modifiers | | | | IOM Reference |
|---|---|---|---|---|---|---|---|---|
| **D7340** | N/A | I | - | N/A | N/A | N/A | N/A | None |
| **D7350** | N/A | I | - | N/A | N/A | N/A | N/A | |

* with documentation

## Terms To Know

**vestibuloplasty.** Surgical procedure in which the vestibule of the mouth is deepened for the purpose of increasing the height of the alveolar ridge.

# D7410-D7412

**D7410** excision of benign lesion up to 1.25 cm

**D7411** excision of benign lesion greater than 1.25 cm

**D7412** excision of benign lesion, complicated

*Requires extensive undermining with advancement or rotational flap closure.*

## Explanation

A benign lesion is removed from soft tissue by surgical excision. This includes scar tissue, localized congenital and inflammatory lesions, and nonodontogenic cysts. After administering a local anesthetic, the dentist makes a full-thickness incision, usually in an elliptical shape around and under the lesion, and removes it with the margins. The wound may be sutured simply. Report D7410 for a lesion up to 1.25 cm and D7411 for a lesion greater than 1.25 cm. The lesion size is measured by the greatest diameter of the lesion apparent together with the margin allowance needed for complete excision. Report D7412 if the excision and removal of the benign lesion is complicated and requires a more extensive undermining for removal and closure with a created flap that is advanced or rotated into place to cover the defect.

## Coding Tips

Local anesthesia and routine postoperative care is included. Any evaluation or radiograph is reported separately. Correct code selection is dependent upon the size of the lesion. Lesion size should not be determined from the pathology report, but from the medical record documentation. Pathology exam of tissue with interpretation is reported separately. When reporting code D7411 or D7412, please note that some payers may require that the pathology report be attached to the claim. To report excision of malignant lesion of the soft tissue, see D7413–D7415. To report removal of benign intraosseous lesions, see D7450–D7461.

## Reimbursement Tips

When selecting the procedure or service that accurately identifies the service performed, dentists must use the most accurate code. If the CDT code more accurately identifies the service, this should be used rather than the CPT codes. This procedure may be covered by the patient's medical insurance. When covered by medical insurance, the payer may require that the appropriate CPT code be reported on the CMS-1500 claim form.

## Associated CPT Codes

| | |
|---|---|
| 21030 | Excision of benign tumor or cyst of maxilla or zygoma by enucleation and curettage |
| 21040 | Excision of benign tumor or cyst of mandible, by enucleation and/or curettage |
| 21047 | Excision of benign tumor or cyst of mandible; requiring extra-oral osteotomy and partial mandibulectomy (eg, locally aggressive or destructive lesion[s]) |
| 40810 | Excision of lesion of mucosa and submucosa, vestibule of mouth; without repair |
| 40812 | Excision of lesion of mucosa and submucosa, vestibule of mouth; with simple repair |
| 40814 | Excision of lesion of mucosa and submucosa, vestibule of mouth; with complex repair |
| 40816 | Excision of lesion of mucosa and submucosa, vestibule of mouth; complex, with excision of underlying muscle |
| 41110 | Excision of lesion of tongue without closure |
| 41112 | Excision of lesion of tongue with closure; anterior two-thirds |
| 41113 | Excision of lesion of tongue with closure; posterior one-third |
| 41114 | Excision of lesion of tongue with closure; with local tongue flap |

41116 Excision, lesion of floor of mouth

41825 Excision of lesion or tumor (except listed above), dentoalveolar structures; without repair

42104 Excision, lesion of palate, uvula; without closure

42106 Excision, lesion of palate, uvula; with simple primary closure

42107 Excision, lesion of palate, uvula; with local flap closure

## ICD-10-CM Diagnostic Codes

D10.0 Benign neoplasm of lip

D10.1 Benign neoplasm of tongue

D10.2 Benign neoplasm of floor of mouth

D10.39 Benign neoplasm of other parts of mouth

## Relative Value Units/Medicare Edits

| Non-Facility RVU | Work | PE | MP | Total |
|---|---|---|---|---|
| **D7410** | 3.73 | 3.29 | 0.77 | 7.79 |
| **D7411** | 5.94 | 5.24 | 1.22 | 12.40 |
| **D7412** | 6.76 | 5.96 | 1.39 | 14.11 |
| **Facility RVU** | **Work** | **PE** | **MP** | **Total** |
| **D7410** | 3.73 | 3.29 | 0.77 | 7.79 |
| **D7411** | 5.94 | 5.24 | 1.22 | 12.40 |
| **D7412** | 6.76 | 5.96 | 1.39 | 14.11 |

| | FUD | Status | MUE | Modifiers | | | | IOM Reference |
|---|---|---|---|---|---|---|---|---|
| **D7410** | N/A | I | - | N/A | N/A | N/A | N/A | None |
| **D7411** | N/A | I | - | N/A | N/A | N/A | N/A | |
| **D7412** | N/A | I | - | N/A | N/A | N/A | N/A | |

* with documentation

## Terms To Know

**benign lesion.** Neoplasm or change in tissue that is not cancerous (nonmalignant).

**congenital.** Present at birth, occurring through heredity or an influence during gestation up to the moment of birth.

**excision.** Surgical removal of an organ or tissue.

**flap.** Mass of flesh and skin partially excised from its location but retaining its blood supply that is moved to another site to repair adjacent or distant defects.

**intraosseous.** Within a bone.

**scar tissue.** Fibrous connective tissue that forms around a wounded area or injury, composed mainly of fibroblasts or collagenous fibers.

# D7413-D7415

**D7413** excision of malignant lesion up to 1.25 cm

**D7414** excision of malignant lesion greater than 1.25 cm

**D7415** excision of malignant lesion, complicated

*Requires extensive undermining with advancement or rotational flap closure.*

## Explanation

A malignant lesion is removed from soft tissue by surgical excision. After administering a local anesthetic, the dentist makes a full-thickness incision, usually in an elliptical shape around and under the lesion, and removes it with the margins. The wound may be sutured simply. Report D7413 for a lesion up to 1.25 cm and D7414 for a lesion greater than 1.25 cm. The lesion size is measured by the greatest diameter of the lesion apparent together with the margin allowance needed for complete excision. Report D7415 if the excision and removal of the malignant lesion is complicated and requires a more extensive undermining for removal and closure with a created flap that is advanced or rotated into place to cover the defect.

## Coding Tips

Anesthesia and routine postoperative care are included. Any evaluation or radiograph is reported separately. Correct code selection was dependent upon the size of the lesion. For excision of benign lesions of the soft tissue, see D7410–D7412. For removal of malignant intraosseous tumor, see D7440–D7441. Pathology exam of tissue with interpretation is reported separately. Some payers may require that the pathology report be attached to the claim.

## Reimbursement Tips

When selecting the procedure or service that accurately identifies the service performed, dentists must use the most accurate code. If the CDT code more accurately identifies the service, this should be used rather than the CPT codes. When the condition is the result of an accident, the dental insurer may require that the medical insurance be billed first. When covered by the patient's medical insurance, the payer may require that the appropriate CPT code be reported on the CMS-1500 claim form.

## Associated CPT Codes

21015 Radical resection of tumor (eg, sarcoma), soft tissue of face or scalp; less than 2 cm

21016 Radical resection of tumor (eg, sarcoma), soft tissue of face or scalp; 2 cm or greater

21034 Excision of malignant tumor of maxilla or zygoma

21044 Excision of malignant tumor of mandible;

21045 Excision of malignant tumor of mandible; radical resection

40500 Vermilionectomy (lip shave), with mucosal advancement

40810 Excision of lesion of mucosa and submucosa, vestibule of mouth; without repair

40812 Excision of lesion of mucosa and submucosa, vestibule of mouth; with simple repair

40814 Excision of lesion of mucosa and submucosa, vestibule of mouth; with complex repair

41110 Excision of lesion of tongue without closure

41112 Excision of lesion of tongue with closure; anterior two-thirds

41113 Excision of lesion of tongue with closure; posterior one-third

41114 Excision of lesion of tongue with closure; with local tongue flap

41116 Excision, lesion of floor of mouth

41825 Excision of lesion or tumor (except listed above), dentoalveolar structures; without repair

| | |
|---|---|
| 41827 | Excision of lesion or tumor (except listed above), dentoalveolar structures; with complex repair |
| 42104 | Excision, lesion of palate, uvula; without closure |
| 42106 | Excision, lesion of palate, uvula; with simple primary closure |
| 42107 | Excision, lesion of palate, uvula; with local flap closure |

## ICD-10-CM Diagnostic Codes

| | |
|---|---|
| C03.0 | Malignant neoplasm of upper gum |
| C03.1 | Malignant neoplasm of lower gum |
| C04.0 | Malignant neoplasm of anterior floor of mouth |
| C04.1 | Malignant neoplasm of lateral floor of mouth |
| C04.8 | Malignant neoplasm of overlapping sites of floor of mouth |
| C05.0 | Malignant neoplasm of hard palate |
| C05.1 | Malignant neoplasm of soft palate |
| C05.2 | Malignant neoplasm of uvula |
| C05.8 | Malignant neoplasm of overlapping sites of palate |
| C06.0 | Malignant neoplasm of cheek mucosa |
| C06.1 | Malignant neoplasm of vestibule of mouth |
| C06.2 | Malignant neoplasm of retromolar area |
| C07 | Malignant neoplasm of parotid gland |
| C08.0 | Malignant neoplasm of submandibular gland |
| C08.1 | Malignant neoplasm of sublingual gland |

## Relative Value Units/Medicare Edits

| Non-Facility RVU | Work | PE | MP | Total |
|---|---|---|---|---|
| **D7413** | 4.81 | 4.24 | 0.99 | 10.04 |
| **D7414** | 7.11 | 6.28 | 1.46 | 14.85 |
| **D7415** | 7.79 | 6.87 | 1.60 | 16.26 |
| **Facility RVU** | **Work** | **PE** | **MP** | **Total** |
| **D7413** | 4.81 | 4.24 | 0.99 | 10.04 |
| **D7414** | 7.11 | 6.28 | 1.46 | 14.85 |
| **D7415** | 7.79 | 6.87 | 1.60 | 16.26 |

| | FUD | Status | MUE | Modifiers | | | | IOM Reference |
|---|---|---|---|---|---|---|---|---|
| **D7413** | N/A | I | - | N/A | N/A | N/A | N/A | None |
| **D7414** | N/A | I | - | N/A | N/A | N/A | N/A | |
| **D7415** | N/A | I | - | N/A | N/A | N/A | N/A | |

* with documentation

## Terms To Know

**excision.** Surgical removal of an organ or tissue.

**flap.** Mass of flesh and skin partially excised from its location but retaining its blood supply that is moved to another site to repair adjacent or distant defects.

**malignant.** Any condition tending to progress toward death, specifically an invasive tumor with a loss of cellular differentiation that has the ability to spread or metastasize to other body areas.

**malignant neoplasm.** Any cancerous tumor or lesion exhibiting uncontrolled tissue growth that can progressively invade other parts of the body with its disease-generating cells.

# D7440-D7441

**D7440** excision of malignant tumor - lesion diameter up to 1.25 cm

**D7441** excision of malignant tumor - lesion diameter greater than 1.25 cm

## Explanation

The oral surgeon excises a malignant tumor of the bone. Incisions include transoral (e.g., maxillary buccal vestibular) and facial (e.g., Weber-Ferguson) depending on the location of the tumor. The bony mass is excised with the use of drills, saws, and osteotomes. The tumor is removed to "free margins" as determined with intraoperative tissue specimens sent to the pathologist for immediate microscopic examination. The oral surgeon may remove teeth and overlying mucosa. Some surgical defects may require immediate soft tissue reconstruction (e.g., myocutaneous flaps). Transoral incisions are closed in a single layer and facial incisions are closed in layers. Intraoral surgical splints may be used. Report code D7440 when tumor is 1.25 cm or smaller, report D7441 when lesion is larger than 1.25 cm.

## Coding Tips

Correct code selection is dependent upon the size of the lesion. For removal of benign odontogenic cyst or tumor, see D7450–D7461. To report excision of malignant lesions of soft tissue, see D7413–D7415.

## Reimbursement Tips

When selecting the procedure or service that accurately identifies the service performed, dentists must use the most accurate code. If the CDT code more accurately identifies the service, this should be used rather than the CPT codes. Some payers may require that the specific site of the tumor be identified and that the operative and pathology reports be attached to the claim. When the condition is the result of an accident, the dental insurer may require that the medical insurance be billed first. When covered by the patient's medical insurance, the payer may require that the appropriate CPT code be reported on the CMS-1500 claim form.

## Associated CPT Codes

| | |
|---|---|
| 21034 | Excision of malignant tumor of maxilla or zygoma |
| 21044 | Excision of malignant tumor of mandible; |
| 21045 | Excision of malignant tumor of mandible; radical resection |
| 41116 | Excision, lesion of floor of mouth |
| 41825 | Excision of lesion or tumor (except listed above), dentoalveolar structures; without repair |
| 41826 | Excision of lesion or tumor (except listed above), dentoalveolar structures; with simple repair |
| 41827 | Excision of lesion or tumor (except listed above), dentoalveolar structures; with complex repair |
| 42140 | Uvulectomy, excision of uvula |

## ICD-10-CM Diagnostic Codes

| | |
|---|---|
| C03.0 | Malignant neoplasm of upper gum |
| C03.1 | Malignant neoplasm of lower gum |
| C04.0 | Malignant neoplasm of anterior floor of mouth |
| C04.1 | Malignant neoplasm of lateral floor of mouth |
| C04.8 | Malignant neoplasm of overlapping sites of floor of mouth |
| C05.0 | Malignant neoplasm of hard palate |
| C05.1 | Malignant neoplasm of soft palate |
| C05.2 | Malignant neoplasm of uvula |
| C05.8 | Malignant neoplasm of overlapping sites of palate |
| C06.0 | Malignant neoplasm of cheek mucosa |
| C06.1 | Malignant neoplasm of vestibule of mouth |

| | |
|---|---|
| C06.2 | Malignant neoplasm of retromolar area |
| C07 | Malignant neoplasm of parotid gland |
| C08.0 | Malignant neoplasm of submandibular gland |
| C08.1 | Malignant neoplasm of sublingual gland |

## Relative Value Units/Medicare Edits

| Non-Facility RVU | Work | PE | MP | Total |
|---|---|---|---|---|
| **D7440** | 5.90 | 5.21 | 1.21 | 12.32 |
| **D7441** | 9.17 | 8.10 | 1.89 | 19.16 |
| **Facility RVU** | **Work** | **PE** | **MP** | **Total** |
| **D7440** | 5.90 | 5.21 | 1.21 | 12.32 |
| **D7441** | 9.17 | 8.10 | 1.89 | 19.16 |

| | FUD | Status | MUE | Modifiers | | | | IOM Reference |
|---|---|---|---|---|---|---|---|---|
| **D7440** | N/A | I | - | N/A | N/A | N/A | N/A | None |
| **D7441** | N/A | I | - | N/A | N/A | N/A | N/A | |

* with documentation

## Terms To Know

**excision.** Surgical removal of an organ or tissue.

**malignant.** Any condition tending to progress toward death, specifically an invasive tumor with a loss of cellular differentiation that has the ability to spread or metastasize to other body areas.

# D7450-D7461

**D7450** removal of benign odontogenic cyst or tumor - lesion diameter up to 1.25 cm

**D7451** removal of benign odontogenic cyst or tumor - lesion diameter greater than 1.25 cm

**D7460** removal of benign nonodontogenic cyst or tumor - lesion diameter up to 1.25 cm

**D7461** removal of benign nonodontogenic cyst or tumor - lesion diameter greater than 1.25 cm

## Explanation

The oral surgeon removes a lesion or tumor of the odontgenic or tooth-forming tissues. If the lesion is within the mucosa, the provider makes incisions around the lesion and dissects it away from adjacent structures. The lesion is removed from the bone and the incision closed with layered sutures. Report code D7450 if the odontogenic lesion is up to 1.25 cm, code D7451 if odontogenic lesion is over 1.25 cm in size. Report D7460 if the nonodontogenic lesion is up to 1.25 cm, code D7461 if the nonodontogenic lesion is over 1.25 cm in size.

## Coding Tips

Some payers may require that the specific site of the tumor be identified and that the operative and pathology reports be attached to the claim. To report excision of malignant intraosseous lesion, see codes D7440–D7441. To report excision of benign lesion of soft tissue, see codes from the D7410–D7412 range.

## Reimbursement Tips

When selecting the procedure or service that accurately identifies the service performed, dentists must use the most accurate code. If the CDT code more accurately identifies the service, this should be used rather than the CPT codes. Some payers may require that the specific site of the tumor be identified and that the operative and pathology reports be attached to the claim. This procedure may be covered by the patient's medical insurance. When covered by medical insurance, the payer may require that the appropriate CPT code be reported on the CMS-1500 claim form.

## Associated CPT Codes

| | |
|---|---|
| 21029 | Removal by contouring of benign tumor of facial bone (eg, fibrous dysplasia) |
| 21030 | Excision of benign tumor or cyst of maxilla or zygoma by enucleation and curettage |
| 21040 | Excision of benign tumor or cyst of mandible, by enucleation and/or curettage |
| 41825 | Excision of lesion or tumor (except listed above), dentoalveolar structures; without repair |
| 41826 | Excision of lesion or tumor (except listed above), dentoalveolar structures; with simple repair |
| 41827 | Excision of lesion or tumor (except listed above), dentoalveolar structures; with complex repair |
| 42408 | Excision of sublingual salivary cyst (ranula) |
| 42409 | Marsupialization of sublingual salivary cyst (ranula) |

## ICD-10-CM Diagnostic Codes

| | |
|---|---|
| D10.0 | Benign neoplasm of lip |
| D10.1 | Benign neoplasm of tongue |
| D10.2 | Benign neoplasm of floor of mouth |
| D10.39 | Benign neoplasm of other parts of mouth |

## Relative Value Units/Medicare Edits

| Non-Facility RVU | Work | PE | MP | Total |
|---|---|---|---|---|
| **D7450** | 3.93 | 3.47 | 0.81 | 8.21 |
| **D7451** | 5.31 | 4.69 | 1.09 | 11.09 |
| **D7460** | 3.91 | 3.45 | 0.81 | 8.17 |
| **D7461** | 5.39 | 4.75 | 1.11 | 11.25 |
| **Facility RVU** | **Work** | **PE** | **MP** | **Total** |
| **D7450** | 3.93 | 3.47 | 0.81 | 8.21 |
| **D7451** | 5.31 | 4.69 | 1.09 | 11.09 |
| **D7460** | 3.91 | 3.45 | 0.81 | 8.17 |
| **D7461** | 5.39 | 4.75 | 1.11 | 11.25 |

| | FUD | Status | MUE | Modifiers | | | | IOM Reference |
|---|---|---|---|---|---|---|---|---|
| **D7450** | N/A | I | - | N/A | N/A | N/A | N/A | None |
| **D7451** | N/A | I | - | N/A | N/A | N/A | N/A | |
| **D7460** | N/A | I | - | N/A | N/A | N/A | N/A | |
| **D7461** | N/A | I | - | N/A | N/A | N/A | N/A | |

* with documentation

## Terms To Know

**benign.** Mild or nonmalignant in nature.

**excision.** Surgical removal of an organ or tissue.

**fissure.** Deep furrow, groove, or cleft in tissue structures.

**granuloma.** Abnormal, dense collections of cells forming a mass or nodule of chronically inflamed tissue with granulations that is usually associated with an infective process.

**leukoplakia.** Thickened white patches or lesions appearing on a mucous membrane, such as oral mucosa or tongue.

**mucosa.** Moist tissue lining the mouth (buccal mucosa), stomach (gastric mucosa), intestines, and respiratory tract.

# D7465

**D7465** destruction of lesion(s) by physical or chemical method, by report

*Examples include using cryo, laser or electro surgery.*

## Explanation

The dentist or oral surgeon destroys a lesion, particularly of the oral soft tissue without excision, but by physical or chemical methods. These include different techniques of lesion destruction. Electrocautery may be used to burn the lesion, cryotherapy to freeze the lesion, chemical injections or topical applications may be used to destroy the lesion, or a laser, which produces high-intensity light, may be used to destroy the lesion. No suturing is required and the resultant surgical wound is left to heal secondarily.

## Coding Tips

This is an out-of-sequence code and will not display in numeric order in the CDT manual. Any evaluation or radiograph is reported separately. Pathology exam of tissue with interpretation is reported separately.

## Reimbursement Tips

When selecting the procedure or service that accurately identifies the service performed, dentists must use the most accurate code. If the CDT code more accurately identifies the service, this should be used rather than the CPT codes. Pertinent documentation to evaluate medical appropriateness should be included when this code is reported. Some payers may require that the pathology report be attached to the claim when performed. This procedure may be covered by the patient's medical insurance. When covered by medical insurance, the payer may require that the appropriate CPT code be reported on the CMS-1500 claim form.

## Associated CPT Codes

| | |
|---|---|
| 40820 | Destruction of lesion or scar of vestibule of mouth by physical methods (eg, laser, thermal, cryo, chemical) |
| 41850 | Destruction of lesion (except excision), dentoalveolar structures |

## ICD-10-CM Diagnostic Codes

| | |
|---|---|
| D10.0 | Benign neoplasm of lip |
| D10.1 | Benign neoplasm of tongue |
| D10.2 | Benign neoplasm of floor of mouth |
| D10.39 | Benign neoplasm of other parts of mouth |

## Relative Value Units/Medicare Edits

| Non-Facility RVU | Work | PE | MP | Total |
|---|---|---|---|---|
| **D7465** | 2.30 | 2.03 | 0.47 | 4.80 |
| **Facility RVU** | **Work** | **PE** | **MP** | **Total** |
| **D7465** | 2.30 | 2.03 | 0.47 | 4.80 |

| | FUD | Status | MUE | Modifiers | | | | IOM Reference |
|---|---|---|---|---|---|---|---|---|
| **D7465** | N/A | I | - | N/A | N/A | N/A | N/A | None |

* with documentation

## Terms To Know

**cryotherapy.** Any surgical procedure that uses intense cold for treatment.

**destruction.** Ablation or eradication of a structure or tissue.

**electrocautery.** Division or cutting of tissue using high-frequency electrical current to produce heat, which destroys cells.

# D7471

**D7471** removal of lateral exostosis (maxilla or mandible)

## Explanation

A lateral exostosis, also known as buccal exostosis, is a bony spur found only on the facial surface of either the upper or lower jaw. To remove the exostosis, the dentist makes an incision to expose the exostosis under the gum. The bone is cut into sections and the pieces are removed. The surface is then smoothed using a diamond bur on a hand piece. The gum is then closed over and sutures are placed.

## Coding Tips

Any evaluation, radiograph, or restoration service is reported separately. Local anesthesia is generally considered part of any surgical procedure.

## Documentation Tips

The following information should be documented on a tooth chart: treatment/location of caries, endodontic procedures, prosthetic services, preventive services, treatment of lesions and dental disease, or other special procedures. A tooth chart may also be used to identify structure and rationale of disease process, and the type of service performed on intraoral structures other than teeth.

## Reimbursement Tips

The third-party payer may require an x-ray or x-ray report before processing the claim.

## ICD-10-CM Diagnostic Codes

M27.8 Other specified diseases of jaws

## Relative Value Units/Medicare Edits

| Non-Facility RVU | Work | PE | MP | Total |
|---|---|---|---|---|
| D7471 | 4.87 | 4.30 | 1.00 | 10.17 |
| **Facility RVU** | **Work** | **PE** | **MP** | **Total** |
| D7471 | 4.87 | 4.30 | 1.00 | 10.17 |

| | FUD | Status | MUE | Modifiers | | | | IOM Reference |
|---|---|---|---|---|---|---|---|---|
| D7471 | N/A | I | - | N/A | N/A | N/A | N/A | None |

* with documentation

## Terms To Know

**buccal.** Relating to or toward the cheek.

**exostosis.** Abnormal formation of a benign bony growth.

**incision.** Act of cutting into tissue or an organ.

**lateral.** On/to the side.

**local anesthesia.** Induced loss of feeling or sensation restricted to a certain area of the body, including topical, local tissue infiltration, field block, or nerve block methods.

**mandible.** Lower jawbone giving structure to the floor of the oral cavity.

**maxilla.** Pyramidally-shaped bone forming the upper jaw, part of the eye orbit, nasal cavity, and palate and lodging the upper teeth.

**removal.** Process of moving out of or away from, or the fact of being removed.

# D7472-D7473

**D7472** removal of torus palatinus
**D7473** removal of torus mandibularis

## Explanation

The physician removes the bony overgrowth of either the palate (D7472) or the floor of the mouth (D7473). An incision is made over the bony overgrowth to expose it. The provider removes small sections of the bone until the entire growth is removed. The area is smoothed using a diamond bur. The incision is closed using sutures.

## Coding Tips

Local anesthesia is included in these services. Any evaluation, radiograph, or restoration service is reported separately.

## Associated CPT Codes

21031 Excision of torus mandibularis
21032 Excision of maxillary torus palatinus

## ICD-10-CM Diagnostic Codes

M27.0 Developmental disorders of jaws

## Relative Value Units/Medicare Edits

| Non-Facility RVU | Work | PE | MP | Total |
|---|---|---|---|---|
| D7472 | 5.83 | 5.15 | 1.20 | 12.18 |
| D7473 | 5.20 | 4.59 | 1.07 | 10.86 |
| **Facility RVU** | **Work** | **PE** | **MP** | **Total** |
| D7472 | 5.83 | 5.15 | 1.20 | 12.18 |
| D7473 | 5.20 | 4.59 | 1.07 | 10.86 |

| | FUD | Status | MUE | Modifiers | | | | IOM Reference |
|---|---|---|---|---|---|---|---|---|
| D7472 | N/A | I | - | N/A | N/A | N/A | N/A | None |
| D7473 | N/A | I | - | N/A | N/A | N/A | N/A | |

* with documentation

## Terms To Know

**osseous tuberosities.** Nodule or tubercle that is related to, consisting of, or resembling bone.

**torus mandibularis.** Developmental disorder of the jaw with bony projection or overgrowth of normal bone usually found on the floor of the mouth under the tongue.

# D7485

**D7485** reduction of osseous tuberosity

## Explanation

The dentist removes the osseous tissue from the tuberosities of dentoalveolar structures, producing more favorable bone contours. The dentist makes an incision through the mucosa of the tuberosity and exposes the underlying bone. Drills, osteotomes, or files are used to remove and contour the bone. The tissue is then sutured directly over the bone. Some soft tissue may be excised prior to closure for adaptation over the newly contoured bone.

## Coding Tips

Local anesthesia is included in this service. Any evaluation, radiograph, or restoration service is reported separately.

## Reimbursement Tips

When selecting the procedure or service that accurately identifies the service performed, dentists must use the most accurate code. If the CDT code more accurately identifies the service, this should be used rather than the CPT codes. Coverage guidelines vary by payer and by patient contract. Some third-party payers may require that this service be reported using the CMS-1500 claim form and the appropriate CPT code(s). Patients are often responsible for copayments or they may reach contract limitations. Check with the payer to determine coverage policies and patient responsibility.

## Associated CPT Codes

41823 Excision of osseous tuberosities, dentoalveolar structures

## ICD-10-CM Diagnostic Codes

M27.8 Other specified diseases of jaws

## Relative Value Units/Medicare Edits

| Non-Facility RVU | Work | PE | MP | Total |
|---|---|---|---|---|
| D7485 | 4.80 | 4.24 | 0.99 | 10.03 |
| **Facility RVU** | **Work** | **PE** | **MP** | **Total** |
| D7485 | 4.80 | 4.24 | 0.99 | 10.03 |

| | FUD | Status | MUE | Modifiers | | | | IOM Reference |
|---|---|---|---|---|---|---|---|---|
| D7485 | N/A | I | - | N/A | N/A | N/A | N/A | None |

* with documentation

## Terms To Know

**anomaly.** Irregularity in the structure or position of an organ or tissue.

**dentoalveolar structure.** Area of alveolar bone surrounding the teeth and adjacent tissue.

**excision.** Surgical removal of an organ or tissue.

**gingiva.** Soft tissues surrounding the crowns of unerupted teeth and necks of erupted teeth.

**osseous.** Related to, consisting of, or resembling bone.

**osteotome.** Tool used for cutting bone.

**periodontal.** Relating to the tissues that support and surround the teeth.

**periodontitis.** Inflammation of the tissue structures supporting the teeth leading to a loss of connective tissue attachments.

# D7510-D7521

**D7510** incision and drainage of abscess - intraoral soft tissue

*Involves incision through mucosa, including periodontal origins.*

**D7511** incision and drainage of abscess - intraoral soft tissue - complicated (includes drainage of multiple fascial spaces)

*Incision is made intraorally and dissection is extended into adjacent fascial space(s) to provide adequate drainage of abscess/cellulitis.*

**D7520** incision and drainage of abscess - extraoral soft tissue

*Involves incision through skin.*

**D7521** incision and drainage of abscess - extraoral soft tissue - complicated (includes drainage of multiple fascial spaces)

*Incision is made extraorally and dissection is extended into adjacent fascial space(s) to provide adequate drainage of abscess/cellulitis.*

## Explanation

Incision of the abscess and drainage of the accumulated pus and bacteria are primary in managing odontogenic infections, which most commonly take the form of a necrotic pulp or deep periodontal pocket. Once the area has been anesthetized with a regional block or local infiltration, the dentist inserts a large gauge needle into the abscess cavity to collect a specimen for laboratory analysis. The subsequent incision into the cavity to drain the pus from the infection is made through the mucosa and submucosa; pus remaining in the cavity is removed. Once all areas of the abscess cavity have been emptied and the pus is aspirated through suction from the patient's mouth, a small drain is prepared and sutured into viable tissue to prevent its loss; the drain remains in place, from two to five days, and removal is done by cutting the suture and slipping the drain from the wound. Report D7511 or D7521 for an incision and a drainage that involves multiple fascial spaces. Report D7520 or D7521 when the drainage incision is made through the skin of the face or neck rather than through oral mucosa.

## Coding Tips

Any evaluation of specimen or radiograph is reported separately. Local anesthesia is generally considered part of these services.

## Documentation Tips

The following information should be documented on a tooth chart: treatment/location of caries, endodontic procedures, prosthetic services, preventive services, treatment of lesions and dental disease, or other special procedures. A tooth chart may also be used to identify structure and rationale of disease process, and the type of service performed on intraoral structures other than teeth.

## Reimbursement Tips

When selecting the procedure or service that accurately identifies the service performed, dentists must use the most accurate code. If the CDT code more accurately identifies the service, this should be used rather than the CPT codes. This procedure may be covered by the patient's medical insurance. When covered by medical insurance, the payer may require that the appropriate CPT code be reported on the CMS-1500 claim form.

## Associated CPT Codes

10008 Fine needle aspiration biopsy, including fluoroscopic guidance; each additional lesion (List separately in addition to code for primary procedure)

10009 Fine needle aspiration biopsy, including CT guidance; first lesion

| | |
|---|---|
| 10010 | Fine needle aspiration biopsy, including CT guidance; each additional lesion (List separately in addition to code for primary procedure) |
| 10011 | Fine needle aspiration biopsy, including MR guidance; first lesion |
| 10012 | Fine needle aspiration biopsy, including MR guidance; each additional lesion (List separately in addition to code for primary procedure) |
| 11102 | Tangential biopsy of skin (eg, shave, scoop, saucerize, curette); single lesion |
| 11103 | Tangential biopsy of skin (eg, shave, scoop, saucerize, curette); each separate/additional lesion (List separately in addition to code for primary procedure) |
| 11104 | Punch biopsy of skin (including simple closure, when performed); single lesion |
| 11105 | Punch biopsy of skin (including simple closure, when performed); each separate/additional lesion (List separately in addition to code for primary procedure) |
| 11106 | Incisional biopsy of skin (eg, wedge) (including simple closure, when performed); single lesion |
| 11107 | Incisional biopsy of skin (eg, wedge) (including simple closure, when performed); each separate/additional lesion (List separately in addition to code for primary procedure) |
| 38300 | Drainage of lymph node abscess or lymphadenitis; simple |
| 38305 | Drainage of lymph node abscess or lymphadenitis; extensive |
| 40800 | Drainage of abscess, cyst, hematoma, vestibule of mouth; simple |
| 40801 | Drainage of abscess, cyst, hematoma, vestibule of mouth; complicated |
| 41000 | Intraoral incision and drainage of abscess, cyst, or hematoma of tongue or floor of mouth; lingual |
| 41005 | Intraoral incision and drainage of abscess, cyst, or hematoma of tongue or floor of mouth; sublingual, superficial |
| 41006 | Intraoral incision and drainage of abscess, cyst, or hematoma of tongue or floor of mouth; sublingual, deep, supramylohyoid |
| 41007 | Intraoral incision and drainage of abscess, cyst, or hematoma of tongue or floor of mouth; submental space |
| 41008 | Intraoral incision and drainage of abscess, cyst, or hematoma of tongue or floor of mouth; submandibular space |
| 41009 | Intraoral incision and drainage of abscess, cyst, or hematoma of tongue or floor of mouth; masticator space |
| 41010 | Incision of lingual frenum (frenotomy) |
| 41015 | Extraoral incision and drainage of abscess, cyst, or hematoma of floor of mouth; sublingual |
| 41016 | Extraoral incision and drainage of abscess, cyst, or hematoma of floor of mouth; submental |
| 41017 | Extraoral incision and drainage of abscess, cyst, or hematoma of floor of mouth; submandibular |
| 41018 | Extraoral incision and drainage of abscess, cyst, or hematoma of floor of mouth; masticator space |
| 41800 | Drainage of abscess, cyst, hematoma from dentoalveolar structures |

## ICD-10-CM Diagnostic Codes

| | |
|---|---|
| K12.2 | Cellulitis and abscess of mouth |
| K12.30 | Oral mucositis (ulcerative), unspecified |
| K12.31 | Oral mucositis (ulcerative) due to antineoplastic therapy |
| K12.32 | Oral mucositis (ulcerative) due to other drugs |
| K12.33 | Oral mucositis (ulcerative) due to radiation |
| K12.39 | Other oral mucositis (ulcerative) |

## Relative Value Units/Medicare Edits

| Non-Facility RVU | Work | PE | MP | Total |
|---|---|---|---|---|
| **D7510** | 1.44 | 1.27 | 0.30 | 3.01 |
| **D7511** | 2.20 | 1.94 | 0.45 | 4.59 |
| **D7520** | 6.08 | 5.37 | 1.25 | 12.70 |
| **D7521** | 6.78 | 5.98 | 1.40 | 14.16 |
| **Facility RVU** | **Work** | **PE** | **MP** | **Total** |
| **D7510** | 1.44 | 1.27 | 0.30 | 3.01 |
| **D7511** | 2.20 | 1.94 | 0.45 | 4.59 |
| **D7520** | 6.08 | 5.37 | 1.25 | 12.70 |
| **D7521** | 6.78 | 5.98 | 1.40 | 14.16 |

| | FUD | Status | MUE | Modifiers | | | | IOM Reference |
|---|---|---|---|---|---|---|---|---|
| **D7510** | N/A | I | - | N/A | N/A | N/A | N/A | None |
| **D7511** | N/A | R | - | N/A | N/A | N/A | N/A | |
| **D7520** | N/A | I | - | N/A | N/A | N/A | N/A | |
| **D7521** | N/A | R | - | N/A | N/A | N/A | N/A | |

* with documentation

## Terms To Know

**cellulitis.** Infection of the skin and subcutaneous tissues, most often caused by Staphylococcus or Streptococcus bacteria secondary to a cutaneous lesion. Progression of the inflammation may lead to abscess and tissue death, or even systemic infection-like bacteremia.

**incision and drainage.** Cutting open body tissue for the removal of tissue fluids or infected discharge from a wound or cavity.

**mucosa.** Moist tissue lining the mouth (buccal mucosa), stomach (gastric mucosa), intestines, and respiratory tract.

**oral soft tissue.** Subcutaneous fat layers beneath oral mucosa or gingiva; excludes bone and teeth.

**periodontal.** Relating to the tissues that support and surround the teeth.

**periodontitis.** Inflammation of the tissue structures supporting the teeth leading to a loss of connective tissue attachments.

**pulp.** Living connective tissue within the tooth's root canal space that supplies blood vessels and nerves to the tooth.

# D7530

**D7530** removal of foreign body from mucosa, skin, or subcutaneous alveolar tissue

## Explanation

The dentist or oral surgeon removes a foreign body that has become imbedded in the mucosa, skin, or subcutaneous alveolar tissue. When in the skin, the dentist makes a simple incision in the skin extraorally overlying the foreign body and retrieves it using hemostats or forceps. The skin may be sutured or allowed to heal secondarily. If the foreign body is in the gingival mucosa or subcutaneous dentoalveolar tissue, the dentist may simply be able to grasp the object with an instrument and remove it, or if the object is further embedded, incisions may be made in the soft tissue within the mouth near the object to remove it. Sutures may or may not be necessary.

## Coding Tips

Any evaluation or radiograph is reported separately.

## Reimbursement Tips

When selecting the procedure or service that accurately identifies the service performed, dentists must use the most accurate code. If the CDT code more accurately identifies the service, this should be used rather than the CPT codes. Third-party payers may require clinical documentation and/or x-rays before making payment determination. Check with the payer to determine their specific requirements for coverage. This procedure may be covered by the patient's medical insurance. When covered by medical insurance, the payer may require that the appropriate CPT code be reported on the CMS-1500 claim form.

## Associated CPT Codes

41805 Removal of embedded foreign body from dentoalveolar structures; soft tissues

## ICD-10-CM Diagnostic Codes

S00.552A Superficial foreign body of oral cavity, initial encounter

## Relative Value Units/Medicare Edits

| Non-Facility RVU | Work | PE | MP | Total |
|---|---|---|---|---|
| D7530 | 2.42 | 2.13 | 0.50 | 5.05 |
| **Facility RVU** | **Work** | **PE** | **MP** | **Total** |
| D7530 | 2.42 | 2.13 | 0.50 | 5.05 |

| | FUD | Status | MUE | Modifiers | | | | IOM Reference |
|---|---|---|---|---|---|---|---|---|
| D7530 | N/A | I | - | N/A | N/A | N/A | N/A | None |

* with documentation

## Terms To Know

**dentoalveolar structure.** Area of alveolar bone surrounding the teeth and adjacent tissue.

**foreign body.** Any object or substance found in an organ and tissue that does not belong under normal circumstances.

**oral soft tissue.** Subcutaneous fat layers beneath oral mucosa or gingiva; excludes bone and teeth.

**packing.** Material placed into a cavity or wound, such as gels, gauze, pads, and sponges.

# D7540

**D7540** removal of reaction producing foreign bodies, musculoskeletal system

*May include, but is not limited to, removal of splinters, pieces of wire, etc., from muscle and/or bone.*

## Explanation

The dentist removes a reaction-producing foreign body within the musculoskeletal system. The denticst removes a foreign body, such as a splinter or a piece of wire, embedded in the bone of dentoalveolar structures or in muscle tissue that is causing an abscess, infection, or hematoma. The dentist may be able to simply grasp the object with an instrument and remove it. If the object is further embedded, mucosal incisions may be made to reach the foreign body in the bone or muscle and remove it, possibly with an osteotome or with the aid of separately reportable radiographic imaging, as necessary. The incision may be packed if contaminated by the object and left to drain with later closure or healing by granulation.

## Coding Tips

Any evaluation or radiograph is reported separately. Third-party payers may require clinical documentation and/or x-rays before making payment determination. Check with payers to determine their specific requirements. Some third-party payers may require that this service be reported using the CMS-1500 claim form and the appropriate CPT code(s).

## Reimbursement Tips

When selecting the procedure or service that accurately identifies the service performed, dentists must use the most accurate code. If the CDT code more accurately identifies the service, this should be used rather than the CPT codes. When the condition is the result of an accident, the dental insurer may require that the medical insurance be billed first. When covered by medical insurance, the payer may require that the appropriate CPT code be reported on the CMS-1500 claim form.

## Associated CPT Codes

20520 Removal of foreign body in muscle or tendon sheath; simple

## ICD-10-CM Diagnostic Codes

S00.552A Superficial foreign body of oral cavity, initial encounter

T84.318A Breakdown (mechanical) of other bone devices, implants and grafts, initial encounter

T84.328A Displacement of other bone devices, implants and grafts, initial encounter

T84.410A Breakdown (mechanical) of muscle and tendon graft, initial encounter

T84.418A Breakdown (mechanical) of other internal orthopedic devices, implants and grafts, initial encounter

T84.60XA Infection and inflammatory reaction due to internal fixation device of unspecified site, initial encounter

T84.7XXA Infection and inflammatory reaction due to other internal orthopedic prosthetic devices, implants and grafts, initial encounter

Z47.1 Aftercare following joint replacement surgery

## Relative Value Units/Medicare Edits

| Non-Facility RVU | Work | PE | MP | Total |
|---|---|---|---|---|
| D7540 | 3.10 | 2.74 | 0.64 | 6.48 |
| Facility RVU | Work | PE | MP | Total |
| D7540 | 3.10 | 2.74 | 0.64 | 6.48 |

| | FUD | Status | MUE | Modifiers | | | | IOM Reference |
|---|---|---|---|---|---|---|---|---|
| D7540 | N/A | I | - | N/A | N/A | N/A | N/A | None |

* with documentation

## Terms To Know

**abscess.** Circumscribed collection of pus resulting from bacteria, frequently associated with swelling and other signs of inflammation.

**dentoalveolar structure.** Area of alveolar bone surrounding the teeth and adjacent tissue.

**foreign body.** Any object or substance found in an organ and tissue that does not belong under normal circumstances.

**incision and drainage.** Cutting open body tissue for the removal of tissue fluids or infected discharge from a wound or cavity.

**oral soft tissue.** Subcutaneous fat layers beneath oral mucosa or gingiva; excludes bone and teeth.

**packing.** Material placed into a cavity or wound, such as gels, gauze, pads, and sponges.

# D7560

**D7560** maxillary sinusotomy for removal of tooth fragment or foreign body

## Explanation

When displacement of an upper third molar (wisdom tooth) into the maxillary sinus occurs during extraction, the tooth or fragment requires removal. In some situations, the cavity of the sinus is irrigated with saline and retrieved through the existing opening. In other situations, a window must be created into the sinus at the canine fossa (Caldwell Luc procedure) to access and remove the foreign body.

## Coding Tips

Topical vasoconstrictive agents, local anesthesia, and nasal packing are not reported separately. For Caldwell-Luc sinusotomy, see CPT codes 31030 and 31032.

## ICD-10-CM Diagnostic Codes

J01.00 Acute maxillary sinusitis, unspecified

T17.0XXA Foreign body in nasal sinus, initial encounter

## Relative Value Units/Medicare Edits

| Non-Facility RVU | Work | PE | MP | Total |
|---|---|---|---|---|
| D7560 | 12.15 | 10.73 | 2.50 | 25.38 |
| Facility RVU | Work | PE | MP | Total |
| D7560 | 12.15 | 10.73 | 2.50 | 25.38 |

| | FUD | Status | MUE | Modifiers | | | | IOM Reference |
|---|---|---|---|---|---|---|---|---|
| D7560 | N/A | I | - | N/A | N/A | N/A | N/A | None |

* with documentation

## Terms To Know

**foreign body.** Any object or substance found in an organ and tissue that does not belong under normal circumstances.

**paranasal sinuses.** Air-filled spaces in the cranial bones lined with mucosa and opening into the nasal cavity and include the maxillary, frontal, ethmoid, and sphenoid sinuses.

# D7910

**D7910** suture of recent small wounds up to 5 cm

## Explanation

The dentist sutures recent small wounds of a traumatic nature in the oral mucosa totaling up to 5 cm. A local anesthetic may be given around the laceration and the wound is cleansed, explored, and often irrigated with a saline or antimicrobial solution. The dentist sutures the wounds in a simple repair fashion that does not require complicated suturing techniques or undermining of tissues for closure.

## Coding Tips

Any evaluation or radiograph is reported separately. This code is not to be used for closure of surgical incisions.

## Reimbursement Tips

When selecting the procedure or service that accurately identifies the service performed, dentists must use the most accurate code. If the CDT code more accurately identifies the service, this should be used rather than the CPT codes. When the condition is the result of an accident, the dental insurer may require that the medical insurance be billed first. When covered by the patient's medical insurance, the payer may require that the appropriate CPT code be reported on the CMS-1500 claim form.

## Associated CPT Codes

12011 Simple repair of superficial wounds of face, ears, eyelids, nose, lips and/or mucous membranes; 2.5 cm or less
12013 Simple repair of superficial wounds of face, ears, eyelids, nose, lips and/or mucous membranes; 2.6 cm to 5.0 cm
40830 Closure of laceration, vestibule of mouth; 2.5 cm or less
40831 Closure of laceration, vestibule of mouth; over 2.5 cm or complex

## ICD-10-CM Diagnostic Codes

S01.511A Laceration without foreign body of lip, initial encounter
S01.512A Laceration without foreign body of oral cavity, initial encounter
S01.521A Laceration with foreign body of lip, initial encounter
S01.522A Laceration with foreign body of oral cavity, initial encounter
S01.531A Puncture wound without foreign body of lip, initial encounter
S01.532A Puncture wound without foreign body of oral cavity, initial encounter
S01.541A Puncture wound with foreign body of lip, initial encounter
S01.542A Puncture wound with foreign body of oral cavity, initial encounter
S01.551A Open bite of lip, initial encounter
S01.552A Open bite of oral cavity, initial encounter

## Relative Value Units/Medicare Edits

| Non-Facility RVU | Work | PE | MP | Total |
|---|---|---|---|---|
| D7910 | 2.20 | 1.94 | 0.45 | 4.59 |
| **Facility RVU** | **Work** | **PE** | **MP** | **Total** |
| D7910 | 2.20 | 1.94 | 0.45 | 4.59 |

| | FUD | Status | MUE | Modifiers | | | | IOM Reference |
|---|---|---|---|---|---|---|---|---|
| D7910 | N/A | I | - | N/A | N/A | N/A | N/A | None |

* with documentation

# D7911-D7912

**D7911** complicated suture - up to 5 cm
**D7912** complicated suture - greater than 5 cm

## Explanation

The dentist repairs wounds of the oral tissues requiring complicated suturing, delicate handling of tissues, and wide undermining for meticulous closure. A local anesthetic may be injected around the laceration and the wound is thoroughly cleansed, explored, and often irrigated with a saline or an antimicrobial solution. Extensive cleaning or removal of foreign matter may be necessary. Due to deeper or more complex lacerations, deep layered suturing techniques with wide undermining is required. Report D7911 for complicated suturing up to 5 cm and D7912 for greater than 5 cm. These codes are not to be reported for the closure of surgical incisions.

## Coding Tips

Any evaluation or radiograph is reported separately. These codes are not to be used for closure of surgical incisions. For code D7912 third-party payers may require clinical documentation and/or x-rays before making payment determination.

## Documentation Tips

The following information should be documented on a tooth chart: treatment/location of caries, endodontic procedures, prosthetic services, preventive services, treatment of lesions and dental disease, or other special procedures. A tooth chart may also be used to identify structure and rationale of disease process, and the type of service performed on intraoral structures other than teeth.

## Reimbursement Tips

When selecting the procedure or service that accurately identifies the service performed, dentists must use the most accurate code. If the CDT code more accurately identifies the service, this should be used rather than the CPT codes. When the condition is the result of an accident, the dental insurer may require that the medical insurance be billed first. When covered by medical insurance, the payer may require that the appropriate CPT code be reported on the CMS-1500 claim form.

## Associated CPT Codes

12051 Repair, intermediate, wounds of face, ears, eyelids, nose, lips and/or mucous membranes; 2.5 cm or less
12052 Repair, intermediate, wounds of face, ears, eyelids, nose, lips and/or mucous membranes; 2.6 cm to 5.0 cm
13132 Repair, complex, forehead, cheeks, chin, mouth, neck, axillae, genitalia, hands and/or feet; 2.6 cm to 7.5 cm
40831 Closure of laceration, vestibule of mouth; over 2.5 cm or complex
42900 Suture pharynx for wound or injury

## ICD-10-CM Diagnostic Codes

S01.511A Laceration without foreign body of lip, initial encounter
S01.512A Laceration without foreign body of oral cavity, initial encounter
S01.521A Laceration with foreign body of lip, initial encounter
S01.522A Laceration with foreign body of oral cavity, initial encounter
S01.531A Puncture wound without foreign body of lip, initial encounter
S01.532A Puncture wound without foreign body of oral cavity, initial encounter
S01.541A Puncture wound with foreign body of lip, initial encounter
S01.542A Puncture wound with foreign body of oral cavity, initial encounter
S01.551A Open bite of lip, initial encounter

S01.552A Open bite of oral cavity, initial encounter

## Relative Value Units/Medicare Edits

| Non-Facility RVU | Work | PE | MP | Total |
|---|---|---|---|---|
| D7911 | 4.93 | 4.35 | 1.02 | 10.30 |
| D7912 | 8.69 | 7.67 | 1.79 | 18.15 |
| **Facility RVU** | **Work** | **PE** | **MP** | **Total** |
| D7911 | 4.93 | 4.35 | 1.02 | 10.30 |
| D7912 | 8.69 | 7.67 | 1.79 | 18.15 |

| | FUD | Status | MUE | Modifiers | | | | IOM Reference |
|---|---|---|---|---|---|---|---|---|
| D7911 | N/A | I | - | N/A | N/A | N/A | N/A | None |
| D7912 | N/A | I | - | N/A | N/A | N/A | N/A | |

* with documentation

## Terms To Know

**buccal mucosa.** Tissue from the mucous membrane on the inside of the cheek.

**debride.** To remove all foreign objects and devitalized or infected tissue from a burn or wound to prevent infection and promote healing.

**mucosa.** Moist tissue lining the mouth (buccal mucosa), stomach (gastric mucosa), intestines, and respiratory tract.

**oral soft tissue.** Subcutaneous fat layers beneath oral mucosa or gingiva; excludes bone and teeth.

# D7921

**D7921** collection and application of autologous blood concentrate product

## Explanation

Platelet-rich plasma (PRP) is an autologous product that is derived from whole blood through the process of gradient density centrifugation. It is used in dental implant and bone augmentation procedures to increase bone maturation rate and improve bone density when added to small bony defects or to larger defects that use autogenous bone as the grafting material. The provider withdraws 350-450 mL of blood. The blood is then processed using a gradient density cell separator. The PRP is then either mixed with grafting material or applied to the defect.

## Coding Tips

This code is reported in addition to other procedures performed during the encounter.

## Documentation Tips

Treatment plan documentation should reflect any treatment failure, change in diagnosis, and/or a change in treatment plan. There should also be evidence of any initiation or reinstatement of a drug regime, which requires close and continuous skilled medical observation.

## Reimbursement Tips

When the condition is the result of an accident, the dental insurer may require that the medical insurance be billed first. When covered by medical insurance, the payer may require that the appropriate CPT code be reported on the CMS-1500 claim form.

## ICD-10-CM Diagnostic Codes

This/these CPT code(s) are add-on code(s). See the primary procedure code that this code is performed with for your ICD-10-CM code selections.

## Relative Value Units/Medicare Edits

| Non-Facility RVU | Work | PE | MP | Total |
|---|---|---|---|---|
| D7921 | 1.31 | 1.15 | 0.27 | 2.73 |
| **Facility RVU** | **Work** | **PE** | **MP** | **Total** |
| D7921 | 1.31 | 1.15 | 0.27 | 2.73 |

| | FUD | Status | MUE | Modifiers | | | | IOM Reference |
|---|---|---|---|---|---|---|---|---|
| D7921 | N/A | I | - | N/A | N/A | N/A | N/A | None |

* with documentation

## Terms To Know

**autologous.** Tissue, cells, or structure obtained from the same individual.

# D7922

**D7922** placement of intra-socket biological dressing to aid in hemostasis or clot stabilization, per site

*This procedure can be performed at time and/or after extraction to aid in hemostasis. The socket is packed with a hemostatic agent to aid in hemostasis and or clot stabilization.*

## Explanation

The provider places a biological dressing into the socket at the time of extracting a tooth or other oral surgical procedure to assist in hemostasis. A gauze dressing covered with a hemostatic agent (e.g., CollaPlug, CollaTape, and Helistat) is placed directly into the extraction site. This is used for the prevention of bleeding at the site).

## Coding Tips

Report this code in addition to the surgical procedure performed.

## ICD-10-CM Diagnostic Codes

The application of this code is too broad to adequately present ICD-10-CM diagnostic code links here. Refer to your ICD-10-CM book.

## Relative Value Units/Medicare Edits

| Non-Facility RVU | Work | PE | MP | Total |
|---|---|---|---|---|
| D7922 | 1.49 | 1.32 | 0.31 | 3.12 |
| **Facility RVU** | **Work** | **PE** | **MP** | **Total** |
| D7922 | 1.49 | 1.32 | 0.31 | 3.12 |

| | FUD | Status | MUE | Modifiers | | | | IOM Reference |
|---|---|---|---|---|---|---|---|---|
| D7922 | N/A | I | - | N/A | N/A | N/A | N/A | None |

* with documentation

## Terms To Know

**dressing.** Material applied to a wound or surgical site for protection, absorption, or drainage of the area.

**dry socket.** In dentistry, painful condition occurring when the blood clot disintegrates after tooth extraction, leaving the socket exposed to the air and infection; it may involve osteitis.

**extraction.** Removal of a tooth and tooth fragments from the alveolus.

**hemostasis.** Interruption of blood flow or the cessation or arrest of bleeding.

# D7953

**D7953** bone replacement graft for ridge preservation - per site

*Graft is placed in an extraction or implant removal site at the time of the extraction or removal to preserve ridge integrity (e.g., clinically indicated in preparation for implant reconstruction or where alveolar contour is critical to planned prosthetic reconstruction). oes not include obtaining graft material. Membrane, if used should be reported separately.*

## Explanation

Grafting material is implanted into the extraction socket following tooth extraction for the protection of the contours of the ridge bone and soft tissue. This service is usually performed when an implant will be placed in the future. After removal of the tooth, the provider inserts donor bone into the tooth socket. This procedure may be performed immediately following extraction or within a two-week period following extraction.

## Coding Tips

Report this code when a bone graft is placed in an extraction site at the time of an extraction. This code is appropriate when billed at the same time as an extraction or in an implant removal site. When the graft is used to augment or reconstruct an edentulous ridge see D7950. When bone grafting is performed and the tooth is present, see D4263. Third-party payers consider bone grafts a covered service only when they are medically necessary for the success of the procedure being performed, or when normal healing cannot be expected to eliminate a bony defect. For this reason, many payers may require that current full-mouth preoperative radiographs and/or panoramic radiograph and a narrative describing the planned prosthetic reconstruction accompany the claim.

## Reimbursement Tips

When provided purely for cosmetic reasons, this service will be denied as not medically necessary by most payers. Most payers will only cover this service when the benefit contract provides coverage for implant services. Some third-party payers may require that this service be reported using the CMS-1500 claim form and the appropriate CPT code(s).

## ICD-10-CM Diagnostic Codes

The application of this code is too broad to adequately present ICD-10-CM diagnostic code links here. Refer to your ICD-10-CM book.

## Relative Value Units/Medicare Edits

| Non-Facility RVU | Work | PE | MP | Total |
|---|---|---|---|---|
| D7953 | 2.99 | 2.64 | 0.62 | 6.25 |
| **Facility RVU** | **Work** | **PE** | **MP** | **Total** |
| D7953 | 2.99 | 2.64 | 0.62 | 6.25 |

| | FUD | Status | MUE | Modifiers | | | | IOM Reference |
|---|---|---|---|---|---|---|---|---|
| D7953 | N/A | N | - | N/A | N/A | N/A | N/A | None |

* with documentation

## Terms To Know

**extraction.** Removal of a tooth and tooth fragments from the alveolus.

**graft.** Tissue implant from another part of the body or another person.

# D7961-D7962

**D7961** buccal/labial frenectomy (frenulectomy)
**D7962** lingual frenectomy (frenulectomy)

## Explanation

The surgeon removes the labial, buccal, or lingual frenum (frenectomy). The buccal frenum is a band of mucosal membrane that connects the alveolar (dental) ridge to the cheek and separates the lip vestibule from the cheek vestibule. The labial frenum is a connecting fold of mucous membrane that joins the lip to the gums at the inside mid center. The lingual frenum is a connecting fold of mucous membrane that joins the tongue to the floor of the mouth on the mid center of the tongue underside. Incisions are made around the frenum and through the mucosa and submucosa. The underlying muscle may be removed as well. The excision may extend to the interincisal papilla for the buccal and labial frenum. The mucosa is closed simply, or the dental surgeon may rearrange the tissue in z-plasty technique. Report D7961 for buccal or labial frenectomy and D7962 for lingual frenectomy.

## Coding Tips

Local anesthesia is generally considered part of these services. These procedures are not usually separately reimbursed when done at the time of a more complex procedure. Check the guidelines for the more complex procedure or consult third-party payers for specific guidelines.

## Reimbursement Tips

When selecting the procedure or service that accurately identifies the service performed, dentists must use the most accurate code. If the CDT code more accurately identifies the service, this should be used rather than the CPT codes. When covered by medical insurance, the payer may require that the appropriate CPT code be reported on the CMS-1500 claim form.

## Associated CPT Codes

| | |
|---|---|
| 40806 | Incision of labial frenum (frenotomy) |
| 40819 | Excision of frenum, labial or buccal (frenumectomy, frenulectomy, frenectomy) |
| 41010 | Incision of lingual frenum (frenotomy) |
| 41115 | Excision of lingual frenum (frenectomy) |

## ICD-10-CM Diagnostic Codes

| | |
|---|---|
| K06.1 | Gingival enlargement |
| K06.2 | Gingival and edentulous alveolar ridge lesions associated with trauma |
| K06.8 | Other specified disorders of gingiva and edentulous alveolar ridge |
| K14.0 | Glossitis |
| K14.6 | Glossodynia |
| Q38.1 | Ankyloglossia |
| Q38.3 | Other congenital malformations of tongue |
| Q38.6 | Other congenital malformations of mouth |

## Relative Value Units/Medicare Edits

| Non-Facility RVU | Work | PE | MP | Total |
|---|---|---|---|---|
| D7961 | | | | |
| D7962 | | | | |
| **Facility RVU** | **Work** | **PE** | **MP** | **Total** |
| D7961 | | | | |
| D7962 | | | | |

| | FUD | Status | MUE | Modifiers | | | | IOM Reference |
|---|---|---|---|---|---|---|---|---|
| D7961 | N/A | | - | N/A | N/A | N/A | N/A | |
| D7962 | N/A | | - | N/A | N/A | N/A | N/A | |

* with documentation

## Terms To Know

**buccal frenum.** Band of mucosal membrane that connects the alveolar (dental) ridge to the cheek, separating the lip vestibule from the cheek vestibule.

**frenulectomy.** Excision of the labial, buccal, or lingual frenum.

**labial frenum.** Connecting fold of mucous membrane that joins the upper or lower lip to the gums at the inside midcenter.

# D7970

**D7970** excision of hyperplastic tissue - per arch

## Explanation

The periodontist excises hyperplastic or excessive mucosa from the alveolus. Incisions are made in the hyperplastic tissue, separating it from the normal mucosa. The excessive tissue is removed; the resultant defect may be directly sutured or left to heal without suturing. With large amounts of excess tissue, more than one surgical section may be required to eliminate all of the tissue. Use this code for each specified quadrant excised.

## Coding Tips

Local anesthesia is generally considered part of this service. Payers may require that the provider identify the arch treated as either upper (U) or lower (L) or both on the claim form.

## Documentation Tips

Third-party payers may require clinical documentation and/or x-rays before making payment determination. Check with payers to determine specific requirements.

## Reimbursement Tips

When selecting the procedure or service that accurately identifies the service performed, dentists must use the most accurate code. If the CDT code more accurately identifies the service, this should be used rather than the CPT codes. When covered by medical insurance, the payer may require that the appropriate CPT code be reported on the CMS-1500 claim form.

## Associated CPT Codes

41828 Excision of hyperplastic alveolar mucosa, each quadrant (specify)

## ICD-10-CM Diagnostic Codes

D00.03 Carcinoma in situ of gingiva and edentulous alveolar ridge
D16.5 Benign neoplasm of lower jaw bone
K05.5 Other periodontal diseases
K06.1 Gingival enlargement
K06.2 Gingival and edentulous alveolar ridge lesions associated with trauma
K06.8 Other specified disorders of gingiva and edentulous alveolar ridge
K09.0 Developmental odontogenic cysts
K13.21 Leukoplakia of oral mucosa, including tongue
K13.29 Other disturbances of oral epithelium, including tongue
K13.4 Granuloma and granuloma-like lesions of oral mucosa
K13.6 Irritative hyperplasia of oral mucosa
K13.79 Other lesions of oral mucosa
M26.00 Unspecified anomaly of jaw size
M26.59 Other dentofacial functional abnormalities
M26.71 Alveolar maxillary hyperplasia
M26.72 Alveolar mandibular hyperplasia
M26.79 Other specified alveolar anomalies
M26.89 Other dentofacial anomalies

## Relative Value Units/Medicare Edits

| Non-Facility RVU | Work | PE | MP | Total |
|---|---|---|---|---|
| D7970 | 3.00 | 2.65 | 0.62 | 6.27 |
| **Facility RVU** | **Work** | **PE** | **MP** | **Total** |
| D7970 | 3.00 | 2.65 | 0.62 | 6.27 |

| | FUD | Status | MUE | Modifiers | | | | IOM Reference |
|---|---|---|---|---|---|---|---|---|
| D7970 | N/A | I | - | N/A | N/A | N/A | N/A | None |

* with documentation

## Terms To Know

**benign.** Mild or nonmalignant in nature.

**coronal.** Relating to the top of a tooth or the crown of the head.

**gingiva.** Soft tissues surrounding the crowns of unerupted teeth and necks of erupted teeth.

**hyperplasia.** Abnormal proliferation in the number of normal cells in regular tissue arrangement.

**local anesthesia.** Induced loss of feeling or sensation restricted to a certain area of the body, including topical, local tissue infiltration, field block, or nerve block methods.

**periodontal.** Relating to the tissues that support and surround the teeth.

# D7971

**D7971** excision of pericoronal gingiva

*Removal of inflammatory or hypertrophied tissues surrounding partially erupted/impacted teeth.*

## Explanation

An excision of pericoronal gingiva is the surgical removal of inflammatory or hypertrophied tissues surrounding partially erupted/impacted teeth. The periodontist uses a scalpel, laser, or electrocautery to excise the tissue and establish normal gingival contours around the tooth. A periodontal dressing may be applied.

## Coding Tips

Local anesthesia is generally considered part of this service. When performed at the time of a restoration, this procedure is usually included and, therefore, not separately billable.

## Reimbursement Tips

When selecting the procedure or service that accurately identifies the service performed, dentists must use the most accurate code. If the CDT code more accurately identifies the service, this should be used rather than the CPT codes. When covered by medical insurance, the payer may require that the appropriate CPT code be reported on the CMS-1500 claim form. Some payers may require that CDT codes D7910–D7912 are reported for this procedure using the ADA claim form.

## Associated CPT Codes

| | |
|---|---|
| 41821 | Operculectomy, excision pericoronal tissues |

## ICD-10-CM Diagnostic Codes

| | |
|---|---|
| D16.5 | Benign neoplasm of lower jaw bone |
| K00.6 | Disturbances in tooth eruption |
| K00.8 | Other disorders of tooth development |
| K01.0 | Embedded teeth |
| K01.1 | Impacted teeth |
| K03.5 | Ankylosis of teeth |
| K05.5 | Other periodontal diseases |
| K06.1 | Gingival enlargement |
| Z18.32 | Retained tooth |

## Relative Value Units/Medicare Edits

| Non-Facility RVU | Work | PE | MP | Total |
|---|---|---|---|---|
| D7971 | 1.17 | 1.03 | 0.24 | 2.44 |
| **Facility RVU** | **Work** | **PE** | **MP** | **Total** |
| D7971 | 1.17 | 1.03 | 0.24 | 2.44 |

| | FUD | Status | MUE | Modifiers | | | | IOM Reference |
|---|---|---|---|---|---|---|---|---|
| D7971 | N/A | I | - | N/A | N/A | N/A | N/A | None |

* with documentation

# D7972

**D7972** surgical reduction of fibrous tuberosity

## Explanation

A fibrous tuberosity is a rounded area at the back of the upper teeth. In this procedure the periodontist excises fibrous soft tissue overlying the tuberosities of dentoalveolar structures, reducing the size of the tuberosity. Elliptically or wedge-shaped incisions are made through the soft tissue of the tuberosity; the tissue is removed, and the surgical wound is sutured directly.

## Coding Tips

Local anesthesia is generally considered part of this service. Third-party payers may bundle this service into the fees for the following procedures: D4210, D4211, D4260, and D4261.

## Reimbursement Tips

When selecting the procedure or service that accurately identifies the service performed, dentists must use the most accurate code. If the CDT code more accurately identifies the service, this should be used rather than the CPT codes. Third-party payers may bundle this service into the fees for the following procedures: D4210, D4211, D4260, and D4261. This procedure may be covered by the patient's medical insurance. When covered by medical insurance, the payer may require that the appropriate CPT code be reported on the CMS-1500 claim form.

## Associated CPT Codes

| | |
|---|---|
| 41822 | Excision of fibrous tuberosities, dentoalveolar structures |

## ICD-10-CM Diagnostic Codes

| | |
|---|---|
| K00.4 | Disturbances in tooth formation |
| K00.5 | Hereditary disturbances in tooth structure, not elsewhere classified |
| K00.6 | Disturbances in tooth eruption |
| K00.8 | Other disorders of tooth development |
| K00.9 | Disorder of tooth development, unspecified |
| K01.0 | Embedded teeth |
| K01.1 | Impacted teeth |
| K05.00 | Acute gingivitis, plaque induced |
| K05.01 | Acute gingivitis, non-plaque induced |
| K05.10 | Chronic gingivitis, plaque induced |
| K05.11 | Chronic gingivitis, non-plaque induced |
| K05.311 | Chronic periodontitis, localized, slight |
| K05.312 | Chronic periodontitis, localized, moderate |
| K05.313 | Chronic periodontitis, localized, severe |
| K05.319 | Chronic periodontitis, localized, unspecified severity |
| K05.321 | Chronic periodontitis, generalized, slight |
| K05.322 | Chronic periodontitis, generalized, moderate |
| K05.323 | Chronic periodontitis, generalized, severe |
| K05.329 | Chronic periodontitis, generalized, unspecified severity |
| K05.4 | Periodontosis |
| K05.5 | Other periodontal diseases |
| K06.011 | Localized gingival recession, minimal |
| K06.012 | Localized gingival recession, moderate |
| K06.013 | Localized gingival recession, severe |
| K06.021 | Generalized gingival recession, minimal |
| K06.022 | Generalized gingival recession, moderate |
| K06.023 | Generalized gingival recession, severe |

| | |
|---|---|
| K06.1 | Gingival enlargement |
| K06.2 | Gingival and edentulous alveolar ridge lesions associated with trauma |
| K06.8 | Other specified disorders of gingiva and edentulous alveolar ridge |
| K08.81 | Primary occlusal trauma |
| K08.82 | Secondary occlusal trauma |
| K08.9 | Disorder of teeth and supporting structures, unspecified |
| M26.70 | Unspecified alveolar anomaly |
| M26.79 | Other specified alveolar anomalies |
| M26.89 | Other dentofacial anomalies |
| M26.9 | Dentofacial anomaly, unspecified |
| M27.8 | Other specified diseases of jaws |

## Relative Value Units/Medicare Edits

| Non-Facility RVU | Work | PE | MP | Total |
|---|---|---|---|---|
| D7972 | 4.10 | 3.62 | 0.84 | 8.56 |
| **Facility RVU** | **Work** | **PE** | **MP** | **Total** |
| D7972 | 4.10 | 3.62 | 0.84 | 8.56 |

| | FUD | Status | MUE | Modifiers | | | | IOM Reference |
|---|---|---|---|---|---|---|---|---|
| D7972 | N/A | I | - | N/A | N/A | N/A | N/A | None |

* with documentation

## Terms To Know

**gingivitis.** Inflamed gingiva (oral mucosa) that surrounds the teeth.

**local anesthesia.** Induced loss of feeling or sensation restricted to a certain area of the body, including topical, local tissue infiltration, field block, or nerve block methods.

**periodontitis.** Inflammation of the tissue structures supporting the teeth leading to a loss of connective tissue attachments.

**tubercle.** Small rough prominence or rounded nodule on a bone.

# D7979

**D7979** non - surgical sialolithotomy

*A sialolith is removed from the gland or ductal portion of the gland without surgical incision into the gland or the duct of the gland; for example via manual manipulation, ductal dilation, or any other non-surgical method.*

## Explanation

The provider removes calculus from a salivary gland without making an incision. This can be performed either by dilating the duct and removing the calculus, expressing the stone via manual manipulation, or other methods that do not involve a surgical incision.

## Coding Tips

Local anesthesia is generally considered to be part of this procedure. Surgical sialolithotomy is report with D7980.

## ICD-10-CM Diagnostic Codes

| | |
|---|---|
| K11.21 | Acute sialoadenitis |
| K11.22 | Acute recurrent sialoadenitis |
| K11.23 | Chronic sialoadenitis |
| K11.3 | Abscess of salivary gland |
| K11.4 | Fistula of salivary gland |
| K11.5 | Sialolithiasis |

## Relative Value Units/Medicare Edits

| Non-Facility RVU | Work | PE | MP | Total |
|---|---|---|---|---|
| D7979 | 1.53 | 1.35 | 0.32 | 3.20 |
| **Facility RVU** | **Work** | **PE** | **MP** | **Total** |
| D7979 | 1.53 | 1.35 | 0.32 | 3.20 |

| | FUD | Status | MUE | Modifiers | | | | IOM Reference |
|---|---|---|---|---|---|---|---|---|
| D7979 | N/A | N | - | N/A | N/A | N/A | N/A | None |

* with documentation

## Terms To Know

**calculus.** Abnormal, stone-like concretion of calcium, cholesterol, mineral salts, or other substances that forms in any part of the body.

**fistula.** Abnormal tube-like passage between two body cavities or organs or from an organ to the outside surface.

**salivary gland.** One of several glands that secrete saliva into the oral cavity.

**sialolithiasis.** Stone or concretion in the salivary duct.

# D7993-D7994

**D7993** surgical placement of craniofacial implant - extra oral

*Surgical placement of a craniofacial implant to aid in retention of an auricular, nasal, or orbital prosthesis.*

**D7994** surgical placement: zygomatic implant

*An implant placed in the zygomatic bone and exiting through the maxillary mucosal tissue providing support and attachment of a maxillary dental prosthesis.*

## Explanation

Prior to the surgical procedure, a surgical guide is created using conventional impressions or through computerized virtual planning to aid in placement of craniofacial or zygomatic implants. The area skin over the designated implant placement is excised. The skin and muscles are reflected exposing the bone. An osteotomy is created in the bone. The implants are placed in the craniofacial or zygomatic bone using the surgical guide. Skin is closed in layers and a dressing is applied. The prostheses are applied after adequate healing. Report D7993 for craniofacial implants and D7994 for zygomatic implants.

## Coding Tips

This code includes any allogenic material used in the grafting. Prostheses are separately reported, see D5911-D5999.

## Reimbursement Tips

When covered by the patient's medical insurance, report the appropriate CPT code. Coverage of this procedure varies by payer. Check with the payer for specific coverage guidelines.

## Associated CPT Codes

21125 Augmentation, mandibular body or angle; prosthetic material
21127 Augmentation, mandibular body or angle; with bone graft, onlay or interpositional (includes obtaining autograft)
21210 Graft, bone; nasal, maxillary or malar areas (includes obtaining graft)
21215 Graft, bone; mandible (includes obtaining graft)
21270 Malar augmentation, prosthetic material

## ICD-10-CM Diagnostic Codes

C41.0 Malignant neoplasm of bones of skull and face
C76.0 Malignant neoplasm of head, face and neck
D16.4 Benign neoplasm of bones of skull and face
M26.02 Maxillary hypoplasia
M26.09 Other specified anomalies of jaw size
M26.11 Maxillary asymmetry
M26.12 Other jaw asymmetry
M26.19 Other specified anomalies of jaw-cranial base relationship
M87.08 Idiopathic aseptic necrosis of bone, other site
M87.180 Osteonecrosis due to drugs, jaw
Q67.4 Other congenital deformities of skull, face and jaw
Q75.4 Mandibulofacial dysostosis
Q75.5 Oculomandibular dysostosis
Q75.8 Other specified congenital malformations of skull and face bones
Q87.0 Congenital malformation syndromes predominantly affecting facial appearance
S02.40CA Maxillary fracture, right side, initial encounter for closed fracture ☑
S02.40CB Maxillary fracture, right side, initial encounter for open fracture ☑
S02.40DA Maxillary fracture, left side, initial encounter for closed fracture ☑
S02.40DB Maxillary fracture, left side, initial encounter for open fracture ☑
S02.40EA Zygomatic fracture, right side, initial encounter for closed fracture ☑
S02.40EB Zygomatic fracture, right side, initial encounter for open fracture ☑
S02.40FA Zygomatic fracture, left side, initial encounter for closed fracture ☑
S02.40FB Zygomatic fracture, left side, initial encounter for open fracture ☑
S02.411A LeFort I fracture, initial encounter for closed fracture
S02.411B LeFort I fracture, initial encounter for open fracture
S02.412A LeFort II fracture, initial encounter for closed fracture
S02.412B LeFort II fracture, initial encounter for open fracture
S02.413A LeFort III fracture, initial encounter for closed fracture
S02.413B LeFort III fracture, initial encounter for open fracture
S02.42XA Fracture of alveolus of maxilla, initial encounter for closed fracture
S02.42XB Fracture of alveolus of maxilla, initial encounter for open fracture
S07.0XXA Crushing injury of face, initial encounter
Z41.1 Encounter for cosmetic surgery
Z42.8 Encounter for other plastic and reconstructive surgery following medical procedure or healed injury

## Relative Value Units/Medicare Edits

| Non-Facility RVU | Work | PE | MP | Total |
|---|---|---|---|---|
| D7993 | | | | |
| D7994 | | | | |
| **Facility RVU** | **Work** | **PE** | **MP** | **Total** |
| D7993 | | | | |
| D7994 | | | | |

| | FUD | Status | MUE | Modifiers | | | | IOM Reference |
|---|---|---|---|---|---|---|---|---|
| D7993 | N/A | | - | N/A | N/A | N/A | N/A | |
| D7994 | N/A | | - | N/A | N/A | N/A | N/A | |

* with documentation

## Terms To Know

**allograft.** Graft from one individual to another of the same species.

**craniofacial.** Relating to skull and facial bones.

**implant.** Material or device inserted or placed within the body for therapeutic, reconstructive, or diagnostic purposes.

**prosthesis.** Man-made substitute for a missing body part.

**zygomatic arch.** Part of the temporal bone of the skull that forms the prominence of the cheek.

# D7997

**D7997** appliance removal (not by dentist who placed appliance), includes removal of archbar

## Explanation

The appliance is removed once the patient has resumed a normal range of jaw movement and the teeth continue to bite into the splint or occlusion. Before removal, the wires holding the device are cleaned where they enter the mucosa and are cut beneath the mucosa by forcing the appliance down around the wire. This prevents possible infection. Removal is performed using light sedation or local anesthesia. Postsurgical orthodontic procedures can begin within 48 hours from removal of the appliance.

## Coding Tips

Local anesthesia is generally considered part of this service.

## ICD-10-CM Diagnostic Codes

Z46.3 Encounter for fitting and adjustment of dental prosthetic device

## Relative Value Units/Medicare Edits

| Non-Facility RVU | Work | PE | MP | Total |
|---|---|---|---|---|
| D7997 | 1.66 | 1.46 | 0.34 | 3.46 |
| **Facility RVU** | **Work** | **PE** | **MP** | **Total** |
| D7997 | 1.66 | 1.46 | 0.34 | 3.46 |

| | FUD | Status | MUE | Modifiers | | | | IOM Reference |
|---|---|---|---|---|---|---|---|---|
| D7997 | N/A | N | - | N/A | N/A | N/A | N/A | None |

* with documentation

## Terms To Know

**prosthesis.** Man-made substitute for a missing body part.

# D7998

**D7998** intraoral placement of a fixation device not in conjunction with a fracture

*The placement of intermaxillary fixation appliance for documented medically accepted treatments not in association with fractures.*

## Explanation

Arch bars are placed onto the patient's upper and lower dental arches with individual wire ligatures around the teeth to secure the mouth in a stable, proper occlusion.

## Coding Tips

For placement of an intraoral fixation performed in conjunction with fracture treatment, see the appropriate fracture code.

## Reimbursement Tips

When selecting the procedure or service that accurately identifies the service performed, dentists must use the most accurate code. If the CDT code more accurately identifies the service, this should be used rather than the CPT codes. Coverage of this procedure varies by payer. Check with payers for specific coverage guidelines. Pertinent documentation to evaluate the medical appropriateness may be required.

## Associated CPT Codes

21110 Application of interdental fixation device for conditions other than fracture or dislocation, includes removal

## ICD-10-CM Diagnostic Codes

The application of this code is too broad to adequately present ICD-10-CM diagnostic code links here. Refer to your ICD-10-CM book.

## Relative Value Units/Medicare Edits

| Non-Facility RVU | Work | PE | MP | Total |
|---|---|---|---|---|
| D7998 | 8.49 | 7.50 | 1.75 | 17.74 |
| **Facility RVU** | **Work** | **PE** | **MP** | **Total** |
| D7998 | 8.49 | 7.50 | 1.75 | 17.74 |

| | FUD | Status | MUE | Modifiers | | | | IOM Reference |
|---|---|---|---|---|---|---|---|---|
| D7998 | N/A | N | - | N/A | N/A | N/A | N/A | None |

* with documentation

## Terms To Know

**fixation.** Act or condition of being attached, secured, fastened, or held in position.

**intraoral.** Within the mouth.

# D8010-D8040

**D8010** limited orthodontic treatment of the primary dentition
**D8020** limited orthodontic treatment of the transitional dentition
**D8030** limited orthodontic treatment of the adolescent dentition
**D8040** limited orthodontic treatment of the adult dentition

## Explanation

Limited orthodontic treatment focuses on one particular problem as a limited objective and does not involve all of the dentition. It may involve fixing only one existing problem or one part of a much bigger problem where it is necessary to concentrate efforts there first before more comprehensive therapy may be undertaken or when a decision is made to defer or forego the comprehensive therapy entirely. Examples include limited treatment to open spaces or upright a falsely positioned tooth in order for a bridge or implant to be placed, correcting crowding in one arch only, or partial treatment to close space in one part of the mouth. Report D8010 for limited orthodontic treatment of the primary dentition or "baby teeth," which will later be replaced by adult teeth. Report D8020 for treatment of the transitional dentition, or teeth in the last phase of transition from first teeth to permanent teeth, when the deciduous molars and canines are in the process of shedding and the adult replacements are emerging. Report D8030 for treatment of adolescent dentition, or teeth that are present after the normal loss of primary teeth but before growth that would affect orthodontic treatment has stopped; and D8040 for limited orthodontic treatment on adult dentition, after affective growth has ceased.

## Coding Tips

Limited orthodontic treatment uses simple appliances and simple movements such as simple singular tooth movement with a retainer. Initial evaluation and radiographs are reported separately. Services related to orthodontic treatment are usually benefits of a patient's diagnostic or basic coverage, even when the program provides orthodontic coverage. Such procedures may include examination, x-rays, and extractions.

## Documentation Tips

The following information should be documented on a tooth chart: treatment/location of caries, endodontic procedures, prosthetic services, preventive services, treatment of lesions and dental disease, or other special procedures. A tooth chart may also be used to identify structure and rationale of disease process, and the type of service performed on intraoral structures other than teeth.

## Reimbursement Tips

Medically necessary orthodontia services are mandated under the Affordable Care Act (ACA) for those patients who have a severe handicapping malocclusion related to a medical condition. Medical record documentation must support the severity of the malocclusion and the medical condition. Some payers may require a standardized assessment, such as the Salzmann Evaluation Index be completed and that a specific score (for example 42 or higher) be documented.

## ICD-10-CM Diagnostic Codes

M26.30 Unspecified anomaly of tooth position of fully erupted tooth or teeth
M26.31 Crowding of fully erupted teeth
M26.32 Excessive spacing of fully erupted teeth
M26.33 Horizontal displacement of fully erupted tooth or teeth
M26.34 Vertical displacement of fully erupted tooth or teeth
M26.35 Rotation of fully erupted tooth or teeth
M26.36 Insufficient interocclusal distance of fully erupted teeth (ridge)
M26.37 Excessive interocclusal distance of fully erupted teeth
M26.39 Other anomalies of tooth position of fully erupted tooth or teeth

## Relative Value Units/Medicare Edits

| Non-Facility RVU | Work | PE | MP | Total |
|---|---|---|---|---|
| D8010 | 4.76 | 9.43 | 0.57 | 14.76 |
| D8020 | 5.62 | 11.14 | 0.67 | 17.43 |
| D8030 | 7.57 | 15.00 | 0.91 | 23.48 |
| D8040 | 7.35 | 14.57 | 0.88 | 22.80 |
| **Facility RVU** | **Work** | **PE** | **MP** | **Total** |
| D8010 | 4.76 | 9.43 | 0.57 | 14.76 |
| D8020 | 5.62 | 11.14 | 0.67 | 17.43 |
| D8030 | 7.57 | 15.00 | 0.91 | 23.48 |
| D8040 | 7.35 | 14.57 | 0.88 | 22.80 |

| | FUD | Status | MUE | Modifiers | | | | IOM Reference |
|---|---|---|---|---|---|---|---|---|
| D8010 | N/A | N | - | N/A | N/A | N/A | N/A | None |
| D8020 | N/A | N | - | N/A | N/A | N/A | N/A | |
| D8030 | N/A | N | - | N/A | N/A | N/A | N/A | |
| D8040 | N/A | N | - | N/A | N/A | N/A | N/A | |

* with documentation

## Terms To Know

**deciduous tooth.** Any of 20 teeth that usually erupt between the ages of 6 and 24 months and are later shed as the permanent, adult teeth displace them.

**permanent tooth.** One of 32 adult teeth that usually erupt between 6 years and adulthood with the third molar.

**primary tooth.** Any of 20 deciduous teeth that usually erupt between the ages of 6 and 24 months.

# D8070-D8090

**D8070** comprehensive orthodontic treatment of the transitional dentition
**D8080** comprehensive orthodontic treatment of the adolescent dentition
**D8090** comprehensive orthodontic treatment of the adult dentition

## Explanation

Comprehensive orthodontic treatment includes incorporating multiple phases of treatment provided at different stages of development, with specific objectives to be met at the various stages. These codes report the diagnosis and treatment meant to improve the patient's craniofacial dysfunction and/or dentofacial deformities, including aesthetic as well as functional relationships. Comprehensive treatment usually entails using fixed orthodontic appliances. Examples include two-stage procedures, such as using an activator in stage one and placing fixed appliances during a second stage of a two-stage treatment. Both phases are reported as comprehensive treatment, with the correct choice for the appropriate stage of the patient's dental development. Report D8070 for comprehensive orthodontic treatment of the transitional dentition, or teeth in the last phase of transition from first teeth to permanent teeth, when the deciduous molars and canines are in the process of shedding and the adult replacements are emerging. Report D8080 for treatment of adolescent dentition, or teeth that are present after the normal loss of primary teeth but before growth that would affect orthodontic treatment has stopped. Report D8090 for comprehensive orthodontic treatment on adult dentition, after affective growth has ceased.

## Coding Tips

Initial evaluation and radiographs are reported separately. Services related to orthodontic treatment are usually benefits of a patient's diagnostic or basic coverage, even when the program provides orthodontic coverage. Such procedures may include examination, x-rays, and extractions.

## Reimbursement Tips

Medically necessary orthodontia services are mandated under the Affordable Care Act (ACA) for those patients who have a severe handicapping malocclusion related to a medical condition. Medical record documentation must support the severity of the malocclusion and the medical condition. Some payers may require a standardized assessment, such as the Salzmann Evaluation Index be completed and that a specific score (for example 42 or higher) be documented.

## ICD-10-CM Diagnostic Codes

| | |
|---|---|
| M26.30 | Unspecified anomaly of tooth position of fully erupted tooth or teeth |
| M26.31 | Crowding of fully erupted teeth |
| M26.32 | Excessive spacing of fully erupted teeth |
| M26.33 | Horizontal displacement of fully erupted tooth or teeth |
| M26.34 | Vertical displacement of fully erupted tooth or teeth |
| M26.35 | Rotation of fully erupted tooth or teeth |
| M26.36 | Insufficient interocclusal distance of fully erupted teeth (ridge) |
| M26.37 | Excessive interocclusal distance of fully erupted teeth |
| M26.39 | Other anomalies of tooth position of fully erupted tooth or teeth |

## Relative Value Units/Medicare Edits

| Non-Facility RVU | Work | PE | MP | Total |
|---|---|---|---|---|
| **D8070** | 23.56 | 46.72 | 2.83 | 73.11 |
| **D8080** | 19.67 | 39.00 | 2.36 | 61.03 |
| **D8090** | 20.54 | 40.72 | 2.47 | 63.73 |
| **Facility RVU** | **Work** | **PE** | **MP** | **Total** |
| **D8070** | 23.56 | 46.72 | 2.83 | 73.11 |
| **D8080** | 19.67 | 39.00 | 2.36 | 61.03 |
| **D8090** | 20.54 | 40.72 | 2.47 | 63.73 |

| | FUD | Status | MUE | Modifiers | | | | IOM Reference |
|---|---|---|---|---|---|---|---|---|
| **D8070** | N/A | N | - | N/A | N/A | N/A | N/A | None |
| **D8080** | N/A | N | - | N/A | N/A | N/A | N/A | |
| **D8090** | N/A | N | - | N/A | N/A | N/A | N/A | |

* with documentation

## Terms To Know

**deciduous tooth.** Any of 20 teeth that usually erupt between the ages of 6 and 24 months and are later shed as the permanent, adult teeth displace them.

**orthodontia.** Treatment of malocclusion and other neuromuscular and skeletal abnormalities of the teeth and their surrounding structures.

**permanent tooth.** One of 32 adult teeth that usually erupt between 6 years and adulthood with the third molar.

**primary tooth.** Any of 20 deciduous teeth that usually erupt between the ages of 6 and 24 months.

Dental - Orthodontics

# D8210-D8220

**D8210** removable appliance therapy

*Removable indicates patient can remove; includes appliances for thumb sucking and tongue thrusting.*

**D8220** fixed appliance therapy

*Fixed indicates patient cannot remove appliance; includes appliances for thumb sucking and tongue thrusting.*



## Explanation

Removal and fixed appliance therapy to treat harmful habits are used for conditions of thumb-sucking and tongue thrusting. These appliances do not interfere with normal oral functioning, but serve as a reminder to keep the thumb out, or to hold the tongue in proper position while swallowing. Oral shields can be used to correct thumb sucking, or a lingual archwire with short spurs soldered at strategic locations. Tongue thrusting may be complex or simple. Simple tongue thrust is one with a teeth-together swallow and a usual malocclusion of a well-circumscribed open bite in the anterior region. A complex tongue thrust is one with a teeth-apart swallow and a usual malocclusion of a poor occlusal fit prompting sliding into occlusion, and a generalized open bite anteriorly. A maxillary soldered, lingual archwire with short, sharp, strategically placed spurs is used in such therapy. These appliances may be used as a retainer that the patient can remove (D8210) or cemented into the mouth as a fixed appliance (D8220). However, such appliances should never be applied as the first step, only after conscious efforts of training and practicing with the patient have been done first to help the patient accept the need for the appliance.

## Coding Tips

Initial evaluation and radiographs are reported separately. Services related to orthodontic treatment are usually benefits of a patient's diagnostic or basic coverage, even when the program provides orthodontic coverage. Such procedures may include examination, x-rays, and extractions.

## ICD-10-CM Diagnostic Codes

| | |
|---|---|
| F98.8 | Other specified behavioral and emotional disorders with onset usually occurring in childhood and adolescence P |

## Relative Value Units/Medicare Edits

| Non-Facility RVU | Work | PE | MP | Total |
|---|---|---|---|---|
| **D8210** | 2.57 | 5.10 | 0.31 | 7.98 |
| **D8220** | 3.09 | 6.13 | 0.37 | 9.59 |
| **Facility RVU** | **Work** | **PE** | **MP** | **Total** |
| **D8210** | 2.57 | 5.10 | 0.31 | 7.98 |
| **D8220** | 3.09 | 6.13 | 0.37 | 9.59 |

| | FUD | Status | MUE | Modifiers | | | | IOM Reference |
|---|---|---|---|---|---|---|---|---|
| **D8210** | N/A | N | - | N/A | N/A | N/A | N/A | None |
| **D8220** | N/A | N | - | N/A | N/A | N/A | N/A | |

* with documentation

# D8660-D8670

**D8660** pre-orthodontic treatment examination to monitor growth and development

*Periodic observation of patient dentition, at intervals established by the dentist, to determine when orthodontic treatment should begin. Diagnostic procedures are documented separately.*

**D8670** periodic orthodontic treatment visit

## Explanation

Report D8660 when the oral care giver provides treatment in a visit specifically for care before an orthodontic treatment regimen is begun and report D8670 when the treatment is given as part of a contracted periodic orthodontic treatment visit.

## Coding Tips

Any radiograph is reported separately. Services related to orthodontic treatment are usually benefits of a patient's diagnostic or basic coverage, even when the program provides orthodontic coverage. Such procedures may include examination, x-rays, and extractions.

## Reimbursement Tips

Coverage of these procedures varies by payer. Check with the payer for specific coverage guidelines.

## ICD-10-CM Diagnostic Codes

| | |
|---|---|
| M26.31 | Crowding of fully erupted teeth |
| M26.32 | Excessive spacing of fully erupted teeth |
| M26.33 | Horizontal displacement of fully erupted tooth or teeth |
| M26.34 | Vertical displacement of fully erupted tooth or teeth |
| M26.35 | Rotation of fully erupted tooth or teeth |
| M26.36 | Insufficient interocclusal distance of fully erupted teeth (ridge) |
| M26.37 | Excessive interocclusal distance of fully erupted teeth |
| M26.39 | Other anomalies of tooth position of fully erupted tooth or teeth |

## Relative Value Units/Medicare Edits

| Non-Facility RVU | Work | PE | MP | Total |
|---|---|---|---|---|
| **D8660** | 0.78 | 1.54 | 0.09 | 2.41 |
| **D8670** | 0.58 | 1.16 | 0.07 | 1.81 |
| **Facility RVU** | **Work** | **PE** | **MP** | **Total** |
| **D8660** | 0.78 | 1.54 | 0.09 | 2.41 |
| **D8670** | 0.58 | 1.16 | 0.07 | 1.81 |

| | FUD | Status | MUE | Modifiers | | | | IOM Reference |
|---|---|---|---|---|---|---|---|---|
| **D8660** | N/A | N | - | N/A | N/A | N/A | N/A | None |
| **D8670** | N/A | N | - | N/A | N/A | N/A | N/A | |

* with documentation

# D8680-D8681

**D8680** orthodontic retention (removal of appliances, construction and placement of retainer(s))
**D8681** removable orthodontic retainer adjustment

## Explanation

The orthodontic retention, also referred to as the orthodontic contention is the stabilization or retention period minimizing unwanted dental movements and maintaining the corrections obtained during the initial period following the removal of the braces or other appliances used for correction. The retention period is for a period of at least six months. Code D8680 describes the removal of the fixed appliance and the creation of a retainer. Removal of the previously placed appliance is dependent upon the brace used. After the removal the provider constructs and places a retainer(s), which is dependent upon the retainer used. Code D8681 describes the adjustment of the retainer provided during the orthodontic retention period.

## Coding Tips

To report periodic orthodontic treatment visit, see D8670.

## Documentation Tips

Some payers may require that x-rays and/or x-ray reports be submitted with the claim.

## ICD-10-CM Diagnostic Codes

| | |
|---|---|
| K00.6 | Disturbances in tooth eruption |
| K08.421 | Partial loss of teeth due to periodontal diseases, class I |
| K08.422 | Partial loss of teeth due to periodontal diseases, class II |
| K08.423 | Partial loss of teeth due to periodontal diseases, class III |
| K08.424 | Partial loss of teeth due to periodontal diseases, class IV |
| K08.431 | Partial loss of teeth due to caries, class I |
| K08.432 | Partial loss of teeth due to caries, class II |
| K08.433 | Partial loss of teeth due to caries, class III |
| K08.434 | Partial loss of teeth due to caries, class IV |
| M26.31 | Crowding of fully erupted teeth |
| M26.32 | Excessive spacing of fully erupted teeth |
| M26.33 | Horizontal displacement of fully erupted tooth or teeth |
| M26.34 | Vertical displacement of fully erupted tooth or teeth |
| M26.35 | Rotation of fully erupted tooth or teeth |
| M26.36 | Insufficient interocclusal distance of fully erupted teeth (ridge) |
| M26.37 | Excessive interocclusal distance of fully erupted teeth |

## Relative Value Units/Medicare Edits

| Non-Facility RVU | Work | PE | MP | Total |
|---|---|---|---|---|
| D8680 | 1.81 | 3.60 | 0.22 | 5.63 |
| D8681 | 0.70 | 1.39 | 0.08 | 2.17 |
| **Facility RVU** | **Work** | **PE** | **MP** | **Total** |
| D8680 | 1.81 | 3.60 | 0.22 | 5.63 |
| D8681 | 0.70 | 1.39 | 0.08 | 2.17 |

| | FUD | Status | MUE | Modifiers | | | | IOM Reference |
|---|---|---|---|---|---|---|---|---|
| D8680 | N/A | N | - | N/A | N/A | N/A | N/A | None |
| D8681 | N/A | N | - | N/A | N/A | N/A | N/A | |

* with documentation

# D8695

**D8695** removal of fixed orthodontic appliances for reasons other than completion of treatment

## Explanation

The provider removes the fixed orthodontic appliance prior to the completion of treatment. The specific service provided depends upon the type of fixed orthodontic appliance. Examples of fixed appliances include braces, fixed lingual retainer, and fan type expander.

## Coding Tips

Removal of the orthodontic appliance at the patient's request is an example of the reason for removal of the appliance. When the orthodontic appliance is removed at the conclusion of active treatment, see D8680. Local anesthesia is generally considered to be part of this procedure.

## Documentation Tips

The medical record should include the complication, condition, or other reason that caused the provider to remove the appliance prior to the completion of the treatment.

## ICD-10-CM Diagnostic Codes

| | |
|---|---|
| Z46.4 | Encounter for fitting and adjustment of orthodontic device |

## Relative Value Units/Medicare Edits

| Non-Facility RVU | Work | PE | MP | Total |
|---|---|---|---|---|
| D8695 | 0.86 | 1.71 | 0.10 | 2.67 |
| **Facility RVU** | **Work** | **PE** | **MP** | **Total** |
| D8695 | 0.86 | 1.71 | 0.10 | 2.67 |

| | FUD | Status | MUE | Modifiers | | | | IOM Reference |
|---|---|---|---|---|---|---|---|---|
| D8695 | N/A | N | - | N/A | N/A | N/A | N/A | None |

* with documentation

## Terms To Know

**orthodontia.** Treatment of malocclusion and other neuromuscular and skeletal abnormalities of the teeth and their surrounding structures.

# D8696-D8697

**D8696** repair of orthodontic appliance - maxillary

*Does not include bracket and standard fixed orthodontic appliances. It does include functional appliances and palatal expanders.*

**D8697** repair of orthodontic appliance - mandibular

*Does not include bracket and standard fixed orthodontic appliances. It does include functional appliances and palatal expanders.*

## Explanation

The provider repairs an orthodontic appliance such as Hawley, Barrer/Spring, Begg/Wraparound, or vacuum/pressure formed retainers of the upper (D8696) or lower (D8697) jaw. The repair is dependent upon the need. The provider examines the appliance for fit, wear, and/or breakage. The type of repair performed is dependent upon the type of damage. This code should not be reported for the repair or replacement of a bracket and standard fixed orthodontic appliances; however, it does include the repair of functional appliances or palatal expanders.

## Coding Tips

This does not include the repair of a bracket or a standard fixed orthodontic appliance; see D8999.

## ICD-10-CM Diagnostic Codes

Z97.2 Presence of dental prosthetic device (complete) (partial)

## Relative Value Units/Medicare Edits

| Non-Facility RVU | Work | PE | MP | Total |
|---|---|---|---|---|
| D8696 | 0.70 | 1.39 | 0.08 | 2.17 |
| D8697 | 0.70 | 1.39 | 0.08 | 2.17 |
| **Facility RVU** | **Work** | **PE** | **MP** | **Total** |
| D8696 | 0.70 | 1.39 | 0.08 | 2.17 |
| D8697 | 0.70 | 1.39 | 0.08 | 2.17 |

| | FUD | Status | MUE | Modifiers | | | | IOM Reference |
|---|---|---|---|---|---|---|---|---|
| D8696 | N/A | N | - | N/A | N/A | N/A | N/A | None |
| D8697 | N/A | N | - | N/A | N/A | N/A | N/A | |

* with documentation

## Terms To Know

**mandibular.** Having to do with the lower jaw.

**maxilla.** Pyramidally-shaped bone forming the upper jaw, part of the eye orbit, nasal cavity, and palate and lodging the upper teeth.

**orthodontia.** Treatment of malocclusion and other neuromuscular and skeletal abnormalities of the teeth and their surrounding structures.

# D8698-D8699

**D8698** re-cement or re-bond fixed retainer - maxillary

**D8699** re-cement or re-bond fixed retainer - mandibular

## Explanation

A fixed retainer is used in orthodontic care to prevent relapses in alignment or rotation of the teeth. Fixed retainers are sometimes used as the primary treatment in orthodontics because they are placed behind the teeth and are invisible to others. The most common problem is for the retainer to become loose. If the retainer needs to be rebonded the provider will remove the old bonding material from the back of the teeth using the high speed drill. Once the bonding material is removed, the teeth are isolated and acid etched. A coat of bonding solution is then applied to the back of the teeth and hardened using manufacturer guidelines. A composite material is then applied and the retainer is positioned. The composite material is then cured. Report D8698 for a retainer of the upper jaw and D8699 when performed on a lower jaw.

## Coding Tips

To report the repair of a fixed retainer, see D8694. Coverage for this procedure varies by payer and by individual contract bonding. Check with payers for their specific coverage guidelines.

## ICD-10-CM Diagnostic Codes

Z97.2 Presence of dental prosthetic device (complete) (partial)

## Relative Value Units/Medicare Edits

| Non-Facility RVU | Work | PE | MP | Total |
|---|---|---|---|---|
| D8698 | 0.73 | 1.46 | 0.09 | 2.28 |
| D8699 | 0.73 | 1.46 | 0.09 | 2.28 |
| **Facility RVU** | **Work** | **PE** | **MP** | **Total** |
| D8698 | 0.73 | 1.46 | 0.09 | 2.28 |
| D8699 | 0.73 | 1.46 | 0.09 | 2.28 |

| | FUD | Status | MUE | Modifiers | | | | IOM Reference |
|---|---|---|---|---|---|---|---|---|
| D8698 | N/A | N | - | N/A | N/A | N/A | N/A | None |
| D8699 | N/A | N | - | N/A | N/A | N/A | N/A | |

* with documentation

## Terms To Know

**bonding.** In dentistry, two or more components connected by chemical adhesion or mechanical means.

**cement.** Any substance that solidly bonds two objects or surfaces together.

**malocclusion.** Condition in which the teeth are misaligned. Underlying causes may include accessory, impacted, or missing teeth; dentofacial abnormalities; thumb sucking; or sleeping positions.

**orthodontia.** Treatment of malocclusion and other neuromuscular and skeletal abnormalities of the teeth and their surrounding structures.

**retainer.** In dentistry, portion of a fixed partial denture that attaches an artificial tooth to the abutment tooth or implant.

# D8701-D8702

**D8701** repair of fixed retainer, includes reattachment - maxillary
**D8702** repair of fixed retainer, includes reattachment - mandibular

## Explanation

The provider repairs a fixed retainer of the upper or lower jaw. The provider removes residual composite and wire from the front of the tooth surface using a fluted tungsten bar. The enamel is then etched with 35 percent phosphoric acid. The area is rinsed and dried. After placing moisture control, the etched surface is painted with unfilled resin. The wire retainer is bonded to the tooth using high filler composite. The composite is light cured and any excess composite is removed. Report D8701 for the upper fixed retainer and D8702 for lower fixed retainer.

## Coding Tips

To report re-cement or re-bond fixed retainer, see D8698–D8699. To report replacement of lost or broken retainer, see D8703–D8704.

## ICD-10-CM Diagnostic Codes

Z97.2 Presence of dental prosthetic device (complete) (partial)

## Relative Value Units/Medicare Edits

| Non-Facility RVU | Work | PE | MP | Total |
|---|---|---|---|---|
| **D8701** | 1.08 | 2.14 | 0.13 | 3.35 |
| **D8702** | 1.08 | 2.14 | 0.13 | 3.35 |
| **Facility RVU** | **Work** | **PE** | **MP** | **Total** |
| **D8701** | 1.08 | 2.14 | 0.13 | 3.35 |
| **D8702** | 1.08 | 2.14 | 0.13 | 3.35 |

| | FUD | Status | MUE | Modifiers | | | | IOM Reference |
|---|---|---|---|---|---|---|---|---|
| **D8701** | N/A | N | - | N/A | N/A | N/A | N/A | None |
| **D8702** | N/A | N | - | N/A | N/A | N/A | N/A | |

* with documentation

## Terms To Know

**retainer.** In dentistry, portion of a fixed partial denture that attaches an artificial tooth to the abutment tooth or implant.

# D8703-D8704

**D8703** replacement of lost or broken retainer - maxillary
**D8704** replacement of lost or broken retainer - mandibular

## Explanation

The provider replaces a lost or broken retainer. Depending on the age of the retainer, it may be necessary for the provider to determine if a fitting is required. Report D8703 for an upper retainer; report D8702 for a lower retainer.

## Coding Tips

To report re-cement or re-bond fixed retainer, see D8698–D8699. To report repair of a fixed retainer, see D8701–D8702.

## ICD-10-CM Diagnostic Codes

Z97.2 Presence of dental prosthetic device (complete) (partial)

## Relative Value Units/Medicare Edits

| Non-Facility RVU | Work | PE | MP | Total |
|---|---|---|---|---|
| **D8703** | 1.10 | 2.19 | 0.13 | 3.42 |
| **D8704** | 1.10 | 2.19 | 0.13 | 3.42 |
| **Facility RVU** | **Work** | **PE** | **MP** | **Total** |
| **D8703** | 1.10 | 2.19 | 0.13 | 3.42 |
| **D8704** | 1.10 | 2.19 | 0.13 | 3.42 |

| | FUD | Status | MUE | Modifiers | | | | IOM Reference |
|---|---|---|---|---|---|---|---|---|
| **D8703** | N/A | N | - | N/A | N/A | N/A | N/A | None |
| **D8704** | N/A | N | - | N/A | N/A | N/A | N/A | |

* with documentation

## Terms To Know

**mandibular.** Having to do with the lower jaw.

**maxilla.** Pyramidally-shaped bone forming the upper jaw, part of the eye orbit, nasal cavity, and palate and lodging the upper teeth.

**retainer.** In dentistry, portion of a fixed partial denture that attaches an artificial tooth to the abutment tooth or implant.

# D9110

**D9110** palliative (emergency) treatment of dental pain - minor procedure

*This is typically reported on a "per visit" basis for emergency treatment of dental pain.*

## Explanation

The patient is given palliative treatment on an emergency basis for dental pain. This code is reported on a per visit basis.

## Coding Tips

When the condition is the result of an accident, the dental insurer may require that the medical insurance be billed first. Any radiograph is reported separately. Payment is based per visit, not per tooth. Temporary restorations may be included and, therefore, not separately reimbursable by some payers. Check with third-party payers for their specific guidelines.

## Reimbursement Tips

When covered by medical insurance, the payer may require that the appropriate CPT code be reported on the CMS-1500 claim form.

## ICD-10-CM Diagnostic Codes

| | |
|---|---|
| G89.21 | Chronic pain due to trauma |
| K03.81 | Cracked tooth |
| K03.89 | Other specified diseases of hard tissues of teeth |
| K04.6 | Periapical abscess with sinus |
| M27.2 | Inflammatory conditions of jaws |
| R68.84 | Jaw pain |

## Relative Value Units/Medicare Edits

| Non-Facility RVU | Work | PE | MP | Total |
|---|---|---|---|---|
| D9110 | 0.36 | 0.72 | 0.04 | 1.12 |
| **Facility RVU** | **Work** | **PE** | **MP** | **Total** |
| D9110 | 0.36 | 0.72 | 0.04 | 1.12 |

| | FUD | Status | MUE | Modifiers | | | | IOM Reference |
|---|---|---|---|---|---|---|---|---|
| D9110 | N/A | R | - | N/A | N/A | N/A | 80* | None |

* with documentation

## Terms To Know

**emergent care.** Treatment for a medical or mental health condition or symptom that arises suddenly and requires care and treatment immediately or as soon as possible.

**palliative treatment.** Treatment of symptoms without treating the underlying cause or to maintain current health status.

# D9120

**D9120** fixed partial denture sectioning

*Separation of one or more connections between abutments and/or pontics when some portion of a fixed prosthesis is to remain intact and serviceable following sectioning and extraction or other treatment. Includes all recontouring and polishing of retained portions.*

## Explanation

The dentist separates one or more connections among abutments that are securing artificial teeth in order to split a partial denture into a segment that remains and a segment that is removed. The remaining segment may be recontoured or polished as part of the procedure.

## Coding Tips

When the condition is the result of an accident, the dental insurer may require that the medical insurance be billed first. For maintenance of an FPD including cleaning, debriding, or examination, report D6080 instead. Payers may require documentation including tooth number, preoperative x-ray, narrative, or clinical treatment notes. For repair to restore the FPD to original condition, report D6090.

## Reimbursement Tips

When covered by medical insurance, the payer may require that the appropriate CPT code be reported on the CMS-1500 claim form. Local anesthesia is usually considered part of implant procedures or services.

## ICD-10-CM Diagnostic Codes

| | |
|---|---|
| K08.530 | Fractured dental restorative material without loss of material |
| K08.531 | Fractured dental restorative material with loss of material |
| K08.539 | Fractured dental restorative material, unspecified |
| Z46.3 | Encounter for fitting and adjustment of dental prosthetic device |

## Relative Value Units/Medicare Edits

| Non-Facility RVU | Work | PE | MP | Total |
|---|---|---|---|---|
| D9120 | 0.47 | 0.93 | 0.06 | 1.46 |
| **Facility RVU** | **Work** | **PE** | **MP** | **Total** |
| D9120 | 0.47 | 0.93 | 0.06 | 1.46 |

| | FUD | Status | MUE | Modifiers | | | | IOM Reference |
|---|---|---|---|---|---|---|---|---|
| D9120 | N/A | N | - | N/A | N/A | N/A | N/A | None |

* with documentation

## Terms To Know

**denture.** Manmade substitution of natural teeth and neighboring structures.

**FPD.** Fixed partial denture.

**partial dentures.** In dentistry, artificial teeth composed of a framework with plastic teeth and gum area replacing part but not all of the natural teeth. The framework can either be formed from an acrylic resin base, cast metal or may be made more flexible using thermoplastics.

# D9130

**D9130** temporomandibular joint dysfunction - non-invasive physical therapies

*Therapy including but not limited to massage, diathermy, ultrasound, or cold application to provide relief from muscle spasms, inflammation or pain, intending to improve freedom of motion and joint function. This should be reported on a per session basis.*

## Explanation

Physical therapy modalities are provided to the patient to alleviate temporomandibular joint dysfunction and provide relief from muscle spasm, inflammation, pain, range of motion, and joint function. The modalities include, but are not limited to, massage, diathermy, ultrasound, or cold application.

## Coding Tips

Report this service once per physical therapy session.

## ICD-10-CM Diagnostic Codes

| | |
|---|---|
| M26.211 | Malocclusion, Angle's class I |
| M26.51 | Abnormal jaw closure |
| M26.52 | Limited mandibular range of motion |
| M26.53 | Deviation in opening and closing of the mandible |
| M26.611 | Adhesions and ankylosis of right temporomandibular joint ☑ |
| M26.613 | Adhesions and ankylosis of bilateral temporomandibular joint ☑ |
| M26.621 | Arthralgia of right temporomandibular joint ☑ |
| M26.623 | Arthralgia of bilateral temporomandibular joint ☑ |
| M26.631 | Articular disc disorder of right temporomandibular joint ☑ |
| M26.633 | Articular disc disorder of bilateral temporomandibular joint ☑ |

## Relative Value Units/Medicare Edits

| Non-Facility RVU | Work | PE | MP | Total |
|---|---|---|---|---|
| **D9130** | 0.06 | 0.13 | 0.01 | 0.20 |
| **Facility RVU** | **Work** | **PE** | **MP** | **Total** |
| **D9130** | 0.06 | 0.13 | 0.01 | 0.20 |

| | FUD | Status | MUE | Modifiers | | | | IOM Reference |
|---|---|---|---|---|---|---|---|---|
| **D9130** | N/A | N | - | N/A | N/A | N/A | N/A | None |

* with documentation

## Terms To Know

**physical therapy modality.** Therapeutic agent or regimen applied or used to provide appropriate treatment of the musculoskeletal system.

**temporomandibular joint-pain dysfunction syndrome.** Multiple symptoms including temporomandibular joint dysfunction, hearing difficulty, headache, vertigo, and burning sensations in the ear, nose, tongue, and throat. Underlying causes may include overclosure of the mandible, TMJ lesions, and stress.

# D9210-D9211, D9215

**D9210** local anesthesia not in conjunction with operative or surgical procedures

**D9211** regional block anesthesia

**D9215** local anesthesia in conjunction with operative or surgical procedures

## Explanation

The dentist administers a local anesthetic in D9215 and a local not in conjunction with operative or surgical procedures in D9210. Topical antiseptic and/or topical anesthetic may be applied to the area first. With a sterilized needle and the patient in position, the dentist inserts the needle into mucosa, injects several drops of local anesthetic solution, and begins slowly advancing the needle toward the target. More local anesthetic is injected before the periosteum is touched, and the local anesthetic is slowly deposited and the needle carefully withdrawn. Local anesthetics are given into small nerve endings in the same area in which the incision or dental treatment is made. Report D9211 if the dentist administers a regional anesthetic block through a similar injection process for pain control of a larger area, such as an entire quadrant. Regional nerve blocks are given close to a main nerve trunk at a distance from the operative/treatment site. Examples of regional nerve blocks are nasopalatine injections, posterior superior alveolar, infraorbital, and inferior alveolar injections.

## Coding Tips

Any evaluations, radiographs, prophylaxis, fluoride, restorative, or extraction service is reported separately. Anesthesia is usually considered part of the procedure being performed and, therefore, is not separately billable.

## Associated HCPCS Codes

| | |
|---|---|
| J0670 | Injection, mepivacaine HCl, per 10 ml |
| J2400 | Injection, chloroprocaine HCl, per 30 ml |
| S0020 | Injection, bupivicaine HCl, 30 ml |

## ICD-10-CM Diagnostic Codes

The application of this code is too broad to adequately present ICD-10-CM diagnostic code links here. Refer to your ICD-10-CM book.

## Relative Value Units/Medicare Edits

| Non-Facility RVU | Work | PE | MP | Total |
|---|---|---|---|---|
| **D9210** | 0.15 | 0.29 | 0.02 | 0.46 |
| **D9211** | 0.17 | 0.33 | 0.02 | 0.52 |
| **D9215** | 0.12 | 0.24 | 0.01 | 0.37 |
| **Facility RVU** | **Work** | **PE** | **MP** | **Total** |
| **D9210** | 0.15 | 0.29 | 0.02 | 0.46 |
| **D9211** | 0.17 | 0.33 | 0.02 | 0.52 |
| **D9215** | 0.12 | 0.24 | 0.01 | 0.37 |

| | FUD | Status | MUE | Modifiers | | | | IOM Reference |
|---|---|---|---|---|---|---|---|---|
| **D9210** | N/A | I | - | N/A | N/A | N/A | N/A | None |
| **D9211** | N/A | I | - | N/A | N/A | N/A | N/A | |
| **D9215** | N/A | I | - | N/A | N/A | N/A | N/A | |

* with documentation

## Terms To Know

**local anesthesia.** Induced loss of feeling or sensation restricted to a certain area of the body, including topical, local tissue infiltration, field block, or nerve block methods.

# D9212

**D9212** trigeminal division block anesthesia

## Explanation

The dentist anesthetizes a branch of the trigeminal nerve. The trigeminal nerve supplies sensory and motor fibers to the face, and is usually blocked superficially. The dentist draws a local anesthetic into a syringe and injects it into the branch of the trigeminal nerve to anesthetize it.

## Coding Tips

Any evaluation, radiograph, prophylaxis, fluoride, restorative, or extraction service is reported separately.

## Documentation Tips

Third-party payers may require clinical documentation and/or x-rays before making payment determination. Check with payers to determine specific requirements

## Reimbursement Tips

When selecting the procedure or service that accurately identifies the service performed, dentists must use the most accurate code. If the CDT code more accurately identifies the service, this should be used rather than the CPT codes. Anesthesia is usually considered part of the procedure being performed and, therefore, is not separately billable.

## Associated CPT Codes

64400 Injection(s), anesthetic agent(s) and/or steroid; trigeminal nerve, each branch (ie, ophthalmic, maxillary, mandibular)

## Associated HCPCS Codes

J0670 Injection, mepivacaine HCl, per 10 ml

J2400 Injection, chloroprocaine HCl, per 30 ml

S0020 Injection, bupivicaine HCl, 30 ml

## ICD-10-CM Diagnostic Codes

The application of this code is too broad to adequately present ICD-10-CM diagnostic code links here. Refer to your ICD-10-CM book.

## Relative Value Units/Medicare Edits

| Non-Facility RVU | Work | PE | MP | Total |
|---|---|---|---|---|
| D9212 | 0.35 | 0.70 | 0.04 | 1.09 |
| **Facility RVU** | **Work** | **PE** | **MP** | **Total** |
| D9212 | 0.35 | 0.70 | 0.04 | 1.09 |

| | FUD | Status | MUE | Modifiers | | | | IOM Reference |
|---|---|---|---|---|---|---|---|---|
| D9212 | N/A | I | - | N/A | N/A | N/A | N/A | None |

* with documentation

## Terms To Know

**anesthesia.** Loss of feeling or sensation, usually induced to permit the performance of surgery or other painful procedures.

**local anesthesia.** Induced loss of feeling or sensation restricted to a certain area of the body, including topical, local tissue infiltration, field block, or nerve block methods.

**nerve block.** Regional anesthesia/analgesia administered by injection that prevents sensory nerve impulses from reaching the central nervous system.

# D9219

**D9219** evaluation for moderate sedation, deep sedation or general anesthesia

## Explanation

The dentist examines the patient to determine medical indications/contraindications for moderate or deep sedation, or general anesthesia.

## Coding Tips

To report deep sedation/general anesthesia services, see D9223. To report nonintravenous sedation, see D9248. To report intravenous moderate (conscious) sedation, see D9243.

## Reimbursement Tips

Coverage of this procedure varies by payer. Check with the payer for specific coverage guidelines.

## ICD-10-CM Diagnostic Codes

Z01.818 Encounter for other preprocedural examination

## Relative Value Units/Medicare Edits

| Non-Facility RVU | Work | PE | MP | Total |
|---|---|---|---|---|
| D9219 | 0.43 | 0.85 | 0.05 | 1.33 |
| **Facility RVU** | **Work** | **PE** | **MP** | **Total** |
| D9219 | 0.43 | 0.85 | 0.05 | 1.33 |

| | FUD | Status | MUE | Modifiers | | | | IOM Reference |
|---|---|---|---|---|---|---|---|---|
| D9219 | N/A | I | - | N/A | N/A | N/A | N/A | None |

* with documentation

## Terms To Know

**deep sedation.** Drug-induced state of depressed consciousness in which the patient cannot be easily aroused but can respond purposely following repeated or painful stimulation. Independent airway function may be impaired and the patient may require assistance in maintaining airway and respiration.

**moderate sedation.** Medically controlled state of depressed consciousness, with or without analgesia, while maintaining the patient's airway, protective reflexes, and ability to respond to stimulation or verbal commands.

# D9222-D9223

**D9222** deep sedation/general anesthesia - first 15 minutes

*Anesthesia time begins when the doctor administering the anesthetic agent initiates the appropriate anesthesia and non-invasive monitoring protocol and remains in continuous attendance of the patient. Anesthesia services are considered completed when the patient may be safely left under the observation of trained personnel and the doctor may safely leave the room to attend to other patients or duties.*

**D9223** deep sedation/general anesthesia - each subsequent 15 minute increment

## Explanation

Deep sedation or general anesthesia, regardless of the administration method is provided. The dentist administers medication that puts the patient completely asleep. The time is calculated starting when the doctor begins the appropriate protocol for administering the agent and monitoring the patient, remaining present and in continuous attendance, until the patient may be safely left in the care and observation of trained personnel and ends when the doctor may leave the room. Report D9222 for the first 15 minutes and D9223 once for each subsequent 15 minute increment.

## Coding Tips

Code D9223 is reported in 15-minute increments. For intravenous moderate (conscious) sedation, see D9243. For nonintravenous conscious sedation, see D9248. Pre-anesthesia evaluation is reported using D9219.

## Reimbursement Tips

Payers have varying policies regarding the reporting partial time increments. Some dental payers may allow an additional time increment to be billed regardless of the amount of time into the next increment. Other payers may require that at least seven minutes must elapse before reporting an additional 15-minute increment of time, while others may require that more time elapse. Check with third-party payers for specific guidelines on reporting time increments, as well as line item versus units reporting.

## Associated CPT Codes

| | |
|---|---|
| 00170 | Anesthesia for intraoral procedures, including biopsy; not otherwise specified |
| 00172 | Anesthesia for intraoral procedures, including biopsy; repair of cleft palate |
| 00174 | Anesthesia for intraoral procedures, including biopsy; excision of retropharyngeal tumor |
| 00176 | Anesthesia for intraoral procedures, including biopsy; radical surgery |

## ICD-10-CM Diagnostic Codes

The application of this code is too broad to adequately present ICD-10-CM diagnostic code links here. Refer to your ICD-10-CM book.

## Relative Value Units/Medicare Edits

| Non-Facility RVU | Work | PE | MP | Total |
|---|---|---|---|---|
| **D9222** | 0.28 | 0.56 | 0.03 | 0.87 |
| **D9223** | 0.28 | 0.56 | 0.03 | 0.87 |
| **Facility RVU** | **Work** | **PE** | **MP** | **Total** |
| **D9222** | 0.28 | 0.56 | 0.03 | 0.87 |
| **D9223** | 0.28 | 0.56 | 0.03 | 0.87 |

| | FUD | Status | MUE | Modifiers | | | | IOM Reference |
|---|---|---|---|---|---|---|---|---|
| **D9222** | N/A | N | - | N/A | N/A | N/A | N/A | None |
| **D9223** | N/A | N | - | N/A | N/A | N/A | N/A | |

* with documentation

## Terms To Know

**anesthesia.** Loss of feeling or sensation, usually induced to permit the performance of surgery or other painful procedures.

**deep sedation.** Drug-induced state of depressed consciousness in which the patient cannot be easily aroused but can respond purposely following repeated or painful stimulation. Independent airway function may be impaired and the patient may require assistance in maintaining airway and respiration.

**general anesthesia.** State of unconsciousness produced by an anesthetic agent or agents, inducing amnesia by blocking the awareness center in the brain, and rendering the patient unable to control protective reflexes, such as breathing.

**sedation.** Induced state of calmness or tranquilized consciousness.

# D9230

**D9230** inhalation of nitrous oxide/analgesia, anxiolysis

## Explanation

The dentist administers an analgesia, anxiolytic agent, through the inhalation of nitrous oxide. Commonly called laughing gas, it is colorless and has a sweet smell. It produces giddiness, relaxation, floating sensations, auditory and visual hallucinations, and is used as an analgesia for minor dental and oral surgery procedures. The effect is almost immediate and also dissipates rapidly upon ceasing inhalation because the gas does not combine with hemoglobin in the blood, but is carried free through the body and excreted in an unchanged state via the lungs.

## Coding Tips

Any evaluation, radiograph, prophylaxis, fluoride, restorative, or extraction service is reported separately.

## Reimbursement Tips

Coverage for this procedure varies by payer and by individual contract. Check with payers for specific coverage guidelines.

## ICD-10-CM Diagnostic Codes

The application of this code is too broad to adequately present ICD-10-CM diagnostic code links here. Refer to your ICD-10-CM book.

## Relative Value Units/Medicare Edits

| Non-Facility RVU | Work | PE | MP | Total |
|---|---|---|---|---|
| D9230 | 0.21 | 0.42 | 0.03 | 0.66 |
| **Facility RVU** | **Work** | **PE** | **MP** | **Total** |
| D9230 | 0.21 | 0.42 | 0.03 | 0.66 |

| | FUD | Status | MUE | Modifiers | | | | IOM Reference |
|---|---|---|---|---|---|---|---|---|
| D9230 | N/A | R | - | N/A | N/A | N/A | 80* | None |

* with documentation

## Terms To Know

**analgesia.** Absence of a normal sense of pain without loss of consciousness.

**analgesic.** Agent that relieves pain without causing loss of consciousness.

# D9239-D9243

**D9239** intravenous moderate (conscious) sedation/analgesia- first 15 minutes

*Anesthesia time begins when the doctor administering the anesthetic agent initiates the appropriate anesthesia and non-invasive monitoring protocol and remains in continuous attendance of the patient. Anesthesia services are considered completed when the patient may be safely left under the observation of trained personnel and the doctor may safely leave the room to attend to other patients or duties.*

**D9243** intravenous moderate (conscious) sedation/analgesia - each subsequent 15 minute increment

## Explanation

Intravenous conscious sedation/analgesia is provided. The provider administers medication that allows a decreased level of consciousness but does not put the patient completely asleep. The patient breathes without assistance and response to commands. The sedative/analgesic agent is administered intravenously. The time is calculated when the doctor begins the appropriate protocol for administering the agent and monitoring the patient, remaining present and in continuous attendance until the patient may be safely left in the care and observation of trained personnel and the doctor may leave the room. Report D9239 for the first 15 minutes and D9243 once for each subsequent 15-minute increment.

## Coding Tips

Code D9243 is reported once for each additional 15-minute increment. For nonintravenous conscious sedation, see D9248. For deep sedation or general anesthesia, see D9222–D9223.

## ICD-10-CM Diagnostic Codes

The application of this code is too broad to adequately present ICD-10-CM diagnostic code links here. Refer to your ICD-10-CM book.

## Relative Value Units/Medicare Edits

| Non-Facility RVU | Work | PE | MP | Total |
|---|---|---|---|---|
| D9239 | 0.26 | 0.51 | 0.03 | 0.80 |
| D9243 | 0.26 | 0.51 | 0.03 | 0.80 |
| **Facility RVU** | **Work** | **PE** | **MP** | **Total** |
| D9239 | 0.26 | 0.51 | 0.03 | 0.80 |
| D9243 | 0.26 | 0.51 | 0.03 | 0.80 |

| | FUD | Status | MUE | Modifiers | | | | IOM Reference |
|---|---|---|---|---|---|---|---|---|
| D9239 | N/A | N | - | N/A | N/A | N/A | N/A | None |
| D9243 | N/A | N | - | N/A | N/A | N/A | N/A | |

* with documentation

## Terms To Know

**conscious sedation.** Medically controlled state of depressed consciousness, with or without analgesia, while maintaining the patient's airway, protective reflexes, and ability to respond to stimulation or verbal commands.

**moderate sedation.** Medically controlled state of depressed consciousness, with or without analgesia, while maintaining the patient's airway, protective reflexes, and ability to respond to stimulation or verbal commands.

# D9248

**D9248** non-intravenous conscious sedation

*This includes non-IV minimal and moderate sedation. A medically controlled state of depressed consciousness while maintaining the patient's airway, protective reflexes and the ability to respond to stimulation or verbal commands. It includes non-intravenous administration of sedative and/or analgesic agent(s) and appropriate monitoring. The level of anesthesia is determined by the anesthesia provider's documentation of the anesthetic's effects upon the central nervous system and not dependent upon the route of administration.*

## Explanation

Nonintravenous conscious sedation is given to the patient.The patient breathes without assistance and responds to commands. The time is calculated when the doctor begins the appropriate protocol for administering the agent and monitoring the patient, remaining in the room and in continuous attendance until the patient may be safely left in the care and observation of trained personnel.

## Coding Tips

To report intravenous moderate (conscious) sedation, see D9243. To report deep sedation/general anesthesia, see D9223.

## Reimbursement Tips

Check with third-party payers for specific guidelines on reporting time increments as well as line item versus units reporting.

## Associated HCPCS Codes

| | |
|---|---|
| J2250 | Injection, midazolam HCl, per 1 mg |
| J2515 | Injection, pentobarbital sodium, per 50 mg |
| J3360 | Injection, diazepam, up to 5 mg |

## ICD-10-CM Diagnostic Codes

The application of this code is too broad to adequately present ICD-10-CM diagnostic code links here. Refer to your ICD-10-CM book.

## Relative Value Units/Medicare Edits

| Non-Facility RVU | Work | PE | MP | Total |
|---|---|---|---|---|
| D9248 | 0.45 | 0.89 | 0.05 | 1.39 |
| **Facility RVU** | **Work** | **PE** | **MP** | **Total** |
| D9248 | 0.45 | 0.89 | 0.05 | 1.39 |

| | FUD | Status | MUE | Modifiers | | | | IOM Reference |
|---|---|---|---|---|---|---|---|---|
| D9248 | N/A | R | - | N/A | N/A | N/A | N/A | None |

* with documentation

## Terms To Know

**analgesia.** Absence of a normal sense of pain without loss of consciousness.

**analgesic.** Agent that relieves pain without causing loss of consciousness.

**anesthesia.** Loss of feeling or sensation, usually induced to permit the performance of surgery or other painful procedures.

**monitored anesthesia care.** Sedation, with or without analgesia, used to achieve a medically controlled state of depressed consciousness while maintaining the patient's airway, protective reflexes, and ability to respond to stimulation or verbal commands. In dental conscious sedation, the patient is rendered free of fear, apprehension, and anxiety through the use of pharmacological agents.

# D9310

**D9310** consultation - diagnostic service provided by dentist or physician other than requesting dentist or physician

*A patient encounter with a practitioner whose opinion or advice regarding evaluation and/or management of a specific problem; may be requested by another practitioner or appropriate source. The consultation includes an oral evaluation. The consulted practitioner may initiate diagnostic and/or therapeutic services.*

## Explanation

This code is a consultation service requested by the providing dentist, physician, or other appropriate professional. Another dentist or dental specialist's opinion and advice regarding the evaluation and care treatment plan of the patient's specific problem is given. The consulting dentist or specialist may initiate diagnostic and therapeutic procedures, but is not the practitioner providing the treatment.

## Coding Tips

Any radiograph, diagnostic, or therapeutic procedure initiated is reported separately. Any oral evaluations performed are included in this procedure and, therefore, are not separately billable. To report problem-focused examinations of a patient who is not referred by another provider, see D0140 or D0160. Initial examinations of a patient who is not referred by another provider is reported using D0150 or D0180. To report the oral evaluation of a patient under 3 years of age including counseling of the primary caregiver, see D0145.

## Documentation Tips

Third-party payers may require clinical documentation and/or x-rays before making payment determination. Check with payers to determine specific requirements.

## Reimbursement Tips

Coverage of this procedure varies by payer. Check with the payer for specific coverage guidelines.

## ICD-10-CM Diagnostic Codes

The application of this code is too broad to adequately present ICD-10-CM diagnostic code links here. Refer to your ICD-10-CM book.

## Relative Value Units/Medicare Edits

| Non-Facility RVU | Work | PE | MP | Total |
|---|---|---|---|---|
| D9310 | 0.64 | 1.27 | 0.08 | 1.99 |
| **Facility RVU** | **Work** | **PE** | **MP** | **Total** |
| D9310 | 0.64 | 1.27 | 0.08 | 1.99 |

| | FUD | Status | MUE | Modifiers | | | | IOM Reference |
|---|---|---|---|---|---|---|---|---|
| D9310 | N/A | I | - | N/A | N/A | N/A | N/A | None |

* with documentation

## Terms To Know

**dental consultation.** Advice or an opinion rendered by a dentist or dental specialist who is not the treating doctor provided at the request of the providing dentist, physician, or other appropriate professional.

**diagnostic dental procedure.** Procedure performed to evaluate the patient's complaints or symptoms and help the dentist establish the nature of the patient's disease or condition so that definitive care can be provided.

# D9311

**D9311** consultation with a medical health care professional

*Treating dentist consults with a medical health care professional concerning medical issues that may affect patient's planned dental treatment.*

## Explanation

Code D9311 is provided when consulting with a medical health care professional to discuss medical issues affecting a planned dental treatment. Another dentist or dental specialist's opinion and advice regarding the evaluation and care treatment plan of the patient's specific problem is given. The consulting dentist or specialist may initiate diagnostic and therapeutic procedures, but is not the practitioner providing the treatment.

## Coding Tips

Any radiograph, diagnostic, or therapeutic procedure initiated is reported separately. Any oral evaluations performed are included in this procedure and, therefore, are not separately billable. To report problem-focused examinations of a patient who is not referred by another provider, see D0140 or D0160. Initial examination of a patient who is not referred by another provider is reported using D0150 or D0180. To report the oral evaluation of a patient under 3 years of age, including counseling of the primary caregiver, see D0145.

## ICD-10-CM Diagnostic Codes

The application of this code is too broad to adequately present ICD-10-CM diagnostic code links here. Refer to your ICD-10-CM book.

## Relative Value Units/Medicare Edits

| Non-Facility RVU | Work | PE | MP | Total |
|---|---|---|---|---|
| D9311 | 0.19 | 0.38 | 0.02 | 0.59 |
| **Facility RVU** | **Work** | **PE** | **MP** | **Total** |
| D9311 | 0.19 | 0.38 | 0.02 | 0.59 |

| | FUD | Status | MUE | Modifiers | | | | IOM Reference |
|---|---|---|---|---|---|---|---|---|
| D9311 | N/A | N | - | N/A | N/A | N/A | N/A | None |

* with documentation

## Terms To Know

**dental consultation.** Advice or an opinion rendered by a dentist or dental specialist who is not the treating doctor provided at the request of the providing dentist, physician, or other appropriate professional.

# D9410-D9420

**D9410** house/extended care facility call

*Includes visits to nursing homes, long-term care facilities, hospice sites, institutions, etc. Report in addition to reporting appropriate code numbers for actual services performed.*

**D9420** hospital or ambulatory surgical center call

*Care provided outside the dentist's office to a patient who is in a hospital or ambulatory surgical center. Services delivered to the patient on the date of service are documented separately using the applicable procedure codes.*

## Explanation

Use these codes to report visits made to a patient's place of residence or to the hospital. Code D9410 is for a house/extended care facility call and includes nursing homes, hospice care centers, and other institutions that may be considered the patient's home, though not a traditional house call to a private home setting. Code D9420 is used when providing treatment in a hospital or ambulatory surgical center. Both of these codes are submitted in addition to the appropriate codes for the actual services performed there.

## Coding Tips

As add-on codes, D9410 and D9420 are not subject to multiple procedure rules. No reimbursement reduction or modifier 51 is applied. Add-on codes describe additional intraservice work associated with the primary procedure. They are performed by the same dentist on the same date of service as the primary service/procedure, and must never be reported as stand-alone codes.

## Reimbursement Tips

Coverage of these procedures varies by payer. Check with the payer for specific coverage guidelines.

## ICD-10-CM Diagnostic Codes

| | |
|---|---|
| Z01.20 | Encounter for dental examination and cleaning without abnormal findings |
| Z01.21 | Encounter for dental examination and cleaning with abnormal findings |

## Relative Value Units/Medicare Edits

| Non-Facility RVU | Work | PE | MP | Total |
|---|---|---|---|---|
| D9410 | 0.79 | 1.56 | 0.09 | 2.44 |
| D9420 | 1.19 | 2.36 | 0.14 | 3.69 |
| **Facility RVU** | **Work** | **PE** | **MP** | **Total** |
| D9410 | 0.79 | 1.56 | 0.09 | 2.44 |
| D9420 | 1.19 | 2.36 | 0.14 | 3.69 |

| | FUD | Status | MUE | Modifiers | | | | IOM Reference |
|---|---|---|---|---|---|---|---|---|
| D9410 | N/A | I | - | N/A | N/A | N/A | N/A | None |
| D9420 | N/A | I | - | N/A | N/A | N/A | N/A | |

* with documentation

# D9430

**D9430** office visit for observation (during regularly scheduled hours) - no other services performed

## Explanation

This code reports office visits. It is used for an office visit for observation only when no other identifiable services are performed during the regularly scheduled office hours.

## Coding Tips

This code is not reported with any other services.

## Reimbursement Tips

Coverage of this procedure varies by payer. Check with the payer for specific coverage guidelines.

## ICD-10-CM Diagnostic Codes

| | |
|---|---|
| Z01.20 | Encounter for dental examination and cleaning without abnormal findings |
| Z01.21 | Encounter for dental examination and cleaning with abnormal findings |

## Relative Value Units/Medicare Edits

| Non-Facility RVU | Work | PE | MP | Total |
|---|---|---|---|---|
| D9430 | 0.13 | 0.26 | 0.02 | 0.41 |
| **Facility RVU** | **Work** | **PE** | **MP** | **Total** |
| D9430 | 0.13 | 0.26 | 0.02 | 0.41 |

| | FUD | Status | MUE | Modifiers | | | | IOM Reference |
|---|---|---|---|---|---|---|---|---|
| D9430 | N/A | I | - | N/A | N/A | N/A | N/A | None |

* with documentation

## Terms To Know

**observation.** Perception of events.

# D9440

**D9440** office visit - after regularly scheduled hours

## Explanation

This code reports office visits. It is used for an office visit occurring after the regularly scheduled hours.

## Coding Tips

As an add-on code, D9440 is not subject to multiple procedure rules. No reimbursement reduction or modifier 51 is applied. Add-on codes describe additional intraservice work associated with the primary procedure. They are performed by the same dentist on the same date of service as the primary service/procedure, and must never be reported as stand-alone codes. Third-party payers may require clinical documentation and/or x-rays before making payment determination. Check with payers to determine their specific requirements.

## Reimbursement Tips

When selecting the procedure or service that accurately identifies the service performed, dentists must use the most accurate code. If the CDT code more accurately identifies the service, this should be used rather than the CPT codes. Coverage of this procedure varies by payer. Check with the payer for specific coverage guidelines.

## Associated CPT Codes

| | |
|---|---|
| 99050 | Services provided in the office at times other than regularly scheduled office hours, or days when the office is normally closed (eg, holidays, Saturday or Sunday), in addition to basic service |

## ICD-10-CM Diagnostic Codes

This/these CDT code(s) are add-on code(s). See the primary procedure code that this code is performed with for your ICD-10-CM code selections. Diagnostic code(s) would be the same as the actual procedure performed.

## Relative Value Units/Medicare Edits

| Non-Facility RVU | Work | PE | MP | Total |
|---|---|---|---|---|
| D9440 | 0.45 | 0.89 | 0.05 | 1.39 |
| **Facility RVU** | **Work** | **PE** | **MP** | **Total** |
| D9440 | 0.45 | 0.89 | 0.05 | 1.39 |

| | FUD | Status | MUE | Modifiers | | | | IOM Reference |
|---|---|---|---|---|---|---|---|---|
| D9440 | N/A | I | - | N/A | N/A | N/A | N/A | None |

* with documentation

# D9450

**D9450** case presentation, detailed and extensive treatment planning

*Established patient. Not performed on same day as evaluation.*

## Explanation

This code is reported for a detailed and extensive treatment plan case presentation of an established patient when the case presentation is not performed on the same day that the evaluation is done.

## Coding Tips

Do not report this code on the same day as an evaluation.

## Reimbursement Tips

Coverage of this procedure varies by payer. Check with the payer for specific coverage guidelines.

## ICD-10-CM Diagnostic Codes

The application of this code is too broad to adequately present ICD-10-CM diagnostic code links here. Refer to your ICD-10-CM book.

## Relative Value Units/Medicare Edits

| Non-Facility RVU | Work | PE | MP | Total |
|---|---|---|---|---|
| D9450 | 0.26 | 0.52 | 0.03 | 0.81 |
| Facility RVU | Work | PE | MP | Total |
| D9450 | 0.26 | 0.52 | 0.03 | 0.81 |

| | FUD | Status | MUE | Modifiers | | | | IOM Reference |
|---|---|---|---|---|---|---|---|---|
| D9450 | N/A | I | - | N/A | N/A | N/A | N/A | None |

* with documentation

## Terms To Know

**dental consultation.** Advice or an opinion rendered by a dentist or dental specialist who is not the treating doctor provided at the request of the providing dentist, physician, or other appropriate professional.

# D9610-D9612

**D9610** therapeutic parenteral drug, single administration

*Includes single administration of antibiotics, steroids, anti-inflammatory drugs, or other therapeutic medications. This code should not be used to report administration of sedative, anesthetic or reversal agents.*

**D9612** therapeutic parenteral drugs, two or more administrations, different medications

*Includes multiple administrations of antibiotics, steroids, anti-inflammatory drugs or other therapeutic medications. This code should not be used to report administration of sedatives, anesthetic or reversal agents. This code should be reported when two or more different medications are necessary and should not be reported in addition to code D9610 on the same date.*

## Explanation

A therapeutic drug is given to the patient. Therapeutic parental drug administration is for the purpose of curing or alleviating a present condition, not for prevention measures. This administration can be by many methods including but not limited to oral, sublingual, inhalation, topical, injection, or intravenous methods. Code D9610 reports a single administration and D9612 reports two or more administrations of different medicines.

## Coding Tips

Use an additional J code to indicate the substance administered. Pertinent documentation to evaluate medical appropriateness should be included when this code is reported. For code D9612, third-party payers may require clinical documentation and/or x-rays before making payment determination. Check with payers to determine their specific requirements. For administration of anesthesia, see D9210–D9223. To report moderate (conscious) sedation, see D9239–D9239. To report non-intravenous conscious sedation, see D9248. To report inhalation of nitrous oxide, see D9230. To report drugs or medicaments provided in the office for home use, see code D9630.

## Documentation Tips

Pertinent documentation to evaluate the medical appropriateness should be included with the claim when these codes are reported.

## Reimbursement Tips

Coverage of these procedures varies by payer. Check with the payer for specific coverage guidelines.

## ICD-10-CM Diagnostic Codes

The application of this code is too broad to adequately present ICD-10-CM diagnostic code links here. Refer to your ICD-10-CM book.

## Relative Value Units/Medicare Edits

| Non-Facility RVU | Work | PE | MP | Total |
|---|---|---|---|---|
| **D9610** | 0.11 | 0.21 | 0.01 | 0.33 |
| **D9612** | 0.27 | 0.53 | 0.03 | 0.83 |
| **Facility RVU** | **Work** | **PE** | **MP** | **Total** |
| **D9610** | 0.11 | 0.21 | 0.01 | 0.33 |
| **D9612** | 0.27 | 0.53 | 0.03 | 0.83 |

| | FUD | Status | MUE | Modifiers | | | | IOM Reference |
|---|---|---|---|---|---|---|---|---|
| **D9610** | N/A | I | - | N/A | N/A | N/A | N/A | None |
| **D9612** | N/A | N | - | N/A | N/A | N/A | N/A | |

* with documentation

## Terms To Know

**injection.** Forcing a liquid substance into a body part such as a joint or muscle.

# D9613

▲ **D9613** infiltration of sustained release therapeutic drug, per quadrant

*Infiltration of a sustained release pharmacologic agent for long acting surgical site pain control. Not for local anesthesia purposes.*

## Explanation

The provider infiltrates a sustained release nonopioid pharmacologic agent for long acting surgical site pain control.

## Coding Tips

This code is not to be used for local anesthesia. Use an additional J code to indicate the substance administered. To report other therapeutic substances, see D9610–D9612.

## Documentation Tips

Pertinent documentation to evaluate the medical appropriateness and medical necessity should be recorded.

## Reimbursement Tips

Payers may require clinical documentation before making payment determinations. Check with payers to determine their specific requirements.

## ICD-10-CM Diagnostic Codes

G89.18 Other acute postprocedural pain

G89.28 Other chronic postprocedural pain

## Relative Value Units/Medicare Edits

| Non-Facility RVU | Work | PE | MP | Total |
|---|---|---|---|---|
| **D9613** | 0.09 | 0.17 | 0.01 | 0.27 |
| **Facility RVU** | **Work** | **PE** | **MP** | **Total** |
| **D9613** | 0.09 | 0.17 | 0.01 | 0.27 |

| | FUD | Status | MUE | Modifiers | | | | IOM Reference |
|---|---|---|---|---|---|---|---|---|
| **D9613** | N/A | N | - | N/A | N/A | N/A | N/A | None |

* with documentation

## Terms To Know

**injection.** Forcing a liquid substance into a body part such as a joint or muscle.

# D9910-D9911

**D9910** application of desensitizing medicament

*Includes in-office treatment for root sensitivity. Typically reported on a "per visit" basis for application of topical fluoride. This code is not to be used for bases, liners or adhesives used under restorations.*

**D9911** application of desensitizing resin for cervical and/or root surface, per tooth

*Typically reported on a "per tooth" basis for application of adhesive resins. This code is not to be used for bases, liners, or adhesives used under restorations.*

## Explanation

When the patient presents with a complaint of tooth or root sensitivity, that may be due to receding gums or even brushing with too much force with a hard-bristled brush, a desensitizing medicament is painted on to the affected teeth that reduced or removed the sensitivity completely. Report D9910 on a per-visit basis. This may be a topical fluoride application for sensitivity. Report D9911 for application of desensitizing resin for cervical and/or root surface on a per-tooth basis. The material may be like that used under other restorative work, but neither code is to be reported for bases, liners, or adhesives when applied to be used under restorations.

## Coding Tips

These codes should not be used for bases, liners, or adhesives that are used with restorations. Report D9910 on a per-visit basis and D9911 on a per-tooth basis. According to the ADA, code D9910 may be reported when a fluoride varnish is used to desensitize a tooth. Check with third-party payers for their specific guidelines. Generally, these services are not covered when provided with another service on the same day.

## Reimbursement Tips

Coverage of these procedures varies by payer. Check with the payer for specific coverage guidelines.

## ICD-10-CM Diagnostic Codes

| | |
|---|---|
| K05.00 | Acute gingivitis, plaque induced |
| K05.01 | Acute gingivitis, non-plaque induced |
| K05.10 | Chronic gingivitis, plaque induced |
| K05.11 | Chronic gingivitis, non-plaque induced |
| K05.211 | Aggressive periodontitis, localized, slight |
| K05.212 | Aggressive periodontitis, localized, moderate |
| K05.213 | Aggressive periodontitis, localized, severe |
| K05.221 | Aggressive periodontitis, generalized, slight |
| K05.222 | Aggressive periodontitis, generalized, moderate |
| K05.223 | Aggressive periodontitis, generalized, severe |
| K05.311 | Chronic periodontitis, localized, slight |
| K05.312 | Chronic periodontitis, localized, moderate |
| K05.313 | Chronic periodontitis, localized, severe |
| K05.321 | Chronic periodontitis, generalized, slight |
| K05.322 | Chronic periodontitis, generalized, moderate |
| K05.323 | Chronic periodontitis, generalized, severe |
| K05.4 | Periodontosis |
| K05.5 | Other periodontal diseases |
| K06.011 | Localized gingival recession, minimal |
| K06.012 | Localized gingival recession, moderate |
| K06.013 | Localized gingival recession, severe |
| K06.021 | Generalized gingival recession, minimal |
| K06.022 | Generalized gingival recession, moderate |
| K06.023 | Generalized gingival recession, severe |

## Relative Value Units/Medicare Edits

| Non-Facility RVU | Work | PE | MP | Total |
|---|---|---|---|---|
| **D9910** | 0.16 | 0.33 | 0.02 | 0.51 |
| **D9911** | 0.23 | 0.45 | 0.03 | 0.71 |
| **Facility RVU** | **Work** | **PE** | **MP** | **Total** |
| **D9910** | 0.16 | 0.33 | 0.02 | 0.51 |
| **D9911** | 0.23 | 0.45 | 0.03 | 0.71 |

| | FUD | Status | MUE | Modifiers | | | | IOM Reference |
|---|---|---|---|---|---|---|---|---|
| **D9910** | N/A | N | - | N/A | N/A | N/A | N/A | None |
| **D9911** | N/A | N | - | N/A | N/A | N/A | N/A | |

* with documentation

## Terms To Know

**bonding.** In dentistry, two or more components connected by chemical adhesion or mechanical means.

**desensitization.** In dentistry, application of medication to decrease the symptoms, usually pain, associated with a dental condition or disease.

**fluoride.** Compound of the gaseous element fluorine that can be incorporated into bone and teeth and provides some protection in reducing dental decay.

# D9912

● **D9912** pre-visit patient screening

*Capture and documentation of a patient's health status prior to or on the scheduled date of service to evaluate risk of infectious disease transmission if the patient is to be treated within the dental practice.*

## Explanation

Code D9912 reports additional supplies, materials, and clinical staff time necessary to perform safety protocols during a public health emergency (PHE) due to respiratory-transmitted infectious disease. Extra precautions, over and above those usually included in an office visit or other non-facility services, are taken to ensure the safety of patients and health care professionals during in-person interactions while allowing for the provision of evaluation, treatment, or procedural services. Use of this code does not depend on a specific patient diagnosis.

## Coding Tips

Use this code to report clinical staff time spent in patient symptom checks in person (on arrival) and over the phone. This code includes any required additional supplies, materials, and increased sanitation measures (surgical masks, cleaning supplies, hand sanitizer, disinfecting wipes, sprays, and cleansers) related to the public health emergency (PHE) over and above those usually associated with a patient encounter.

## Associated CPT Codes

99072 Additional supplies, materials, and clinical staff time over and above those usually included in an office visit or other nonfacility service(s), when performed during a Public Health Emergency, as defined by law, due to respiratory-transmitted infectious disease

## ICD-10-CM Diagnostic Codes

The application of this code is too broad to adequately present ICD-10-CM diagnostic code links here. Refer to your ICD-10-CM book.

## Relative Value Units/Medicare Edits

| Non-Facility RVU | Work | PE | MP | Total |
|---|---|---|---|---|
| D9912 | | | | |
| **Facility RVU** | **Work** | **PE** | **MP** | **Total** |
| D9912 | | | | |

| | FUD | Status | MUE | Modifiers | | | | IOM Reference |
|---|---|---|---|---|---|---|---|---|
| D9912 | N/A | | - | N/A | N/A | N/A | N/A | |

* with documentation

## Terms To Know

**COVID-19.** First diagnosed in December 2019 in China, coronavirus disease 2019 (COVID-19) is a respiratory infection caused by a newly identified (novel) virus not previously seen in humans, known as severe acute respiratory syndrome coronavirus 2 (SARS-CoV-2). Symptoms of this lower respiratory illness include fever, dry cough, loss of taste and/or smell, skin lesions of toes, gastrointestinal disturbances, and tiredness that may progress to include difficulty breathing and ventilator assistance. Older patients and those with high blood pressure, heart problems, diabetes, and obesity are more likely to develop serious symptoms of the illness, which may result in death of the patient.

# D9920

**D9920** behavior management, by report

*May be reported in addition to treatment provided. Should be reported in 15-minute increments.*

## Explanation

Behavior management can be reported in addition to the treatment provided and should be used in 15-minute increments, by report.

## Coding Tips

Report once for each 15 minutes or significant portion. To report dental case management services, see D9991–D9994.

## Documentation Tips

Documentation should include the total time spent counseling the patient as well as a detailed account of the counseling provided.

## Reimbursement Tips

Coverage of this procedure varies by payer. Check with the payer for specific coverage guidelines.

## ICD-10-CM Diagnostic Codes

Z71.3 Dietary counseling and surveillance
Z71.51 Drug abuse counseling and surveillance of drug abuser
Z71.6 Tobacco abuse counseling
Z71.9 Counseling, unspecified

## Relative Value Units/Medicare Edits

| Non-Facility RVU | Work | PE | MP | Total |
|---|---|---|---|---|
| D9920 | 0.17 | 0.34 | 0.02 | 0.53 |
| **Facility RVU** | **Work** | **PE** | **MP** | **Total** |
| D9920 | 0.17 | 0.34 | 0.02 | 0.53 |

| | FUD | Status | MUE | Modifiers | | | | IOM Reference |
|---|---|---|---|---|---|---|---|---|
| D9920 | N/A | N | - | N/A | N/A | N/A | N/A | None |

* with documentation

## Terms To Know

**behavior management.** Education and modification techniques or methodologies aimed at helping a patient change undesirable habits or behaviors.

# D9930

**D9930** treatment of complications (post-surgical) - unusual circumstances, by report

*For example, treatment of a dry socket following extraction or removal of bony sequestrum.*

## Explanation

Report this code with the report for treatment of post-surgical complications that are unusual, not normally expected after surgery, and require extra attention from the oral health caregiver. This could be treatment of a dry socket after tooth extraction or removal of sequestrum from the jaw bone.

## Coding Tips

Report this service on a daily treatment basis.

## Documentation Tips

Documentation should clearly specify the complication.

## Reimbursement Tips

This procedure may be bundled into the surgical service and not separately reimbursed.

## ICD-10-CM Diagnostic Codes

| | |
|---|---|
| G89.18 | Other acute postprocedural pain |
| G89.28 | Other chronic postprocedural pain |
| M27.3 | Alveolitis of jaws |
| T81.31XA | Disruption of external operation (surgical) wound, not elsewhere classified, initial encounter |
| T81.32XA | Disruption of internal operation (surgical) wound, not elsewhere classified, initial encounter |
| T81.41XA | Infection following a procedure, superficial incisional surgical site, initial encounter |
| T81.42XA | Infection following a procedure, deep incisional surgical site, initial encounter |

## Relative Value Units/Medicare Edits

| Non-Facility RVU | Work | PE | MP | Total |
|---|---|---|---|---|
| **D9930** | 0.18 | 0.36 | 0.02 | 0.56 |
| **Facility RVU** | **Work** | **PE** | **MP** | **Total** |
| **D9930** | 0.18 | 0.36 | 0.02 | 0.56 |

| | FUD | Status | MUE | Modifiers | | | | IOM Reference |
|---|---|---|---|---|---|---|---|---|
| **D9930** | N/A | R | - | N/A | N/A | N/A | 80* | 100-02,1,70; 100-04,4,20.5 |

* with documentation

## Terms To Know

**dental complication.** Problem arising after observation and treatment in dental care has begun.

**dry socket.** In dentistry, painful condition occurring when the blood clot disintegrates after tooth extraction, leaving the socket exposed to the air and infection; it may involve osteitis.

# D9932-D9933

**D9932** cleaning and inspection of removable complete denture, maxillary

*This procedure does not include any adjustments.*

**D9933** cleaning and inspection of removable complete denture, mandibular

*This procedure does not include any adjustments.*

## Explanation

A removable complete denture is cleaned and inspected. The denture is cleaned using ultrasound, and stubborn stains and/or calculus are removed. The dentist examines the denture to determine any wear or damage to the denture. Report D9932 for upper denture, D9933 for lower denture.

## Coding Tips

To report the cleaning and inspection of a partial denture, see D9934–D9935. Correct code selection is dependent upon the type of denture. Any adjustments are reported separately.

## Documentation Tips

Documentation should include notation that the dentures are cleaned and inspected, and any findings such as abrasions or wear should be noted. Also document any adjustments that are required.

## Reimbursement Tips

Coverage guidelines vary by payer and by patient contract. Check with the payer to determine coverage policies.

## ICD-10-CM Diagnostic Codes

| | |
|---|---|
| Z01.20 | Encounter for dental examination and cleaning without abnormal findings |
| Z46.3 | Encounter for fitting and adjustment of dental prosthetic device |

## Relative Value Units/Medicare Edits

| Non-Facility RVU | Work | PE | MP | Total |
|---|---|---|---|---|
| **D9932** | 0.09 | 0.17 | 0.01 | 0.27 |
| **D9933** | 0.09 | 0.17 | 0.01 | 0.27 |
| **Facility RVU** | **Work** | **PE** | **MP** | **Total** |
| **D9932** | 0.09 | 0.17 | 0.01 | 0.27 |
| **D9933** | 0.09 | 0.17 | 0.01 | 0.27 |

| | FUD | Status | MUE | Modifiers | | | | IOM Reference |
|---|---|---|---|---|---|---|---|---|
| **D9932** | N/A | N | - | N/A | N/A | N/A | N/A | None |
| **D9933** | N/A | N | - | N/A | N/A | N/A | N/A | |

* with documentation

## Terms To Know

**denture.** Manmade substitution of natural teeth and neighboring structures.

# D9934-D9935

**D9934** cleaning and inspection of removable partial denture, maxillary

*This procedure does not include any adjustments.*

**D9935** cleaning and inspection of removable partial denture, mandibular

*This procedure does not include any adjustments.*

## Explanation

A removable partial denture is cleaned and inspected. The denture is cleaned using ultrasound and stubborn stains and/or calculus are removed. The dentist examines the denture to determine any wear or damage to the denture. Report D9934 for upper denture, D9935 for lower denture.

## Coding Tips

To report the cleaning and inspection of a complete denture, see D9932–D9933. Correct code selection is dependent upon the type of denture. Any adjustments are reported separately.

## Documentation Tips

Documentation should include notation that the dentures are cleaned and inspected, and any findings such as abrasions or wear should be noted. Also document any adjustments that are required or repairs to framework or clasps.

## Reimbursement Tips

Coverage guidelines vary by payer and by patient contract. Check with the payer to determine coverage policies.

## ICD-10-CM Diagnostic Codes

Z01.20 Encounter for dental examination and cleaning without abnormal findings

Z46.3 Encounter for fitting and adjustment of dental prosthetic device

## Relative Value Units/Medicare Edits

| Non-Facility RVU | Work | PE | MP | Total |
|---|---|---|---|---|
| D9934 | 0.09 | 0.17 | 0.01 | 0.27 |
| D9935 | 0.09 | 0.17 | 0.01 | 0.27 |
| **Facility RVU** | **Work** | **PE** | **MP** | **Total** |
| D9934 | 0.09 | 0.17 | 0.01 | 0.27 |
| D9935 | 0.09 | 0.17 | 0.01 | 0.27 |

| | FUD | Status | MUE | Modifiers | | | | IOM Reference |
|---|---|---|---|---|---|---|---|---|
| D9934 | N/A | N | - | N/A | N/A | N/A | N/A | None |
| D9935 | N/A | N | - | N/A | N/A | N/A | N/A | |

* with documentation

## Terms To Know

**denture.** Manmade substitution of natural teeth and neighboring structures.

# D9941

**D9941** fabrication of athletic mouthguard

## Explanation

The provider constructs a custom mouth guard to be worn during a sport activity. There are different types of athletic mouth guards including intraoral, extraoral, or combined and selection of the type of mouth guard is dependent upon which offers the most protection for the sport played. The steps for fabrication are dependent upon the type of mouth guard being provided. Most frequently, the mouth guard is fabricated over a dental cast. The most commonly used materials include EVA copolymers, soft acrylic resin, and polyvinylchloride. The fabrication is complex and often requires several visits to complete.

## Coding Tips

When documentation indicates that a guard is prescribed to protect the teeth from stresses that may result in cracking or abnormal wear, to protect the temporomandibular joints from excessive bite forces, or to reduce the heavy forces generated by the jaw closing muscles, see D9944–D9946.

## ICD-10-CM Diagnostic Codes

Z46.3 Encounter for fitting and adjustment of dental prosthetic device

## Relative Value Units/Medicare Edits

| Non-Facility RVU | Work | PE | MP | Total |
|---|---|---|---|---|
| D9941 | 0.49 | 0.96 | 0.06 | 1.51 |
| **Facility RVU** | **Work** | **PE** | **MP** | **Total** |
| D9941 | 0.49 | 0.96 | 0.06 | 1.51 |

| | FUD | Status | MUE | Modifiers | | | | IOM Reference |
|---|---|---|---|---|---|---|---|---|
| D9941 | N/A | N | - | N/A | N/A | N/A | N/A | None |

* with documentation

## Terms To Know

**extraoral.** Outside of the mouth or oral cavity.

**intraoral.** Within the mouth.

# D9942

**D9942** repair and/or reline of occlusal guard

## Explanation

The provider repairs or relines an occlusal guard. Occlusal guards are used to evenly distribute bite forces to protect the teeth from stresses that may result in cracking or abnormal wear, protect the temporomandibular joints from excessive bite forces, or reduce the heavy forces generated by the jaw closing muscles. Occlusal guards may also be used to prevent the grinding of teeth at night. The procedure for repair is dependent upon the exact nature of the damage but is usually for chips or cracks. A reline is performed to improve fit, retention or wear characteristics. Base material is added to the tooth side of the guard, resurfacing the area.

## Coding Tips

For fabrication of an athletic mouth guard, see D9941.

## ICD-10-CM Diagnostic Codes

Z46.3 Encounter for fitting and adjustment of dental prosthetic device

## Relative Value Units/Medicare Edits

| Non-Facility RVU | Work | PE | MP | Total |
|---|---|---|---|---|
| D9942 | 0.58 | 1.15 | 0.07 | 1.80 |
| **Facility RVU** | **Work** | **PE** | **MP** | **Total** |
| D9942 | 0.58 | 1.15 | 0.07 | 1.80 |

| | FUD | Status | MUE | Modifiers | | | | IOM Reference |
|---|---|---|---|---|---|---|---|---|
| D9942 | N/A | N | - | N/A | N/A | N/A | N/A | None |

* with documentation

## Terms To Know

**occlusal.** Biting surfaces of premolar and molar teeth or the areas of contact between opposing teeth in the maxilla and mandible.

**reline.** Adjust the fit of a denture by filling in or resurfacing the part that makes contact with mucosal tissue.

# D9943

**D9943** occlusal guard adjustment

## Explanation

The dentist makes necessary adjustments to an occlusal guard. An occlusal guard is used to minimize the effects of bruxism (grinding teeth) or other occlusal factors such a malocclusion or excessive chewing on one side. The dentist inspects the occlusal guard for fit and for wear. With the guard inserted the patient is asked to bite down, slide forward and back and squeeze. Articulating paper may be used. If adjustments are necessary these are made using an acrylic burr or rubber cone as necessary.

## Coding Tips

To report adjustments to occlusal orthotic devices, such as a TMJ appliance, see D7881. To report the provision of an occlusal guard, see D9944–D9946.

## Documentation Tips

Documentation should clearly identify why the adjustments were necessary to support the reporting of this service.

## Reimbursement Tips

Coverage guidelines vary by payer and by patient contract. Check with the payer to determine coverage policies.

## ICD-10-CM Diagnostic Codes

F45.8 Other somatoform disorders

G47.63 Sleep related bruxism

## Relative Value Units/Medicare Edits

| Non-Facility RVU | Work | PE | MP | Total |
|---|---|---|---|---|
| D9943 | 0.34 | 0.68 | 0.04 | 1.06 |
| **Facility RVU** | **Work** | **PE** | **MP** | **Total** |
| D9943 | 0.34 | 0.68 | 0.04 | 1.06 |

| | FUD | Status | MUE | Modifiers | | | | IOM Reference |
|---|---|---|---|---|---|---|---|---|
| D9943 | N/A | N | - | N/A | N/A | N/A | N/A | None |

* with documentation

## Terms To Know

**bruxism.** Involuntary clenching or grinding of the teeth, usually while asleep, often stemming from repressed anger, tension, stress, fear, or frustration. Bruxism results in symptoms of temporomandibular joint disease such as jaw pain, headaches, earaches, and damaged teeth.

Dental - Adjunctive Services

# D9944-D9946

**D9944** occlusal guard - hard appliance, full arch

*Removable dental appliance designed to minimize the effects of bruxism or other occlusal factors. Not to be reported for any type of sleep apnea, snoring or TMD appliances.*

**D9945** occlusal guard - soft appliance, full arch

*Removable dental appliance designed to minimize the effects of bruxism or other occlusal factors. Not to be reported for any type of sleep apnea, snoring or TMD appliances.*

**D9946** occlusal guard - hard appliance, partial arch

*Removable dental appliance designed to minimize the effects of bruxism or other occlusal factors. Provides only partial occlusal coverage such as anterior deprogrammer. Not to be reported for any type of sleep apnea, snoring or TMD appliances.*

## Explanation

Occlusal guards are used to evenly distribute bite forces to protect the teeth from stresses that may result in cracking or abnormal wear, protect the temporomandibular joints from excessive bite forces, or reduce the heavy forces generated by the jaw closing muscles. They are also often used to prevent grinding of the teeth at night. The lower jaw is manipulated into a stable position (centric relation). After documenting the interocclusal record, impressions are made of the teeth, and a cast is created. The cast is then placed on an articulator with the teeth positioned according to the interocclusal record. An impression of the cast is made, which is then used to create the occlusal guard. Once the occlusal guard is hardened, sharp edges removed, and polished, the provider fits the guard and makes any necessary adjustments. The patient is provided instructions on wearing and caring for the guard. Report D9944 for hard appliance for the full arch, D9945 for soft appliance of the full arch, and D9446 for hard appliance for the partial arch.

## Coding Tips

This service may also be referred to as a night guard, bite guard, or occlusal splint. For occlusal orthotic devices used to treat TMJ dysfunctions, see D7880. For athletic mouth guards, see D9941. For repair or reline of occlusal guard, see D9942.

## ICD-10-CM Diagnostic Codes

| | |
|---|---|
| F45.8 | Other somatoform disorders |
| G47.63 | Sleep related bruxism |

## Relative Value Units/Medicare Edits

| Non-Facility RVU | Work | PE | MP | Total |
|---|---|---|---|---|
| **D9944** | 0.92 | 1.83 | 0.11 | 2.86 |
| **D9945** | 0.76 | 1.51 | 0.09 | 2.36 |
| **D9946** | 0.70 | 1.38 | 0.08 | 2.16 |
| **Facility RVU** | **Work** | **PE** | **MP** | **Total** |
| **D9944** | 0.92 | 1.83 | 0.11 | 2.86 |
| **D9945** | 0.76 | 1.51 | 0.09 | 2.36 |
| **D9946** | 0.70 | 1.38 | 0.08 | 2.16 |

| | FUD | Status | MUE | Modifiers | | | | IOM Reference |
|---|---|---|---|---|---|---|---|---|
| **D9944** | N/A | N | - | N/A | N/A | N/A | N/A | None |
| **D9945** | N/A | N | - | N/A | N/A | N/A | N/A | |
| **D9946** | N/A | N | - | N/A | N/A | N/A | N/A | |

* with documentation

## Terms To Know

**bruxism.** Involuntary clenching or grinding of the teeth, usually while asleep, often stemming from repressed anger, tension, stress, fear, or frustration. Bruxism results in symptoms of temporomandibular joint disease such as jaw pain, headaches, earaches, and damaged teeth.

# D9947-D9949

- **D9947** custom sleep apnea appliance fabrication and placement
- **D9948** adjustment of custom sleep apnea appliance
- **D9949** repair of custom sleep apnea appliance

## Explanation

Patients with mild to moderate obstructive sleep apnea and those who cannot tolerate CPAP machines may benefit from an oral sleep apnea appliance. The patient is evaluated for sleep apnea prior to treatment. Impressions are made of the upper and lower jaw. The provider determines the best angle, degree of movement, and advancement of the lower jaw to provide sleep apnea relief. The appliance is then constructed to the specifications of the physician and the patient is fitted with any additional adjustments when reporting D9947. Adjustment of the appliance is reported with code D9948 and repair of the appliance with code D9949

## Coding Tips

For an occlusal guard, see D9944-D9946. For adjustment of an occlusal guard, see D9943. For repair of an occlusal guard, see D9942.

## Documentation Tips

Sleep apnea testing with a positive diagnosis of obstructive sleep apnea may be required by some payers.

## Reimbursement Tips

This service may not be a covered service under dental and/or medical insurance.

## ICD-10-CM Diagnostic Codes

G47.30 Sleep apnea, unspecified
G47.33 Obstructive sleep apnea (adult) (pediatric)
G47.39 Other sleep apnea

## Relative Value Units/Medicare Edits

| Non-Facility RVU | Work | PE | MP | Total |
|---|---|---|---|---|
| **D9947** | | | | |
| **D9948** | | | | |
| **D9949** | | | | |
| **Facility RVU** | **Work** | **PE** | **MP** | **Total** |
| **D9947** | | | | |
| **D9948** | | | | |
| **D9949** | | | | |

| | FUD | Status | MUE | Modifiers | | | | IOM Reference |
|---|---|---|---|---|---|---|---|---|
| **D9947** | N/A | | - | N/A | N/A | N/A | N/A | |
| **D9948** | N/A | | - | N/A | N/A | N/A | N/A | |
| **D9949** | N/A | | - | N/A | N/A | N/A | N/A | |

* with documentation

## Terms To Know

**appliance.** Device providing function to a body part.

**sleep apnea.** Intermittent cessation of breathing during sleep that may cause hypoxemia and pulmonary arterial hypertension.

# D9950

**D9950** occlusion analysis - mounted case

*Includes, but is not limited to, facebow, interocclusal records tracings, and diagnostic wax-up; for diagnostic casts, see D0470.*

## Explanation

Primarily performed to evaluate malocclusion or abnormal bite forces, there are two methods that can be employed to accomplish this procedure. In the first method, the provider takes casts of both the maxillary and mandibular bite. These casts are then transferred to an articulator. The articulator is used to record and map the bite looking for abnormal forces or malocclusion. The second method employs a computerized system. After placing electrodes in the appropriate positions on the face and jaw, the patient is instructed to bite on a sensor. The information received by the sensor is transferred to a computerized program, which maps the forces of the bite, identifies malocclusion, and generates a three-dimensional model.

## Coding Tips

To report diagnostic casts, see D0470.

## ICD-10-CM Diagnostic Codes

Z46.3 Encounter for fitting and adjustment of dental prosthetic device

## Relative Value Units/Medicare Edits

| Non-Facility RVU | Work | PE | MP | Total |
|---|---|---|---|---|
| **D9950** | 0.88 | 1.74 | 0.11 | 2.73 |
| **Facility RVU** | **Work** | **PE** | **MP** | **Total** |
| **D9950** | 0.88 | 1.74 | 0.11 | 2.73 |

| | FUD | Status | MUE | Modifiers | | | | IOM Reference |
|---|---|---|---|---|---|---|---|---|
| **D9950** | N/A | R | - | N/A | N/A | N/A | 80* | 100-04,4,20.5 |

* with documentation

## Terms To Know

**analysis.** Study of body fluid, tissue, section, or parts.

**cast.** In dentistry, model or reproduction made from an impression or mold.

**occlusion.** Constriction, closure, or blockage of a passage.

# D9951-D9952

**D9951** occlusal adjustment - limited

*May also be known as equilibration; reshaping the occlusal surfaces of teeth to create harmonious contact relationships between the maxillary and mandibular teeth. Presently includes discing/odontoplasty/enamoplasty. Typically reported on a "per visit" basis. This should not be reported when the procedure only involves bite adjustment in the routine post-delivery care for a direct/indirect restoration or fixed/removable prosthodontics.*

**D9952** occlusal adjustment - complete

*Occlusal adjustment may require several appointments of varying length, and sedation may be necessary to attain adequate relaxation of the musculature. Study casts mounted on an articulating instrument may be utilized for analysis of occlusal disharmony. It is designed to achieve functional relationships and masticatory efficiency in conjunction with restorative treatment, orthodontics, orthognathic surgery, or jaw trauma when indicated. Occlusal adjustment enhances the healing potential of tissues affected by the lesions of occlusal trauma.*

## Explanation

Occlusal adjustment is making corrections in the bite from loose or shifting teeth, or teeth that are biting too hard against each other. Occlusal adjustment redistributes the forces applied to teeth in biting and chewing and relieves the excessive pressures on gums and other supporting tissues. The dentist determines which points on which teeth are to be adjusted. The teeth are marked with indicator tape while biting and grinding and then reshaping is done with carbide or diamond tips and a hand drill instrument. Report D9951 for limited occlusal adjustment, done in one area of the mouth, and D9952 for complete occlusal adjustment of the entire mouth.

## Coding Tips

Code D9951 is reported on a per-visit basis.

## Reimbursement Tips

Coverage of these procedures varies by payer. Check with the payer for specific coverage guidelines.

## ICD-10-CM Diagnostic Codes

Z46.4 Encounter for fitting and adjustment of orthodontic device

## Relative Value Units/Medicare Edits

| Non-Facility RVU | Work | PE | MP | Total |
|---|---|---|---|---|
| **D9951** | 0.41 | 0.81 | 0.05 | 1.27 |
| **D9952** | 1.79 | 3.54 | 0.21 | 5.54 |
| **Facility RVU** | **Work** | **PE** | **MP** | **Total** |
| **D9951** | 0.41 | 0.81 | 0.05 | 1.27 |
| **D9952** | 1.79 | 3.54 | 0.21 | 5.54 |

| | FUD | Status | MUE | Modifiers | | | | IOM Reference |
|---|---|---|---|---|---|---|---|---|
| **D9951** | N/A | R | - | N/A | N/A | N/A | 80* | 100-02,1,70; 100-04,4,20.5 |
| **D9952** | N/A | R | - | N/A | N/A | N/A | 80* | |

* with documentation

# D9961

**D9961** duplicate/copy patient's records

## Explanation

This code is adjunct to basic services rendered. The dentist reports this code to indicate the duplication and/or copying of the patient's records.

## Coding Tips

To report the detailed and extensive treatment planning and case presentation, see D9450.

## Reimbursement Tips

Most third-party payers will not reimburse for this service. Federal statutes allow that "the identification of labor costs for copying protected health information (PHI), whether in paper or electronic form, which can include a reasonable cost-based fee for time spent creating and copying the file." Most states have specific guidelines regarding the amount a patient or authorized representative, attorney, or insurer may be charged for this service. Check with specific state statutes for specific guidelines.

## ICD-10-CM Diagnostic Codes

The application of this code is too broad to adequately present ICD-10-CM diagnostic code links here. Refer to your ICD-10-CM book.

## Relative Value Units/Medicare Edits

| Non-Facility RVU | Work | PE | MP | Total |
|---|---|---|---|---|
| **D9961** | 0.21 | 0.42 | 0.03 | 0.66 |
| **Facility RVU** | **Work** | **PE** | **MP** | **Total** |
| **D9961** | 0.21 | 0.42 | 0.03 | 0.66 |

| | FUD | Status | MUE | Modifiers | | | | IOM Reference |
|---|---|---|---|---|---|---|---|---|
| **D9961** | N/A | N | - | N/A | N/A | N/A | N/A | None |

* with documentation

# D9970

**D9970** enamel microabrasion

*The removal of discolored surface enamel defects resulting from altered mineralization or decalcification of the superficial enamel layer. Submit per treatment visit.*

## Explanation

After isolating the teeth to be treated with a rubber dam, the provider carefully rubs the tooth surface with a special compound of hydrochloric acid and abrasive compounds to remove surface stains and discoloration.

## Coding Tips

This code is reported once for each time the microabrasion is performed. To report scaling, see D4341–D4346. To report the removal of plaque, calculus and stains, report D1110–D1120.

## ICD-10-CM Diagnostic Codes

| | |
|---|---|
| K00.3 | Mottled teeth |

## Relative Value Units/Medicare Edits

| Non-Facility RVU | Work | PE | MP | Total |
|---|---|---|---|---|
| D9970 | 0.28 | 0.56 | 0.03 | 0.87 |
| **Facility RVU** | **Work** | **PE** | **MP** | **Total** |
| D9970 | 0.28 | 0.56 | 0.03 | 0.87 |

| | FUD | Status | MUE | Modifiers | | | | IOM Reference |
|---|---|---|---|---|---|---|---|---|
| D9970 | N/A | N | - | N/A | N/A | N/A | N/A | None |

* with documentation

## Terms To Know

**calculus.** Abnormal, stone-like concretion of calcium, cholesterol, mineral salts, or other substances that forms in any part of the body.

**plaque.** Accumulation of a soft sticky substance on the teeth largely composed of bacteria and its byproducts.

**superficial.** On the skin surface or near the surface of any involved structure or field of interest.

# D9971

**D9971** odontoplasty - per tooth

*Removal/reshaping of enamel surfaces or projections.*

## Explanation

Odontoplasty, also known as enamel shaping, enameloplasty, and recontouring or stripping, is the process of shaping natural teeth to improve their appearance. This is done when teeth acquire projections in the enamel, become uneven, or have rough incisal edges. Anesthesia is not required. The enamel of the teeth is removed and/or contoured by the dentist to achieve a more balanced, aesthetic look in the mouth. This is done cautiously as enamel can never be replaced.

## Coding Tips

Report D9971 per tooth treated. Documentation may indicate that the provider enlarged occlusal pits and fissures using a bur and may be referred to as a fissurotomy and reported with code D9971. Any radiograph is reported separately.

## Documentation Tips

The following information should be documented on a tooth chart: treatment/location of caries, endodontic procedures, prosthetic services, preventive services, treatment of lesions and dental disease, or other special procedures. A tooth chart may also be used to identify structure and rationale of disease process, and the type of service performed on intraoral structures other than teeth.

## Reimbursement Tips

Coverage of this procedure varies by payer. Check with the payer for specific coverage guidelines.

## ICD-10-CM Diagnostic Codes

| | |
|---|---|
| K00.2 | Abnormalities of size and form of teeth |
| K00.3 | Mottled teeth |
| K00.4 | Disturbances in tooth formation |
| K00.5 | Hereditary disturbances in tooth structure, not elsewhere classified |
| K03.6 | Deposits [accretions] on teeth |
| K03.7 | Posteruptive color changes of dental hard tissues |

## Relative Value Units/Medicare Edits

| Non-Facility RVU | Work | PE | MP | Total |
|---|---|---|---|---|
| D9971 | 0.33 | 0.65 | 0.04 | 1.02 |
| **Facility RVU** | **Work** | **PE** | **MP** | **Total** |
| D9971 | 0.33 | 0.65 | 0.04 | 1.02 |

| | FUD | Status | MUE | Modifiers | | | | IOM Reference |
|---|---|---|---|---|---|---|---|---|
| D9971 | N/A | N | - | N/A | N/A | N/A | N/A | None |

* with documentation

## Terms To Know

**odontoplasty.** Adjustment of tooth shape, size, or length.

Dental - Adjunctive Services

# D9972-D9974

**D9972** external bleaching - per arch - performed in office
**D9973** external bleaching - per tooth
**D9974** internal bleaching - per tooth

## Explanation

When the dentist applies tooth whitening materials, the oral tissues are first covered in a protective gel or a rubber shield is placed. The bleaching agent is then applied to the teeth. Occasionally, laser light is used in the tooth whitening procedure to enhance the whitening action of the bleaching agent. Bleaching agents that contain peroxide (usually 10 percent carbamide peroxide for home-applied products and up to 35 percent hydrogen peroxide for professionally applied products) will bleach the enamel of the teeth, removing deep, intrinsic stains and actually changing the color of the tooth. Non-bleaching whitening products rely on physical or chemical chelation action to remove the external, surface stains only. Report D9972 per arch of external bleaching, D9973 for each tooth externally bleached, and D9974 for internal bleaching per tooth.

## Coding Tips

Any evaluation or radiograph is reported separately. These procedures include use of D3910 tooth isolation with rubber dam. In the case of D9972–D9974, "external" refers to the outer (buccal) aspect of the teeth. For the provision of an external bleaching kit for home use, see D9975.

## Reimbursement Tips

When performed for cosmetic purposes, these services are likely not covered by third-party payers.

## ICD-10-CM Diagnostic Codes

| | |
|---|---|
| K00.2 | Abnormalities of size and form of teeth |
| K00.3 | Mottled teeth |
| K00.4 | Disturbances in tooth formation |
| K00.5 | Hereditary disturbances in tooth structure, not elsewhere classified |
| K03.6 | Deposits [accretions] on teeth |
| K03.7 | Posteruptive color changes of dental hard tissues |

## Relative Value Units/Medicare Edits

| Non-Facility RVU | Work | PE | MP | Total |
|---|---|---|---|---|
| **D9972** | 0.97 | 1.92 | 0.12 | 3.01 |
| **D9973** | 0.28 | 0.56 | 0.03 | 0.87 |
| **D9974** | 0.81 | 1.60 | 0.10 | 2.51 |
| **Facility RVU** | **Work** | **PE** | **MP** | **Total** |
| **D9972** | 0.97 | 1.92 | 0.12 | 3.01 |
| **D9973** | 0.28 | 0.56 | 0.03 | 0.87 |
| **D9974** | 0.81 | 1.60 | 0.10 | 2.51 |

| | FUD | Status | MUE | Modifiers | | | | IOM Reference |
|---|---|---|---|---|---|---|---|---|
| **D9972** | N/A | N | - | N/A | N/A | N/A | N/A | None |
| **D9973** | N/A | N | - | N/A | N/A | N/A | N/A | |
| **D9974** | N/A | N | - | N/A | N/A | N/A | N/A | |

* with documentation

# D9986-D9987

**D9986** missed appointment
**D9987** cancelled appointment

## Explanation

The patient missed an appointment without prior notification in D9986. In D9987, the patient cancels a previously scheduled appointment with the dentist.

## Coding Tips

These codes may not be reimbursed by third-party payers but may be used for administrative and patient billing purposes.

## Documentation Tips

It is advisable to document in the medical record when a patient cancels or misses an appointment.

## Reimbursement Tips

This service is usually a noncovered service.

## ICD-10-CM Diagnostic Codes

The application of this code is too broad to adequately present ICD-10-CM diagnostic code links here. Refer to your ICD-10-CM book.

## Relative Value Units/Medicare Edits

| Non-Facility RVU | Work | PE | MP | Total |
|---|---|---|---|---|
| **D9986** | 0.00 | 0.00 | 0.00 | 0.00 |
| **D9987** | 0.00 | 0.00 | 0.00 | 0.00 |
| **Facility RVU** | **Work** | **PE** | **MP** | **Total** |
| **D9986** | 0.00 | 0.00 | 0.00 | 0.00 |
| **D9987** | 0.00 | 0.00 | 0.00 | 0.00 |

| | FUD | Status | MUE | Modifiers | | | | IOM Reference |
|---|---|---|---|---|---|---|---|---|
| **D9986** | N/A | I | - | N/A | N/A | N/A | N/A | None |
| **D9987** | N/A | I | - | N/A | N/A | N/A | N/A | |

* with documentation

## Terms To Know

**third-party payer.** Public or private organization that pays for or underwrites coverage for health care expenses for another entity, usually an employer (e.g., Blue Cross Blue Shield, Medicare, Medicaid, commercial insurers).

# D9990

**D9990** certified translation or sign-language services - per visit

## Explanation

Communication assistance by either a certified translator or sign-language professional to assist in the communication and treatment of the patient.

## Coding Tips

This service should be reported once per visit.

## Reimbursement Tips

Coverage of this procedure varies by payer. Check with the payer for specific coverage guidelines.

## ICD-10-CM Diagnostic Codes

The application of this code is too broad to adequately present ICD-10-CM diagnostic code links here. Refer to your ICD-10-CM book.

## Relative Value Units/Medicare Edits

| Non-Facility RVU | Work | PE | MP | Total |
|---|---|---|---|---|
| D9990 | 0.11 | 0.21 | 0.01 | 0.33 |
| **Facility RVU** | **Work** | **PE** | **MP** | **Total** |
| D9990 | 0.11 | 0.21 | 0.01 | 0.33 |

| | FUD | Status | MUE | Modifiers | | | | IOM Reference |
|---|---|---|---|---|---|---|---|---|
| D9990 | N/A | N | - | N/A | N/A | N/A | N/A | None |

* with documentation

# D9991-D9994

**D9991** dental case management - addressing appointment compliance barriers

*Individualized efforts to assist a patient to maintain scheduled appointments by solving transportation challenges or other barriers.*

**D9992** dental case management - care coordination

*Assisting in a patient's decisions regarding the coordination of oral health care services across multiple providers, provider types, specialty areas of treatment, health care settings, health care organizations and payment systems. This is the additional time and resources expended to provide experience or expertise beyond that possessed by the patient.*

**D9993** dental case management - motivational interviewing

*Patient-centered, personalized counseling using methods such as Motivational Interviewing (MI) to identify and modify behaviors interfering with positive oral health outcomes. This is a separate service from traditional nutritional or tobacco counseling.*

**D9994** dental case management - patient education to improve oral health literacy

*Individual, customized communication of information to assist the patient in making appropriate health decisions designed to improve oral health literacy, explained in a manner acknowledging economic circumstances and different cultural beliefs, values, attitudes, traditions and language preferences, and adopting information and services to these differences, which requires the expenditure of time and resources beyond that of an oral evaluation or case presentation.*

## Explanation

These codes are used to report dental case management services including issues keeping appointments, coordination with other caregivers, motivation, or education regarding oral health.

## Coding Tips

Third-party payers may not provide coverage for these services.

## ICD-10-CM Diagnostic Codes

The application of this code is too broad to adequately present ICD-10-CM diagnostic code links here. Refer to your ICD-10-CM book.

## Relative Value Units/Medicare Edits

| Non-Facility RVU | Work | PE | MP | Total |
|---|---|---|---|---|
| D9991 | 0.05 | 0.11 | 0.01 | 0.17 |
| D9992 | 0.11 | 0.21 | 0.01 | 0.33 |
| D9993 | 0.05 | 0.11 | 0.01 | 0.17 |
| D9994 | 0.05 | 0.11 | 0.01 | 0.17 |
| **Facility RVU** | **Work** | **PE** | **MP** | **Total** |
| D9991 | 0.05 | 0.11 | 0.01 | 0.17 |
| D9992 | 0.11 | 0.21 | 0.01 | 0.33 |
| D9993 | 0.05 | 0.11 | 0.01 | 0.17 |
| D9994 | 0.05 | 0.11 | 0.01 | 0.17 |

| | FUD | Status | MUE | Modifiers | | | | IOM Reference |
|---|---|---|---|---|---|---|---|---|
| D9991 | N/A | N | - | N/A | N/A | N/A | N/A | None |
| D9992 | N/A | N | - | N/A | N/A | N/A | N/A | |
| D9993 | N/A | N | - | N/A | N/A | N/A | N/A | |
| D9994 | N/A | N | - | N/A | N/A | N/A | N/A | |

* with documentation

## Terms To Know

**case management services.** Physician case management is a process of involving direct patient care as well as coordinating and controlling access to the patient or initiating and/or supervising other necessary health care services.

**coordination of care.** Care provided concurrently with counseling that includes treatment instructions to the patient or caregiver; special accommodations for home, work, school, vacation, or other locations; coordination with other providers and agencies; and living arrangements.

**patient.** Individual who is receiving or who has received health care services. This could include a person who is deceased.

# D9995-D9996

**D9995** teledentistry - synchronous; real-time encounter

*Reported in addition to other procedures (e.g., diagnostic) delivered to the patient on the date of service.*

**D9996** teledentistry - asynchronous; information stored and forwarded to dentist for subsequent review

*Reported in addition to other procedures (e.g., diagnostic) delivered to the patient on the date of service.*

## Explanation

The provider provides synchronous real-time telemedicine services to the patient. The service involves electronic communication using interactive telecommunications equipment that includes at a minimum audio and video. Report D9995 when the telemedicine communication is provided in real-time. Report D9996 when the telemedicine communication is stored and provided for review at a subsequent time.

## Coding Tips

These services are reported in addition to other services provided to the patient at the same encounter.

## ICD-10-CM Diagnostic Codes

The application of this code is too broad to adequately present ICD-10-CM diagnostic code links here. Refer to your ICD-10-CM book.

## Relative Value Units/Medicare Edits

| Non-Facility RVU | Work | PE | MP | Total |
|---|---|---|---|---|
| D9995 | 0.00 | 0.00 | 0.00 | 0.00 |
| D9996 | 0.00 | 0.00 | 0.00 | 0.00 |
| **Facility RVU** | **Work** | **PE** | **MP** | **Total** |
| D9995 | 0.00 | 0.00 | 0.00 | 0.00 |
| D9996 | 0.00 | 0.00 | 0.00 | 0.00 |

| | FUD | Status | MUE | Modifiers | | | | IOM Reference |
|---|---|---|---|---|---|---|---|---|
| D9995 | N/A | N | - | N/A | N/A | N/A | N/A | None |
| D9996 | N/A | N | - | N/A | N/A | N/A | N/A | |

* with documentation

## Terms To Know

**telemedicine.** Medical information exchanged from site to site via electronic communication. Examples include patient evaluation and consultation, monitoring, education and other clinical services.

# D9997

▲ **D9997** dental case management - patients with special health care needs

*Special treatment considerations for patients/individuals with physical, medical, developmental, or cognitive conditions resulting in substantial functional limitations or incapacitation, which require that modifications be made to delivery of treatment to provide customized or comprehensive oral health care services.*

## Explanation

The provider uses special techniques when communicating and treating patients with physical, medical, developmental, or cognitive conditions.

## Coding Tips

Third-party payers may not provide coverage for these services.

## Documentation Tips

The provider should document the special health needs and the accommodation services provided.

## ICD-10-CM Diagnostic Codes

The application of this code is too broad to adequately present ICD-10-CM diagnostic code links here. Refer to your ICD-10-CM book.

## Relative Value Units/Medicare Edits

| Non-Facility RVU | Work | PE | MP | Total |
|---|---|---|---|---|
| D9997 | 0.00 | 0.00 | 0.00 | 0.00 |
| **Facility RVU** | **Work** | **PE** | **MP** | **Total** |
| D9997 | 0.00 | 0.00 | 0.00 | 0.00 |

| | FUD | Status | MUE | Modifiers | | | | IOM Reference |
|---|---|---|---|---|---|---|---|---|
| D9997 | N/A | I | - | N/A | N/A | N/A | N/A | None |

* with documentation

## Terms To Know

**cognitive.** Being aware by drawing from knowledge, such as judgment, reason, perception, and memory.

**developmental delay disorders.** Various disorders manifested by a delay in development based on that anticipated for a certain age level or period of development. Both biological and nonbiological factors may be involved. Originating before age 18, these impairments may continue indefinitely.

## D5931-D5932, D5936

**D5931** obturator prosthesis, surgical

**D5932** obturator prosthesis, definitive

**D5936** obturator prosthesis, interim

### Explanation

Facial trauma, as well as surgery to the maxilla, maxillary sinus, palate, and alveolus, particularly for cancer, can result in severe impairment of speech and swallowing. Postoperatively, the patient is fitted with a series of obturators depending on the particular needs to restore function, as well as for aesthetic purposes. An immediate surgical obturator (D5931) is placed, usually in the operating room, and helps to restore oral function and aesthetics, as well as to support healing and prevent the formation of scarring and hold packing in place. When the packing is removed, this device is replaced by an interim obturator prosthesis (D5936). This device is used during the healing phase and requires frequent modification while it is in place. Once the defect is stable, a definitive obturator prosthesis (D5932) is fabricated that further augments oral function and aesthetic appearance.

### Relative Value Units/Medicare Edits

| Non-Facility RVU | Work | PE | MP | Total |
|---|---|---|---|---|
| D5931 | | | | |
| D5932 | | | | |
| D5936 | | | | |
| **Facility RVU** | **Work** | **PE** | **MP** | **Total** |
| D5931 | | | | |
| D5932 | | | | |
| D5936 | | | | |

## D5937

**D5937** trismus appliance (not for TMD treatment)

### Explanation

Trismus is the inability to fully open the mouth due to jaw muscle spasms, an underlying condition such as tetanus, trauma, surgery, radiation, or due to abnormally short jaw muscles, as seen in Hecht syndrome. This condition affects all functions including eating and speech, oral hygiene, and may also impact the patient's physical appearance. There are several different types of appliances available, based on the needs of the patient (e.g., internal or external, elastic, etc.).

### Relative Value Units/Medicare Edits

| Non-Facility RVU | Work | PE | MP | Total |
|---|---|---|---|---|
| D5937 | | | | |
| **Facility RVU** | **Work** | **PE** | **MP** | **Total** |
| D5937 | | | | |

## D5952-D5953, D5960

**D5952** speech aid prosthesis, pediatric

**D5953** speech aid prosthesis, adult

**D5960** speech aid prosthesis, modification

### Relative Value Units/Medicare Edits

| Non-Facility RVU | Work | PE | MP | Total |
|---|---|---|---|---|
| D5952 | | | | |
| D5953 | | | | |
| D5960 | | | | |
| **Facility RVU** | **Work** | **PE** | **MP** | **Total** |
| D5952 | | | | |
| D5953 | | | | |
| D5960 | | | | |

## D5954

**D5954** palatal augmentation prosthesis

### Explanation

This device aids in speech and swallowing by reconfiguring the hard palate to enhance contact with the tongue. This may be necessary due to trauma, cancer surgery, or neurological diseases that prevent this from occurring normally.

### Relative Value Units/Medicare Edits

| Non-Facility RVU | Work | PE | MP | Total |
|---|---|---|---|---|
| D5954 | | | | |
| **Facility RVU** | **Work** | **PE** | **MP** | **Total** |
| D5954 | | | | |

## D5955-D5959

**D5955** palatal lift prosthesis, definitive

**D5958** palatal lift prosthesis, interim

**D5959** palatal lift prosthesis, modification

### Explanation

In addition to trauma, cleft palate, and surgery for other conditions, a palatal lift prosthesis may be used to compensate for velopharyngeal muscles that are weak or uncoordinated (e.g., cerebral palsy). The device may be used on a permanent or temporary basis, depending on the severity of the condition and the needs of the patient. An interim prosthesis (D5958) may be fabricated until the patient is ready to fit with a definitive or long-term device (D5955). Modifications may be necessary in accordance with the patient's needs, such as healing of a surgical site, patient growth, etc. (D5959).

### Relative Value Units/Medicare Edits

| Non-Facility RVU | Work | PE | MP | Total |
|---|---|---|---|---|
| D5955 | | | | |
| D5958 | | | | |
| D5959 | | | | |
| **Facility RVU** | **Work** | **PE** | **MP** | **Total** |
| D5955 | | | | |
| D5958 | | | | |
| D5959 | | | | |

## D5982

**D5982** surgical stent

### Explanation

A surgical guide stent, which is made of acrylic material, is used in the placement and stabilization of grafts and the accurate insertion of transosteal and endosteal implants by helping to establish the correct relationship between the ridge and the implant.

### Relative Value Units/Medicare Edits

| Non-Facility RVU | Work | PE | MP | Total |
|---|---|---|---|---|
| D5982 | | | | |
| Facility RVU | Work | PE | MP | Total |
| D5982 | | | | |

## D5986

**D5986** fluoride gel carrier

### Explanation

A prosthesis is placed by the provider over the dental arch to cover the teeth in order to apply topical fluoride over tooth enamel and dentin. This is also referred to as a fluoride applicator.

### Relative Value Units/Medicare Edits

| Non-Facility RVU | Work | PE | MP | Total |
|---|---|---|---|---|
| D5986 | | | | |
| Facility RVU | Work | PE | MP | Total |
| D5986 | | | | |

## D5987

**D5987** commissure splint

### Explanation

If the patient sustains a thermal or chemical burn to the mouth and/or lips, or undergoes surgical procedures, severe contractures of the lips and mouth may occur. Contractures are classified as anterior (most often caused by electrical burns; involve the oral commissure, lips, anterior part of the tongue, and anterior buccal sulcus and surrounding mucosa), posterior (caused by ingestion of caustic agents and involve the posterior buccal mucosa, posterior tongue, retro-molar area, and oropharynx), and total (caused by the ingestion of lye and involving the lips, tongue, oral cavity, and oropharyngeal mucosa).

### Relative Value Units/Medicare Edits

| Non-Facility RVU | Work | PE | MP | Total |
|---|---|---|---|---|
| D5987 | | | | |
| Facility RVU | Work | PE | MP | Total |
| D5987 | | | | |

## D5988

**D5988** surgical splint

### Explanation

The fabrication of a surgical splint is often necessary after surgery or trauma to the bones of the face as a means of supporting and stabilizing the repair until healing takes place.

### Relative Value Units/Medicare Edits

| Non-Facility RVU | Work | PE | MP | Total |
|---|---|---|---|---|
| D5988 | | | | |
| Facility RVU | Work | PE | MP | Total |
| D5988 | | | | |

## D7260

**D7260** oroantral fistula closure

### Explanation

The physician closes an opening between the mouth and the maxillary sinus. The communication is through the maxillary bone and this tract is lined with epithelium. Local anesthesia is injected into the mucosa. The provider uses a scalpel to excise the epithelized tract. An incision is made into the palatal mucosa and a local mucosal flap is developed. The flap is sutured in multiple layers, covering the oromaxillary tract. Careful postoperative instructions are given to limit sinus pressure by not allowing nose blowing which would reopen the tract and impair healing.

### Relative Value Units/Medicare Edits

| Non-Facility RVU | Work | PE | MP | Total |
|---|---|---|---|---|
| D7260 | | | | |
| Facility RVU | Work | PE | MP | Total |
| D7260 | | | | |

## D7261

**D7261** primary closure of a sinus perforation

### Explanation

After the surgical extraction of a tooth the sinus may be exposed. It may be necessary for the physician to close an oroantral or oronasal communication. The physician exposes the communication and sutures it closed.

### Relative Value Units/Medicare Edits

| Non-Facility RVU | Work | PE | MP | Total |
|---|---|---|---|---|
| D7261 | | | | |
| Facility RVU | Work | PE | MP | Total |
| D7261 | | | | |

## D7490

**D7490** radical resection of maxilla or mandible

### Explanation

The physician removes a malignant tumor from the mandible. Through an intraoral and/or extraoral approach, the physician isolates and dissects the mandibular tumor. The tumor and surrounding tissues are removed. The tissues are closed with layered sutures or may be packed and left open. A reconstructive procedure, such as bone harvesting, may be necessary and is reported separately

### Relative Value Units/Medicare Edits

| Non-Facility RVU | Work | PE | MP | Total |
|---|---|---|---|---|
| D7490 | | | | |
| Facility RVU | Work | PE | MP | Total |
| D7490 | | | | |

## D7550

**D7550** partial ostectomy/sequestrectomy for removal of non-vital bone

### Explanation

The physician removes a portion of the alveolus that is loose or sloughed-off as the result of infection or reduced blood supply. Incisions are made through the mucosa to expose the alveolar bone. Curettes, drills, or osteotomes are used to remove the diseased alveolar bone or sequestrum. The mucosa may be sutured directly over the surgical wound, or it may be packed and allowed to heal secondarily.

### Relative Value Units/Medicare Edits

| Non-Facility RVU | Work | PE | MP | Total |
|---|---|---|---|---|
| D7550 | | | | |
| Facility RVU | Work | PE | MP | Total |
| D7550 | | | | |

## D7840

**D7840** condylectomy

### Explanation

The physician removes the condyle of the mandible, the posterior, rounded projection on the angled branch of the jaw that articulates with the temporal bone. An incision is usually made in the skin anterior to the contour of the ear. The physician dissects the tissue layers until the condyle is exposed. The condyle is cut with drills or saws from the mandible and removed. An additional incision just under the angle of the mandible may be required. The area can be reconstructed with bone and cartilage, or a prosthetic condyle may be inserted. The skin incision is closed with layered sutures and a pressure dressing may be applied.

### Relative Value Units/Medicare Edits

| Non-Facility RVU | Work | PE | MP | Total |
|---|---|---|---|---|
| D7840 | | | | |
| Facility RVU | Work | PE | MP | Total |
| D7840 | | | | |

## D7880

**D7880** occlusal orthotic device, by report

### Explanation

The physician fits the patient for an occlusal orthotic device including a splint.

### Relative Value Units/Medicare Edits

| Non-Facility RVU | Work | PE | MP | Total |
|---|---|---|---|---|
| D7880 | | | | |
| Facility RVU | Work | PE | MP | Total |
| D7880 | | | | |

## D7881

**D7881** occlusal orthotic device adjustment

### Explanation

The provider makes adjustments to a previously provided occlusal orthotic device. An occlusal orthotic device or splint is a device specifically fitted for people who have a history of temporomandibular joint pain or other conditions. Usually made of an acrylic resin, the provider may need to make adjustments to the device for a better fit by heating, filing, or other methods.

### Relative Value Units/Medicare Edits

| Non-Facility RVU | Work | PE | MP | Total |
|---|---|---|---|---|
| D7881 | | | | |
| Facility RVU | Work | PE | MP | Total |
| D7881 | | | | |

## D7899

**D7899** unspecified TMD therapy, by report

### Explanation

This code is used to report TMD therapy procedures for which there is no other code that specifically describes the procedure.

### Relative Value Units/Medicare Edits

| Non-Facility RVU | Work | PE | MP | Total |
|---|---|---|---|---|
| D7899 | | | | |
| Facility RVU | Work | PE | MP | Total |
| D7899 | | | | |

## D7920

**D7920** skin graft (identify defect covered, location and type of graft)

### Explanation

The physician repairs a defect by applying a skin graft. There are numerous types of skin grafting procedures from split thickness to a full thickness grafts. These procedures involve the removal of the full layer of epidermis and a thin layer of dermis from the donor site and attaching it to cover the defect. Skin substitutes and replacement may also be used.

### Relative Value Units/Medicare Edits

| Non-Facility RVU | Work | PE | MP | Total |
|---|---|---|---|---|
| D7920 | | | | |
| Facility RVU | Work | PE | MP | Total |
| D7920 | | | | |

## D7941-D7945

**D7941** osteotomy - mandibular rami

**D7943** osteotomy - mandibular rami with bone graft; includes obtaining the graft

**D7944** osteotomy - segmented or subapical

**D7945** osteotomy - body of mandible

### Explanation

The physician reconstructs the mandible. In D7941 and D7943 the mandibular ramus is lengthened, set back, or rotated. Approach can be either intra- or extraoral. When an intraoral approach is used, the physician makes an incision overlying the external oblique ridge, through the mucosa near the second mandibular molars. For an extraoral approach, the physician makes a skin incision below the angle of the mandible. In both approaches, the mandibular ramus is exposed. Drills, saws, and/or osteotomes are used to cut the mandible along the inside, top, and outside surfaces of the bone, but not completely through. The physician uses osteotomes and/or other instruments to pry the mandible apart along the bone cuts in a sagittal plane. Once separated, the physician moves the mandible into the desired position and holds the bone in reduction using wires. An osteotomy with a bone graft is used in D7943. A segmented or subapical osteotomy (D7944) is primarily used in the treatment of maxillary protrusion to achieve functional occlusion and to improve the facial profile. Drills, saws, and/or osteotomes are used to cut the mandible between the apices of the anterior teeth. In D7945 the procedure is performed on the body of the mandible.

### Relative Value Units/Medicare Edits

| Non-Facility RVU | Work | PE | MP | Total |
|---|---|---|---|---|
| D7941 | | | | |
| D7943 | | | | |
| D7944 | | | | |
| D7945 | | | | |
| **Facility RVU** | **Work** | **PE** | **MP** | **Total** |
| D7941 | | | | |
| D7943 | | | | |
| D7944 | | | | |
| D7945 | | | | |

## D7955

**D7955** repair of maxillofacial soft and/or hard tissue defect

### Explanation

The physician repairs maxillofacial defects resulting from trauma, previous surgeries, or congenital defects. Procedures performed as reconstruction of the edentulous maxilla and/or mandible prior to prosthetic devices are not reported using this procedure code; however, reconstruction of the facial bones to return form and function are. Techniques vary depending upon the type of defect being repaired. An example of a procedure reported using this code would be the reconstruction of the midface to correct developmental or traumatic skeletal deformities. Reconstruction includes both osteotomies and bone grafts. The physician may use a variety of incisions, including a bicoronal scalp flap, eyelid, and transoral incisions. Through the incisions, the physician performs osteotomies as necessary of the midface with saws, burs, or osteotomes. The osteotomies performed here do not follow the standard LeFort surgical fracture lines. Bone grafts are harvested from the patient's hip, rib, or skull and the surgically created wound is closed. The interpositional bone grafts are placed between the bony interfaces of the repositioned maxilla and midface. Internal fixation devices such as wires, plates, and screws are used to hold the reduction securely in place. The transoral incisions are closed in a single layer. Eyelid and scalp incisions are closed in layers. Intermaxillary fixation may be applied.

### Relative Value Units/Medicare Edits

| Non-Facility RVU | Work | PE | MP | Total |
|---|---|---|---|---|
| D7955 | | | | |
| **Facility RVU** | **Work** | **PE** | **MP** | **Total** |
| D7955 | | | | |

## D7981

**D7981** excision of salivary gland, by report

### Explanation

The physician removes a diseased, infected, blocked, or injured salivary gland. Technique is dependent upon the salivary gland being removed. When removal is of the submandibular gland the physician makes an incision in the skin of the neck below the inferior border of the mandible and near the angle of the mandible. The underlying tissues are dissected to the submandibular gland. The gland is exposed, freed from the surrounding tissue, and removed. The incision is closed with sutures. When the parotid gland is excised the physician makes a preauricular incision with a curved cervical extension to the midpoint of the mandible. The anterior and posterior skin flaps are retracted and the tissues are retracted to expose the parotid gland, leaving the fascia over the gland intact.

### Relative Value Units/Medicare Edits

| Non-Facility RVU | Work | PE | MP | Total |
|---|---|---|---|---|
| D7981 | | | | |
| **Facility RVU** | **Work** | **PE** | **MP** | **Total** |
| D7981 | | | | |

## D7982

**D7982** sialodochoplasty

### Explanation

The physician repairs a salivary duct by inserting a hollow plastic or silicone tube into the duct. The tube is threaded through the duct. The duct is allowed to heal and may be sutured around the tube. The tube is later removed and patency is restored.

### Relative Value Units/Medicare Edits

| Non-Facility RVU | Work | PE | MP | Total |
|---|---|---|---|---|
| D7982 | | | | |
| **Facility RVU** | **Work** | **PE** | **MP** | **Total** |
| D7982 | | | | |

## D7983

**D7983** closure of salivary fistula

### Explanation

The physician closes a salivary fistula. The physician makes an incision around the fistula and excises the fistula down to the level of the duct. After excision of the fistula, the incision is closed directly.

### Relative Value Units/Medicare Edits

| Non-Facility RVU | Work | PE | MP | Total |
|---|---|---|---|---|
| D7983 | | | | |
| **Facility RVU** | **Work** | **PE** | **MP** | **Total** |
| D7983 | | | | |

## D7990

**D7990** emergency tracheotomy

### Explanation

The physician creates a tracheotomy in an emergent situation. The physician makes a horizontal neck incision and dissects the muscles to expose the trachea. The thyroid isthmus is cut if necessary. The trachea is incised and an airway is inserted.

### Relative Value Units/Medicare Edits

| Non-Facility RVU | Work | PE | MP | Total |
|---|---|---|---|---|
| D7990 | | | | |
| **Facility RVU** | **Work** | **PE** | **MP** | **Total** |
| D7990 | | | | |

## D7991

**D7991** coronoidectomy

### Explanation

The physician removes the diseased or fractured coronoid process of the mandible, the anterior projection on the angled branch of the jaw to which the temporal muscle is attached. The physician makes an incision intraorally along the external oblique ridge of the mandible. The tissue is reflected from the bone, exposing the coronoid process. Using drills and/or osteotomes, the coronoid process is clamped and sectioned from the mandible. The muscle attachments are cut from the coronoid process and will retract, forming scar tissue. The coronoid process is removed. The mucosal incision is closed primarily.

### Relative Value Units/Medicare Edits

| Non-Facility RVU | Work | PE | MP | Total |
|---|---|---|---|---|
| D7991 | | | | |
| **Facility RVU** | **Work** | **PE** | **MP** | **Total** |
| D7991 | | | | |

## D7995

**D7995** synthetic graft - mandible or facial bones, by report

### Explanation

The physician reconstructs the mandible or facial bone with a synthetic bone graft to correct defects due to injury, infection, or tumor resection. The procedure may also be performed to augment atrophic or thin mandibles or other facial bone abnormalities. Depending on the site being treated, the physician may perform the procedure intraorally or extraorally.

### Relative Value Units/Medicare Edits

| Non-Facility RVU | Work | PE | MP | Total |
|---|---|---|---|---|
| D7995 | | | | |
| **Facility RVU** | **Work** | **PE** | **MP** | **Total** |
| D7995 | | | | |

## D7996

**D7996** implant-mandible for augmentation purposes (excluding alveolar ridge), by report

### Explanation

The physician uses prosthetic material to augment the mandible. The physician may use an intraoral approach or may make skin incisions extraorally below the body or angle of the mandible. The physician dissects tissues away and the bone of the body or angle is exposed. A synthetic material is placed on the mandible to augment the contours. The graft is secured and the incisions are closed.

### Relative Value Units/Medicare Edits

| Non-Facility RVU | Work | PE | MP | Total |
|---|---|---|---|---|
| D7996 | | | | |
| **Facility RVU** | **Work** | **PE** | **MP** | **Total** |
| D7996 | | | | |

# 99202-99205

**★99202** Office or other outpatient visit for the evaluation and management of a new patient, which requires a medically appropriate history and/or examination and straightforward medical decision making. When using time for code selection, 15-29 minutes of total time is spent on the date of the encounter.

**★99203** Office or other outpatient visit for the evaluation and management of a new patient, which requires a medically appropriate history and/or examination and low level of medical decision making. When using time for code selection, 30-44 minutes of total time is spent on the date of the encounter.

**★99204** Office or other outpatient visit for the evaluation and management of a new patient, which requires a medically appropriate history and/or examination and moderate level of medical decision making. When using time for code selection, 45-59 minutes of total time is spent on the date of the encounter.

**★99205** Office or other outpatient visit for the evaluation and management of a new patient, which requires a medically appropriate history and/or examination and high level of medical decision making. When using time for code selection, 60-74 minutes of total time is spent on the date of the encounter.

## Explanation

Providers report these codes for new patients being seen in the doctor's office, a multispecialty group clinic, or other outpatient environment. All require a medically appropriate history and/or examination. Code selection is based on the level of medical decision making (MDM) or total time personally spent by the physician and/or other qualified health care professional(s) on the date of the encounter. Factors to be considered in MDM include the number and complexity of problems addressed during the encounter, amount and complexity of data requiring review and analysis, and the risk of complications and/or morbidity or mortality associated with patient management. The most basic service is represented by 99202, which entails straightforward MDM. If time is used for code selection, 15 to 29 minutes of total time is spent on the day of encounter. Report 99203 for a visit requiring a low level of MDM or 30 to 44 minutes of total time; 99204 for a visit requiring a moderate level of MDM or 45 to 59 minutes of total time; and 99205 for a visit requiring a high level of MDM or 60 to 74 minutes of total time.

## Coding Tips

These codes are used to report office or other outpatient services for a new patient. A medically appropriate history and physical examination, as determined by the treating provider, should be documented. The level of history and physical examination are no longer used when determining the level of service. Codes should be selected based upon the current CPT Medical Decision Making table. Alternately, time alone may be used to select the appropriate level of service. Total time for reporting these services includes face-to-face and non-face-to-face time personally spent by the physician or other qualified health care professional on the date of the encounter. For office or other outpatient services for an established patient, see 99211-99215. For observation care services, see 99217-99226. For patients admitted and discharged from observation or inpatient status on the same date, see 99234-99236. Telemedicine services may be reported by the performing provider by adding modifier 95 to these procedure codes and using the appropriate place of service. Services at the origination site are reported with HCPCS Level II code Q3014.

## Documentation Tips

Documentation should include the history and exam performed in addition to the medical decision making performed. When time is the determinant for code selection, total time should be documented. Medical necessity must be clearly stated and support the level of service reported.

## Reimbursement Tips

The place-of-service (POS) codes used for reporting these services are the same as those for a new patient: POS code 11 represents the clinician's office environment and POS code 22 represents the outpatient setting. When a separately identifiable E/M service is reported at the same time as another procedure or service, modifier 25 should be appended to the E/M service to indicate the service is distinct from the other service performed.

## ICD-10-CM Diagnostic Codes

The application of this code is too broad to adequately present ICD-10-CM diagnostic code links here. Refer to your ICD-10-CM book.

**AMA:** **99202** 2020,Sep,14; 2020,Sep,3; 2020,Oct,14; 2020,Nov,3; 2020,May,3; 2020,Jun,3; 2020,Jan,3; 2020,Feb,3; 2020,Dec,11; 2019,Oct,10; 2019,Jan,3; 2019,Feb,3; 2018,Sep,14; 2018,Mar,7; 2018,Jan,8; 2018,Apr,9; 2018,Apr,10; 2017,Jun,6; 2017,Jan,8; 2017,Aug,3; 2016,Sep,6; 2016,Mar,10; 2016,Jan,7; 2016,Jan,13; 2016,Dec,11; 2015,Oct,3; 2015,Jan,12; 2015,Jan,16; 2015,Dec,3 **99203** 2020,Sep,3; 2020,Sep,14; 2020,Oct,14; 2020,Nov,3; 2020,May,3; 2020,Jun,3; 2020,Jan,3; 2020,Feb,3; 2019,Oct,10; 2019,Jan,3; 2019,Feb,3; 2018,Sep,14; 2018,Mar,7; 2018,Jan,8; 2018,Apr,10; 2018,Apr,9; 2017,Jun,6; 2017,Jan,8; 2017,Aug,3; 2016,Sep,6; 2016,Mar,10; 2016,Jan,7; 2016,Jan,13; 2016,Dec,11; 2015,Oct,3; 2015,Jan,12; 2015,Jan,16; 2015,Dec,3 **99204** 2020,Sep,14; 2020,Sep,3; 2020,Oct,14; 2020,Nov,12; 2020,Nov,3; 2020,May,3; 2020,Jun,3; 2020,Jan,3; 2020,Feb,3; 2019,Oct,10; 2019,Jan,3; 2019,Feb,3; 2018,Sep,14; 2018,Mar,7; 2018,Jan,8; 2018,Apr,9; 2018,Apr,10; 2017,Jun,6; 2017,Jan,8; 2017,Aug,3; 2016,Sep,6; 2016,Mar,10; 2016,Jan,7; 2016,Jan,13; 2016,Dec,11; 2015,Oct,3; 2015,Jan,16; 2015,Jan,12; 2015,Dec,3 **99205** 2020,Sep,14; 2020,Sep,3; 2020,Oct,14; 2020,Nov,12; 2020,Nov,3; 2020,May,3; 2020,Jun,3; 2020,Jan,3; 2020,Feb,3; 2019,Oct,10; 2019,Jan,3; 2019,Feb,3; 2018,Sep,14; 2018,Mar,7; 2018,Jan,8; 2018,Apr,9; 2018,Apr,10; 2017,Jun,6; 2017,Jan,8; 2017,Aug,3; 2016,Sep,6; 2016,Mar,10; 2016,Jan,7; 2016,Jan,13; 2016,Dec,11; 2015,Oct,3; 2015,Jan,12; 2015,Jan,16; 2015,Dec,3

## Relative Value Units/Medicare Edits

| Non-Facility RVU | Work | PE | MP | Total |
|---|---|---|---|---|
| **99202** | 0.93 | 1.10 | 0.09 | 2.12 |
| **99203** | 1.60 | 1.51 | 0.15 | 3.26 |
| **99204** | 2.60 | 2.04 | 0.23 | 4.87 |
| **99205** | 3.50 | 2.62 | 0.31 | 6.43 |
| **Facility RVU** | **Work** | **PE** | **MP** | **Total** |
| **99202** | 0.93 | 0.41 | 0.09 | 1.43 |
| **99203** | 1.60 | 0.67 | 0.15 | 2.42 |
| **99204** | 2.60 | 1.11 | 0.23 | 3.94 |
| **99205** | 3.50 | 1.54 | 0.31 | 5.35 |

| | FUD | Status | MUE | Modifiers | | | | IOM Reference |
|---|---|---|---|---|---|---|---|---|
| **99202** | N/A | A | 1(2) | N/A | N/A | N/A | 80* | 100-04,11,40.1.3; 100-04,12,100.1.1; 100-04,12,190.3; 100-04,12,190.6; 100-04,12,190.6.1; 100-04,12,190.7; 100-04,12,230; 100-04,12,230.1; 100-04,12,230.2; 100-04,12,230.3; 100-04,12,30.6.10; 100-04,12,30.6.15.1; 100-04,12,30.6.4; 100-04,12,30.6.7; 100-04; 100-04,11,40.1.3; 100-04,12,190.3; 100-04,12,190.6; 100-04,12,190.6.1; 100-04,12,190.7; 100-04,12,230; 100-04,12,230.1; 100-04,12,230.2; 100-04,12,230.3; 100-04,12,30.6.10; 100-04,12,30.6.15.1; 100-04,12,30.6.4; 100-04,12,30.6.7; 100-04,12,40.3; 100-04,12 |
| **99203** | N/A | A | 1(2) | N/A | N/A | N/A | 80* | |
| **99204** | N/A | A | 1(2) | N/A | N/A | N/A | 80* | |
| **99205** | N/A | A | 1(2) | N/A | N/A | N/A | 80* | |

* with documentation

# 99211-99215

**▲★99211** Office or other outpatient visit for the evaluation and management of an established patient that may not require the presence of a physician or other qualified health care professional

**★99212** Office or other outpatient visit for the evaluation and management of an established patient, which requires a medically appropriate history and/or examination and straightforward medical decision making. When using time for code selection, 10-19 minutes of total time is spent on the date of the encounter.

**★99213** Office or other outpatient visit for the evaluation and management of an established patient, which requires a medically appropriate history and/or examination and low level of medical decision making. When using time for code selection, 20-29 minutes of total time is spent on the date of the encounter.

**★99214** Office or other outpatient visit for the evaluation and management of an established patient, which requires a medically appropriate history and/or examination and moderate level of medical decision making. When using time for code selection, 30-39 minutes of total time is spent on the date of the encounter.

**★99215** Office or other outpatient visit for the evaluation and management of an established patient, which requires a medically appropriate history and/or examination and high level of medical decision making. When using time for code selection, 40-54 minutes of total time is spent on the date of the encounter.

## Explanation

Providers report these codes for established patients being seen in the doctor's office, a multispecialty group clinic, or other outpatient environment. All require a medically appropriate history and/or examination excluding the most basic service represented by 99211 that describes an encounter that may not require the presence of a physician or other qualified health care professional. For the remainder of codes within this range, code selection is based on the level of medical decision making (MDM) or total time personally spent by the physician and/or other qualified health care professional(s) on the date of the encounter. Factors to be considered in MDM include the number and complexity of problems addressed during the encounter, amount and complexity of data requiring review and analysis, and the risk of complications and/or morbidity or mortality associated with patient management. Report 99212 for a visit that entails straightforward MDM. If time is used for code selection, 10 to 19 minutes of total time is spent on the day of encounter. Report 99213 for a visit requiring a low level of MDM or 20 to 29 minutes of total time; 99214 for a moderate level of MDM or 30 to 39 minutes of total time; and 99215 for a high level of MDM or 40 to 54 minutes of total time.

## Coding Tips

These codes are used to report office or other outpatient services for an established patient. A medically appropriate history and physical examination, as determined by the treating provider, should be documented. The level of history and physical examination are no longer used when determining the level of service. Codes should be selected based upon the current CPT Medical Decision Making table. Alternately, time alone may be used to select the appropriate level of service. Total time for reporting these services includes face-to-face and non-face-to-face time personally spent by the physician or other qualified health care professional on the date of the encounter. Code 99211 does not require the presence of a physician or other qualified health care professional. For office or other outpatient services for a new patient, see 99202-99205. For observation care services, see 99217-99226. For patients admitted and discharged from observation or inpatient status on the same date, see 99234-99236. Medicare has identified 99211 as a telehealth/telemedicine service. Commercial payers should be contacted regarding their coverage guidelines. Telemedicine services may be reported by the performing provider by adding modifier 95 to these procedure codes and using the appropriate place of service. Services at the origination site are reported with HCPCS Level II code Q3014.

## Documentation Tips

Documentation should include the history and exam performed in addition to the medical decision making performed. When time is the determinant for code selection, total time should be documented. Medical necessity must be clearly stated and support the level of service reported.

## Reimbursement Tips

The place-of-service (POS) codes used for reporting these services are the same as those for a new patient: POS code 11 represents the clinician's office environment and POS code 22 represents the outpatient setting. When a separately identifiable E/M service is reported at the same time as another procedure or service, modifier 25 should be appended to the E/M service to indicate the service is distinct from the other service performed.

## ICD-10-CM Diagnostic Codes

The application of this code is too broad to adequately present ICD-10-CM diagnostic code links here. Refer to your ICD-10-CM book.

**AMA:** **99211** 2020,Sep,14; 2020,Sep,3; 2020,Oct,14; 2020,Nov,3; 2020,Nov,12; 2020,May,3; 2020,Jun,3; 2020,Jan,3; 2020,Feb,3; 2019,Oct,10; 2019,Jan,3; 2019,Feb,3; 2018,Sep,14; 2018,Mar,7; 2018,Jan,8; 2018,Apr,10; 2018,Apr,9; 2017,Mar,10; 2017,Jun,6; 2017,Jan,8; 2017,Aug,3; 2016,Sep,6; 2016,Mar,10; 2016,Jan,7; 2016,Jan,13; 2016,Dec,11; 2015,Oct,3; 2015,Jan,12; 2015,Jan,16; 2015,Dec,3 **99212** 2020,Sep,14; 2020,Sep,3; 2020,Oct,14; 2020,Nov,3; 2020,May,3; 2020,Jun,3; 2020,Jan,3; 2020,Feb,3; 2019,Oct,10; 2019,Jan,3; 2019,Feb,3; 2018,Sep,14; 2018,Mar,7; 2018,Jan,8; 2018,Apr,9; 2018,Apr,10; 2017,Oct,5; 2017,Jun,6; 2017,Jan,8; 2017,Aug,3; 2016,Sep,6; 2016,Mar,10; 2016,Jan,13; 2016,Jan,7; 2016,Dec,11; 2015,Oct,3; 2015,Jan,12; 2015,Jan,16; 2015,Dec,3 **99213** 2020,Sep,14; 2020,Sep,3; 2020,Oct,14; 2020,Nov,3; 2020,May,3; 2020,Jun,3; 2020,Jan,3; 2020,Feb,3; 2019,Oct,10; 2019,Jan,3; 2019,Feb,3; 2018,Sep,14; 2018,Mar,7; 2018,Jan,8; 2018,Apr,10; 2018,Apr,9; 2017,Jun,6; 2017,Jan,8; 2017,Aug,3; 2016,Sep,6; 2016,Mar,10; 2016,Jan,7; 2016,Jan,13; 2016,Dec,11; 2015,Oct,3; 2015,Jan,12; 2015,Jan,16; 2015,Dec,3 **99214** 2020,Sep,14; 2020,Sep,3; 2020,Oct,14; 2020,Nov,3; 2020,Nov,12; 2020,May,3; 2020,Jun,3; 2020,Jan,3; 2020,Feb,3; 2019,Oct,10; 2019,Jan,3; 2019,Feb,3; 2018,Sep,14; 2018,Mar,7; 2018,Jan,8; 2018,Apr,10; 2018,Apr,9; 2017,Jun,6; 2017,Jan,8; 2017,Aug,3; 2016,Sep,6; 2016,Mar,10; 2016,Jan,7; 2016,Jan,13; 2016,Dec,11; 2015,Oct,3; 2015,Jan,16; 2015,Jan,12; 2015,Dec,3 **99215** 2020,Sep,3; 2020,Sep,14; 2020,Oct,14; 2020,Nov,3; 2020,Nov,12; 2020,May,3; 2020,Jun,3; 2020,Jan,3; 2020,Feb,3; 2019,Oct,10; 2019,Jan,3; 2019,Feb,3; 2018,Sep,14; 2018,Mar,7; 2018,Jan,8; 2018,Apr,9; 2018,Apr,10; 2017,Jun,6; 2017,Jan,8; 2017,Aug,3; 2016,Sep,6; 2016,Mar,10; 2016,Jan,7; 2016,Jan,13; 2016,Dec,11; 2015,Oct,3; 2015,Jan,12; 2015,Jan,16; 2015,Dec,3

## Relative Value Units/Medicare Edits

| Non-Facility RVU | Work | PE | MP | Total |
|---|---|---|---|---|
| **99211** | 0.18 | 0.47 | 0.01 | 0.66 |
| **99212** | 0.70 | 0.88 | 0.05 | 1.63 |
| **99213** | 1.30 | 1.25 | 0.10 | 2.65 |
| **99214** | 1.92 | 1.70 | 0.14 | 3.76 |
| **99215** | 2.80 | 2.24 | 0.21 | 5.25 |
| **Facility RVU** | **Work** | **PE** | **MP** | **Total** |
| **99211** | 0.18 | 0.07 | 0.01 | 0.26 |
| **99212** | 0.70 | 0.29 | 0.05 | 1.04 |
| **99213** | 1.30 | 0.55 | 0.10 | 1.95 |
| **99214** | 1.92 | 0.82 | 0.14 | 2.88 |
| **99215** | 2.80 | 1.23 | 0.21 | 4.24 |

| | FUD | Status | MUE | Modifiers | | | | IOM Reference |
|---|---|---|---|---|---|---|---|---|
| **99211** | N/A | A | 1(3) | N/A | N/A | N/A | 80* | 100-04,11,40.1.3; 100-04,12,100.1.1; 100-04,12,190.3; 100-04,12,190.6; 100-04,12,190.6.1; 100-04,12,190.7; 100-04,12,230; 100-04,12,230.1; 100-04,12,230.2; 100-04,12,230.3; 100-04,12,30.6.10; 100-04,12,30.6.15.1; 100-04,12,30.6.17; 100-04,12,30.6.4; 100-0; 100-04,11,40.1.3; 100-04,12,190.3; 100-04,12,190.6; 100-04,12,190.6.1; 100-04,12,190.7; 100-04,12,230; 100-04,12,230.1; 100-04,12,230.2; 100-04,12,230.3; 100-04,12,30.6.10; 100-04,12,30.6.15.1; 100-04,12,30.6.4; 100-04,12,30.6.7; 100-04,12,40.3; 100-04,12 |
| **99212** | N/A | A | 2(3) | N/A | N/A | N/A | 80* | |
| **99213** | N/A | A | 2(3) | N/A | N/A | N/A | 80* | |
| **99214** | N/A | A | 2(3) | N/A | N/A | N/A | 80* | |
| **99215** | N/A | A | 1(3) | N/A | N/A | N/A | 80* | |

* with documentation

# 99221-99223

**99221** Initial hospital care, per day, for the evaluation and management of a patient, which requires these 3 key components: A detailed or comprehensive history; A detailed or comprehensive examination; and Medical decision making that is straightforward or of low complexity. Counseling and/or coordination of care with other physicians, other qualified health care professionals, or agencies are provided consistent with the nature of the problem(s) and the patient's and/or family's needs. Usually, the problem(s) requiring admission are of low severity. Typically, 30 minutes are spent at the bedside and on the patient's hospital floor or unit.

**99222** Initial hospital care, per day, for the evaluation and management of a patient, which requires these 3 key components: A comprehensive history; A comprehensive examination; and Medical decision making of moderate complexity. Counseling and/or coordination of care with other physicians, other qualified health care professionals, or agencies are provided consistent with the nature of the problem(s) and the patient's and/or family's needs. Usually, the problem(s) requiring admission are of moderate severity. Typically, 50 minutes are spent at the bedside and on the patient's hospital floor or unit.

**99223** Initial hospital care, per day, for the evaluation and management of a patient, which requires these 3 key components: A comprehensive history; A comprehensive examination; and Medical decision making of high complexity. Counseling and/or coordination of care with other physicians, other qualified health care professionals, or agencies are provided consistent with the nature of the problem(s) and the patient's and/or family's needs. Usually, the problem(s) requiring admission are of high severity. Typically, 70 minutes are spent at the bedside and on the patient's hospital floor or unit.

## Explanation

Initial hospital inpatient service codes describe the first encounter with the patient by the admitting physician or qualified clinician. For initial encounters by a physician other than the admitting physician, see the initial inpatient consultation codes or subsequent inpatient care codes. When the patient is admitted to the hospital under inpatient status during the course of another encounter from a different site of service, such as the physician's office, a nursing home, or the emergency department, all of the E/M services rendered by the supervising clinician as part of the inpatient admission status are considered part of the initial inpatient care services when they are performed on the same day. The level of initial inpatient care reported by the clinician should incorporate the other services related to the hospital admission that were provided in any other sites of services as well as those provided in the actual inpatient setting. Codes are reported per day and do not differentiate between new or established patients. Under the initial inpatient care category, there are three levels represented by 99221, 99222, and 99223. All of these levels require all three key components, history, exam, and medical decision-making (MDM), to be documented. The lowest level of care within this category, 99221, requires a detailed or comprehensive history and exam as well as straightforward or low complexity medical decision-making with approximately 30 minutes time being spent at the patient's bedside and on the patient's floor or unit. For the mid-level and highest level initial inpatient care codes, a comprehensive history and examination are required. MDM is the differentiating factor for these two levels; for moderate complexity, report 99222 and for initial inpatient care requiring MDM of high complexity, report 99223. The clinician typically spends 50 (99222) to 70 (99223) minutes at the patient's bedside or on the unit accordingly. Note that these codes include services provided to patients in a "partial hospital" setting.

## Coding Tips

These codes are used to report initial hospital inpatient services. All three key components (history, exam, and medical decision making) must be met or exceeded for the level of service selected. Time may be used to select the level of service when counseling and coordination of care are documented as at least half of the floor/unit time spent with the patient. Evaluation and management services provided by the clinician leading up to the initiation of observation status or inpatient admission are part of the patient's initial hospital care when performed on the same date of service. Codes may be selected based upon the 1995 or the 1997 Evaluation and Management Guidelines. CPT guidelines indicate these services are reported only by the admitting/supervising provider; all other providers should report 99231-99233 or 99251-99255. Medicare and some payers may allow providers of different specialties to report initial hospital services and require the admitting/supervising provider to append modifier AI. For subsequent inpatient care, see 99231-99233. For discharge from an inpatient stay on a different date of service than the admission, see 99238-99239. For patients admitted and discharged from observation or inpatient status on the same date, see 99234-99236. Medicare has provisionally identified these codes as telehealth/telemedicine services. Current Medicare coverage guidelines should be reviewed. Commercial payers should be contacted regarding their coverage guidelines. Telemedicine services may be reported by the performing provider by adding modifier 95 to these procedure codes and using the appropriate place of service. Services at the origination site are reported with HCPCS Level II code Q3014.

## Reimbursement Tips

Medicare and some payers may require the admitting provider to append modifier AI. Report place-of-service code 21 for the inpatient setting.

## ICD-10-CM Diagnostic Codes

The application of this code is too broad to adequately present ICD-10-CM diagnostic code links here. Refer to your ICD-10-CM book.

**AMA:** **99221** 2020,Sep,3; 2020,Oct,14; 2018,Jan,8; 2018,Dec,8; 2018,Dec,8; 2017,Jun,6; 2017,Jan,8; 2017,Aug,3; 2016,Mar,10; 2016,Jan,13; 2016,Jan,7; 2016,Dec,11; 2015,Jul,3; 2015,Jan,16; 2015,Dec,3; 2015,Dec,18 **99222** 2020,Sep,3; 2020,Oct,14; 2018,Jan,8; 2018,Dec,8; 2018,Dec,8; 2017,Jun,6; 2017,Jan,8; 2017,Aug,3; 2016,Mar,10; 2016,Jan,7; 2016,Jan,13; 2016,Dec,11; 2015,Mar,3; 2015,Jul,3; 2015,Jan,16; 2015,Dec,3; 2015,Dec,18 **99223** 2020,Sep,3; 2020,Oct,14; 2018,Jan,8; 2018,Dec,8; 2018,Dec,8; 2017,Jun,6; 2017,Jan,8; 2017,Aug,3; 2016,Mar,10; 2016,Jan,13; 2016,Jan,7; 2016,Dec,11; 2015,Jul,3; 2015,Jan,16; 2015,Dec,18; 2015,Dec,3

## Relative Value Units/Medicare Edits

| Non-Facility RVU | Work | PE | MP | Total |
|---|---|---|---|---|
| **99221** | 1.92 | 0.78 | 0.20 | 2.90 |
| **99222** | 2.61 | 1.08 | 0.21 | 3.90 |
| **99223** | 3.86 | 1.60 | 0.28 | 5.74 |
| **Facility RVU** | **Work** | **PE** | **MP** | **Total** |
| **99221** | 1.92 | 0.78 | 0.20 | 2.90 |
| **99222** | 2.61 | 1.08 | 0.21 | 3.90 |
| **99223** | 3.86 | 1.60 | 0.28 | 5.74 |

| | FUD | Status | MUE | Modifiers | | | | IOM Reference |
|---|---|---|---|---|---|---|---|---|
| **99221** | N/A | A | 1(3) | N/A | N/A | N/A | 80* | 100-04,11,40.1.3; |
| **99222** | N/A | A | 1(3) | N/A | N/A | N/A | 80* | 100-04,12,100; |
| **99223** | N/A | A | 1(3) | N/A | N/A | N/A | 80* | 100-04,12,30.6.10; |
| | | | | | | | | 100-04,12,30.6.15.1; |
| | | | | | | | | 100-04,12,30.6.4; |
| | | | | | | | | 100-04,12,30.6.9; |
| | | | | | | | | 100-04,12,30.6.9; |
| | | | | | | | | 100-04,12,30.6.9; |
| | | | | | | | | 100-04,12,30.6.9.1; |
| | | | | | | | | 100-04,12,40.3; |
| | | | | | | | | 100-04,12,90.4.5; |
| | | | | | | | | 100-04,23,20.9.1.1; |
| | | | | | | | | 100-04,6,20.1.1.2; |
| | | | | | | | | 100-04,6,30.4.1; |

* with documentation

## Terms To Know

**inpatient.** Time period in which a patient is housed in a hospital or facility offering medical, surgical, and/or psychiatric services, usually without interruption.



# 99231-99233

**★99231** Subsequent hospital care, per day, for the evaluation and management of a patient, which requires at least 2 of these 3 key components: A problem focused interval history; A problem focused examination; Medical decision making that is straightforward or of low complexity. Counseling and/or coordination of care with other physicians, other qualified health care professionals, or agencies are provided consistent with the nature of the problem(s) and the patient's and/or family's needs. Usually, the patient is stable, recovering or improving. Typically, 15 minutes are spent at the bedside and on the patient's hospital floor or unit.

**★99232** Subsequent hospital care, per day, for the evaluation and management of a patient, which requires at least 2 of these 3 key components: An expanded problem focused interval history; An expanded problem focused examination; Medical decision making of moderate complexity. Counseling and/or coordination of care with other physicians, other qualified health care professionals, or agencies are provided consistent with the nature of the problem(s) and the patient's and/or family's needs. Usually, the patient is responding inadequately to therapy or has developed a minor complication. Typically, 25 minutes are spent at the bedside and on the patient's hospital floor or unit.

**★99233** Subsequent hospital care, per day, for the evaluation and management of a patient, which requires at least 2 of these 3 key components: A detailed interval history; A detailed examination; Medical decision making of high complexity. Counseling and/or coordination of care with other physicians, other qualified health care professionals, or agencies are provided consistent with the nature of the problem(s) and the patient's and/or family's needs. Usually, the patient is unstable or has developed a significant complication or a significant new problem. Typically, 35 minutes are spent at the bedside and on the patient's hospital floor or unit.

## Explanation

Subsequent hospital inpatient service codes describe visits that occur after the first encounter of the patient's inpatient hospital admission by the supervising physician or qualified clinician. Codes are reported per day and do not differentiate between new or established patients. Under the subsequent inpatient care category, there are three levels represented by 99231, 99232, and 99233. All of these levels require at least two out of the three key components—history, exam, and medical decision making—to be documented. The lowest level of care within this category, 99231, describes a problem-focused interval history as well as a problem-focused examination with straightforward or low complexity medical decision making and involves approximately 15 minutes of time by the provider at the patient's bedside or on the unit. For the mid-level subsequent inpatient care code, 99232, an expanded problem-focused history and examination are required with moderate medical decision making. Time associated with this level usually involves 25 minutes at the bedside or on the patient's floor. The third and highest level of subsequent inpatient care, 99233, requires a detailed history and exam as well as medical decision making of high complexity. For this level of care, the provider typically spends around 35 minutes with the patient or on the unit. All three levels of subsequent inpatient care involve the clinician reviewing the patient's medical record, results from diagnostic studies, as well as any changes to the patient's status such as physical condition, response to treatments, or changes in health history since the last assessment.

## Coding Tips

These codes are used to report subsequent hospital inpatient services. Two of the three key components (history, exam, and medical decision making) must be met or exceeded for the level of service selected. Time may be used to select the level of service when counseling and coordination of care are documented as at least half of the floor/unit time spent with the patient. Codes may be selected based upon the 1995 or the 1997 Evaluation and Management Guidelines. Subsequent inpatient care services include review of the medical record, including all diagnostic studies, as well as changes noted in the patient's condition and response to treatment since the last evaluation. For initial inpatient care, see 99221-99223. For discharge from an inpatient stay on a different date of service than the admission, see 99238-99239. For patients admitted and discharged from observation or inpatient status on the same date, see 99234-99236. Telemedicine services may be reported by the performing providér by adding modifier 95 to these procedure codes and using the appropriate place of service. Services at the origination site are reported with HCPCS Level II code Q3014.

## Documentation Tips

Medicare allows only the medically necessary portion of the visit. Even if a complete note is generated, only the necessary services for the condition of the patient at the time of the visit can be considered in determining the level of an E/M code. Medical necessity must be clearly stated and support the level of service reported.

## Reimbursement Tips

Report place-of-service code 21 for the inpatient setting.

## ICD-10-CM Diagnostic Codes

The application of this code is too broad to adequately present ICD-10-CM diagnostic code links here. Refer to your ICD-10-CM book.

**AMA: 99231** 2020,Sep,3; 2018,Jan,8; 2018,Dec,8; 2018,Dec,8; 2017,Jun,6; 2017,Jan,8; 2017,Aug,3; 2016,Jan,7; 2016,Jan,13; 2016,Dec,11; 2015,Jul,3; 2015,Jan,16; 2015,Dec,3 **99232** 2020,Sep,3; 2018,Jan,8; 2018,Dec,8; 2018,Dec,8; 2017,Jun,6; 2017,Jan,8; 2017,Aug,3; 2016,Oct,8; 2016,Jan,7; 2016,Jan,13; 2016,Dec,11; 2015,Jul,3; 2015,Jan,16; 2015,Dec,3 **99233** 2020,Sep,3; 2018,Jan,8; 2018,Dec,8; 2018,Dec,8; 2017,Jun,6; 2017,Jan,8; 2017,Aug,3; 2016,Oct,8; 2016,Jan,13; 2016,Jan,7; 2016,Dec,11; 2015,Jul,3; 2015,Jan,16; 2015,Dec,3

## Relative Value Units/Medicare Edits

| Non-Facility RVU | Work | PE | MP | Total |
|---|---|---|---|---|
| **99231** | 0.76 | 0.29 | 0.05 | 1.10 |
| **99232** | 1.39 | 0.57 | 0.10 | 2.06 |
| **99233** | 2.00 | 0.82 | 0.14 | 2.96 |
| **Facility RVU** | **Work** | **PE** | **MP** | **Total** |
| **99231** | 0.76 | 0.29 | 0.05 | 1.10 |
| **99232** | 1.39 | 0.57 | 0.10 | 2.06 |
| **99233** | 2.00 | 0.82 | 0.14 | 2.96 |

| | FUD | Status | MUE | Modifiers | | | | IOM Reference |
|---|---|---|---|---|---|---|---|---|
| **99231** | N/A | A | 1(3) | N/A | N/A | N/A | 80* | 100-04,11,40.1.3; 100-04,12,100; 100-04,12,190.3; 100-04,12,190.3.5; 100-04,12,190.6; 100-04,12,190.6.1; 100-04,12,190.7; 100-04,12,30.6.10; 100-04,12,30.6.15.1; 100-04,12,30.6.4; 100-04,12,30.6.9; 100-04,12,30.6.9; 100-04,12,30.6.9; 100-04,12,30.6.9.1; 1; 100-04,11,40.1.3; 100-04,12,100; 100-04,12,190.3; 100-04,12,190.3.5; 100-04,12,190.6; 100-04,12,190.6.1; 100-04,12,190.7; 100-04,12,30.6.10; 100-04,12,30.6.15.1; 100-04,12,30.6.4; 100-04,12,30.6.9; 100-04,12,30.6.9; 100-04,12,30.6.9; 100-04,12,30.6.9.2; 1 |
| **99232** | N/A | A | 1(3) | N/A | N/A | N/A | 80* | |
| **99233** | N/A | A | 1(3) | N/A | N/A | N/A | 80* | |

* with documentation

## Terms To Know

**subsequent care.** All evaluation and instructions for care rendered subsequent to the inpatient admission by the admitting provider and all other providers.

# 99238-99239

**99238** Hospital discharge day management; 30 minutes or less
**99239** more than 30 minutes

## Explanation

Hospital discharge services are time-based codes that, when reported, describe the amount of time spent by the qualified clinician during all final steps involved in the discharge of a patient from the hospital on a date that differs from the date of admission, including the last patient exam, discussing the hospital stay, instructions for ongoing care as it relates to all pertinent caregivers, as well as preparing the medical discharge records, prescriptions, and/or referrals as applicable. Time reported should be for the total duration of time spent by the provider even when the time spent on that date is not continuous. For a hospital discharge duration of 30 minutes or less, report 99238; for a duration of greater than 30 minutes, report 99239. There are no key components associated with these services.

## Coding Tips

These codes are used to report all discharge day services for the hospital inpatient, including patient examination, discharge and follow-up care instructions, and preparation of all medical records. These are time-based codes and time spent with the patient must be documented in the medical record. For observation discharge on a different date of service than the admission, see 99217. For patients admitted and discharged from observation or inpatient status on the same date, see 99234–99236. Medicare has provisionally identified these codes as telehealth/telemedicine services. Current Medicare coverage guidelines should be reviewed. Commercial payers should be contacted regarding their coverage guidelines. Telemedicine services may be reported by the performing provider by adding modifier 95 to these procedure codes and using the appropriate place of service. Services at the origination site are reported with HCPCS Level II code Q3014.

## Documentation Tips

Medicare allows only the medically necessary portion of the visit. Even if a complete note is generated, only the necessary services for the condition of the patient at the time of the visit can be considered in determining the level of an E/M code. Medical necessity must be clearly stated and support the level of service reported.

## Reimbursement Tips

Report place-of-service code 21 for the inpatient setting.

## ICD-10-CM Diagnostic Codes

The application of this code is too broad to adequately present ICD-10-CM diagnostic code links here. Refer to your ICD-10-CM book.

**AMA:** **99238** 2018,Jan,8; 2018,Dec,8; 2018,Dec,8; 2017,Jun,6; 2017,Jan,8; 2017,Aug,3; 2016,Jan,13; 2016,Dec,11; 2015,Jan,16 **99239** 2018,Jan,8; 2018,Dec,8; 2018,Dec,8; 2017,Jun,6; 2017,Jan,8; 2017,Aug,3; 2016,Jan,13; 2016,Dec,11; 2015,Jan,16

## Relative Value Units/Medicare Edits

| Non-Facility RVU | Work | PE | MP | Total |
|---|---|---|---|---|
| **99238** | 1.28 | 0.70 | 0.09 | 2.07 |
| **99239** | 1.90 | 1.02 | 0.13 | 3.05 |
| **Facility RVU** | **Work** | **PE** | **MP** | **Total** |
| **99238** | 1.28 | 0.70 | 0.09 | 2.07 |
| **99239** | 1.90 | 1.02 | 0.13 | 3.05 |

| | FUD | Status | MUE | Modifiers | | | | IOM Reference |
|---|---|---|---|---|---|---|---|---|
| **99238** | N/A | A | 1(3) | N/A | N/A | N/A | 80* | 100-04,11,40.1.3; 100-04,12,100; 100-04,12,30.6.4; 100-04,12,30.6.9; 100-04,12,30.6.9; 100-04,12,30.6.9; 100-04,12,30.6.9.1; 100-04,12,30.6.9.2; 100-04,12,30.6.9.2; 100-04,12,40.3; 100-04,12,90.4.5; 100-04,13,70.2; 100-04,23,20.9.1.1; 100-04,6,20.1.1.2; 1; 100-04,11,40.1.3; 100-04,12,100; 100-04,12,30.6.4; 100-04,12,30.6.9; 100-04,12,30.6.9; 100-04,12,30.6.9; 100-04,12,30.6.9.1; 100-04,12,30.6.9.2; 100-04,12,30.6.9.2; 100-04,12,40.3; 100-04,12,90.4.5; 100-04,23,20.9.1.1; 100-04,6,20.1.1.2; 100-04,6,30.4.1; |
| **99239** | N/A | A | 1(3) | N/A | N/A | N/A | 80* | |

* with documentation

## Terms To Know

**discharge date.** For medical facilities, the date the patient is formally released, expires, or is transferred. In other situations, the date that medical care or treatment ended.

# 99281-99285

**99281** Emergency department visit for the evaluation and management of a patient, which requires these 3 key components: A problem focused history; A problem focused examination; and Straightforward medical decision making. Counseling and/or coordination of care with other physicians, other qualified health care professionals, or agencies are provided consistent with the nature of the problem(s) and the patient's and/or family's needs. Usually, the presenting problem(s) are self limited or minor.

**99282** Emergency department visit for the evaluation and management of a patient, which requires these 3 key components: An expanded problem focused history; An expanded problem focused examination; and Medical decision making of low complexity. Counseling and/or coordination of care with other physicians, other qualified health care professionals, or agencies are provided consistent with the nature of the problem(s) and the patient's and/or family's needs. Usually, the presenting problem(s) are of low to moderate severity.

**99283** Emergency department visit for the evaluation and management of a patient, which requires these 3 key components: An expanded problem focused history; An expanded problem focused examination; and Medical decision making of moderate complexity. Counseling and/or coordination of care with other physicians, other qualified health care professionals, or agencies are provided consistent with the nature of the problem(s) and the patient's and/or family's needs. Usually, the presenting problem(s) are of moderate severity.

**99284** Emergency department visit for the evaluation and management of a patient, which requires these 3 key components: A detailed history; A detailed examination; and Medical decision making of moderate complexity. Counseling and/or coordination of care with other physicians, other qualified health care professionals, or agencies are provided consistent with the nature of the problem(s) and the patient's and/or family's needs. Usually, the presenting problem(s) are of high severity, and require urgent evaluation by the physician, or other qualified health care professionals but do not pose an immediate significant threat to life or physiologic function.

**99285** Emergency department visit for the evaluation and management of a patient, which requires these 3 key components within the constraints imposed by the urgency of the patient's clinical condition and/or mental status: A comprehensive history; A comprehensive examination; and Medical decision making of high complexity. Counseling and/or coordination of care with other physicians, other qualified health care professionals, or agencies are provided consistent with the nature of the problem(s) and the patient's and/or family's needs. Usually, the presenting problem(s) are of high severity and pose an immediate significant threat to life or physiologic function.

## Explanation

Emergency department services codes describe E/M services provided to patients in the emergency department (ED). ED codes are typically reported per day and do not differentiate between new or established patients. Under the emergency department services category, there are five levels represented by 99281-99285. All levels require the three key components (history, exam, and medical decision-making [MDM]) to be documented. The lowest level of care, 99281, requires a problem-focused history and exam with straightforward medical decision-making involving a minor or self-limiting complaint. Mid-level services describe an expanded problem-focused history and exam with MDM of low or moderate complexity as represented by 99282 and 99283, respectively. At these levels of service, the encounter typically addresses low to moderate severity health concerns. The last two levels of service in this category represent high-severity problems. Code 99284 describes a high-severity health concern that does not pose an immediate threat to life or physiologic function; a detailed history and exam in conjunction with moderate complexity MDM are required for reporting this level of service. The highest level of service, 99285, requires a comprehensive history and examination with high complexity MDM for high-severity health issues that pose an immediate threat to the life or physiologic function of the patient. Time is not listed as a component in the code descriptors for emergency department services as these types of services are provided based on the varying intensity of the patient's condition and may involve emergency providers caring for several patients over an extended period of time involving multiple encounters, making it difficult for the clinician to accurately detail the amount of time spent face-to-face with the patient.

## Coding Tips

These codes are used to report emergency department services for the new or established patient. All three key components (history, exam, and medical decision making) must be met or exceeded for the level of service selected. Time is not a factor when selecting this E/M service. An emergency department is typically described as an organized hospital-based facility available 24 hours a day, providing unscheduled episodic services to patients in need of urgent medical attention. For critical care services provided in the emergency department, see 99291-99292. For observation care services provided to a patient located in the emergency department, see 99217-99220. For patients admitted and discharged from observation or inpatient status on the same date, see 99234-99236. Report place of service code 23 for services provided in the hospital emergency room. Medicare has provisionally identified these codes as telehealth/telemedicine services. Current Medicare coverage guidelines should be reviewed. Commercial payers should be contacted regarding their coverage guidelines. Telemedicine services may be reported by the performing provider by adding modifier 95 to these procedure codes and using the appropriate place of service. Services at the origination site are reported with HCPCS Level II code Q3014.

## Documentation Tips

Medicare allows only the medically necessary portion of the visit. Even if a complete note is generated, only the necessary services for the condition of the patient at the time of the visit can be considered in determining the level of an E/M code. Medical necessity must be clearly stated and support the level of service reported.

## Reimbursement Tips

Report place-of-service code 23 for services provided in the hospital emergency room.

## ICD-10-CM Diagnostic Codes

The application of this code is too broad to adequately present ICD-10-CM diagnostic code links here. Refer to your ICD-10-CM book.

**AMA:** **99281** 2020,Oct,13; 2020,Jul,13; 2019,Jul,10; 2018,Jan,8; 2017,Jun,6; 2017,Jan,8; 2017,Aug,3; 2016,Jan,7; 2016,Jan,13; 2015,Jan,12; 2015,Jan,16 **99282** 2020,Oct,13; 2020,Jul,13; 2019,Jul,10; 2018,Jan,8; 2017,Jun,6; 2017,Jan,8; 2017,Aug,3; 2016,Jan,7; 2016,Jan,13; 2015,Jan,12; 2015,Jan,16 **99283** 2020,Oct,13; 2020,Jul,13; 2019,Jul,10; 2018,Jan,8; 2017,Jun,6; 2017,Jan,8; 2017,Aug,3; 2016,Jan,7; 2016,Jan,13; 2015,Jan,12; 2015,Jan,16 **99284** 2020,Oct,13; 2020,Jul,13; 2019,Jul,10; 2018,Jan,8; 2017,Jun,6; 2017,Jan,8; 2017,Aug,3; 2016,Jan,7; 2016,Jan,13; 2015,Jan,12; 2015,Jan,16 **99285** 2020,Oct,13; 2020,Jul,13; 2020,Jan,12; 2019,Jul,10; 2018,Jan,8; 2017,Jun,6; 2017,Jan,8; 2017,Aug,3; 2016,Jan,7; 2016,Jan,13; 2015,Jan,12; 2015,Jan,16

## Relative Value Units/Medicare Edits

| Non-Facility RVU | Work | PE | MP | Total |
|---|---|---|---|---|
| **99281** | 0.48 | 0.11 | 0.05 | 0.64 |
| **99282** | 0.93 | 0.21 | 0.10 | 1.24 |
| **99283** | 1.60 | 0.33 | 0.16 | 2.09 |
| **99284** | 2.74 | 0.54 | 0.27 | 3.55 |
| **99285** | 4.00 | 0.75 | 0.43 | 5.18 |
| **Facility RVU** | **Work** | **PE** | **MP** | **Total** |
| **99281** | 0.48 | 0.11 | 0.05 | 0.64 |
| **99282** | 0.93 | 0.21 | 0.10 | 1.24 |
| **99283** | 1.60 | 0.33 | 0.16 | 2.09 |
| **99284** | 2.74 | 0.54 | 0.27 | 3.55 |
| **99285** | 4.00 | 0.75 | 0.43 | 5.18 |

| | FUD | Status | MUE | Modifiers | | | | IOM Reference |
|---|---|---|---|---|---|---|---|---|
| **99281** | N/A | A | 1(3) | N/A | N/A | N/A | 80* | 100-04,11,40.1.3; 100-04,12,100; 100-04,12,30.6.11; 100-04,12,30.6.4; 100-04,12,30.6.9.1; 100-04,12,40.3; 100-04,12,90.4.5; 100-04,13,70.2; 100-04,23,20.9.1.1; 100-04,4,160; 100-04,4,290.5.3; 100-04,11,40.1.3; 100-04,12,100; 100-04,12,30.6.11; 100-04,12,30.6.4; 100-04,12,30.6.9.1; 100-04,12,40.3; 100-04,12,90.4.5; 100-04,13,70.2; 100-04,23,20.9.1.1; 100-04,4,160; 100-04,4,290.5.1; 100-04,4,290.5.3 |
| **99282** | N/A | A | 1(3) | N/A | N/A | N/A | 80* | |
| **99283** | N/A | A | 1(3) | N/A | N/A | N/A | 80* | |
| **99284** | N/A | A | 1(3) | N/A | N/A | N/A | 80* | |
| **99285** | N/A | A | 1(3) | N/A | N/A | N/A | 80* | |

* with documentation

CPT-E/M Services

# 12020-12021

**12020** Treatment of superficial wound dehiscence; simple closure
**12021** with packing

## Explanation

There has been a breakdown of the healing skin either before or after suture removal. The skin margins have opened. The dentist cleanses the wound with irrigation and antimicrobial solutions. The skin margins may be trimmed to initiate bleeding surfaces. Report 12020 if the wound is sutured in a single layer. Report 12021 if the wound is left open and packed with gauze strips due to the presence of infection. This allows infection to drain from the wound and the skin closure will be delayed until the infection is resolved.

## Coding Tips

For extensive or complicated secondary wound closure, see 13160. For wound closure by tissue adhesive(s) only, see HCPCS Level II code G0168. To report extensive debridement of soft tissue and/or bone, not associated with open fractures and/or dislocations, resulting from penetrating and/or blunt trauma, see 11042–11047. Surgical trays, A4550, are not separately reimbursed by Medicare; however, other third-party payers may cover them. Check with the specific payer to determine coverage. When the condition is the result of an accident, the dental insurer may require that the medical insurance be billed first. When covered by the medical insurance, the payer may require that the appropriate CPT code be reported on the CMS-1500 claim form.

## Documentation Tips

The following information should be documented on a tooth chart: treatment/location of caries, endodontic procedures, prosthetic services, preventive services, treatment of lesions and dental disease, or other special procedures. A tooth chart may also be used to identify structure and rationale of disease process, and the type of service performed on intraoral structures other than teeth.

## Reimbursement Tips

These procedures may be covered by medical insurances. When covered by medical insurance, the payer may require that the appropriate CPT code be reported on the CMS-1500 claim form.

## ICD-10-CM Diagnostic Codes

T81.31XA Disruption of external operation (surgical) wound, not elsewhere classified, initial encounter
T81.32XA Disruption of internal operation (surgical) wound, not elsewhere classified, initial encounter
T81.33XA Disruption of traumatic injury wound repair, initial encounter

**AMA:** **12020** 2019,Nov,3; 2018,Jan,8; 2017,Jan,8; 2016,Jan,13; 2015,Jan,16
**12021** 2019,Nov,3; 2018,Jan,8; 2017,Jan,8; 2016,Jan,13; 2015,Jan,16

## Relative Value Units/Medicare Edits

| Non-Facility RVU | Work | PE | MP | Total |
|---|---|---|---|---|
| **12020** | 2.67 | 5.82 | 0.43 | 8.92 |
| **12021** | 1.89 | 2.97 | 0.30 | 5.16 |
| **Facility RVU** | **Work** | **PE** | **MP** | **Total** |
| **12020** | 2.67 | 2.43 | 0.43 | 5.53 |
| **12021** | 1.89 | 1.91 | 0.30 | 4.10 |

| | FUD | Status | MUE | Modifiers | | | | IOM Reference |
|---|---|---|---|---|---|---|---|---|
| **12020** | 10 | A | 2(3) | N/A | 51 | N/A | 80 | 100-04,12,90.4.5 |
| **12021** | 10 | A | 3(3) | N/A | 51 | N/A | 80 | |

* with documentation

## Terms To Know

**dehiscence.** Complication of healing in which the surgical wound ruptures or bursts open, superficially or through multiple layers.

**infection.** Presence of microorganisms in body tissues that may result in cellular damage.

**irrigate.** Washing out, lavage.

**packing.** Material placed into a cavity or wound, such as gels, gauze, pads, and sponges.

CPT - Integumentary

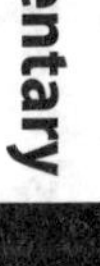

# 21031

**21031** Excision of torus mandibularis

## Explanation

The dentist removes a benign outgrowth of bone (torus mandibularis) most commonly from the lingual (tongue) side of the mandible. Using an intraoral approach, the dentist makes an incision in the mucosa overlying the outgrowth of bone and reflects the tissue. The excess bone is removed with a drill or osteotome. The mucosal incision is closed with sutures.

## Coding Tips

This code is used when the payer requires a CPT code to report the procedure. See also code D7473. This is a unilateral procedure. If performed bilaterally, some payers require that the service be reported twice with modifier 50 appended to the second code, while others require identification of the service only once with modifier 50 appended. Check with individual payers. Modifier 50 identifies a procedure performed identically on the opposite side of the body (mirror image). If specimen is transported to an outside laboratory, report 99000 for handling or conveyance. Payers may require that this service be reported using D7473 on the ADA dental claim form. Check with the payer to determine requirements. For excision of the maxillary torus palatinus, see code 21032 or D7472.

## Documentation Tips

The following information should be documented on a tooth chart: treatment/location of caries, endodontic procedures, prosthetic services, preventive services, treatment of lesions and dental disease, or other special procedures. A tooth chart may also be used to identify structure and rationale of disease process, and the type of service performed on intraoral structures other than teeth.

## Associated HCPCS Codes

D7473 removal of torus mandibularis

## ICD-10-CM Diagnostic Codes

M27.0 Developmental disorders of jaws

**AMA:** **21031** 2018,Sep,7

## Relative Value Units/Medicare Edits

| Non-Facility RVU | Work | PE | MP | Total |
|---|---|---|---|---|
| 21031 | 3.30 | 7.89 | 0.30 | 11.49 |
| **Facility RVU** | **Work** | **PE** | **MP** | **Total** |
| 21031 | 3.30 | 4.43 | 0.30 | 8.03 |

| | FUD | Status | MUE | Modifiers | | | | IOM Reference |
|---|---|---|---|---|---|---|---|---|
| 21031 | 90 | A | 2(3) | 50 | 51 | N/A | 80 | 100-04,12,90.4.5 |

* with documentation

## Terms To Know

**torus mandibularis.** Developmental disorder of the jaw with bony projection or overgrowth of normal bone usually found on the floor of the mouth under the tongue.

# 21032

**21032** Excision of maxillary torus palatinus

## Explanation

The dentist excises a torus palatinus (a bony protuberance), usually found at the junction of the intermaxillary and transverse palatine structures, by making an incision through the mucosa overlying the protuberance. The torus is exposed. Drills, osteotomes, or files are used to remove and contour the bone. The tissue is sutured directly over the bone. Some soft tissue may be excised prior to closure for adaptation over the newly contoured bone.

## Coding Tips

This procedure code is used when the payer requires the CPT code. See also D7472. This procedure includes the removal of tori, osseous tuberosities, and other osseous protuberances. If significant additional time and effort is documented, append modifier 22 and submit a cover letter and operative report. An excisional biopsy is not reported separately if a therapeutic excision is performed during the same surgical session. Local anesthesia is included in the service. If specimen is transported to an outside laboratory, report 99000 for handling or conveyance. Payers may require that this service be reported using D7472 on the ADA dental claim form. Check with the payer to determine their requirements. For biopsy only, see codes from range 20220-20245 or D7285.

## Documentation Tips

The following information should be documented on a tooth chart: treatment/location of caries, endodontic procedures, prosthetic services, preventive services, treatment of lesions and dental disease, or other special procedures. A tooth chart may also be used to identify structure and rationale of disease process, and the type of service performed on intraoral structures other than teeth.

## Associated HCPCS Codes

D7472 removal of torus palatinus

## ICD-10-CM Diagnostic Codes

M27.0 Developmental disorders of jaws

**AMA:** **21032** 2018,Sep,7

## Relative Value Units/Medicare Edits

| Non-Facility RVU | Work | PE | MP | Total |
|---|---|---|---|---|
| 21032 | 3.34 | 7.74 | 0.32 | 11.40 |
| **Facility RVU** | **Work** | **PE** | **MP** | **Total** |
| 21032 | 3.34 | 4.16 | 0.32 | 7.82 |

| | FUD | Status | MUE | Modifiers | | | | IOM Reference |
|---|---|---|---|---|---|---|---|---|
| 21032 | 90 | A | 1(3) | N/A | 51 | N/A | 80 | 100-04,12,90.4.5 |

* with documentation

## Terms To Know

**torus palatinus.** Developmental disorder of the jaw with bony overgrowth or projection found on the roof of the mouth (palate).

# 40804-40805

**40804** Removal of embedded foreign body, vestibule of mouth; simple
**40805** complicated

## Explanation

The dentist removes a foreign body embedded in the vestibule of the mouth. The vestibule consists of the mucosal and submucosal tissue of the lips and cheeks within the oral cavity, not including the dentoalveolar structures. The dentist may simply grasp the object with an instrument and remove it or incisions may be made to free the object and remove it. Complicated removal of a large foreign body or one that is difficult to access is done in 40805. Closure of the wound may be needed.

## Coding Tips

Drain placement and removal are not reported separately. Note that 40805 is used when removal of the embedded foreign body is complicated. If multiple foreign bodies are removed, report 40804 or 40805 for each incision site and append modifier 59 to additional codes. Local anesthesia is included in the service. If a specimen is transported to an outside laboratory, report 99000 for handling or conveyance. For removal of an embedded foreign body from dentoalveolar structures, soft tissue, see 41805; bone, see 41806.

## Documentation Tips

When multiple foreign bodies are documented, this may support the use of the complicated removal of embedded foreign body code (40804).

## Associated HCPCS Codes

| | |
|---|---|
| D7530 | removal of foreign body from mucosa, skin, or subcutaneous alveolar tissue |
| D7540 | removal of reaction producing foreign bodies, musculoskeletal system |

## ICD-10-CM Diagnostic Codes

| | |
|---|---|
| S00.552A | Superficial foreign body of oral cavity, initial encounter |
| S01.522A | Laceration with foreign body of oral cavity, initial encounter |
| S01.542A | Puncture wound with foreign body of oral cavity, initial encounter |
| T18.0XXA | Foreign body in mouth, initial encounter |

**AMA:** **40804** 2014,Jan,11 **40805** 2014,Jan,11

## Relative Value Units/Medicare Edits

| Non-Facility RVU | Work | PE | MP | Total |
|---|---|---|---|---|
| **40804** | 1.30 | 4.34 | 0.15 | 5.79 |
| **40805** | 2.79 | 5.54 | 0.25 | 8.58 |
| **Facility RVU** | **Work** | **PE** | **MP** | **Total** |
| **40804** | 1.30 | 1.89 | 0.15 | 3.34 |
| **40805** | 2.79 | 2.81 | 0.25 | 5.85 |

| | FUD | Status | MUE | Modifiers | | | | IOM Reference |
|---|---|---|---|---|---|---|---|---|
| **40804** | 10 | A | 1(3) | N/A | 51 | N/A | 80* | 100-04,12,90.4.5 |
| **40805** | 10 | A | 2(3) | N/A | 51 | N/A | 80* | |

* with documentation

# 40806

**40806** Incision of labial frenum (frenotomy)

## Explanation

The dentist performs a frenotomy by incising the labial frenum. The labial frenum is a connecting fold of mucous membrane that joins the lip to the gums at the inside midcenter. This procedure is often performed to release tension on the frenum and surrounding tissues. The frenum is simply incised and not removed.

## Coding Tips

When the labial frenum is attached close to the crest of the alveolar ridge, it can interfere with tooth eruption or wearing of an upper denture. Local anesthesia is included in this service. For excision of frenum (frenectomy), see 40819. Surgical trays (A4550) are not separately reimbursed by Medicare; however, other third-party payers may cover them. Check with the specific payer to determine coverage. See also codes D7961 and D7962. A frenotomy is often bundled into other more comprehensive dental services and, therefore, is not separately billable.

## Associated HCPCS Codes

| | |
|---|---|
| D7961 | buccal/labial frenectomy (frenulectomy) |
| D7962 | lingual frenectomy (frenulectomy) |

## ICD-10-CM Diagnostic Codes

| | |
|---|---|
| K13.0 | Diseases of lips |
| Q38.0 | Congenital malformations of lips, not elsewhere classified |
| Q38.1 | Ankyloglossia |

**AMA:** **40806** 2014,Jan,11

## Relative Value Units/Medicare Edits

| Non-Facility RVU | Work | PE | MP | Total |
|---|---|---|---|---|
| **40806** | 0.31 | 2.67 | 0.04 | 3.02 |
| **Facility RVU** | **Work** | **PE** | **MP** | **Total** |
| **40806** | 0.31 | 0.48 | 0.04 | 0.83 |

| | FUD | Status | MUE | Modifiers | | | | IOM Reference |
|---|---|---|---|---|---|---|---|---|
| **40806** | 0 | A | 2(2) | N/A | 51 | N/A | 80* | 100-04,12,90.4.5 |

* with documentation

## Terms To Know

**frenulectomy.** Excision of the labial, buccal, or lingual frenum.

# 40808

**40808** Biopsy, vestibule of mouth

## Explanation

The physician performs a biopsy on a lesion in the vestibule of the mouth. The vestibule consists of the mucosal and submucosal tissue of the lips and cheeks within the oral cavity, not including the dentoalveolar structures. The physician makes an incision in the area of the vestibule to be biopsied and removes a portion of the lesion and some surrounding tissue. The incision is closed simply.

## Coding Tips

This procedure is for a biopsy of the vestibule of the mouth. If an entire lesion is removed, use the appropriate excision code. If multiple areas are biopsied, report 40808 for each site taken and append modifier 51 to additional codes. Local anesthesia is included in this service. For excision of a lesion of the mucosa and submucosa, vestibule of mouth, see 40810–40812. For excision of lesions from the lips and mucous membranes, see 11440–11446. Payers may require that this service be reported using D7286 on the ADA dental claim form. Surgical trays (A4550) may be separately reimbursed by third-party payers. Check with the specific payer to determine coverage.

## Reimbursement Tips

Some payers may require that this service be reported using the appropriate CDT code.

## Associated HCPCS Codes

D7286 incisional biopsy of oral tissue-soft

## ICD-10-CM Diagnostic Codes

C06.1 Malignant neoplasm of vestibule of mouth
D10.39 Benign neoplasm of other parts of mouth
K12.1 Other forms of stomatitis
K12.2 Cellulitis and abscess of mouth
K12.39 Other oral mucositis (ulcerative)
K13.21 Leukoplakia of oral mucosa, including tongue
K13.24 Leukokeratosis nicotina palati
K13.29 Other disturbances of oral epithelium, including tongue
K13.4 Granuloma and granuloma-like lesions of oral mucosa
K13.5 Oral submucous fibrosis
K13.6 Irritative hyperplasia of oral mucosa
K13.79 Other lesions of oral mucosa

## AMA: **40808** 2019,Jan,9

## Relative Value Units/Medicare Edits

| Non-Facility RVU | Work | PE | MP | Total |
|---|---|---|---|---|
| 40808 | 1.05 | 3.81 | 0.13 | 4.99 |
| **Facility RVU** | **Work** | **PE** | **MP** | **Total** |
| 40808 | 1.05 | 1.36 | 0.13 | 2.54 |

| | FUD | Status | MUE | Modifiers | | | | IOM Reference |
|---|---|---|---|---|---|---|---|---|
| 40808 | 10 | A | 2(3) | N/A | 51 | N/A | 80 | 100-04,12,90.4.5 |

* with documentation

# 40810-40812

**40810** Excision of lesion of mucosa and submucosa, vestibule of mouth; without repair
**40812** with simple repair

## Explanation

The physician removes a lesion in the vestibule of the mouth. The vestibule consists of the mucosal and submucosal tissue of the lips and cheeks within the oral cavity, not including the dentoalveolar structures. The physician makes an incision around the lesion and through submucosal tissue, removing the lesion. No repair of the wound is done in 40810. Simple repair of the wound is done in 40812, such as a sutured closure.

## Coding Tips

If only a portion of the lesion is removed, report code 40808 for biopsy of the vestibule of the mouth. An excisional biopsy is not reported separately if a therapeutic excision is performed during the same surgical session. Local anesthesia is included in the service. Note that 40812 is identified when a lesion of the mucosa or submucosa, vestibule of mouth is excised with a simple repair. For the excision of a lesion of the vestibule of the mouth with complex repair, see 40814. To report an excision of a lesion of the mucosa and submucosa, vestibule of the mouth, complex, with an excision of the underlying muscle, see code 40816. For excision of lesions from the lips and mucous membranes, see codes 11440–11446. Surgical trays (A4550) may be separately reimbursed by third-party payers. Check with the specific payer to determine coverage.

## Documentation Tips

Documentation should include a copy of the pathology report. Examine the documentation to verify the type of repair required.

## Reimbursement Tips

Payers may require that this service be reported using the appropriate code from the D7410-D7414 range on the ADA dental claim form. Check with payers to determine their requirements. Local anesthesia is generally considered part of the procedure. These procedures may be covered by medical insurances. When covered by medical insurance, the payer may require that the appropriate CPT code be reported on the CMS-1500 claim form.

## Associated HCPCS Codes

D7410 excision of benign lesion up to 1.25 cm
D7411 excision of benign lesion greater than 1.25 cm
D7413 excision of malignant lesion up to 1.25 cm
D7414 excision of malignant lesion greater than 1.25 cm

## ICD-10-CM Diagnostic Codes

C06.1 Malignant neoplasm of vestibule of mouth
D10.39 Benign neoplasm of other parts of mouth
D37.09 Neoplasm of uncertain behavior of other specified sites of the oral cavity
K09.8 Other cysts of oral region, not elsewhere classified
K12.1 Other forms of stomatitis
K12.2 Cellulitis and abscess of mouth
K12.39 Other oral mucositis (ulcerative)
K13.21 Leukoplakia of oral mucosa, including tongue
K13.22 Minimal keratinized residual ridge mucosa
K13.23 Excessive keratinized residual ridge mucosa
K13.24 Leukokeratosis nicotina palati
K13.29 Other disturbances of oral epithelium, including tongue

K13.4 Granuloma and granuloma-like lesions of oral mucosa
K13.5 Oral submucous fibrosis
K13.6 Irritative hyperplasia of oral mucosa
K13.70 Unspecified lesions of oral mucosa
K13.79 Other lesions of oral mucosa

**AMA:** **40810** 2014,Jan,11 **40812** 2014,Jan,11

## Relative Value Units/Medicare Edits

| Non-Facility RVU | Work | PE | MP | Total |
|---|---|---|---|---|
| **40810** | 1.36 | 4.94 | 0.15 | 6.45 |
| **40812** | 2.37 | 5.96 | 0.25 | 8.58 |
| **Facility RVU** | **Work** | **PE** | **MP** | **Total** |
| **40810** | 1.36 | 2.06 | 0.15 | 3.57 |
| **40812** | 2.37 | 2.85 | 0.25 | 5.47 |

| | FUD | Status | MUE | Modifiers | | | | IOM Reference |
|---|---|---|---|---|---|---|---|---|
| **40810** | 10 | A | 2(3) | N/A | 51 | N/A | 80 | 100-04,12,90.4.5 |
| **40812** | 10 | A | 2(3) | N/A | 51 | N/A | 80 | |

* with documentation

## Terms To Know

**excision.** Surgical removal of an organ or tissue.

# 40819

**40819** Excision of frenum, labial or buccal (frenumectomy, frenulectomy, frenectomy)

## Explanation

The dentist removes the labial or buccal frenum. The buccal frenum is a band of mucosal membrane that connects the alveolar (dental) ridge to the cheek and separates the lip vestibule from the cheek vestibule. The labial frenum is a connecting fold of mucous membrane that joins the lip to the gums at the inside midcenter. Incisions are made around the frenum and through the mucosa and submucosa. The underlying muscle is removed as well. The excision may extend to the interincisal papilla. The mucosa is closed simply, or the dentist may rearrange the tissue as in a Z-plasty technique.

## Coding Tips

When the labial frenum is attached close to the crest of the alveolar ridge, it can interfere with tooth eruption or wearing of an upper denture. Local anesthesia is included in this service. For incision of the labial frenum (frenotomy), see 40806. For incision or excision of the lingual frenum, see 41010 or 41115, respectively. This service may also be reported using HCPCS Level II code D7961. This procedure is often included in a more comprehensive service and, therefore, should not be billed separately. Check with third-party payers for specific guidelines.

## Reimbursement Tips

Some payers may require that this service be reported using the appropriate CDT code.

## Associated HCPCS Codes

D7961 buccal/labial frenectomy (frenulectomy)

## ICD-10-CM Diagnostic Codes

K13.0 Diseases of lips
K13.79 Other lesions of oral mucosa
Q38.0 Congenital malformations of lips, not elsewhere classified
Q38.1 Ankyloglossia
Q38.6 Other congenital malformations of mouth

**AMA:** **40819** 2020,Aug,14

## Relative Value Units/Medicare Edits

| Non-Facility RVU | Work | PE | MP | Total |
|---|---|---|---|---|
| **40819** | 2.51 | 5.41 | 0.21 | 8.13 |
| **Facility RVU** | **Work** | **PE** | **MP** | **Total** |
| **40819** | 2.51 | 3.19 | 0.21 | 5.91 |

| | FUD | Status | MUE | Modifiers | | | | IOM Reference |
|---|---|---|---|---|---|---|---|---|
| **40819** | 90 | A | 2(2) | N/A | 51 | N/A | 80* | 100-04,12,90.4.5 |

* with documentation

## Terms To Know

**frenulectomy.** Excision of the labial, buccal, or lingual frenum.

**frenum.** Small, connected piece of skin or mucous membrane that serves to restrain, curb, or limit movement of the attached part.

**labial frenum.** Connecting fold of mucous membrane that joins the upper or lower lip to the gums at the inside midcenter.

# 40830-40831

**40830** Closure of laceration, vestibule of mouth; 2.5 cm or less
**40831** over 2.5 cm or complex

## Explanation

The physician sutures a laceration of the vestibule of the mouth measuring 2.5 cm or less in length. The physician performs a simple closure without submucosal sutures or tissue rearrangement in 40830. Extensive tissue damage or crushing, requiring complex closure, such as retention sutures, or the closure of a laceration more than 2.5 cm is done in 40831.

## Coding Tips

Local anesthesia is included in these services. For complex closure of a laceration, vestibule of mouth, see 40831. For vestibuloplasty, see 40840–40845. For repair of a laceration of lips and/or mucous membranes, simple, see 12011; intermediate, see 12051–12052. Surgical trays (A4550) are not separately reimbursed by Medicare; however, other third-party payers may cover them. Check with the specific payer to determine coverage. Payers may require that this service be reported using the appropriate code from range D7910–D7912 on the ADA dental claim form. Check with payers to determine their requirements.

## Reimbursement Tips

When 40830 or 40831 is performed with another separately identifiable procedure, the highest dollar value code is listed as the primary procedure and subsequent procedures are appended with modifier 51.

## Associated HCPCS Codes

| | |
|---|---|
| D7910 | suture of recent small wounds up to 5 cm |
| D7911 | complicated suture - up to 5 cm |
| D7912 | complicated suture - greater than 5 cm |

## ICD-10-CM Diagnostic Codes

| | |
|---|---|
| S01.511A | Laceration without foreign body of lip, initial encounter |
| S01.512A | Laceration without foreign body of oral cavity, initial encounter |
| S01.521A | Laceration with foreign body of lip, initial encounter |
| S01.522A | Laceration with foreign body of oral cavity, initial encounter |
| S01.551A | Open bite of lip, initial encounter |
| S01.552A | Open bite of oral cavity, initial encounter |

**AMA: 40830** 2014,Jan,11 **40831** 2014,Jan,11

## Relative Value Units/Medicare Edits

| Non-Facility RVU | Work | PE | MP | Total |
|---|---|---|---|---|
| 40830 | 1.82 | 6.27 | 0.31 | 8.40 |
| 40831 | 2.57 | 7.61 | 0.43 | 10.61 |
| **Facility RVU** | **Work** | **PE** | **MP** | **Total** |
| 40830 | 1.82 | 2.73 | 0.31 | 4.86 |
| 40831 | 2.57 | 3.70 | 0.43 | 6.70 |

| | FUD | Status | MUE | Modifiers | | | | IOM Reference |
|---|---|---|---|---|---|---|---|---|
| 40830 | 10 | A | 2(3) | N/A | 51 | N/A | 80* | 100-04,12,90.4.5 |
| 40831 | 10 | A | 2(3) | N/A | 51 | N/A | 80* | |

* with documentation

# 40840-40843

**40840** Vestibuloplasty; anterior
**40842** posterior, unilateral
**40843** posterior, bilateral

## Explanation

The dentist performs a vestibuloplasty and deepens the vestibule of the mouth by any series of surgical procedures for the purpose of increasing the height of the alveolar ridge, allowing a complete denture to be worn. The vestibule refers to the mucosal and submucosal tissue of the inner lips and cheeks, the part of the oral cavity outside of the dentoalveolar structures. This procedure may be performed in several ways. The dentist may rearrange the patient's own tissue or the submucosal tissue may be dissected and freed from the bone. The mucosa is moved deeper into the vestibule. Soft tissues may also be grafted into the mouth. An anterior procedure is performed in 40840; a one-sided procedure is done on the posterior portion of the mouth in 40842; and a posterior procedure is done on both sides of the mouth in 40843.

## Coding Tips

When 40840 is performed with another separately identifiable procedure, the highest dollar value code is listed as the primary procedure and subsequent procedures are appended with modifier 51. If significant additional time and effort is documented, append modifier 22 and submit a cover letter and operative report. Local anesthesia is included in the service. This service may also be reported using D7340. For vestibuloplasty of the entire arch, see 40844 or D7340; complex (including ridge extension, muscle repositioning), see 40845 or D7350.

## Reimbursement Tips

When the condition is the result of an accident, the dental insurer may require that the medical insurance be billed first. When covered by medical insurance, the payer may require that the appropriate CPT code be reported on the CMS-1500 claim form.

## Associated HCPCS Codes

| | |
|---|---|
| D7340 | vestibuloplasty - ridge extension (secondary epithelialization) |

## ICD-10-CM Diagnostic Codes

| | |
|---|---|
| K08.23 | Severe atrophy of the mandible |
| K08.26 | Severe atrophy of the maxilla |
| K08.51 | Open restoration margins of tooth |
| K08.81 | Primary occlusal trauma |
| K08.82 | Secondary occlusal trauma |
| K08.89 | Other specified disorders of teeth and supporting structures |
| M26.09 | Other specified anomalies of jaw size |
| M26.12 | Other jaw asymmetry |
| M26.19 | Other specified anomalies of jaw-cranial base relationship |
| M26.29 | Other anomalies of dental arch relationship |
| M26.50 | Dentofacial functional abnormalities, unspecified |
| M26.59 | Other dentofacial functional abnormalities |
| M26.79 | Other specified alveolar anomalies |
| M26.89 | Other dentofacial anomalies |
| Q38.6 | Other congenital malformations of mouth |
| S07.0XXA | Crushing injury of face, initial encounter |
| T20.29XA | Burn of second degree of multiple sites of head, face, and neck, initial encounter |
| T20.39XA | Burn of third degree of multiple sites of head, face, and neck, initial encounter |

T20.69XA Corrosion of second degree of multiple sites of head, face, and neck, initial encounter
T20.79XA Corrosion of third degree of multiple sites of head, face, and neck, initial encounter
T28.0XXA Burn of mouth and pharynx, initial encounter
Z42.8 Encounter for other plastic and reconstructive surgery following medical procedure or healed injury

**AMA:** **40840** 2014,Jan,11 **40842** 2014,Jan,11 **40843** 2014,Jan,11

## Relative Value Units/Medicare Edits

| Non-Facility RVU | Work | PE | MP | Total |
|---|---|---|---|---|
| **40840** | 9.15 | 14.67 | 1.30 | 25.12 |
| **40842** | 9.15 | 16.71 | 1.62 | 27.48 |
| **40843** | 12.79 | 20.49 | 2.26 | 35.54 |
| **Facility RVU** | **Work** | **PE** | **MP** | **Total** |
| **40840** | 9.15 | 7.87 | 1.30 | 18.32 |
| **40842** | 9.15 | 9.10 | 1.62 | 19.87 |
| **40843** | 12.79 | 10.59 | 2.26 | 25.64 |

| | FUD | Status | MUE | Modifiers | | | | IOM Reference |
|---|---|---|---|---|---|---|---|---|
| **40840** | 90 | R | 1(2) | N/A | 51 | N/A | N/A | 100-04,12,90.4.5 |
| **40842** | 90 | R | 1(2) | N/A | 51 | N/A | 80* | |
| **40843** | 90 | R | 1(2) | N/A | 51 | N/A | N/A | |

* with documentation

## Terms To Know

**vestibuloplasty.** Surgical procedure in which the vestibule of the mouth is deepened for the purpose of increasing the height of the alveolar ridge.

# 40844

**40844** Vestibuloplasty; entire arch

## Explanation

The dentist performs a vestibuloplasty and deepens the vestibule of the mouth by any series of surgical procedures for the purpose of increasing the height of the alveolar ridge, allowing a complete denture to be worn. The vestibule refers to the mucosal and submucosal tissue of the inner lips and cheeks, the part of the oral cavity outside of the dentoalveolar structures. This procedure may be performed in several ways. The dentist may rearrange the patient's own tissue or the submucosal tissue may be dissected and freed from the bone. The mucosa is moved deeper into the vestibule. Soft tissues may also be grafted into the mouth. Report 40844 when this procedure is done over the arch of the mouth.

## Coding Tips

When 40844 is performed with another separately identifiable procedure, the highest dollar value code is listed as the primary procedure and subsequent procedures are appended with modifier 51. If significant additional time and effort is documented, append modifier 22 and submit a cover letter and operative report. Local anesthesia is included in the service. For posterior vestibuloplasty, unilateral, see 40842; bilateral, see 40843. Some payers may require code D7340.

## Reimbursement Tips

If significant additional time and effort are documented, append modifier 22 and submit a cover letter and operative report.

## Associated HCPCS Codes

D7340 vestibuloplasty - ridge extension (secondary epithelialization)

## ICD-10-CM Diagnostic Codes

K08.23 Severe atrophy of the mandible
K08.26 Severe atrophy of the maxilla
K08.51 Open restoration margins of tooth
K08.81 Primary occlusal trauma
K08.82 Secondary occlusal trauma
K08.89 Other specified disorders of teeth and supporting structures
M26.09 Other specified anomalies of jaw size
M26.12 Other jaw asymmetry
M26.19 Other specified anomalies of jaw-cranial base relationship
M26.29 Other anomalies of dental arch relationship
M26.50 Dentofacial functional abnormalities, unspecified
M26.59 Other dentofacial functional abnormalities
M26.79 Other specified alveolar anomalies
M26.89 Other dentofacial anomalies
Q38.6 Other congenital malformations of mouth
S07.0XXA Crushing injury of face, initial encounter
T20.29XA Burn of second degree of multiple sites of head, face, and neck, initial encounter
T20.39XA Burn of third degree of multiple sites of head, face, and neck, initial encounter
T20.69XA Corrosion of second degree of multiple sites of head, face, and neck, initial encounter
T20.79XA Corrosion of third degree of multiple sites of head, face, and neck, initial encounter
T28.0XXA Burn of mouth and pharynx, initial encounter

| | |
|---|---|
| Z42.8 | Encounter for other plastic and reconstructive surgery following medical procedure or healed injury |

**AMA:** **40844** 2014,Jan,11

## Relative Value Units/Medicare Edits

| Non-Facility RVU | Work | PE | MP | Total |
|---|---|---|---|---|
| **40844** | 16.80 | 24.69 | 2.97 | 44.46 |
| **Facility RVU** | **Work** | **PE** | **MP** | **Total** |
| **40844** | 16.80 | 14.82 | 2.97 | 34.59 |

| | FUD | Status | MUE | Modifiers | | | | IOM Reference |
|---|---|---|---|---|---|---|---|---|
| **40844** | 90 | R | 1(2) | N/A | 51 | N/A | N/A | 100-04,12,90.4.5 |

* with documentation

## Terms To Know

**vestibuloplasty.** Surgical procedure in which the vestibule of the mouth is deepened for the purpose of increasing the height of the alveolar ridge.

# 40845

**40845** Vestibuloplasty; complex (including ridge extension, muscle repositioning)

## Explanation

The dentist performs a vestibuloplasty and deepens the vestibule of the mouth by any series of surgical procedures for the purpose of increasing the height of the alveolar ridge, allowing a complete denture to be worn. The vestibule refers to the mucosal and submucosal tissue of the inner lips and cheeks, the part of the oral cavity outside of the dentoalveolar structures. This procedure is performed for complex cases, such as those in which the physician must lower muscle attachments to provide enough space for deepening the vestibule. Soft tissue grafting from other areas of the body into the mouth is often required. Hypertrophied and hyperplastic tissue may need to be trimmed and soft tissue revised by dissecting it from the alveolar ridge and rearranging its attachment.

## Coding Tips

Some payers may require that this procedure be reported using D7350. When 40845 is performed with another separately identifiable procedure, the highest dollar value code is listed as the primary procedure and subsequent procedures are appended with modifier 51. If significant additional time and effort is documented, append modifier 22 and submit a cover letter and operative report. Report any free grafts or flaps separately, see 15004, 15120, and 15240. Local anesthesia is included in the service. For anterior vestibuloplasty, see 40840. For posterior vestibuloplasty, unilateral, see 40842; bilateral, see 40843. For vestibuloplasty of the entire arch, see 40844.

## Reimbursement Tips

Some payers may require that this procedure be reported using code D7350. If significant additional time and effort are documented, append modifier 22 and submit a cover letter and operative report.

## Associated HCPCS Codes

| | |
|---|---|
| D7350 | vestibuloplasty - ridge extension (including soft tissue grafts, muscle reattachment, revision of soft tissue attachment and management of hypertrophied and hyperplastic tissue) |

## ICD-10-CM Diagnostic Codes

| | |
|---|---|
| K08.23 | Severe atrophy of the mandible |
| K08.26 | Severe atrophy of the maxilla |
| K08.51 | Open restoration margins of tooth |
| M26.09 | Other specified anomalies of jaw size |
| M26.12 | Other jaw asymmetry |
| M26.19 | Other specified anomalies of jaw-cranial base relationship |
| M26.29 | Other anomalies of dental arch relationship |
| M26.50 | Dentofacial functional abnormalities, unspecified |
| M26.59 | Other dentofacial functional abnormalities |
| M26.79 | Other specified alveolar anomalies |
| M26.89 | Other dentofacial anomalies |
| S01.411A | Laceration without foreign body of right cheek and temporomandibular area, initial encounter ☑ |
| S01.412A | Laceration without foreign body of left cheek and temporomandibular area, initial encounter ☑ |
| S01.511A | Laceration without foreign body of lip, initial encounter |
| S01.512A | Laceration without foreign body of oral cavity, initial encounter |
| S01.521A | Laceration with foreign body of lip, initial encounter |
| S01.522A | Laceration with foreign body of oral cavity, initial encounter |

| | |
|---|---|
| S01.531A | Puncture wound without foreign body of lip, initial encounter |
| S01.532A | Puncture wound without foreign body of oral cavity, initial encounter |
| S01.541A | Puncture wound with foreign body of lip, initial encounter |
| S01.542A | Puncture wound with foreign body of oral cavity, initial encounter |
| S01.551A | Open bite of lip, initial encounter |
| S01.552A | Open bite of oral cavity, initial encounter |
| S07.0XXA | Crushing injury of face, initial encounter |
| T20.29XA | Burn of second degree of multiple sites of head, face, and neck, initial encounter |
| T20.39XA | Burn of third degree of multiple sites of head, face, and neck, initial encounter |
| T20.69XA | Corrosion of second degree of multiple sites of head, face, and neck, initial encounter |
| T20.79XA | Corrosion of third degree of multiple sites of head, face, and neck, initial encounter |
| T28.0XXA | Burn of mouth and pharynx, initial encounter |
| Z42.8 | Encounter for other plastic and reconstructive surgery following medical procedure or healed injury |

**AMA:** **40845** 2014,Jan,11

## Relative Value Units/Medicare Edits

| Non-Facility RVU | Work | PE | MP | Total |
|---|---|---|---|---|
| **40845** | 19.36 | 21.68 | 2.62 | 43.66 |
| **Facility RVU** | **Work** | **PE** | **MP** | **Total** |
| **40845** | 19.36 | 13.37 | 2.62 | 35.35 |

| | FUD | Status | MUE | Modifiers | | | | IOM Reference |
|---|---|---|---|---|---|---|---|---|
| **40845** | 90 | R | 1(3) | N/A | 51 | N/A | 80* | 100-04,12,90.4.5 |

* with documentation

# 41000-41007

**41000** Intraoral incision and drainage of abscess, cyst, or hematoma of tongue or floor of mouth; lingual

**41005** sublingual, superficial

**41006** sublingual, deep, supramylohyoid

**41007** submental space

## Explanation

The physician makes a small intraoral incision through the mucosa of the tongue or floor of the mouth overlying an abscess, cyst, or hematoma and drains the fluid. The incision and drainage site of the cyst, hematoma, or abscess is on the tongue (lingual) in 41000. In 41005, the lesion is located superficially under the tongue (sublingual) and in 41006, the sublingual lesion is deep to the supramylohyoid muscle. The physician dissects through the anterior floor of the mouth into the supramylohyoid muscle to drain an abscess in the submental space in 41007.

## Coding Tips

Local anesthesia is included in these services. For incision and drainage of a sublingual cyst, see 41005 or 41006. Payers may require that these services be reported using D7510 or D7511 on the ADA dental claim form. Check with payers to determine their requirements.

## Reimbursement Tips

When the condition is the result of an accident, the dental insurer may require that the medical insurance be billed first. When covered by medical insurance, the payer may require that the appropriate CPT code be reported on the CMS-1500 claim form.

## Associated HCPCS Codes

| | |
|---|---|
| D7510 | incision and drainage of abscess - intraoral soft tissue |
| D7511 | incision and drainage of abscess - intraoral soft tissue - complicated (includes drainage of multiple fascial spaces) |

## ICD-10-CM Diagnostic Codes

| | |
|---|---|
| K09.1 | Developmental (nonodontogenic) cysts of oral region |
| K09.8 | Other cysts of oral region, not elsewhere classified |
| K09.9 | Cyst of oral region, unspecified |
| K12.2 | Cellulitis and abscess of mouth |
| K13.29 | Other disturbances of oral epithelium, including tongue |
| K14.0 | Glossitis |
| K14.8 | Other diseases of tongue |
| K14.9 | Disease of tongue, unspecified |
| S00.532A | Contusion of oral cavity, initial encounter |

**AMA:** **41000** 2014,Jan,11 **41005** 2014,Jan,11 **41006** 2014,Jan,11 **41007** 2014,Jan,11

## Relative Value Units/Medicare Edits

| Non-Facility RVU | Work | PE | MP | Total |
|---|---|---|---|---|
| **41000** | 1.35 | 3.17 | 0.16 | 4.68 |
| **41005** | 1.31 | 5.07 | 0.13 | 6.51 |
| **41006** | 3.34 | 6.37 | 0.28 | 9.99 |
| **41007** | 3.20 | 6.35 | 0.26 | 9.81 |
| **Facility RVU** | **Work** | **PE** | **MP** | **Total** |
| **41000** | 1.35 | 1.66 | 0.16 | 3.17 |
| **41005** | 1.31 | 1.80 | 0.13 | 3.24 |
| **41006** | 3.34 | 3.06 | 0.28 | 6.68 |
| **41007** | 3.20 | 3.00 | 0.26 | 6.46 |

| | FUD | Status | MUE | Modifiers | | | | IOM Reference |
|---|---|---|---|---|---|---|---|---|
| **41000** | 10 | A | 1(3) | N/A | 51 | N/A | 80 | 100-04,12,90.4.5 |
| **41005** | 10 | A | 1(3) | N/A | 51 | N/A | 80* | |
| **41006** | 90 | A | 2(3) | N/A | 51 | N/A | 80* | |
| **41007** | 90 | A | 2(3) | N/A | 51 | N/A | 80* | |

* with documentation

## Terms To Know

**abscess.** Circumscribed collection of pus resulting from bacteria, frequently associated with swelling and other signs of inflammation.

**cellulitis.** Infection of the skin and subcutaneous tissues, most often caused by Staphylococcus or Streptococcus bacteria secondary to a cutaneous lesion. Progression of the inflammation may lead to abscess and tissue death, or even systemic infection-like bacteremia.

**cyst.** Elevated encapsulated mass containing fluid, semisolid, or solid material with a membranous lining.

**hematoma.** Tumor-like collection of blood in some part of the body caused by a break in a blood vessel wall, usually as a result of trauma.

**incision and drainage.** Cutting open body tissue for the removal of tissue fluids or infected discharge from a wound or cavity.

# 41008

**41008** Intraoral incision and drainage of abscess, cyst, or hematoma of tongue or floor of mouth; submandibular space

## Explanation

The dentist makes a small intraoral incision through the mucosa of the tongue or floor of the mouth overlying an abscess, cyst, or hematoma and drains the fluid. The dentist incises through the mucosa of the floor of the mouth to the supramylohyoid muscle and carries the dissection deeper into the tissue to reach the submandibular space. The abscess, hematoma, or cyst is opened with a surgical instrument and the fluid is drained. An artificial drain may be placed.

## Coding Tips

Placement and removal of drain are not reported separately. Local anesthesia is included in the service. Payers may require that this service be reported using D7510 or D7511 on the ADA dental claim form. Check with payers to determine their requirements.

## Associated HCPCS Codes

| | |
|---|---|
| D7510 | incision and drainage of abscess - intraoral soft tissue |
| D7511 | incision and drainage of abscess - intraoral soft tissue - complicated (includes drainage of multiple fascial spaces) |

## ICD-10-CM Diagnostic Codes

| | |
|---|---|
| K09.8 | Other cysts of oral region, not elsewhere classified |
| K12.2 | Cellulitis and abscess of mouth |
| K13.29 | Other disturbances of oral epithelium, including tongue |
| K14.0 | Glossitis |
| K14.8 | Other diseases of tongue |
| S00.532A | Contusion of oral cavity, initial encounter |

**AMA: 41008** 2014,Jan,11

## Relative Value Units/Medicare Edits

| Non-Facility RVU | Work | PE | MP | Total |
|---|---|---|---|---|
| **41008** | 3.46 | 7.83 | 0.38 | 11.67 |
| **Facility RVU** | **Work** | **PE** | **MP** | **Total** |
| **41008** | 3.46 | 3.69 | 0.38 | 7.53 |

| | FUD | Status | MUE | Modifiers | | | | IOM Reference |
|---|---|---|---|---|---|---|---|---|
| **41008** | 90 | A | 2(3) | N/A | 51 | N/A | 80* | 100-04,12,90.4.5 |

* with documentation

## Terms To Know

**abscess.** Circumscribed collection of pus resulting from bacteria, frequently associated with swelling and other signs of inflammation.

**incision and drainage.** Cutting open body tissue for the removal of tissue fluids or infected discharge from a wound or cavity.

# 41009

**41009** Intraoral incision and drainage of abscess, cyst, or hematoma of tongue or floor of mouth; masticator space

## Explanation

The dentist makes a small intraoral incision through the mucosa of the tongue or floor of the mouth overlying an abscess, cyst, or hematoma and drains the fluid. The dentist dissects down through the mucosa in the posterior floor of the mouth and into the masticator space, containing the ramus, the posterior part of the mandible, and the masticator muscles to drain the abscess. The abscess, hematoma, or cyst is opened with a surgical instrument and the fluid is drained. An artificial drain may be placed.

## Coding Tips

Placement and removal of drain are not reported separately. Local anesthesia is included in the service. Payers may require that this service be reported using D7510 or D7511 on the ADA dental claim form. Check with payers to determine their requirements. For extraoral approach, see code 41018.

## Reimbursement Tips

When the condition is the result of an accident, the dental insurer may require that the medical insurance be billed first. When covered by dental insurance, the payer may require that the appropriate CDT code be reported on the dental claim form.

## Associated HCPCS Codes

| | |
|---|---|
| D7510 | incision and drainage of abscess - intraoral soft tissue |
| D7511 | incision and drainage of abscess - intraoral soft tissue - complicated (includes drainage of multiple fascial spaces) |

## ICD-10-CM Diagnostic Codes

| | |
|---|---|
| K12.2 | Cellulitis and abscess of mouth |
| K13.29 | Other disturbances of oral epithelium, including tongue |
| K14.0 | Glossitis |
| K14.8 | Other diseases of tongue |

**AMA: 41009** 2014,Jan,11

## Relative Value Units/Medicare Edits

| Non-Facility RVU | Work | PE | MP | Total |
|---|---|---|---|---|
| 41009 | 3.71 | 8.42 | 0.37 | 12.50 |
| Facility RVU | Work | PE | MP | Total |
| 41009 | 3.71 | 4.18 | 0.37 | 8.26 |

| | FUD | Status | MUE | Modifiers | | | | IOM Reference |
|---|---|---|---|---|---|---|---|---|
| 41009 | 90 | A | 2(3) | N/A | 51 | N/A | 80* | 100-04,12,90.4.5 |

* with documentation

## Terms To Know

**incision and drainage.** Cutting open body tissue for the removal of tissue fluids or infected discharge from a wound or cavity.

# 41010

**41010** Incision of lingual frenum (frenotomy)

## Explanation

The dentist makes an incision in the lingual frenum, freeing the tongue and allowing greater range of motion. The lingual frenum is the connecting fold or membrane under the tongue that attaches it to the floor of the mouth. Sutures may be placed. The frenum is simply incised and not removed.

## Coding Tips

Suturing is not reported separately. Local anesthesia is included in the service. For frenoplasty, see 41520. For lingual frenectomy, see 41115. This procedure is often included in a more comprehensive service when performed during the same encounter and, therefore, is not billed separately. Check with third-party payers for their specific guidelines. See also codes D7961-D7962.

## Reimbursement Tips

When the condition is the result of an accident, the dental insurer may require that the medical insurance be billed first. When covered by medical insurance, the payer may require that the appropriate CPT code be reported on the CMS-1500 claim form.

## Associated HCPCS Codes

| | |
|---|---|
| D7961 | buccal/labial frenectomy (frenulectomy) |
| D7962 | lingual frenectomy (frenulectomy) |

## ICD-10-CM Diagnostic Codes

| | |
|---|---|
| F80.0 | Phonological disorder |
| F80.82 | Social pragmatic communication disorder |
| F80.89 | Other developmental disorders of speech and language |
| K14.0 | Glossitis |
| P92.2 | Slow feeding of newborn N |
| P92.3 | Underfeeding of newborn N |
| P92.4 | Overfeeding of newborn N |
| P92.5 | Neonatal difficulty in feeding at breast N |
| P92.8 | Other feeding problems of newborn N |
| Q38.1 | Ankyloglossia |
| Q38.3 | Other congenital malformations of tongue |
| R63.31 | Pediatric feeding disorder, acute P |
| R63.32 | Pediatric feeding disorder, chronic P |
| R63.39 | Other feeding difficulties |

**AMA: 41010** 2020,Aug,14; 2018,Jan,8; 2017,Sep,14; 2017,Nov,10

## Relative Value Units/Medicare Edits

| Non-Facility RVU | Work | PE | MP | Total |
|---|---|---|---|---|
| 41010 | 1.11 | 5.27 | 0.15 | 6.53 |
| Facility RVU | Work | PE | MP | Total |
| 41010 | 1.11 | 1.93 | 0.15 | 3.19 |

| | FUD | Status | MUE | Modifiers | | | | IOM Reference |
|---|---|---|---|---|---|---|---|---|
| 41010 | 10 | A | 1(2) | N/A | 51 | N/A | 80* | 100-04,12,90.4.5 |

* with documentation

# 41015-41016

**41015** Extraoral incision and drainage of abscess, cyst, or hematoma of floor of mouth; sublingual

**41016** submental

## Explanation

The dentist drains an abscess, a cyst, or a hematoma from the floor of the mouth by making an extraoral incision in the skin below the inferior border of the mandible and dissecting through the tissue to reach the affected space. In 41015, the dentist dissects through the supramylohyoid muscle and submental space into the sublingual space below the tongue to drain the abscess. In 41016, dissection is taken to the supramylohyoid muscle to drain an abscess in the submental space.

## Coding Tips

Placement and removal of drain are not reported separately. Local anesthesia is included in these services. Payers may require that these services be reported using D7520 or D7521 on the ADA dental claim form. Check with payers to determine their requirements.

## Documentation Tips

The infectious agent, if known, should be recorded in the medical record documentation. Documentation should note that the approach was through the skin below the location of the lesion.

## Reimbursement Tips

When the condition is the result of an accident, the dental insurer may require that the medical insurance be billed first. When covered by medical insurance, the payer may require that the appropriate CPT code be reported on the CMS-1500 claim form.

## Associated HCPCS Codes

| | |
|---|---|
| D7520 | incision and drainage of abscess - extraoral soft tissue |
| D7521 | incision and drainage of abscess - extraoral soft tissue - complicated (includes drainage of multiple fascial spaces) |

## ICD-10-CM Diagnostic Codes

| | |
|---|---|
| K09.1 | Developmental (nonodontogenic) cysts of oral region |
| K09.8 | Other cysts of oral region, not elsewhere classified |
| K09.9 | Cyst of oral region, unspecified |
| K12.2 | Cellulitis and abscess of mouth |
| K13.29 | Other disturbances of oral epithelium, including tongue |
| K14.0 | Glossitis |
| K14.8 | Other diseases of tongue |
| K14.9 | Disease of tongue, unspecified |

**AMA:** **41015** 2014,Jan,11 **41016** 2014,Jan,11

## Relative Value Units/Medicare Edits

| Non-Facility RVU | Work | PE | MP | Total |
|---|---|---|---|---|
| **41015** | 4.08 | 7.49 | 0.34 | 11.91 |
| **41016** | 4.19 | 9.34 | 0.45 | 13.98 |
| **Facility RVU** | **Work** | **PE** | **MP** | **Total** |
| **41015** | 4.08 | 4.44 | 0.34 | 8.86 |
| **41016** | 4.19 | 5.61 | 0.45 | 10.25 |

| | FUD | Status | MUE | Modifiers | | | | IOM Reference |
|---|---|---|---|---|---|---|---|---|
| **41015** | 90 | A | 2(3) | N/A | 51 | N/A | 80* | 100-04,12,90.4.5 |
| **41016** | 90 | A | 1(3) | N/A | 51 | N/A | 80* | |

* with documentation

## Terms To Know

**abscess.** Circumscribed collection of pus resulting from bacteria, frequently associated with swelling and other signs of inflammation.

**cyst.** Elevated encapsulated mass containing fluid, semisolid, or solid material with a membranous lining.

**glossitis.** Inflammation and swelling of the tongue that may be associated with infection, adverse drug reactions, smoking, or injury.

**hematoma.** Tumor-like collection of blood in some part of the body caused by a break in a blood vessel wall, usually as a result of trauma.

**incision and drainage.** Cutting open body tissue for the removal of tissue fluids or infected discharge from a wound or cavity.

CPT - Digestive

# 41017

**41017** Extraoral incision and drainage of abscess, cyst, or hematoma of floor of mouth; submandibular

## Explanation

The dentist drains an abscess, a cyst, or a hematoma from the floor of the mouth in the submandibular space. The dentist makes an incision under the angle of the mandible, or between the angle and the chin and below the inferior border of the mandible. Dissection is limited to the submandibular space. The fluid is then drained and an artificial drain may be placed. If placed, the drain is later removed.

## Coding Tips

Placement and removal of drain are not reported separately. Local anesthesia is included in the service. Payers may require that this service be reported using D7520 or D7521 on the ADA dental claim form. Check with payers to determine their requirements.

## Documentation Tips

The infectious agent, if known, should be documented in the medical record.

## Reimbursement Tips

Some payers may require that this service be reported using the appropriate CDT code.

## Associated HCPCS Codes

| | |
|---|---|
| D7520 | incision and drainage of abscess - extraoral soft tissue |
| D7521 | incision and drainage of abscess - extraoral soft tissue - complicated (includes drainage of multiple fascial spaces) |

## ICD-10-CM Diagnostic Codes

| | |
|---|---|
| K09.8 | Other cysts of oral region, not elsewhere classified |
| K12.2 | Cellulitis and abscess of mouth |
| K13.29 | Other disturbances of oral epithelium, including tongue |
| K14.0 | Glossitis |
| K14.8 | Other diseases of tongue |

**AMA:** **41017** 2014,Jan,11

## Relative Value Units/Medicare Edits

| Non-Facility RVU | Work | PE | MP | Total |
|---|---|---|---|---|
| **41017** | 4.19 | 9.24 | 0.43 | 13.86 |
| **Facility RVU** | **Work** | **PE** | **MP** | **Total** |
| **41017** | 4.19 | 5.53 | 0.43 | 10.15 |

| | FUD | Status | MUE | Modifiers | | | | IOM Reference |
|---|---|---|---|---|---|---|---|---|
| **41017** | 90 | A | 2(3) | N/A | 51 | N/A | 80* | 100-04,12,90.4.5 |

* with documentation

## Terms To Know

**dissection.** Separating by cutting tissue or body structures apart.

**incision and drainage.** Cutting open body tissue for the removal of tissue fluids or infected discharge from a wound or cavity.

# 41018

**41018** Extraoral incision and drainage of abscess, cyst, or hematoma of floor of mouth; masticator space

## Explanation

The dentist drains an abscess, a cyst, or a hematoma from the floor of the mouth by making an extraoral incision in the skin below the inferior border of the mandible and dissecting up through the tissue to reach the affected space. An incision is made just below the angle of the ramus of the mandible, the posterior part of the mandible, and into the masticator space containing the masticator muscles to drain the abscess, cyst, or hematoma. A drain may be placed to facilitate healing, which is later removed.

## Coding Tips

Placement and removal of drain are not reported separately. Local anesthesia is included in the service. Payers may require that this service be reported using D7520 or D7521 on the ADA dental claim form. Check with payers to determine their requirements.

## Documentation Tips

The infectious agent, if known, should be documented in the medical record.

## Reimbursement Tips

When the condition is the result of an accident, the dental insurer may require that the medical insurance be billed first. When covered by medical insurance, the payer may require that the appropriate CPT code be reported on the CMS-1500 claim form.

## Associated HCPCS Codes

| | |
|---|---|
| D7520 | incision and drainage of abscess - extraoral soft tissue |
| D7521 | incision and drainage of abscess - extraoral soft tissue - complicated (includes drainage of multiple fascial spaces) |

## ICD-10-CM Diagnostic Codes

| | |
|---|---|
| K09.8 | Other cysts of oral region, not elsewhere classified |
| K12.2 | Cellulitis and abscess of mouth |
| K13.29 | Other disturbances of oral epithelium, including tongue |
| K14.0 | Glossitis |
| K14.8 | Other diseases of tongue |

**AMA:** **41018** 2014,Jan,11

## Relative Value Units/Medicare Edits

| Non-Facility RVU | Work | PE | MP | Total |
|---|---|---|---|---|
| **41018** | 5.22 | 9.72 | 0.52 | 15.46 |
| **Facility RVU** | **Work** | **PE** | **MP** | **Total** |
| **41018** | 5.22 | 5.98 | 0.52 | 11.72 |

| | FUD | Status | MUE | Modifiers | | | | IOM Reference |
|---|---|---|---|---|---|---|---|---|
| **41018** | 90 | A | 2(3) | N/A | 51 | N/A | 80* | 100-04,12,90.4.5 |

* with documentation

# 41115

**41115** Excision of lingual frenum (frenectomy)

## Explanation

The dentist removes a tight or short lingual frenum to free the tongue and allow greater range of motion. The lingual frenum is the connecting fold or membrane under the tongue that attaches it to the floor of the mouth. The dentist makes incisions in the frenum both near the tongue and near the mandible, which ultimately connect as they move posteriorly. The frenum is excised. The surgical wound may be sutured.

## Coding Tips

This procedure differs from 41010 in that the frenum is removed (excised) rather than just cut (incised). Suturing is not reported separately. Local anesthesia is included in the service. This service is often included in a more comprehensive service when performed at the same time and, therefore, is not separately billable. Check with third-party payers for their specific guidelines. See also code D7962.

## Associated HCPCS Codes

D7962 lingual frenectomy (frenulectomy)

## ICD-10-CM Diagnostic Codes

F80.0 Phonological disorder
F80.82 Social pragmatic communication disorder
F80.89 Other developmental disorders of speech and language
K14.0 Glossitis
K14.6 Glossodynia
P92.2 Slow feeding of newborn N
P92.3 Underfeeding of newborn N
P92.4 Overfeeding of newborn N
P92.5 Neonatal difficulty in feeding at breast N
P92.8 Other feeding problems of newborn N
Q38.1 Ankyloglossia
Q38.3 Other congenital malformations of tongue
R63.31 Pediatric feeding disorder, acute P
R63.32 Pediatric feeding disorder, chronic P
R63.39 Other feeding difficulties

**AMA: 41115** 2018,Jan,8; 2017,Sep,14; 2017,Nov,10

## Relative Value Units/Medicare Edits

| Non-Facility RVU | Work | PE | MP | Total |
|---|---|---|---|---|
| 41115 | 1.79 | 5.79 | 0.25 | 7.83 |
| **Facility RVU** | **Work** | **PE** | **MP** | **Total** |
| 41115 | 1.79 | 2.23 | 0.25 | 4.27 |

| | FUD | Status | MUE | Modifiers | | | | IOM Reference |
|---|---|---|---|---|---|---|---|---|
| 41115 | 10 | A | 1(2) | N/A | 51 | N/A | 80* | 100-04,12,90.4.5 |

* with documentation

# 41520

**41520** Frenoplasty (surgical revision of frenum, eg, with Z-plasty)

## Explanation

The dentist performs a frenoplasty and surgically alters the frenum by rearranging the tissue, usually with a Z-plasty technique. The lingual frenum is the connecting fold or membrane under the tongue that attaches it to the floor of the mouth. An incision in the shape of a "Z" is made through the frenum and the tissues are reapproximated in a different position and sutured.

## Coding Tips

Some payers may require that this service be reported using D7963. When performed at the time of other, more comprehensive services the frenuloplasty is considered to be an integral part of the more comprehensive service and not separately billable. Check with third-party payers for their specific guidelines. Local anesthesia is included in the service. For frenotomy, see 40806 and 41010 or D7960.

## Reimbursement Tips

When performed at the time of other, more comprehensive services, the frenuloplasty is considered to be an integral part of the more comprehensive service and not separately billable. Check with third-party payers for specific guidelines.

## Associated HCPCS Codes

D7963 frenuloplasty

## ICD-10-CM Diagnostic Codes

K14.0 Glossitis
K14.6 Glossodynia
P92.2 Slow feeding of newborn N
P92.3 Underfeeding of newborn N
P92.4 Overfeeding of newborn N
P92.5 Neonatal difficulty in feeding at breast N
P92.8 Other feeding problems of newborn N
Q38.1 Ankyloglossia
Q38.3 Other congenital malformations of tongue
R63.31 Pediatric feeding disorder, acute P
R63.32 Pediatric feeding disorder, chronic P
R63.39 Other feeding difficulties

**AMA: 41520** 2020,Aug,14; 2018,Jan,8; 2017,Sep,14; 2017,Nov,10

## Relative Value Units/Medicare Edits

| Non-Facility RVU | Work | PE | MP | Total |
|---|---|---|---|---|
| 41520 | 2.83 | 7.63 | 0.39 | 10.85 |
| **Facility RVU** | **Work** | **PE** | **MP** | **Total** |
| 41520 | 2.83 | 4.08 | 0.39 | 7.30 |

| | FUD | Status | MUE | Modifiers | | | | IOM Reference |
|---|---|---|---|---|---|---|---|---|
| 41520 | 90 | A | 1(3) | N/A | 51 | N/A | 80* | 100-04,12,90.4.5 |

* with documentation

# 41820

**41820** Gingivectomy, excision gingiva, each quadrant

## Explanation

The dentist excises or trims hypertrophic (overgrown) gingiva to normal contours. The dentist excises the overgrown gingiva using a scalpel, electrocautery, or a laser. Periodontal dressing or packing is often placed. Use this code for each quadrant of the mouth where gingivectomy is performed.

## Coding Tips

Excision of gingiva from the second, third, or fourth quadrant of the dentition may be reported separately. When 41820 is performed with another separately identifiable procedure, the highest dollar value code is listed as the primary procedure and subsequent procedures are appended with modifier 51. Local anesthesia is included in the service. For gingivoplasty, each quadrant, see code 41872 or codes from range D4210-D4211.

## Documentation Tips

The following information should be documented on a tooth chart: treatment/location of caries, endodontic procedures, prosthetic services, preventive services, treatment of lesions and dental disease, or other special procedures. A tooth chart may also be used to identify structure and rationale of disease process, and the type of service performed on intraoral structures other than teeth.

## Reimbursement Tips

Most payers require that dentists report this procedure using the appropriate ADA code on the dental claim form.

## Associated HCPCS Codes

D4210 gingivectomy or gingivoplasty - four or more contiguous teeth or tooth bounded spaces per quadrant

D4211 gingivectomy or gingivoplasty - one to three contiguous teeth or tooth bounded spaces per quadrant

## ICD-10-CM Diagnostic Codes

C03.1 Malignant neoplasm of lower gum
D00.03 Carcinoma in situ of gingiva and edentulous alveolar ridge
K00.5 Hereditary disturbances in tooth structure, not elsewhere classified
K04.5 Chronic apical periodontitis
K04.6 Periapical abscess with sinus
K04.7 Periapical abscess without sinus
K04.8 Radicular cyst
K04.99 Other diseases of pulp and periapical tissues
K05.00 Acute gingivitis, plaque induced
K05.01 Acute gingivitis, non-plaque induced
K05.10 Chronic gingivitis, plaque induced
K05.11 Chronic gingivitis, non-plaque induced
K05.211 Aggressive periodontitis, localized, slight
K05.212 Aggressive periodontitis, localized, moderate
K05.213 Aggressive periodontitis, localized, severe
K05.221 Aggressive periodontitis, generalized, slight
K05.222 Aggressive periodontitis, generalized, moderate
K05.223 Aggressive periodontitis, generalized, severe
K05.311 Chronic periodontitis, localized, slight
K05.312 Chronic periodontitis, localized, moderate
K05.313 Chronic periodontitis, localized, severe
K05.321 Chronic periodontitis, generalized, slight
K05.322 Chronic periodontitis, generalized, moderate
K05.323 Chronic periodontitis, generalized, severe
K05.5 Other periodontal diseases
K06.011 Localized gingival recession, minimal
K06.012 Localized gingival recession, moderate
K06.013 Localized gingival recession, severe
K06.021 Generalized gingival recession, minimal
K06.022 Generalized gingival recession, moderate
K06.023 Generalized gingival recession, severe
K06.1 Gingival enlargement
K06.2 Gingival and edentulous alveolar ridge lesions associated with trauma
K06.3 Horizontal alveolar bone loss
K06.8 Other specified disorders of gingiva and edentulous alveolar ridge
K08.3 Retained dental root
K08.81 Primary occlusal trauma
K08.82 Secondary occlusal trauma
K08.89 Other specified disorders of teeth and supporting structures
M26.29 Other anomalies of dental arch relationship
M26.31 Crowding of fully erupted teeth
M26.32 Excessive spacing of fully erupted teeth
M26.33 Horizontal displacement of fully erupted tooth or teeth
M26.34 Vertical displacement of fully erupted tooth or teeth
M26.35 Rotation of fully erupted tooth or teeth
M26.36 Insufficient interocclusal distance of fully erupted teeth (ridge)
M26.37 Excessive interocclusal distance of fully erupted teeth
M26.39 Other anomalies of tooth position of fully erupted tooth or teeth
M26.59 Other dentofacial functional abnormalities
M26.79 Other specified alveolar anomalies
M26.89 Other dentofacial anomalies
S02.5XXA Fracture of tooth (traumatic), initial encounter for closed fracture
S02.5XXB Fracture of tooth (traumatic), initial encounter for open fracture
Z18.32 Retained tooth

**AMA:** **41820** 2014,Jan,11

## Relative Value Units/Medicare Edits

| Non-Facility RVU | Work | PE | MP | Total |
|---|---|---|---|---|
| **41820** | 0.00 | 0.00 | 0.00 | 0.00 |
| **Facility RVU** | **Work** | **PE** | **MP** | **Total** |
| **41820** | 0.00 | 0.00 | 0.00 | 0.00 |

| | FUD | Status | MUE | Modifiers | | | | IOM Reference |
|---|---|---|---|---|---|---|---|---|
| **41820** | 0 | R | 4(2) | N/A | 51 | N/A | 80* | 100-04,12,90.4.5 |

* with documentation

## Terms To Know

**gingivectomy.** Surgical excision or trimming of overgrown gum tissue back to normal contours using a scalpel, electrocautery, or a laser.

# 41821

**41821** Operculectomy, excision pericoronal tissues

## Explanation

The dentist removes a small piece of gingiva from the back or top of a tooth. A scalpel, a laser, or electrocautery is used to excise the tissue and establish normal gingival contours around the tooth. A periodontal dressing may be applied.

## Coding Tips

Some third-party payers may require that this service be reported using D7971. When 41821 is performed with another separately identifiable procedure, the highest dollar value code is listed as the primary procedure and subsequent procedures are appended with modifier 51. Local anesthesia is included in the service. For excision of a lesion or tumor, other than those procedures listed in 41820–41823, see 41825–41827. For destruction of a lesion (except excision), dentoalveolar structures, see 41850.

## Documentation Tips

The following information should be documented on a tooth chart: treatment/location of caries, endodontic procedures, prosthetic services, preventive services, treatment of lesions and dental disease, or other special procedures. A tooth chart may also be used to identify structure and rationale of disease process, and the type of service performed on intraoral structures other than teeth.

## Reimbursement Tips

Most third-party payers require that dentists report this procedure using the appropriate ADA code on the dental claim form.

## Associated HCPCS Codes

D7971 excision of pericoronal gingiva

## ICD-10-CM Diagnostic Codes

| | |
|---|---|
| K00.4 | Disturbances in tooth formation |
| K00.5 | Hereditary disturbances in tooth structure, not elsewhere classified |
| K00.6 | Disturbances in tooth eruption |
| K00.8 | Other disorders of tooth development |
| K01.0 | Embedded teeth |
| K01.1 | Impacted teeth |
| K03.5 | Ankylosis of teeth |
| K05.5 | Other periodontal diseases |
| K06.3 | Horizontal alveolar bone loss |
| K06.8 | Other specified disorders of gingiva and edentulous alveolar ridge |
| K08.81 | Primary occlusal trauma |
| K08.82 | Secondary occlusal trauma |
| K08.89 | Other specified disorders of teeth and supporting structures |
| M26.29 | Other anomalies of dental arch relationship |
| M26.31 | Crowding of fully erupted teeth |
| Z18.32 | Retained tooth |

**AMA: 41821** 2014,Jan,11

## Relative Value Units/Medicare Edits

| Non-Facility RVU | Work | PE | MP | Total |
|---|---|---|---|---|
| 41821 | 0.00 | 0.00 | 0.00 | 0.00 |
| **Facility RVU** | **Work** | **PE** | **MP** | **Total** |
| 41821 | 0.00 | 0.00 | 0.00 | 0.00 |

| | FUD | Status | MUE | Modifiers | | | | IOM Reference |
|---|---|---|---|---|---|---|---|---|
| 41821 | 0 | R | 2(3) | N/A | 51 | N/A | 80* | 100-04,12,90.4.5 |

* with documentation

## Terms To Know

**coronal.** Relating to the top of a tooth or the crown of the head.

**gingiva.** Soft tissues surrounding the crowns of unerupted teeth and necks of erupted teeth.

**hypertrophy.** Overgrowth or enlargement of normal cells in tissue.

**leukoplakia.** Thickened white patches or lesions appearing on a mucous membrane, such as oral mucosa or tongue.

**periodontal.** Relating to the tissues that support and surround the teeth.

# 41822

**41822** Excision of fibrous tuberosities, dentoalveolar structures

## Explanation

The dentist excises fibrous soft tissue overlying the tuberosities of dentoalveolar structures, reducing the size of the tuberosity. The dentist makes wedged or elliptically shaped incisions through the soft tissue of the tuberosity. The tissue is removed and the surgical wound is sutured directly.

## Coding Tips

This procedure includes the removal of overlying soft tissue and sufficient bone to provide an acceptable tissue contour. Local anesthesia is included in the service. Third-party payers may require that this service be reported using D7972. Additionally, payers may bundle this service into gingivectomy or other osseous surgical procedures.

## Documentation Tips

The following information should be documented on a tooth chart: treatment/location of caries, endodontic procedures, prosthetic services, preventive services, treatment of lesions and dental disease, or other special procedures. A tooth chart may also be used to identify structure and rationale of disease process, and the type of service performed on intraoral structures other than teeth.

## Reimbursement Tips

Most third-party payers require that dentists report this procedure using the appropriate ADA code on the dental claim form.

## Associated HCPCS Codes

D7972 surgical reduction of fibrous tuberosity

## ICD-10-CM Diagnostic Codes

K00.4 Disturbances in tooth formation
K00.5 Hereditary disturbances in tooth structure, not elsewhere classified
K00.6 Disturbances in tooth eruption
K00.8 Other disorders of tooth development
K01.0 Embedded teeth
K01.1 Impacted teeth
K05.00 Acute gingivitis, plaque induced
K05.01 Acute gingivitis, non-plaque induced
K05.10 Chronic gingivitis, plaque induced
K05.11 Chronic gingivitis, non-plaque induced
K05.211 Aggressive periodontitis, localized, slight
K05.212 Aggressive periodontitis, localized, moderate
K05.213 Aggressive periodontitis, localized, severe
K05.221 Aggressive periodontitis, generalized, slight
K05.222 Aggressive periodontitis, generalized, moderate
K05.223 Aggressive periodontitis, generalized, severe
K05.311 Chronic periodontitis, localized, slight
K05.312 Chronic periodontitis, localized, moderate
K05.313 Chronic periodontitis, localized, severe
K05.321 Chronic periodontitis, generalized, slight
K05.322 Chronic periodontitis, generalized, moderate
K05.323 Chronic periodontitis, generalized, severe
K05.4 Periodontosis
K05.5 Other periodontal diseases
K06.1 Gingival enlargement
K06.2 Gingival and edentulous alveolar ridge lesions associated with trauma
K06.8 Other specified disorders of gingiva and edentulous alveolar ridge
K08.81 Primary occlusal trauma
K08.82 Secondary occlusal trauma
K08.89 Other specified disorders of teeth and supporting structures
M26.07 Excessive tuberosity of jaw
M26.79 Other specified alveolar anomalies
M26.89 Other dentofacial anomalies
M27.8 Other specified diseases of jaws

**AMA:** **41822** 2014,Jan,11

## Relative Value Units/Medicare Edits

| Non-Facility RVU | Work | PE | MP | Total |
|---|---|---|---|---|
| **41822** | 2.41 | 7.75 | 0.43 | 10.59 |
| **Facility RVU** | **Work** | **PE** | **MP** | **Total** |
| **41822** | 2.41 | 3.00 | 0.43 | 5.84 |

| | FUD | Status | MUE | Modifiers | | | | IOM Reference |
|---|---|---|---|---|---|---|---|---|
| **41822** | 10 | R | 1(2) | N/A | 51 | N/A | 80* | 100-04,12,90.4.5 |

* with documentation

## Terms To Know

**anomaly.** Irregularity in the structure or position of an organ or tissue.

**gingivitis.** Inflamed gingiva (oral mucosa) that surrounds the teeth.

**incision.** Act of cutting into tissue or an organ.

**periodontitis.** Inflammation of the tissue structures supporting the teeth leading to a loss of connective tissue attachments.

**tubercle.** Small rough prominence or rounded nodule on a bone.

CPT - Digestive

# 41823

**41823** Excision of osseous tuberosities, dentoalveolar structures

## Explanation

The dentist removes the osseous tissue from the tuberosities of dentoalveolar structures, producing more favorable bone contours. The dentist makes an incision through the mucosa of the tuberosity and exposes the underlying bone. Drills, osteotomes, or files are used to remove and contour the bone. The tissue is sutured directly over the bone. Some soft tissue may be excised prior to closure for adaptation over the newly contoured bone.

## Coding Tips

This procedure includes the removal of tori, osseous tuberosities, and other osseous protuberances. The overlying soft tissue is reflected and sufficient bone is removed to provide an acceptable tissue contour. If there is a fibrous component to the tuberosity and simultaneous reduction of the fibrous portion is performed, the procedure is not reported separately. If significant additional time and effort is documented, append modifier 22 and submit a cover letter and operative report. Local anesthesia is included in the service. Some payers may require that this procedure be reported using either D7471 or D7485.

## Documentation Tips

The following information should be documented on a tooth chart: treatment/location of caries, endodontic procedures, prosthetic services, preventive services, treatment of lesions and dental disease, or other special procedures. A tooth chart may also be used to identify structure and rationale of disease process, and the type of service performed on intraoral structures other than teeth.

## Reimbursement Tips

Most third-party payers require that dentists report this procedure using the appropriate ADA code on the dental claim form.

## Associated HCPCS Codes

D7471 removal of lateral exostosis (maxilla or mandible)
D7485 reduction of osseous tuberosity

## ICD-10-CM Diagnostic Codes

K00.4 Disturbances in tooth formation
K00.5 Hereditary disturbances in tooth structure, not elsewhere classified
K00.6 Disturbances in tooth eruption
K00.8 Other disorders of tooth development
K01.0 Embedded teeth
K01.1 Impacted teeth
K05.211 Aggressive periodontitis, localized, slight
K05.212 Aggressive periodontitis, localized, moderate
K05.213 Aggressive periodontitis, localized, severe
K05.221 Aggressive periodontitis, generalized, slight
K05.222 Aggressive periodontitis, generalized, moderate
K05.223 Aggressive periodontitis, generalized, severe
K05.311 Chronic periodontitis, localized, slight
K05.312 Chronic periodontitis, localized, moderate
K05.313 Chronic periodontitis, localized, severe
K05.321 Chronic periodontitis, generalized, slight
K05.322 Chronic periodontitis, generalized, moderate
K05.323 Chronic periodontitis, generalized, severe
K05.4 Periodontosis
K05.5 Other periodontal diseases
K06.1 Gingival enlargement
K06.2 Gingival and edentulous alveolar ridge lesions associated with trauma
K06.3 Horizontal alveolar bone loss
K06.8 Other specified disorders of gingiva and edentulous alveolar ridge
K08.81 Primary occlusal trauma
K08.82 Secondary occlusal trauma
K08.89 Other specified disorders of teeth and supporting structures
K09.0 Developmental odontogenic cysts
M26.07 Excessive tuberosity of jaw
M26.71 Alveolar maxillary hyperplasia
M26.72 Alveolar mandibular hyperplasia
M26.79 Other specified alveolar anomalies
M26.89 Other dentofacial anomalies
M27.8 Other specified diseases of jaws

**AMA:** **41823** 2014,Jan,11

## Relative Value Units/Medicare Edits

| Non-Facility RVU | Work | PE | MP | Total |
|---|---|---|---|---|
| **41823** | 3.77 | 11.16 | 0.66 | 15.59 |
| **Facility RVU** | **Work** | **PE** | **MP** | **Total** |
| **41823** | 3.77 | 6.16 | 0.66 | 10.59 |

| | FUD | Status | MUE | Modifiers | | | | IOM Reference |
|---|---|---|---|---|---|---|---|---|
| **41823** | 90 | R | 1(2) | N/A | 51 | N/A | 80* | 100-04,12,90.4.5 |

* with documentation

## Terms To Know

**exostosis.** Abnormal formation of a benign bony growth.

**osseous.** Related to, consisting of, or resembling bone.

**osteotome.** Tool used for cutting bone.

**periodontitis.** Inflammation of the tissue structures supporting the teeth leading to a loss of connective tissue attachments.

**tubercle.** Small rough prominence or rounded nodule on a bone.

CPT - Digestive

# 41828

**41828** Excision of hyperplastic alveolar mucosa, each quadrant (specify)

## Explanation

The dentist excises hyperplastic or excessive mucosa from the alveolus. Incisions are made in the hyperplastic tissue, separating it from the normal mucosa. The excessive tissue is removed. The resultant defect may be directly sutured or left to heal without suturing. With large amounts of excess tissue, more than one surgical session may be required to eliminate all of the tissue. Use this code for each specified quadrant excised.

## Coding Tips

Each session required to complete the procedure and tissue grafts is reported separately. Specify the quadrant where the procedure was performed. When 41828 is performed with another separately identifiable procedure, the highest dollar value code is listed as the primary procedure and subsequent procedures are appended with modifier 51. If significant additional time and effort is documented, append modifier 22 and submit a cover letter and operative report. An excisional biopsy is not reported separately if a therapeutic excision is performed during the same surgical session. Local anesthesia is included in the service. Some payers may require that this service be reported using D7970. Check with payers for their specific guidelines.

## Documentation Tips

The following information should be documented on a tooth chart: treatment/location of caries, endodontic procedures, prosthetic services, preventive services, treatment of lesions and dental disease, or other special procedures. A tooth chart may also be used to identify structure and rationale of disease process, and the type of service performed on intraoral structures other than teeth.

## Reimbursement Tips

Most third-party payers require that dentists report this procedure using the appropriate ADA code on the dental claim form.

## Associated HCPCS Codes

D7970 excision of hyperplastic tissue - per arch

## ICD-10-CM Diagnostic Codes

K13.6 Irritative hyperplasia of oral mucosa

**AMA: 41828** 2014,Jan,11

## Relative Value Units/Medicare Edits

| Non-Facility RVU | Work | PE | MP | Total |
|---|---|---|---|---|
| 41828 | 3.14 | 6.83 | 0.56 | 10.53 |
| **Facility RVU** | **Work** | **PE** | **MP** | **Total** |
| 41828 | 3.14 | 2.82 | 0.56 | 6.52 |

| | FUD | Status | MUE | Modifiers | | | | IOM Reference |
|---|---|---|---|---|---|---|---|---|
| 41828 | 10 | R | 4(2) | N/A | 51 | N/A | 80* | 100-04,12,90.4.5 |

* with documentation

## Terms To Know

**alveolar process.** Bony part of the maxilla or mandible that supports the tooth roots and into which the teeth are implanted.

# 41870

**41870** Periodontal mucosal grafting

## Explanation

The dentist takes mucosa from one area of the mouth and grafts it around the teeth to repair areas of gingival recession. The dentist uses a scalpel to remove a small piece of mucosa, usually from the hard palate. After preparing the recipient site, the dentist sutures the graft in the area of gingival recession.

## Coding Tips

When 41870 is performed with another separately identifiable procedure, the highest dollar value code is listed as the primary procedure and subsequent procedures are appended with modifier 51. If significant additional time and effort is documented, append modifier 22 and submit a cover letter and operative report. Local anesthesia is included in the service. See 40818 for excision of the mucosa of the vestibule of the mouth as a donor graft. Soft tissue grafting may also be reported using D4270-D4273 and D4275-D4276.

## Documentation Tips

The following information should be documented on a tooth chart: treatment/location of caries, endodontic procedures, prosthetic services, preventive services, treatment of lesions and dental disease, or other special procedures. A tooth chart may also be used to identify structure and rationale of disease process, and the type of service performed on intraoral structures other than teeth.

## Reimbursement Tips

Most third-party payers require that dentists report this procedure using the appropriate ADA code on the dental claim form.

## Associated HCPCS Codes

D4270 pedicle soft tissue graft procedure

D4273 autogenous connective tissue graft procedure (including donor and recipient surgical sites) first tooth, implant, or edentulous tooth position in graft

D4275 non-autogenous connective tissue graft (including recipient site and donor material) first tooth, implant, or edentulous tooth position in graft

D4276 combined connective tissue and pedicle graft, per tooth

## ICD-10-CM Diagnostic Codes

K00.6 Disturbances in tooth eruption

K05.10 Chronic gingivitis, plaque induced

K05.11 Chronic gingivitis, non-plaque induced

K05.211 Aggressive periodontitis, localized, slight

K05.212 Aggressive periodontitis, localized, moderate

K05.213 Aggressive periodontitis, localized, severe

K05.221 Aggressive periodontitis, generalized, slight

K05.222 Aggressive periodontitis, generalized, moderate

K05.223 Aggressive periodontitis, generalized, severe

K05.311 Chronic periodontitis, localized, slight

K05.312 Chronic periodontitis, localized, moderate

K05.313 Chronic periodontitis, localized, severe

K05.321 Chronic periodontitis, generalized, slight

K05.322 Chronic periodontitis, generalized, moderate

K05.323 Chronic periodontitis, generalized, severe

K05.4 Periodontosis

K05.5 Other periodontal diseases

| | |
|---|---|
| K06.011 | Localized gingival recession, minimal |
| K06.012 | Localized gingival recession, moderate |
| K06.013 | Localized gingival recession, severe |
| K06.021 | Generalized gingival recession, minimal |
| K06.022 | Generalized gingival recession, moderate |
| K06.023 | Generalized gingival recession, severe |
| K06.1 | Gingival enlargement |
| K06.2 | Gingival and edentulous alveolar ridge lesions associated with trauma |
| K06.3 | Horizontal alveolar bone loss |
| K06.8 | Other specified disorders of gingiva and edentulous alveolar ridge |

**AMA:** **41870** 2014,Jan,11

## Relative Value Units/Medicare Edits

| Non-Facility RVU | Work | PE | MP | Total |
|---|---|---|---|---|
| **41870** | 0.00 | 0.00 | 0.00 | 0.00 |
| **Facility RVU** | **Work** | **PE** | **MP** | **Total** |
| **41870** | 0.00 | 0.00 | 0.00 | 0.00 |

| | FUD | Status | MUE | Modifiers | | | | IOM Reference |
|---|---|---|---|---|---|---|---|---|
| **41870** | 0 | R | 2(3) | N/A | 51 | N/A | 80* | 100-04,12,90.4.5 |

* with documentation

## Terms To Know

**allograft.** Graft from one individual to another of the same species.

**graft.** Tissue implant from another part of the body or another person.

**mucosa.** Moist tissue lining the mouth (buccal mucosa), stomach (gastric mucosa), intestines, and respiratory tract.

**pedicle graft.** Mass of flesh and skin partially excised from the donor location, retaining its blood supply through intact blood vessels, and grafted onto another site to repair adjacent or distant defects.

# 41872

**41872** Gingivoplasty, each quadrant (specify)

## Explanation

The dentist alters the contours of the gums by performing gingivoplasty. Areas of gingiva may be excised or incisions may be made through the gingiva to create a gingival flap. The flap may be sutured in a different position, trimmed, or both. Any incisions made are closed with sutures.

## Coding Tips

Gingivoplasty on the second, third, or fourth quadrant of the dentition may be reported separately. If gingivoplasty is completed, per quadrant, during separate sessions, report one quadrant per session. When 41872 is performed with another separately identifiable procedure, the highest dollar value code is listed as the primary procedure and subsequent procedures are appended with modifier 51. Local anesthesia is included in the service. For gingivectomy, each quadrant, see 41820 or D4210-D4211.

## Documentation Tips

The following information should be documented on a tooth chart: treatment/location of caries, endodontic procedures, prosthetic services, preventive services, treatment of lesions and dental disease, or other special procedures. A tooth chart may also be used to identify structure and rationale of disease process, and the type of service performed on intraoral structures other than teeth.

## Reimbursement Tips

Most third-party payers require that dentists report this procedure using the appropriate ADA code on the dental claim form.

## Associated HCPCS Codes

| | |
|---|---|
| D4210 | gingivectomy or gingivoplasty - four or more contiguous teeth or tooth bounded spaces per quadrant |
| D4211 | gingivectomy or gingivoplasty - one to three contiguous teeth or tooth bounded spaces per quadrant |
| D4212 | gingivectomy or gingivoplasty to allow access for restorative procedure, per tooth |

## ICD-10-CM Diagnostic Codes

| | |
|---|---|
| C03.0 | Malignant neoplasm of upper gum |
| C03.1 | Malignant neoplasm of lower gum |
| K00.6 | Disturbances in tooth eruption |
| K01.0 | Embedded teeth |
| K01.1 | Impacted teeth |
| K05.00 | Acute gingivitis, plaque induced |
| K05.01 | Acute gingivitis, non-plaque induced |
| K05.10 | Chronic gingivitis, plaque induced |
| K05.11 | Chronic gingivitis, non-plaque induced |
| K05.211 | Aggressive periodontitis, localized, slight |
| K05.212 | Aggressive periodontitis, localized, moderate |
| K05.213 | Aggressive periodontitis, localized, severe |
| K05.221 | Aggressive periodontitis, generalized, slight |
| K05.222 | Aggressive periodontitis, generalized, moderate |
| K05.223 | Aggressive periodontitis, generalized, severe |
| K05.311 | Chronic periodontitis, localized, slight |
| K05.312 | Chronic periodontitis, localized, moderate |
| K05.313 | Chronic periodontitis, localized, severe |
| K05.321 | Chronic periodontitis, generalized, slight |

| | |
|---|---|
| K05.322 | Chronic periodontitis, generalized, moderate |
| K05.323 | Chronic periodontitis, generalized, severe |
| K05.4 | Periodontosis |
| K05.5 | Other periodontal diseases |
| K06.011 | Localized gingival recession, minimal |
| K06.012 | Localized gingival recession, moderate |
| K06.013 | Localized gingival recession, severe |
| K06.021 | Generalized gingival recession, minimal |
| K06.022 | Generalized gingival recession, moderate |
| K06.023 | Generalized gingival recession, severe |
| K06.1 | Gingival enlargement |
| K06.2 | Gingival and edentulous alveolar ridge lesions associated with trauma |
| K06.3 | Horizontal alveolar bone loss |
| K06.8 | Other specified disorders of gingiva and edentulous alveolar ridge |
| K08.0 | Exfoliation of teeth due to systemic causes |
| K08.111 | Complete loss of teeth due to trauma, class I |
| K08.112 | Complete loss of teeth due to trauma, class II |
| K08.113 | Complete loss of teeth due to trauma, class III |
| K08.114 | Complete loss of teeth due to trauma, class IV |
| K08.121 | Complete loss of teeth due to periodontal diseases, class I |
| K08.122 | Complete loss of teeth due to periodontal diseases, class II |
| K08.123 | Complete loss of teeth due to periodontal diseases, class III |
| K08.124 | Complete loss of teeth due to periodontal diseases, class IV |
| K08.131 | Complete loss of teeth due to caries, class I |
| K08.132 | Complete loss of teeth due to caries, class II |
| K08.133 | Complete loss of teeth due to caries, class III |
| K08.134 | Complete loss of teeth due to caries, class IV |
| K08.191 | Complete loss of teeth due to other specified cause, class I |
| K08.192 | Complete loss of teeth due to other specified cause, class II |
| K08.193 | Complete loss of teeth due to other specified cause, class III |
| K08.194 | Complete loss of teeth due to other specified cause, class IV |
| K08.411 | Partial loss of teeth due to trauma, class I |
| K08.412 | Partial loss of teeth due to trauma, class II |
| K08.413 | Partial loss of teeth due to trauma, class III |
| K08.414 | Partial loss of teeth due to trauma, class IV |
| K08.421 | Partial loss of teeth due to periodontal diseases, class I |
| K08.422 | Partial loss of teeth due to periodontal diseases, class II |
| K08.423 | Partial loss of teeth due to periodontal diseases, class III |
| K08.424 | Partial loss of teeth due to periodontal diseases, class IV |
| K08.431 | Partial loss of teeth due to caries, class I |
| K08.432 | Partial loss of teeth due to caries, class II |
| K08.433 | Partial loss of teeth due to caries, class III |
| K08.434 | Partial loss of teeth due to caries, class IV |
| K08.491 | Partial loss of teeth due to other specified cause, class I |
| K08.492 | Partial loss of teeth due to other specified cause, class II |
| K08.493 | Partial loss of teeth due to other specified cause, class III |
| K08.494 | Partial loss of teeth due to other specified cause, class IV |
| M26.39 | Other anomalies of tooth position of fully erupted tooth or teeth |
| M26.72 | Alveolar mandibular hyperplasia |
| M26.74 | Alveolar mandibular hypoplasia |
| M26.79 | Other specified alveolar anomalies |
| M27.2 | Inflammatory conditions of jaws |
| M27.8 | Other specified diseases of jaws |
| M87.180 | Osteonecrosis due to drugs, jaw |
| S01.552A | Open bite of oral cavity, initial encounter |

**AMA: 41872** 2014,Jan,11

## Relative Value Units/Medicare Edits

| Non-Facility RVU | Work | PE | MP | Total |
|---|---|---|---|---|
| **41872** | 3.01 | 10.28 | 0.53 | 13.82 |
| **Facility RVU** | **Work** | **PE** | **MP** | **Total** |
| **41872** | 3.01 | 5.24 | 0.53 | 8.78 |

| | FUD | Status | MUE | Modifiers | | | | IOM Reference |
|---|---|---|---|---|---|---|---|---|
| **41872** | 90 | R | 4(2) | N/A | 51 | N/A | 80* | 100-04,12,90.4.5 |

* with documentation

## Terms To Know

**gingiva.** Soft tissues surrounding the crowns of unerupted teeth and necks of erupted teeth.

**gingivectomy.** Surgical excision or trimming of overgrown gum tissue back to normal contours using a scalpel, electrocautery, or a laser.

**gingivoplasty.** Repair or reconstruction of the gum tissue, altering the gingival contours by excising areas of gum tissue or making incisions through the gingiva to create a gingival flap.

CPT - Digestive

# 41874

**41874** Alveoloplasty, each quadrant (specify)

## Explanation

The dentist alters the contours of the alveolus by selectively performing alveoloplasty to remove sharp areas or undercuts of alveolar bone. The dentist makes incisions in the mucosa overlying the alveolus, exposing the alveolar bone. Drills, osteotomes, or files are used to contour the bone. The mucosa is sutured in place over the contoured bone.

## Coding Tips

Alveoloplasty on the second, third, or fourth quadrant may be reported separately. If gingivoplasty is completed per quadrant during separate sessions, report one quadrant per session. This procedure is for contouring of the alveolus in up to one-half of an upper or lower arch. When 41874 is performed with another separately identifiable procedure, the highest dollar value code is listed as the primary procedure and subsequent procedures are appended with modifier 51. Local anesthesia is included in this service. Alveoloplasty may also be reported using codes D7310, D7311, D7320, or D7321. For alveolectomy, see 41830. For closure of lacerations, see 40830 or 40831. For segmental osteotomy, see 21198.

## Documentation Tips

The following information should be documented on a tooth chart: treatment/location of caries, endodontic procedures, prosthetic services, preventive services, treatment of lesions and dental disease, or other special procedures. A tooth chart may also be used to identify structure and rationale of disease process and the type of service performed on intraoral structures other than teeth.

## Reimbursement Tips

Most third-party payers require that dentists report this procedure using the appropriate ADA code on the dental claim form.

## Associated HCPCS Codes

| | |
|---|---|
| D7310 | alveoloplasty in conjunction with extractions - four or more teeth or tooth spaces, per quadrant |
| D7311 | alveoloplasty in conjunction with extractions - one to three teeth or tooth spaces, per quadrant |
| D7320 | alveoloplasty not in conjunction with extractions - four or more teeth or tooth spaces, per quadrant |
| D7321 | alveoloplasty not in conjunction with extractions - one to three teeth or tooth spaces, per quadrant |

## ICD-10-CM Diagnostic Codes

| | |
|---|---|
| C03.0 | Malignant neoplasm of upper gum |
| C03.1 | Malignant neoplasm of lower gum |
| C06.2 | Malignant neoplasm of retromolar area |
| C41.1 | Malignant neoplasm of mandible |
| D00.03 | Carcinoma in situ of gingiva and edentulous alveolar ridge |
| D16.4 | Benign neoplasm of bones of skull and face |
| D16.5 | Benign neoplasm of lower jaw bone |
| K01.1 | Impacted teeth |
| K04.1 | Necrosis of pulp |
| K04.4 | Acute apical periodontitis of pulpal origin |
| K04.5 | Chronic apical periodontitis |
| K04.8 | Radicular cyst |
| K05.311 | Chronic periodontitis, localized, slight |
| K05.312 | Chronic periodontitis, localized, moderate |
| K05.313 | Chronic periodontitis, localized, severe |
| K05.321 | Chronic periodontitis, generalized, slight |
| K05.322 | Chronic periodontitis, generalized, moderate |
| K05.323 | Chronic periodontitis, generalized, severe |
| K05.4 | Periodontosis |
| K06.011 | Localized gingival recession, minimal |
| K06.012 | Localized gingival recession, moderate |
| K06.013 | Localized gingival recession, severe |
| K06.021 | Generalized gingival recession, minimal |
| K06.022 | Generalized gingival recession, moderate |
| K06.023 | Generalized gingival recession, severe |
| K08.0 | Exfoliation of teeth due to systemic causes |
| K08.111 | Complete loss of teeth due to trauma, class I |
| K08.112 | Complete loss of teeth due to trauma, class II |
| K08.113 | Complete loss of teeth due to trauma, class III |
| K08.114 | Complete loss of teeth due to trauma, class IV |
| K08.121 | Complete loss of teeth due to periodontal diseases, class I |
| K08.122 | Complete loss of teeth due to periodontal diseases, class II |
| K08.123 | Complete loss of teeth due to periodontal diseases, class III |
| K08.124 | Complete loss of teeth due to periodontal diseases, class IV |
| K08.191 | Complete loss of teeth due to other specified cause, class I |
| K08.192 | Complete loss of teeth due to other specified cause, class II |
| K08.193 | Complete loss of teeth due to other specified cause, class III |
| K08.194 | Complete loss of teeth due to other specified cause, class IV |
| K08.411 | Partial loss of teeth due to trauma, class I |
| K08.412 | Partial loss of teeth due to trauma, class II |
| K08.413 | Partial loss of teeth due to trauma, class III |
| K08.414 | Partial loss of teeth due to trauma, class IV |
| K08.421 | Partial loss of teeth due to periodontal diseases, class I |
| K08.422 | Partial loss of teeth due to periodontal diseases, class II |
| K08.423 | Partial loss of teeth due to periodontal diseases, class III |
| K08.424 | Partial loss of teeth due to periodontal diseases, class IV |
| K08.491 | Partial loss of teeth due to other specified cause, class I |
| K08.492 | Partial loss of teeth due to other specified cause, class II |
| K08.493 | Partial loss of teeth due to other specified cause, class III |
| K08.494 | Partial loss of teeth due to other specified cause, class IV |
| K08.81 | Primary occlusal trauma |
| K08.82 | Secondary occlusal trauma |
| K08.89 | Other specified disorders of teeth and supporting structures |
| M26.39 | Other anomalies of tooth position of fully erupted tooth or teeth |
| M26.59 | Other dentofacial functional abnormalities |
| M26.71 | Alveolar maxillary hyperplasia |
| M26.72 | Alveolar mandibular hyperplasia |
| M26.74 | Alveolar mandibular hypoplasia |
| M26.79 | Other specified alveolar anomalies |
| M26.89 | Other dentofacial anomalies |
| M27.2 | Inflammatory conditions of jaws |
| M27.3 | Alveolitis of jaws |
| M27.8 | Other specified diseases of jaws |
| M87.180 | Osteonecrosis due to drugs, jaw |

**AMA: 41874** 2014,Jan,11

## Relative Value Units/Medicare Edits

| Non-Facility RVU | Work | PE | MP | Total |
|---|---|---|---|---|
| **41874** | 3.19 | 8.11 | 0.31 | 11.61 |
| **Facility RVU** | **Work** | **PE** | **MP** | **Total** |
| **41874** | 3.19 | 3.68 | 0.31 | 7.18 |

| | FUD | Status | MUE | Modifiers | | | | IOM Reference |
|---|---|---|---|---|---|---|---|---|
| **41874** | 90 | R | 4(2) | N/A | 51 | N/A | 80* | 100-04,12,90.4.5 |

* with documentation

## Terms To Know

**alveoloplasty.** Surgical recontouring of the bone to which a tooth is attached, usually performed prior to the fitting of prosthesis.

**caries.** Localized section of tooth decay that begins on the tooth surface with destruction of the calcified enamel, allowing bacterial destruction to continue and form cavities and may extend to the dentin and pulp.

**mucosa.** Moist tissue lining the mouth (buccal mucosa), stomach (gastric mucosa), intestines, and respiratory tract.

**occlusal.** Biting surfaces of premolar and molar teeth or the areas of contact between opposing teeth in the maxilla and mandible.

**recession.** Drawing away or back from the normal position; displacing tissue surgically to a point posterior to the normal location or insertion.

# 99188

**99188** Application of topical fluoride varnish by a physician or other qualified health care professional

## Explanation

The physician, or other qualified health care provider, uses a small piece of gauze to wipe clean and dry the teeth. Once dry, the topical fluoride is "painted" on the entire surface of each tooth using a small brush. The varnish goes on "tacky" but hardens once saliva from the mouth touches it. Topical fluoride varnish is used to prevent tooth decay by going into the tooth enamel and strengthening the tooth. Use of topical fluoride varnish works to stop the formation of new caries, impede or stop existing tooth decay from worsening, and, in early cases of tooth decay, repairs the tooth completely.

## Coding Tips

This service is provided by the dentist or other qualified health care provider such as a dental assistant. When the varnish is applied solely to desensitize the tooth, see also D9910. Any evaluation, radiograph, restorative, or extraction service is reported separately. Removal of coronal plaque is reported separately using D1110 or D1120.

## Documentation Tips

The following information should be documented on a tooth chart: treatment/location of caries, endodontic procedures, prosthetic services, preventive services, treatment of lesions and dental disease, or other special procedures. A tooth chart may also be used to identify structure and rationale of disease process, and the type of service performed on intraoral structures other than teeth.

## Reimbursement Tips

Most dental insurers will require that this service be reported using the appropriate CDT code (D1206–D1208). Check with third-party payers to determine their specific reporting guidelines.

## Associated HCPCS Codes

D1206 topical application of fluoride varnish

## ICD-10-CM Diagnostic Codes

K02.51 Dental caries on pit and fissure surface limited to enamel
K02.52 Dental caries on pit and fissure surface penetrating into dentin
K02.53 Dental caries on pit and fissure surface penetrating into pulp
K02.61 Dental caries on smooth surface limited to enamel
K02.62 Dental caries on smooth surface penetrating into dentin
K02.63 Dental caries on smooth surface penetrating into pulp
M35.0C Sjögren syndrome with dental involvement
Z29.3 Encounter for prophylactic fluoride administration
Z41.8 Encounter for other procedures for purposes other than remedying health state
Z98.810 Dental sealant status

## Relative Value Units/Medicare Edits

| Non-Facility RVU | Work | PE | MP | Total |
|---|---|---|---|---|
| **99188** | 0.20 | 0.14 | 0.02 | 0.36 |
| **Facility RVU** | **Work** | **PE** | **MP** | **Total** |
| **99188** | 0.20 | 0.08 | 0.02 | 0.30 |

| | FUD | Status | MUE | Modifiers | | | | IOM Reference |
|---|---|---|---|---|---|---|---|---|
| **99188** | N/A | N | 1(2) | N/A | N/A | N/A | 80* | 100-04,12,90.4.5 |

* with documentation

## Terms To Know

**caries.** Localized section of tooth decay that begins on the tooth surface with destruction of the calcified enamel, allowing bacterial destruction to continue and form cavities and may extend to the dentin and pulp.

**fluoride.** Compound of the gaseous element fluorine that can be incorporated into bone and teeth and provides some protection in reducing dental decay.

**prophylaxis.** Intervention or protective therapy intended to prevent a disease.

# Correct Coding Initiative Update 27.3



❖Indicates Mutually Exclusive Edit

**12020** 0213T, 0216T, 0543T-0544T, 0545T, 0567T-0574T, 0580T, 0581T, 0582T, 11000-11006, 11042-11047, 11900-11901, 12021, 15772, 15774, 20560-20561, 20700-20701, 36000, 36400-36410, 36420-36430, 36440, 36591-36592, 36600, 36640, 43752, 51701-51703, 64400, 64405-64408, 64415-64435, 64445-64451, 64479-64484, 64490-64505, 64510-64530, 66987-66988, 69990, 92012-92014, 93000-93010, 93040-93042, 93318, 93355, 94002, 94200, 94680-94690, 95812-95816, 95819, 95822, 95829, 95955, 96360-96368, 96372, 96374-96377, 96523, 97597-97598, 97602-97608, 99155, 99156, 99157, 99211-99223, 99231-99255, 99291-99292, 99304-99310, 99315-99316, 99334-99337, 99347-99350, 99374-99375, 99377-99378, 99446-99449, 99451-99452, 99495-99496, G0168, G0463, G0471, J0670, J2001

**12021** 0213T, 0216T, 0543T-0544T, 0567T-0574T, 0580T, 0581T, 0582T, 11042, 11900-11901, 20560-20561, 20700-20701, 36000, 36400-36410, 36420-36430, 36440, 36591-36592, 36600, 36640, 43752, 51701-51703, 64400, 64405-64408, 64415-64435, 64445-64451, 64479-64484, 64490-64505, 64510-64530, 66987-66988, 69990, 92012-92014, 93000-93010, 93040-93042, 93318, 93355, 94002, 94200, 94680-94690, 95812-95816, 95819, 95822, 95829, 95955, 96360-96368, 96372, 96374-96377, 96523, 97597-97598, 97602-97608, 99155, 99156, 99157, 99211-99223, 99231-99255, 99291-99292, 99304-99310, 99315-99316, 99334-99337, 99347-99350, 99374-99375, 99377-99378, 99446-99449, 99451-99452, 99495-99496, G0168, G0463, G0471, J2001

**21031** 00170, 0213T, 0216T, 0596T-0597T, 11000-11006, 11010-11012❖, 11042-11047, 12001-12007, 12011-12057, 13100-13133, 13151-13153, 21050, 21073, 36000, 36400-36410, 36420-36430, 36440, 36591-36592, 36600, 36640, 43752, 51701-51703, 62320-62327, 64400, 64405-64408, 64415-64435, 64445-64454, 64461-64463, 64479-64505, 64510-64530, 69990, 92012-92014, 93000-93010, 93040-93042, 93318, 93355, 94002, 94200, 94680-94690, 95812-95816, 95819, 95822, 95829, 95955, 96360-96368, 96372, 96374-96377, 96523, 97597-97598, 97602, 99155, 99156, 99157, 99211-99223, 99231-99255, 99291-99292, 99304-99310, 99315-99316, 99334-99337, 99347-99350, 99374-99375, 99377-99378, 99446-99449, 99451-99452, 99495-99496, G0463, G0471, J0670, J2001

**21032** 0213T, 0216T, 0596T-0597T, 11000-11006, 11010-11012❖, 11042-11047, 12001-12007, 12011-12057, 13100-13133, 13151-13153, 21050, 36000, 36400-36410, 36420-36430, 36440, 36591-36592, 36600, 36640, 43752, 51701-51703, 62320-62327, 64400, 64405-64408, 64415-64435, 64445-64454, 64461-64463, 64479-64505, 64510-64530, 69990, 92012-92014, 93000-93010, 93040-93042, 93318, 93355, 94002, 94200, 94680-94690, 95812-95816, 95819, 95822, 95829, 95955, 96360-96368, 96372, 96374-96377, 96523, 97597-97598, 97602, 99155, 99156, 99157, 99211-99223, 99231-99255, 99291-99292, 99304-99310, 99315-99316, 99334-99337, 99347-99350, 99374-99375, 99377-99378, 99446-99449, 99451-99452, 99495-99496, G0463, G0471, J0670, J2001

**40804** 00170, 0213T, 0216T, 0596T-0597T, 11000-11006, 11042-11047, 12001-12007, 12011-12057, 13100-13133, 13151-13153, 36000, 36400-36410, 36420-36430, 36440, 36591-36592, 36600, 36640, 43752, 51701-51703, 62320-62327, 64400, 64405-64408, 64415-64435, 64445-64454, 64461-64463, 64479-64505, 64510-64530, 69990, 92012-92014, 92502, 93000-93010, 93040-93042, 93318, 93355, 94002, 94200, 94680-94690, 95812-95816, 95819, 95822, 95829, 95955, 96360-96368, 96372, 96374-96377, 96523, 97597-97598, 97602, 99155, 99156, 99157, 99211-99223, 99231-99255, 99291-99292, 99304-99310, 99315-99316, 99334-99337, 99347-99350, 99374-99375, 99377-99378, 99446-99449, 99451-99452, 99495-99496, G0463, G0471, J0670, J2001

**40805** 00170, 0213T, 0216T, 0596T-0597T, 11000-11006, 11042-11047, 12001-12007, 12011-12057, 13100-13133, 13151-13153, 36000, 36400-36410, 36420-36430, 36440, 36591-36592, 36600, 36640, 40804, 43752, 51701-51703, 62320-62327, 64400, 64405-64408, 64415-64435, 64445-64454, 64461-64463, 64479-64505, 64510-64530, 69990, 92012-92014, 92502, 93000-93010, 93040-93042, 93318, 93355, 94002, 94200, 94680-94690, 95812-95816, 95819, 95822, 95829, 95955, 96360-96368, 96372, 96374-96377, 96523, 97597-97598, 97602, 99155, 99156, 99157, 99211-99223, 99231-99255, 99291-99292, 99304-99310, 99315-99316, 99334-99337, 99347-99350, 99374-99375, 99377-99378, 99446-99449, 99451-99452, 99495-99496, G0463, G0471, J0670, J2001

**40806** 00170, 0213T, 0216T, 0596T-0597T, 11000-11006, 11042-11047, 12001-12007, 12011-12057, 13100-13133, 13151-13153, 36000, 36400-36410, 36420-36430, 36440, 36591-36592, 36600, 36640, 43752, 51701-51703, 62320-62327, 64400, 64405-64408, 64415-64435, 64445-64454, 64461-64463, 64479-64505, 64510-64530, 69990, 92012-92014, 92502, 93000-93010, 93040-93042, 93318, 93355, 94002, 94200, 94680-94690, 95812-95816, 95819, 95822, 95829, 95955, 96360-96368, 96372, 96374-96377, 96523, 97597-97598, 97602, 99155, 99156, 99157, 99211-99223, 99231-99255, 99291-99292, 99304-99310, 99315-99316, 99334-99337, 99347-99350, 99374-99375, 99377-99378, 99446-99449, 99451-99452, 99495-99496, G0463, G0471, J0670, J2001

**40808** 00170, 0213T, 0216T, 0596T-0597T, 10005, 10007, 10009, 10011, 10021, 11102-11107❖, 12001-12007, 12011-12057, 13100-13133, 13151-13153, 36000, 36400-36410, 36420-36430, 36440, 36591-36592, 36600, 36640, 43752, 51701-51703, 62320-62327, 64400, 64405-64408, 64415-64435, 64445-64454, 64461-64463, 64479-64505, 64510-64530, 69990, 92012-92014, 92502, 93000-93010, 93040-93042, 93318, 93355, 94002, 94200, 94680-94690, 95812-95816, 95819, 95822, 95829, 95955, 96360-96368, 96372, 96374-96377, 96523, 99155, 99156, 99157, 99211-99223, 99231-99255, 99291-99292, 99304-99310, 99315-99316, 99334-99337, 99347-99350, 99374-99375, 99377-99378, 99446-99449, 99451-99452, 99495-99496, G0463, G0471, J0670, J2001

**40810** 00170, 0213T, 0216T, 0596T-0597T, 11000-11006, 11042-11047, 12001-12007, 12011-12057, 13100-13133, 13151-13153, 36000, 36400-36410, 36420-36430, 36440, 36591-36592, 36600, 36640, 40808, 43752, 51701-51703, 62320-62327, 64400, 64405-64408, 64415-64435, 64445-64454, 64461-64463, 64479-64505, 64510-64530, 69990, 92012-92014, 92502, 93000-93010, 93040-93042, 93318, 93355, 94002, 94200, 94680-94690, 95812-95816, 95819, 95822, 95829, 95955, 96360-96368, 96372, 96374-96377, 96523, 97597-97598, 97602, 99155, 99156, 99157, 99211-99223, 99231-99255, 99291-99292, 99304-99310, 99315-99316, 99334-99337, 99347-99350, 99374-99375, 99377-99378, 99446-99449, 99451-99452, 99495-99496, G0463, G0471, J0670, J2001

**40812** 00170, 0213T, 0216T, 0596T-0597T, 11000-11006, 11042-11047, 12001-12007, 12011-12057, 13100-13133, 13151-13153, 36000, 36400-36410, 36420-36430, 36440, 36591-36592, 36600, 36640, 40808-40810, 43752, 51701-51703, 62320-62327, 64400, 64405-64408, 64415-64435, 64445-64454, 64461-64463, 64479-64505, 64510-64530, 69990, 92012-92014, 92502, 93000-93010, 93040-93042, 93318, 93355, 94002, 94200, 94680-94690, 95812-95816, 95819, 95822, 95829, 95955, 96360-96368, 96372, 96374-96377, 96523, 97597-97598, 97602, 99155, 99156, 99157, 99211-99223, 99231-99255, 99291-99292, 99304-99310, 99315-99316, 99334-99337, 99347-99350, 99374-99375, 99377-99378, 99446-99449, 99451-99452, 99495-99496, G0463, G0471, J0670, J2001

**40819** 00170, 0213T, 0216T, 0596T-0597T, 11000-11006, 11042-11047, 12001-12007, 12011-12057, 13100-13133, 13151-13153, 36000, 36400-36410, 36420-36430, 36440, 36591-36592, 36600, 36640, 40806, 43752, 51701-51703, 62320-62327, 64400, 64405-64408, 64415-64435, 64445-64454, 64461-64463, 64479-64505, 64510-64530, 69990, 92012-92014, 92502, 93000-93010, 93040-93042, 93318, 93355, 94002, 94200, 94680-94690, 95812-95816, 95819, 95822, 95829, 95955, 96360-96368, 96372, 96374-96377, 96523, 97597-97598, 97602, 99155, 99156, 99157, 99211-99223, 99231-99255, 99291-99292, 99304-99310, 99315-99316, 99334-99337, 99347-99350, 99374-99375, 99377-99378, 99446-99449, 99451-99452, 99495-99496, G0463, G0471, J0670, J2001

**40830** 00170, 0213T, 0216T, 0596T-0597T, 11000-11006, 11042-11047, 12001-12007, 12011-12057, 13100-13133, 13151-13153, 36000, 36400-36410, 36420-36430, 36440, 36591-36592, 36600, 36640, 40831✦, 43752, 51701-51703, 62320-62327, 64400, 64405-64408, 64415-64435, 64445-64454, 64461-64463, 64479-64505, 64510-64530, 69990, 92012-92014, 92502, 93000-93010, 93040-93042, 93318, 93355, 94002, 94200, 94680-94690, 95812-95816, 95819, 95822, 95829, 95955, 96360-96368, 96372, 96374-96377, 96523, 97597-97598, 97602, 99155, 99156, 99157, 99211-99223, 99231-99255, 99291-99292, 99304-99310, 99315-99316, 99334-99337, 99347-99350, 99374-99375, 99377-99378, 99446-99449, 99451-99452, 99495-99496, G0463, G0471, J0670, J2001

**40831** 00170, 0213T, 0216T, 0596T-0597T, 11000-11006, 11042-11047, 12001-12007, 12011-12057, 13100-13133, 13151-13153, 36000, 36400-36410, 36420-36430, 36440, 36591-36592, 36600, 36640, 43752, 51701-51703, 62320-62327, 64400, 64405-64408, 64415-64435, 64445-64454, 64461-64463, 64479-64505, 64510-64530, 69990, 92012-92014, 92502, 93000-93010, 93040-93042, 93318, 93355, 94002, 94200, 94680-94690, 95812-95816, 95819, 95822, 95829, 95955, 96360-96368, 96372, 96374-96377, 96523, 97597-97598, 97602, 99155, 99156, 99157, 99211-99223, 99231-99255, 99291-99292, 99304-99310, 99315-99316, 99334-99337, 99347-99350, 99374-99375, 99377-99378, 99446-99449, 99451-99452, 99495-99496, G0463, G0471, J0670, J2001

**40840** 00170, 0213T, 0216T, 0596T-0597T, 11000-11006, 11042-11047, 12001-12007, 12011-12057, 13100-13133, 13151-13153, 36000, 36400-36410, 36420-36430, 36440, 36591-36592, 36600, 36640, 40842✦, 43752, 51701-51703, 62320-62327, 64400, 64405-64408, 64415-64435, 64445-64454, 64461-64463, 64479-64505, 64510-64530, 69990, 92012-92014, 92502, 93000-93010, 93040-93042, 93318, 93355, 94002, 94200, 94680-94690, 95812-95816, 95819, 95822, 95829, 95955, 96360-96368, 96372, 96374-96377, 96523, 97597-97598, 97602, 99155, 99156, 99157, 99211-99223, 99231-99255, 99291-99292, 99304-99310, 99315-99316, 99334-99337, 99347-99350, 99374-99375, 99377-99378, 99446-99449, 99451-99452, 99495-99496, G0463, G0471, J0670, J2001

**40842** 00170, 0213T, 0216T, 0596T-0597T, 11000-11006, 11042-11047, 12001-12007, 12011-12057, 13100-13133, 13151-13153, 36000, 36400-36410, 36420-36430, 36440, 36591-36592, 36600, 36640, 43752, 51701-51703, 62320-62327, 64400, 64405-64408, 64415-64435, 64445-64454, 64461-64463, 64479-64505, 64510-64530, 69990, 92012-92014, 92502, 93000-93010, 93040-93042, 93318, 93355, 94002, 94200, 94680-94690, 95812-95816, 95819, 95822, 95829, 95955, 96360-96368, 96372, 96374-96377, 96523, 97597-97598, 97602, 99155, 99156, 99157, 99211-99223, 99231-99255, 99291-99292, 99304-99310, 99315-99316, 99334-99337, 99347-99350, 99374-99375, 99377-99378, 99446-99449, 99451-99452, 99495-99496, G0463, G0471, J0670, J2001

**40843** 00170, 0213T, 0216T, 0596T-0597T, 11000-11006, 11042-11047, 12001-12007, 12011-12057, 13100-13133, 13151-13153, 36000, 36400-36410, 36420-36430, 36440, 36591-36592, 36600, 36640, 40840-40842, 43752, 51701-51703, 62320-62327, 64400, 64405-64408, 64415-64435, 64445-64454, 64461-64463, 64479-64505, 64510-64530, 69990, 92012-92014, 92502, 93000-93010, 93040-93042, 93318, 93355, 94002, 94200, 94680-94690, 95812-95816, 95819, 95822, 95829, 95955, 96360-96368, 96372, 96374-96377, 96523, 97597-97598, 97602, 99155, 99156, 99157, 99211-99223, 99231-99255, 99291-99292, 99304-99310, 99315-99316, 99334-99337, 99347-99350, 99374-99375, 99377-99378, 99446-99449, 99451-99452, 99495-99496, G0463, G0471, J0670, J2001

**40844** 00170, 0213T, 0216T, 0596T-0597T, 11000-11006, 11042-11047, 12001-12007, 12011-12057, 13100-13133, 13151-13153, 36000, 36400-36410, 36420-36430, 36440, 36591-36592, 36600, 36640, 40842-40843, 43752, 51701-51703, 62320-62327, 64400, 64405-64408, 64415-64435, 64445-64454, 64461-64463, 64479-64505, 64510-64530, 69990, 92012-92014, 92502, 93000-93010, 93040-93042, 93318, 93355, 94002, 94200, 94680-94690, 95812-95816, 95819, 95822, 95829, 95955, 96360-96368, 96372, 96374-96377, 96523, 97597-97598, 97602, 99155, 99156, 99157, 99211-99223, 99231-99255, 99291-99292, 99304-99310, 99315-99316, 99334-99337, 99347-99350, 99374-99375, 99377-99378, 99446-99449, 99451-99452, 99495-99496, G0463, G0471, J0670, J2001

**40845** 00170, 0213T, 0216T, 0596T-0597T, 11000-11006, 11042-11047, 12001-12007, 12011-12057, 13100-13133, 13151-13153, 36000, 36400-36410, 36420-36430, 36440, 36591-36592, 36600, 36640, 40840-40844, 43752, 51701-51703, 62320-62327, 64400, 64405-64408, 64415-64435, 64445-64454, 64461-64463, 64479-64505, 64510-64530, 69990, 92012-92014, 92502, 93000-93010, 93040-93042, 93318, 93355, 94002, 94200, 94680-94690, 95812-95816, 95819, 95822, 95829, 95955, 96360-96368, 96372, 96374-96377, 96523, 97597-97598, 97602, 99155, 99156, 99157, 99211-99223, 99231-99255, 99291-99292, 99304-99310, 99315-99316, 99334-99337, 99347-99350, 99374-99375, 99377-99378, 99446-99449, 99451-99452, 99495-99496, G0463, G0471, J0670, J2001

**41000** 00170, 0213T, 0216T, 0596T-0597T, 10030, 10060-10061✦, 10160, 12001-12007, 12011-12057, 13100-13133, 13151-13153, 36000, 36400-36410, 36420-36430, 36440, 36591-36592, 36600, 36640, 43752, 49185, 49424, 51701-51703, 62320-62327, 64400, 64405-64408, 64415-64435, 64445-64454, 64461-64463, 64479-64505, 64510-64530, 69990, 92012-92014, 92502, 93000-93010, 93040-93042, 93318, 93355, 94002, 94200, 94680-94690, 95812-95816, 95819, 95822, 95829, 95955, 96360-96368, 96372, 96374-96377, 96523, 99155, 99156, 99157, 99211-99223, 99231-99255, 99291-99292, 99304-99310, 99315-99316, 99334-99337, 99347-99350, 99374-99375, 99377-99378, 99446-99449, 99451-99452, 99495-99496, G0463, G0471, J0670, J2001

**41005** 00170, 0213T, 0216T, 0596T-0597T, 10030, 10060-10061✦, 10160, 12001-12007, 12011-12057, 13100-13133, 13151-13153, 36000, 36400-36410, 36420-36430, 36440, 36591-36592, 36600, 36640, 41015✦, 43752, 49185, 49424, 51701-51703, 62320-62327, 64400, 64405-64408, 64415-64435, 64445-64454, 64461-64463, 64479-64505, 64510-64530, 69990, 92012-92014, 92502, 93000-93010, 93040-93042, 93318, 93355, 94002, 94200, 94680-94690, 95812-95816, 95819, 95822, 95829, 95955, 96360-96368, 96372, 96374-96377, 96523, 99155, 99156, 99157, 99211-99223, 99231-99255, 99291-99292, 99304-99310, 99315-99316, 99334-99337, 99347-99350, 99374-99375, 99377-99378, 99446-99449, 99451-99452, 99495-99496, G0463, G0471, J0670, J2001

**41006** 00170, 0213T, 0216T, 0596T-0597T, 10030, 10060-10061✦, 10160, 12001-12007, 12011-12057, 13100-13133, 13151-13153, 36000,

36400-36410, 36420-36430, 36440, 36591-36592, 36600, 36640, 41005, 41015❖, 43752, 49185, 49424, 51701-51703, 62320-62327, 64400, 64405-64408, 64415-64435, 64445-64454, 64461-64463, 64479-64505, 64510-64530, 69990, 92012-92014, 92502, 93000-93010, 93040-93042, 93318, 93355, 94002, 94200, 94680-94690, 95812-95816, 95819, 95822, 95829, 95955, 96360-96368, 96372, 96374-96377, 96523, 99155, 99156, 99157, 99211-99223, 99231-99255, 99291-99292, 99304-99310, 99315-99316, 99334-99337, 99347-99350, 99374-99375, 99377-99378, 99446-99449, 99451-99452, 99495-99496, G0463, G0471, J0670, J2001

**41007** 00170, 0213T, 0216T, 0596T-0597T, 10030, 10060-10061❖, 10160, 12001-12007, 12011-12057, 13100-13133, 13151-13153, 36000, 36400-36410, 36420-36430, 36440, 36591-36592, 36600, 36640, 41008❖, 41016❖, 43752, 49185, 49424, 51701-51703, 62320-62327, 64400, 64405-64408, 64415-64435, 64445-64454, 64461-64463, 64479-64505, 64510-64530, 69990, 92012-92014, 92502, 93000-93010, 93040-93042, 93318, 93355, 94002, 94200, 94680-94690, 95812-95816, 95819, 95822, 95829, 95955, 96360-96368, 96372, 96374-96377, 96523, 99155, 99156, 99157, 99211-99223, 99231-99255, 99291-99292, 99304-99310, 99315-99316, 99334-99337, 99347-99350, 99374-99375, 99377-99378, 99446-99449, 99451-99452, 99495-99496, G0463, G0471, J0670, J2001

**41008** 00170, 0213T, 0216T, 0596T-0597T, 10030, 10061❖, 10160, 12001-12007, 12011-12057, 13100-13133, 13151-13153, 36000, 36400-36410, 36420-36430, 36440, 36591-36592, 36600, 36640, 43752, 49185, 49424, 51701-51703, 62320-62327, 64400, 64405-64408, 64415-64435, 64445-64454, 64461-64463, 64479-64505, 64510-64530, 69990, 92012-92014, 92502, 93000-93010, 93040-93042, 93318, 93355, 94002, 94200, 94680-94690, 95812-95816, 95819, 95822, 95829, 95955, 96360-96368, 96372, 96374-96377, 96523, 99155, 99156, 99157, 99211-99223, 99231-99255, 99291-99292, 99304-99310, 99315-99316, 99334-99337, 99347-99350, 99374-99375, 99377-99378, 99446-99449, 99451-99452, 99495-99496, G0463, G0471, J0670, J2001

**41009** 00170, 0213T, 0216T, 0596T-0597T, 10030, 10060-10061❖, 10160, 12001-12007, 12011-12057, 13100-13133, 13151-13153, 36000, 36400-36410, 36420-36430, 36440, 36591-36592, 36600, 36640, 41018❖, 43752, 49185, 49424, 51701-51703, 62320-62327, 64400, 64405-64408, 64415-64435, 64445-64454, 64461-64463, 64479-64505, 64510-64530, 69990, 92012-92014, 92502, 93000-93010, 93040-93042, 93318, 93355, 94002, 94200, 94680-94690, 95812-95816, 95819, 95822, 95829, 95955, 96360-96368, 96372, 96374-96377, 96523, 99155, 99156, 99157, 99211-99223, 99231-99255, 99291-99292, 99304-99310, 99315-99316, 99334-99337, 99347-99350, 99374-99375, 99377-99378, 99446-99449, 99451-99452, 99495-99496, G0463, G0471, J0670, J2001

**41010** 00170, 0213T, 0216T, 0596T-0597T, 11000-11006, 11042-11047, 12001-12007, 12011-12057, 13100-13133, 13151-13153, 36000, 36400-36410, 36420-36430, 36440, 36591-36592, 36600, 36640, 43752, 51701-51703, 62320-62327, 64400, 64405-64408, 64415-64435, 64445-64454, 64461-64463, 64479-64505, 64510-64530, 69990, 92012-92014, 92502, 93000-93010, 93040-93042, 93318, 93355, 94002, 94200, 94680-94690, 95812-95816, 95819, 95822, 95829, 95955, 96360-96368, 96372, 96374-96377, 96523, 97597-97598, 97602, 99155, 99156, 99157, 99211-99223, 99231-99255, 99291-99292, 99304-99310, 99315-99316, 99334-99337, 99347-99350, 99374-99375, 99377-99378, 99446-99449, 99451-99452, 99495-99496, G0463, G0471, J0670, J2001

**41015** 00170, 0213T, 0216T, 0596T-0597T, 10030, 10060-10061❖, 10160, 12001-12007, 12011-12057, 13100-13133, 13151-13153, 36000, 36400-36410, 36420-36430, 36440, 36591-36592, 36600, 36640, 43752, 49185, 49424, 51701-51703, 62320-62327, 64400, 64405-64408, 64415-64435, 64445-64454, 64461-64463, 64479-64505, 64510-64530, 69990, 92012-92014, 92502, 93000-93010, 93040-93042, 93318, 93355, 94002, 94200, 94680-94690, 95812-95816, 95819, 95822, 95829, 95955, 96360-96368, 96372, 96374-96377, 96523, 99155, 99156, 99157, 99211-99223, 99231-99255, 99291-99292, 99304-99310, 99315-99316, 99334-99337, 99347-99350, 99374-99375, 99377-99378, 99446-99449, 99451-99452, 99495-99496, G0463, G0471, J0670, J2001

**41016** 00170, 0213T, 0216T, 0596T-0597T, 10030, 10060-10061❖, 10160, 12001-12007, 12011-12057, 13100-13133, 13151-13153, 36000, 36400-36410, 36420-36430, 36440, 36591-36592, 36600, 36640, 43752, 49185, 49424, 51701-51703, 62320-62327, 64400, 64405-64408, 64415-64435, 64445-64454, 64461-64463, 64479-64505, 64510-64530, 69990, 92012-92014, 92502, 93000-93010, 93040-93042, 93318, 93355, 94002, 94200, 94680-94690, 95812-95816, 95819, 95822, 95829, 95955, 96360-96368, 96372, 96374-96377, 96523, 99155, 99156, 99157, 99211-99223, 99231-99255, 99291-99292, 99304-99310, 99315-99316, 99334-99337, 99347-99350, 99374-99375, 99377-99378, 99446-99449, 99451-99452, 99495-99496, G0463, G0471, J0670, J2001

**41017** 00170, 0213T, 0216T, 0596T-0597T, 10030, 10060-10061, 10160, 12001-12007, 12011-12057, 13100-13133, 13151-13153, 36000, 36400-36410, 36420-36430, 36440, 36591-36592, 36600, 36640, 43752, 49185, 49424, 51701-51703, 62320-62327, 64400, 64405-64408, 64415-64435, 64445-64454, 64461-64463, 64479-64505, 64510-64530, 69990, 92012-92014, 92502, 93000-93010, 93040-93042, 93318, 93355, 94002, 94200, 94680-94690, 95812-95816, 95819, 95822, 95829, 95955, 96360-96368, 96372, 96374-96377, 96523, 99155, 99156, 99157, 99211-99223, 99231-99255, 99291-99292, 99304-99310, 99315-99316, 99334-99337, 99347-99350, 99374-99375, 99377-99378, 99446-99449, 99451-99452, 99495-99496, G0463, G0471, J0670, J2001

**41018** 00170, 0213T, 0216T, 0596T-0597T, 10030, 10060-10061❖, 10160, 12001-12007, 12011-12057, 13100-13133, 13151-13153, 36000, 36400-36410, 36420-36430, 36440, 36591-36592, 36600, 36640, 43752, 49185, 49424, 51701-51703, 62320-62327, 64400, 64405-64408, 64415-64435, 64445-64454, 64461-64463, 64479-64505, 64510-64530, 69990, 92012-92014, 92502, 93000-93010, 93040-93042, 93318, 93355, 94002, 94200, 94680-94690, 95812-95816, 95819, 95822, 95829, 95955, 96360-96368, 96372, 96374-96377, 96523, 99155, 99156, 99157, 99211-99223, 99231-99255, 99291-99292, 99304-99310, 99315-99316, 99334-99337, 99347-99350, 99374-99375, 99377-99378, 99446-99449, 99451-99452, 99495-99496, G0463, G0471, J0670, J2001

**41115** 00170, 0213T, 0216T, 0596T-0597T, 11000-11006, 11042-11047, 12001-12007, 12011-12057, 13100-13133, 13151-13153, 36000, 36400-36410, 36420-36430, 36440, 36591-36592, 36600, 36640, 41010, 43752, 51701-51703, 62320-62327, 64400, 64405-64408, 64415-64435, 64445-64454, 64461-64463, 64479-64505, 64510-64530, 69990, 92012-92014, 92502, 93000-93010, 93040-93042, 93318, 93355, 94002, 94200, 94680-94690, 95812-95816, 95819, 95822, 95829, 95955, 96360-96368, 96372, 96374-96377, 96523, 97597-97598, 97602, 99155, 99156, 99157, 99211-99223, 99231-99255, 99291-99292, 99304-99310, 99315-99316, 99334-99337, 99347-99350, 99374-99375, 99377-99378, 99446-99449, 99451-99452, 99495-99496, G0463, G0471, J0670, J2001

**41520** 00170, 0213T, 0216T, 0596T-0597T, 11000-11006, 11042-11047, 12001-12007, 12011-12057, 13100-13133, 13151-13153, 36000, 36400-36410, 36420-36430, 36440, 36591-36592, 36600, 36640, 40806, 41010, 41115, 43752, 51701-51703, 62320-62327, 64400, 64405-64408, 64415-64435, 64445-64454, 64461-64463, 64479-64505, 64510-64530, 69990, 92012-92014, 92502, 93000-93010, 93040-93042, 93318, 93355, 94002, 94200, 94680-94690, 95812-95816, 95819, 95822, 95829,

95955, 96360-96368, 96372, 96374-96377, 96523, 97597-97598, 97602, 99155, 99156, 99157, 99211-99223, 99231-99255, 99291-99292, 99304-99310, 99315-99316, 99334-99337, 99347-99350, 99374-99375, 99377-99378, 99446-99449, 99451-99452, 99495-99496, G0463, G0471, J0670, J2001

**41820** 00170, 0213T, 0216T, 0596T-0597T, 11000-11006, 11042-11047, 12001-12007, 12011-12057, 13100-13133, 13151-13153, 36000, 36400-36410, 36420-36430, 36440, 36591-36592, 36600, 36640, 43752, 51701-51703, 62320-62327, 64400, 64405-64408, 64415-64435, 64445-64454, 64461-64463, 64479-64505, 64510-64530, 69990, 92012-92014, 92502, 93000-93010, 93040-93042, 93318, 93355, 94002, 94200, 94680-94690, 95812-95816, 95819, 95822, 95829, 95955, 96360-96368, 96372, 96374-96377, 96523, 97597-97598, 97602, 99155, 99156, 99157, 99211-99223, 99231-99255, 99291-99292, 99304-99310, 99315-99316, 99334-99337, 99347-99350, 99374-99375, 99377-99378, 99446-99449, 99451-99452, 99495-99496, G0463, G0471

**41821** 00170, 0213T, 0216T, 0596T-0597T, 11000-11006, 11042-11047, 12001-12007, 12011-12057, 13100-13133, 13151-13153, 36000, 36400-36410, 36420-36430, 36440, 36591-36592, 36600, 36640, 43752, 51701-51703, 62320-62327, 64400, 64405-64408, 64415-64435, 64445-64454, 64461-64463, 64479-64505, 64510-64530, 69990, 92012-92014, 92502, 93000-93010, 93040-93042, 93318, 93355, 94002, 94200, 94680-94690, 95812-95816, 95819, 95822, 95829, 95955, 96360-96368, 96372, 96374-96377, 96523, 97597-97598, 97602, 99155, 99156, 99157, 99211-99223, 99231-99255, 99291-99292, 99304-99310, 99315-99316, 99334-99337, 99347-99350, 99374-99375, 99377-99378, 99446-99449, 99451-99452, 99495-99496, G0463, G0471

**41822** 00170, 0213T, 0216T, 0596T-0597T, 11000-11006, 11042-11047, 12001-12007, 12011-12057, 13100-13133, 13151-13153, 36000, 36400-36410, 36420-36430, 36440, 36591-36592, 36600, 36640, 43752, 51701-51703, 62320-62327, 64400, 64405-64408, 64415-64435, 64445-64454, 64461-64463, 64479-64505, 64510-64530, 69990, 92012-92014, 92502, 93000-93010, 93040-93042, 93318, 93355, 94002, 94200, 94680-94690, 95812-95816, 95819, 95822, 95829, 95955, 96360-96368, 96372, 96374-96377, 96523, 97597-97598, 97602, 99155, 99156, 99157, 99211-99223, 99231-99255, 99291-99292, 99304-99310, 99315-99316, 99334-99337, 99347-99350, 99374-99375, 99377-99378, 99446-99449, 99451-99452, 99495-99496, G0463, G0471, J0670, J2001

**41823** 00170, 0213T, 0216T, 0596T-0597T, 11000-11006, 11042-11047, 12001-12007, 12011-12057, 13100-13133, 13151-13153, 36000, 36400-36410, 36420-36430, 36440, 36591-36592, 36600, 36640, 43752, 51701-51703, 62320-62327, 64400, 64405-64408, 64415-64435, 64445-64454, 64461-64463, 64479-64505, 64510-64530, 69990, 92012-92014, 92502, 93000-93010, 93040-93042, 93318, 93355, 94002, 94200, 94680-94690, 95812-95816, 95819, 95822, 95829, 95955, 96360-96368, 96372, 96374-96377, 96523, 97597-97598, 97602, 99155, 99156, 99157, 99211-99223, 99231-99255, 99291-99292, 99304-99310, 99315-99316, 99334-99337, 99347-99350, 99374-99375, 99377-99378, 99446-99449, 99451-99452, 99495-99496, G0463, G0471, J0670, J2001

**41828** 00170, 0213T, 0216T, 0596T-0597T, 11000-11006, 11042-11047, 12001-12007, 12011-12057, 13100-13133, 13151-13153, 36000, 36400-36410, 36420-36430, 36440, 36591-36592, 36600, 36640, 43752, 51701-51703, 62320-62327, 64400, 64405-64408, 64415-64435, 64445-64454, 64461-64463, 64479-64505, 64510-64530, 69990, 92012-92014, 92502, 93000-93010, 93040-93042, 93318, 93355, 94002, 94200, 94680-94690, 95812-95816, 95819, 95822, 95829, 95955, 96360-96368, 96372, 96374-96377, 96523, 97597-97598, 97602, 99155, 99156, 99157, 99211-99223, 99231-99255, 99291-99292, 99304-99310, 99315-99316, 99334-99337, 99347-99350, 99374-99375, 99377-99378, 99446-99449, 99451-99452, 99495-99496, G0463, G0471, J0670, J2001

**41870** 00170, 0213T, 0216T, 0596T-0597T, 12001-12007, 12011-12057, 13100-13133, 13151-13153, 36000, 36400-36410, 36420-36430, 36440, 36591-36592, 36600, 36640, 43752, 51701-51703, 62320-62327, 64400, 64405-64408, 64415-64435, 64445-64454, 64461-64463, 64479-64505, 64510-64530, 69990, 92012-92014, 92502, 93000-93010, 93040-93042, 93318, 93355, 94002, 94200, 94680-94690, 95812-95816, 95819, 95822, 95829, 95955, 96360-96368, 96372, 96374-96377, 96523, 99155, 99156, 99157, 99211-99223, 99231-99255, 99291-99292, 99304-99310, 99315-99316, 99334-99337, 99347-99350, 99374-99375, 99377-99378, 99446-99449, 99451-99452, 99495-99496, G0463, G0471

**41872** 00170, 0213T, 0216T, 0596T-0597T, 11000-11006, 11042-11047, 12001-12007, 12011-12057, 13100-13133, 13151-13153, 36000, 36400-36410, 36420-36430, 36440, 36591-36592, 36600, 36640, 43752, 51701-51703, 62320-62327, 64400, 64405-64408, 64415-64435, 64445-64454, 64461-64463, 64479-64505, 64510-64530, 69990, 92012-92014, 92502, 93000-93010, 93040-93042, 93318, 93355, 94002, 94200, 94680-94690, 95812-95816, 95819, 95822, 95829, 95955, 96360-96368, 96372, 96374-96377, 96523, 97597-97598, 97602, 99155, 99156, 99157, 99211-99223, 99231-99255, 99291-99292, 99304-99310, 99315-99316, 99334-99337, 99347-99350, 99374-99375, 99377-99378, 99446-99449, 99451-99452, 99495-99496, G0463, G0471, J0670, J2001

**41874** 00170, 0213T, 0216T, 0596T-0597T, 11000-11006, 11042-11047, 12001-12007, 12011-12057, 13100-13133, 13151-13153, 36000, 36400-36410, 36420-36430, 36440, 36591-36592, 36600, 36640, 43752, 51701-51703, 62320-62327, 64400, 64405-64408, 64415-64435, 64445-64454, 64461-64463, 64479-64505, 64510-64530, 69990, 92012-92014, 92502, 93000-93010, 93040-93042, 93318, 93355, 94002, 94200, 94680-94690, 95812-95816, 95819, 95822, 95829, 95955, 96360-96368, 96372, 96374-96377, 96523, 97597-97598, 97602, 99155, 99156, 99157, 99211-99223, 99231-99255, 99291-99292, 99304-99310, 99315-99316, 99334-99337, 99347-99350, 99374-99375, 99377-99378, 99446-99449, 99451-99452, 99495-99496, G0463, G0471, J0670, J2001

**99188** 36591-36592, 96523

**99202** 0362T, 0373T, 0469T, 36591-36592, 43752, 80500-80502, 90863, 90940, 92002-92014, 92227-92228, 92531-92532, 93561-93562, 93792, 93793, 94002-94004, 94660-94662, 95851-95852, 96020, 96105, 96116, 96125, 96130, 96132, 96136, 96138, 96146, 96156-96159, 96164-96168, 96523, 97151, 97153-97158, 97169-97172, 97802-97804, 99091, 99172-99173, 99174, 99177, 99211-99215, 99354-99359, 99408-99409, 99421-99423, 99446-99449, 99463❖, 99474, 99605-99606, G0102, G0117-G0118, G0245-G0246, G0248, G0250, G0270-G0271, G0396-G0397, G0406-G0408❖, G0425-G0427❖, G0442-G0447, G0459, G0473, G0508-G0509❖, G2011

**99203** 0362T, 0373T, 0469T, 36591-36592, 43752, 80500-80502, 90863, 90940, 92002-92014, 92227-92228, 92531-92532, 93561-93562, 93792, 93793, 94002-94004, 94660-94662, 95851-95852, 96020, 96105, 96116, 96125, 96130, 96132, 96136, 96138, 96146, 96156-96159, 96164-96168, 96523, 97151, 97153-97158, 97169-97172, 97802-97804, 99091, 99172-99173, 99174, 99177, 99202, 99211-99215, 99354-99359, 99408-99409, 99421-99423, 99446-99449, 99463❖, 99474, 99605-99606, G0102, G0117-G0118, G0245-G0246, G0248, G0250, G0270-G0271, G0396-G0397, G0406-G0408❖, G0425-G0427❖, G0442-G0447, G0459, G0473, G0508-G0509❖, G2011

**99204** 0362T, 0373T, 0469T, 36591-36592, 43752, 80500-80502, 90863, 90940, 92002-92014, 92227-92228, 92531-92532, 93561-93562, 93792, 93793, 94002-94004, 94660-94662, 95851-95852, 96020, 96105, 96116, 96125, 96130, 96132, 96136, 96138, 96146, 96156-96159, 96164-96168,

96523, 97151, 97153-97158, 97169-97172, 97802-97804, 99091, 99172-99173, 99174, 99177, 99202-99203, 99211-99215, 99354-99359, 99408-99409, 99421-99423, 99446-99449, 99463✦, 99474, 99605-99606, G0102, G0117-G0118, G0245-G0246, G0248, G0250, G0270-G0271, G0396-G0397, G0406-G0408✦, G0425-G0427✦, G0442-G0447, G0459, G0473, G0508-G0509✦, G2011

**99205** 0362T, 0373T, 0469T, 36591-36592, 43752, 80500-80502, 90863, 90940, 92002-92014, 92227-92228, 92531-92532, 93561-93562, 93792, 93793, 94002-94004, 94660-94662, 95851-95852, 96020, 96105, 96116, 96125, 96130, 96132, 96136, 96138, 96146, 96156-96159, 96164-96168, 96523, 97151, 97153-97158, 97169-97172, 97802-97804, 99091, 99172-99173, 99174, 99177, 99202-99204, 99211-99215, 99354-99359, 99408-99409, 99421-99423, 99446-99449, 99463✦, 99474, 99605-99606, G0102, G0117-G0118, G0245-G0246, G0248, G0250, G0270-G0271, G0396-G0397, G0406-G0408✦, G0425-G0427✦, G0442-G0447, G0459, G0473, G0508-G0509✦, G2011

**99211** 0362T, 0373T, 0469T, 0543T-0544T, 0567T-0574T, 0580T, 0581T, 0582T, 36591-36592, 43752, 80500-80502, 90863, 90940, 92002-92014, 92227-92228, 92531-92532, 93561-93562, 93792, 93793, 94002-94004, 94660-94662, 95851-95852, 96020, 96105, 96116, 96125, 96130, 96132, 96136, 96138, 96146, 96156-96159, 96164-96168, 96523, 97151, 97153-97158, 97169-97172, 97802-97804, 99091, 99172-99173, 99174, 99177, 99354-99359, 99408-99409, 99415, 99446-99449, 99474, 99605-99606, G0102, G0117-G0118, G0245-G0246, G0248, G0250, G0270-G0271, G0396-G0397, G0406-G0408✦, G0425-G0427✦, G0442-G0447, G0459, G0473, G0508-G0509✦, G2011

**99212** 0362T, 0373T, 0469T, 0543T-0544T, 0567T-0574T, 0580T, 0581T, 0582T, 20560-20561, 36591-36592, 43752, 80500-80502, 90863, 90940, 92002-92014, 92227-92228, 92531-92532, 93561-93562, 93792, 93793, 94002-94004, 94660-94662, 95851-95852, 96020, 96105, 96116, 96125, 96130, 96132, 96136, 96138, 96146, 96156-96159, 96164-96168, 96523, 97151, 97153-97158, 97169-97172, 97802-97804, 99091, 99172-99173, 99174, 99177, 99211, 99354-99359, 99408-99409, 99421, 99446-99449, 99474, 99605-99606, G0102, G0117-G0118, G0245-G0246, G0248, G0250, G0270-G0271, G0396-G0397, G0406-G0408✦, G0425-G0427✦, G0442-G0447, G0459, G0473, G0508-G0509✦, G2011

**99213** 0362T, 0373T, 0469T, 0543T-0544T, 0567T-0574T, 0580T, 0581T, 0582T, 20560-20561, 36591-36592, 43752, 80500-80502, 90863, 90940, 92002-92014, 92227-92228, 92531-92532, 93561-93562, 93792, 93793, 94002-94004, 94660-94662, 95851-95852, 96020, 96105, 96116, 96125, 96130, 96132, 96136, 96138, 96146, 96156-96159, 96164-96168, 96523, 97151, 97153-97158, 97169-97172, 97802-97804, 99091, 99172-99173, 99174, 99177, 99211-99212, 99354-99359, 99408-99409, 99421-99423, 99446-99449, 99463✦, 99474, 99605-99606, G0102, G0117-G0118, G0245-G0246, G0248, G0250, G0270-G0271, G0396-G0397, G0406-G0408✦, G0425-G0427✦, G0442-G0447, G0459, G0473, G0508-G0509✦, G2011

**99214** 0362T, 0373T, 0469T, 0543T-0544T, 0567T-0574T, 0580T, 0581T, 0582T, 20560-20561, 20700-20701, 36591-36592, 43752, 80500-80502, 90863, 90940, 92002-92014, 92227-92228, 92531-92532, 93561-93562, 93792, 93793, 94002-94004, 94660-94662, 95851-95852, 96020, 96105, 96116, 96125, 96130, 96132, 96136, 96138, 96146, 96156-96159, 96164-96168, 96523, 97151, 97153-97158, 97169-97172, 97802-97804, 99091, 99172-99173, 99174, 99177, 99211-99213, 99354-99359, 99408-99409, 99421-99423, 99446-99449, 99463✦, 99474, 99605-99606, G0102, G0117-G0118, G0245-G0246, G0248, G0250, G0270-G0271, G0396-G0397, G0406-G0408✦, G0425-G0427✦, G0442-G0447, G0459, G0473, G0508-G0509✦, G2011

**99215** 0362T, 0373T, 0469T, 0543T-0544T, 0567T-0574T, 0580T, 0581T, 0582T, 20560-20561, 20700-20701, 36591-36592, 43752, 62329, 80500-80502, 90863, 90940, 92002-92014, 92227-92228, 92531-92532, 93561-93562, 93792, 93793, 94002-94004, 94660-94662, 95851-95852, 96020, 96105, 96116, 96125, 96130, 96132, 96136, 96138, 96146, 96156-96159, 96164-96168, 96523, 97151, 97153-97158, 97169-97172, 97802-97804, 99091, 99172-99173, 99174, 99177, 99211-99214, 99354-99359, 99408-99409, 99421-99423, 99446-99449, 99463✦, 99474, 99605-99606, G0102, G0117-G0118, G0245-G0246, G0248, G0250, G0270-G0271, G0396-G0397, G0406-G0408✦, G0425-G0427✦, G0442-G0447, G0459, G0473, G0508-G0509✦, G2011

**99221** 0362T, 0373T, 0469T, 0543T-0544T, 0567T-0574T, 0580T, 0581T, 0582T, 0591T-0593T, 20560-20561, 20700-20701, 36591-36592, 43752, 80500-80502, 90863, 90940, 92002-92014, 92227-92228, 92531-92532, 93792, 93793, 94002-94004, 94644, 94660-94662, 95851-95852, 96020, 96105, 96116, 96125-96130, 96132, 96136, 96138, 96146, 96156-96159, 96164-96168, 96360, 96365, 96369, 96372-96374, 96377, 96401-96406, 96409, 96413, 96416, 96420-96422, 96425-96440, 96446-96450, 96523, 97151, 97153-97158, 97169-97172, 97802-97804, 99091, 99172-99173, 99174, 99177, 99184, 99202-99220, 99224-99233, 99238-99239, 99281-99285, 99304-99310, 99315-99318, 99324-99328, 99334-99337, 99341-99350, 99381-99404, 99408-99412, 99446-99449, 99451-99452, 99460, 99462-99463✦, 99474, 99483, 99497, 99605-99606, G0102, G0245-G0246, G0250, G0270-G0271, G0380-G0384, G0396-G0397, G0406-G0408, G0424-G0427, G0442-G0447, G0459, G0463, G0473, G0498, G0508-G0509, G2011

**99222** 0362T, 0373T, 0469T, 0543T-0544T, 0567T-0574T, 0580T, 0581T, 0582T, 0591T-0593T, 15774, 20560-20561, 20700-20701, 36591-36592, 43752, 62329, 80500-80502, 90863, 90940, 92002-92014, 92227-92228, 92531-92532, 93792, 93793, 94002-94004, 94644, 94660-94662, 95851-95852, 96020, 96105, 96116, 96125-96130, 96132, 96136, 96138, 96146, 96156-96159, 96164-96168, 96360, 96365, 96369, 96372-96374, 96377, 96401-96406, 96409, 96413, 96416, 96420-96422, 96425-96440, 96446-96450, 96523, 97151, 97153-97158, 97169-97172, 97802-97804, 99091, 99172-99173, 99174, 99177, 99184, 99202-99221, 99224-99233, 99238-99239, 99281-99285, 99304-99310, 99315-99318, 99324-99328, 99334-99337, 99341-99350, 99381-99404, 99408-99412, 99446-99449, 99451-99452, 99460, 99462-99463✦, 99474, 99479-99480, 99483, 99497, 99605-99606, G0102, G0245-G0246, G0250, G0270-G0271, G0380-G0384, G0396-G0397, G0406-G0408, G0424-G0427, G0442-G0447, G0459, G0463, G0473, G0498, G0508-G0509, G2011

**99223** 0362T, 0373T, 0469T, 0543T-0544T, 0567T-0574T, 0580T, 0581T, 0582T, 0591T-0593T, 15772, 15774, 20560-20561, 20700-20701, 36591-36592, 43752, 62329, 80500-80502, 90863, 90940, 92002-92014, 92227-92228, 92531-92532, 93792, 93793, 94002-94004, 94644, 94660-94662, 95851-95852, 96020, 96105, 96116, 96125-96130, 96132, 96136, 96138, 96146, 96156-96159, 96164-96168, 96360, 96365, 96369, 96372-96374, 96377, 96401-96406, 96409, 96413, 96416, 96420-96422, 96425-96440, 96446-96450, 96523, 97151, 97153-97158, 97169-97172, 97802-97804, 99091, 99172-99173, 99174, 99177, 99184, 99202-99222, 99224-99233, 99238-99239, 99281-99285, 99304-99310, 99315-99318, 99324-99328, 99334-99337, 99341-99350, 99381-99404, 99408-99412, 99446-99449, 99451-99452, 99460-99463✦, 99474, 99478-99480, 99483, 99497, 99605-99606, G0102, G0245-G0246, G0250, G0270-G0271, G0380-G0384, G0396-G0397, G0406-G0408, G0424-G0427, G0442-G0447, G0459, G0463, G0473, G0498, G0508-G0509, G2011

**99231** 0362T, 0373T, 0469T, 0543T-0544T, 0567T-0574T, 0580T, 0581T, 0582T, 20560-20561, 36591-36592, 43752, 80500-80502, 90863, 90940,

92002-92014, 92227-92228, 92531-92532, 93792, 93793, 94002-94004, 94644, 94660-94662, 95851-95852, 96020, 96105, 96116, 96125-96130, 96132, 96136, 96138, 96146, 96156-96159, 96164-96168, 96360, 96365, 96369, 96372-96374, 96377, 96401-96406, 96409, 96413, 96416, 96420-96422, 96425-96440, 96446-96450, 96523, 97151, 97153-97158, 97169-97172, 97802-97804, 99091, 99172-99173, 99174, 99177, 99184, 99281-99285, 99408-99409, 99446-99449, 99451-99452, 99474, 99605-99606, G0102, G0245-G0246, G0250, G0270-G0271, G0380-G0384, G0396-G0397, G0406-G0408, G0425-G0427, G0442-G0447, G0459, G0473, G0498, G0508-G0509, G2011

**99232** 0362T, 0373T, 0469T, 0543T-0544T, 0567T-0574T, 0580T, 0581T, 0582T, 20560-20561, 20701, 36591-36592, 43752, 80500-80502, 90863, 90940, 92002-92014, 92227-92228, 92531-92532, 93792, 93793, 94002-94004, 94644, 94660-94662, 95851-95852, 96020, 96105, 96116, 96125-96130, 96132, 96136, 96138, 96146, 96156-96159, 96164-96168, 96360, 96365, 96369, 96372-96374, 96377, 96401-96406, 96409, 96413, 96416, 96420-96422, 96425-96440, 96446-96450, 96523, 97151, 97153-97158, 97169-97172, 97802-97804, 99091, 99172-99173, 99174, 99177, 99184, 99231, 99281-99285, 99408-99409, 99446-99449, 99451-99452, 99462, 99474, 99605-99606, G0102, G0245-G0246, G0250, G0270-G0271, G0380-G0384, G0396-G0397, G0406-G0408, G0425-G0427, G0442-G0447, G0459, G0473, G0498, G0508-G0509, G2011

**99233** 0362T, 0373T, 0469T, 0543T-0544T, 0567T-0574T, 0580T, 0581T, 0582T, 20560-20561, 20700-20701, 36591-36592, 43752, 80500-80502, 90863, 90940, 92002-92014, 92227-92228, 92531-92532, 93792, 93793, 94002-94004, 94644, 94660-94662, 95851-95852, 96020, 96105, 96116, 96125-96130, 96132, 96136, 96138, 96146, 96156-96159, 96164-96168, 96360, 96365, 96369, 96372-96374, 96377, 96401-96406, 96409, 96413, 96416, 96420-96422, 96425-96440, 96446-96450, 96523, 97151, 97153-97158, 97169-97172, 97802-97804, 99091, 99172-99173, 99174, 99177, 99184, 99231-99232, 99281-99285, 99408-99409, 99446-99449, 99451-99452, 99460, 99462-99463❖, 99474, 99605-99606, G0102, G0245-G0246, G0250, G0270-G0271, G0380-G0384, G0396-G0397, G0406-G0408, G0425-G0427, G0442-G0447, G0459, G0473, G0498, G0508-G0509, G2011

**99238** 0362T, 0373T, 0469T, 0543T-0544T, 0567T-0574T, 0580T, 0581T, 0582T, 20560-20561, 20701, 36591-36592, 43752, 80500-80502, 90863, 90940, 92002-92014, 92227-92228, 92531-92532, 93792, 93793, 94002-94004, 94644, 94660-94662, 95851-95852, 96020, 96105, 96116, 96125-96130, 96132, 96136, 96138, 96146, 96156-96159, 96164-96168, 96360, 96365, 96369, 96372-96374, 96377, 96401-96406, 96409, 96413, 96416, 96420-96422, 96425-96440, 96446-96450, 96523, 97151, 97153-97158, 97169-97172, 97802-97804, 99091, 99172-99173, 99174, 99177, 99202-99217❖, 99231-99233, 99281-99285, 99408-99409, 99446-99449, 99451-99452, 99474, 99483, 99605-99606, G0102, G0245-G0246, G0250, G0270-G0271, G0380-G0384, G0396-G0397, G0442-G0447, G0459, G0463, G0473, G0498, G2011

**99239** 0362T, 0373T, 0469T, 0543T-0544T, 0567T-0574T, 0580T, 0581T, 0582T, 20560-20561, 20700-20701, 36591-36592, 43752, 80500-80502, 90863, 90940, 92002-92014, 92227-92228, 92531-92532, 93792, 93793, 94002-94004, 94644, 94660-94662, 95851-95852, 96020, 96105, 96116, 96125-96130, 96132, 96136, 96138, 96146, 96156-96159, 96164-96168, 96360, 96365, 96369, 96372-96374, 96377, 96401-96406, 96409, 96413, 96416, 96420-96422, 96425-96440, 96446-96450, 96523, 97151, 97153-97158, 97169-97172, 97802-97804, 99091, 99172-99173, 99174, 99177, 99202-99217❖, 99231-99233, 99238, 99281-99285, 99408-99409, 99446-99449, 99451-99452, 99474, 99483, 99605-99606, G0102, G0245-G0246, G0250, G0270-G0271, G0380-G0384, G0396-G0397, G0442-G0447, G0459, G0463, G0473, G0498, G2011

**99281** 0362T, 0373T, 0469T, 36591-36592, 43752, 90863, 90940, 92002-92014, 92227-92228, 92531-92532, 93792, 93793, 94002-94004, 94660-94662, 95851-95852, 96020, 96105, 96116, 96125-96130, 96132, 96136, 96138, 96146, 96156-96159, 96164-96168, 96360, 96365, 96369, 96372-96374, 96377, 96401-96406, 96409, 96413, 96416, 96420-96422, 96425-96440, 96446-96450, 96523, 97151, 97153-97158, 97169-97172, 97802-97804, 99091, 99172-99173, 99174, 99177, 99408-99409, 99446-99449, 99451-99452, 99474, 99605-99606, G0102, G0245-G0246, G0270-G0271, G0380❖, G0382-G0384❖, G0396-G0397, G0406-G0408, G0425-G0427, G0442-G0447, G0459, G0473, G0498, G0508-G0509, G2011

**99282** 0362T, 0373T, 0469T, 36591-36592, 43752, 90863, 90940, 92002-92014, 92227-92228, 92531-92532, 93792, 93793, 94002-94004, 94660-94662, 95851-95852, 96020, 96105, 96116, 96125-96130, 96132, 96136, 96138, 96146, 96156-96159, 96164-96168, 96360, 96365, 96369, 96372-96374, 96377, 96401-96406, 96409, 96413, 96416, 96420-96422, 96425-96440, 96446-96450, 96523, 97151, 97153-97158, 97169-97172, 97802-97804, 99091, 99172-99173, 99174, 99177, 99281, 99408-99409, 99446-99449, 99451-99452, 99474, 99605-99606, G0102, G0245-G0246, G0270-G0271, G0380-G0384❖, G0396-G0397, G0406-G0408, G0425-G0427, G0442-G0447, G0459, G0473, G0498, G0508-G0509, G2011

**99283** 0362T, 0373T, 0469T, 36591-36592, 43752, 90863, 90940, 92002-92014, 92227-92228, 92531-92532, 93792, 93793, 94002-94004, 94660-94662, 95851-95852, 96020, 96105, 96116, 96125-96130, 96132, 96136, 96138, 96146, 96156-96159, 96164-96168, 96360, 96365, 96369, 96372-96374, 96377, 96401-96406, 96409, 96413, 96416, 96420-96422, 96425-96440, 96446-96450, 96523, 97151, 97153-97158, 97169-97172, 97802-97804, 99091, 99172-99173, 99174, 99177, 99281-99282, 99408-99409, 99446-99449, 99451-99452, 99474, 99605-99606, G0102, G0245-G0246, G0270-G0271, G0380-G0384❖, G0396-G0397, G0406-G0408, G0425-G0427, G0442-G0447, G0459, G0473, G0498, G0508-G0509, G2011

**99284** 0362T, 0373T, 0469T, 36591-36592, 43752, 90863, 90940, 92002-92014, 92227-92228, 92531-92532, 93792, 93793, 94002-94004, 94660-94662, 95851-95852, 96020, 96105, 96116, 96125-96130, 96132, 96136, 96138, 96146, 96156-96159, 96164-96168, 96360, 96365, 96369, 96372-96374, 96377, 96401-96406, 96409, 96413, 96416, 96420-96422, 96425-96440, 96446-96450, 96523, 97151, 97153-97158, 97169-97172, 97802-97804, 99091, 99172-99173, 99174, 99177, 99281-99283, 99408-99409, 99446-99449, 99451-99452, 99463❖, 99474, 99605-99606, G0102, G0245-G0246, G0270-G0271, G0380-G0384❖, G0396-G0397, G0406-G0408, G0425-G0427, G0442-G0447, G0459, G0473, G0498, G0508-G0509, G2011

**99285** 0362T, 0373T, 0469T, 36591-36592, 43752, 90863, 90940, 92002-92014, 92227-92228, 92531-92532, 93792, 93793, 94002-94004, 94660-94662, 95851-95852, 96020, 96105, 96116, 96125-96130, 96132, 96136, 96138, 96146, 96156-96159, 96164-96168, 96360, 96365, 96369, 96372-96374, 96377, 96401-96406, 96409, 96413, 96416, 96420-96422, 96425-96440, 96446-96450, 96523, 97151, 97153-97158, 97169-97172, 97802-97804, 99091, 99172-99173, 99174, 99177, 99281-99284, 99408-99409, 99446-99449, 99451-99452, 99463❖, 99474, 99605-99606, G0102, G0245-G0246, G0270-G0271, G0380-G0384❖, G0396-G0397, G0406-G0408, G0425-G0427, G0442-G0447, G0459, G0473, G0498, G0508-G0509, G2011

**D0120** No CCI edits apply to this code.

**D0140** No CCI edits apply to this code.

**D0145** No CCI edits apply to this code.

**D0150** No CCI edits apply to this code.
**D0160** No CCI edits apply to this code.
**D0170** No CCI edits apply to this code.
**D0171** No CCI edits apply to this code.
**D0180** No CCI edits apply to this code.
**D0190** No CCI edits apply to this code.
**D0191** No CCI edits apply to this code.
**D0210** No CCI edits apply to this code.
**D0220** No CCI edits apply to this code.
**D0230** No CCI edits apply to this code.
**D0240** No CCI edits apply to this code.
**D0250** No CCI edits apply to this code.
**D0270** No CCI edits apply to this code.
**D0272** No CCI edits apply to this code.
**D0273** No CCI edits apply to this code.
**D0274** No CCI edits apply to this code.
**D0277** No CCI edits apply to this code.
**D0310** No CCI edits apply to this code.
**D0320** No CCI edits apply to this code.
**D0321** No CCI edits apply to this code.
**D0322** No CCI edits apply to this code.
**D0330** No CCI edits apply to this code.
**D0340** No CCI edits apply to this code.
**D0350** No CCI edits apply to this code.
**D0351** No CCI edits apply to this code.
**D0364** No CCI edits apply to this code.
**D0365** No CCI edits apply to this code.
**D0366** No CCI edits apply to this code.
**D0367** No CCI edits apply to this code.
**D0368** No CCI edits apply to this code.
**D0369** No CCI edits apply to this code.
**D0370** No CCI edits apply to this code.
**D0371** No CCI edits apply to this code.
**D0380** No CCI edits apply to this code.
**D0381** No CCI edits apply to this code.
**D0382** No CCI edits apply to this code.
**D0383** No CCI edits apply to this code.
**D0384** No CCI edits apply to this code.
**D0385** No CCI edits apply to this code.
**D0386** No CCI edits apply to this code.
**D0391** No CCI edits apply to this code.
**D0393** No CCI edits apply to this code.
**D0394** No CCI edits apply to this code.
**D0411** No CCI edits apply to this code.
**D0412** No CCI edits apply to this code.
**D0414** No CCI edits apply to this code.
**D0415** No CCI edits apply to this code.
**D0416** No CCI edits apply to this code.
**D0417** No CCI edits apply to this code.
**D0418** No CCI edits apply to this code.
**D0419** No CCI edits apply to this code.
**D0422** No CCI edits apply to this code.
**D0423** No CCI edits apply to this code.
**D0431** No CCI edits apply to this code.
**D0460** No CCI edits apply to this code.
**D0470** No CCI edits apply to this code.
**D0472** No CCI edits apply to this code.
**D0473** No CCI edits apply to this code.
**D0474** No CCI edits apply to this code.
**D0475** No CCI edits apply to this code.
**D0476** No CCI edits apply to this code.
**D0477** No CCI edits apply to this code.
**D0478** No CCI edits apply to this code.
**D0479** No CCI edits apply to this code.
**D0480** No CCI edits apply to this code.
**D0481** No CCI edits apply to this code.
**D0482** No CCI edits apply to this code.
**D0483** No CCI edits apply to this code.
**D0484** No CCI edits apply to this code.
**D0485** No CCI edits apply to this code.
**D0486** No CCI edits apply to this code.
**D0502** No CCI edits apply to this code.
**D0600** No CCI edits apply to this code.
**D0601** No CCI edits apply to this code.
**D0602** No CCI edits apply to this code.
**D0603** No CCI edits apply to this code.
**D0604** No CCI edits apply to this code.
**D0605** No CCI edits apply to this code.
**D0606** No CCI edits apply to this code.
**D0701** No CCI edits apply to this code.
**D0702** No CCI edits apply to this code.
**D0703** No CCI edits apply to this code.
**D0704** No CCI edits apply to this code.
**D0705** No CCI edits apply to this code.
**D0706** No CCI edits apply to this code.
**D0707** No CCI edits apply to this code.
**D0708** No CCI edits apply to this code.
**D0709** No CCI edits apply to this code.
**D1110** No CCI edits apply to this code.
**D1120** No CCI edits apply to this code.
**D1206** No CCI edits apply to this code.
**D1208** No CCI edits apply to this code.
**D1310** No CCI edits apply to this code.
**D1320** No CCI edits apply to this code.
**D1321** No CCI edits apply to this code.
**D1330** No CCI edits apply to this code.

**D1351** No CCI edits apply to this code.
**D1352** No CCI edits apply to this code.
**D1353** No CCI edits apply to this code.
**D1354** No CCI edits apply to this code.
**D1355** No CCI edits apply to this code.
**D1510** No CCI edits apply to this code.
**D1516** No CCI edits apply to this code.
**D1517** No CCI edits apply to this code.
**D1520** No CCI edits apply to this code.
**D1526** No CCI edits apply to this code.
**D1527** No CCI edits apply to this code.
**D1551** No CCI edits apply to this code.
**D1552** No CCI edits apply to this code.
**D1553** No CCI edits apply to this code.
**D1556** No CCI edits apply to this code.
**D1557** No CCI edits apply to this code.
**D1558** No CCI edits apply to this code.
**D1701** No CCI edits apply to this code.
**D1702** No CCI edits apply to this code.
**D1703** No CCI edits apply to this code.
**D1704** No CCI edits apply to this code.
**D1705** No CCI edits apply to this code.
**D1706** No CCI edits apply to this code.
**D1707** No CCI edits apply to this code.
**D2140** No CCI edits apply to this code.
**D2150** No CCI edits apply to this code.
**D2160** No CCI edits apply to this code.
**D2161** No CCI edits apply to this code.
**D2330** No CCI edits apply to this code.
**D2331** No CCI edits apply to this code.
**D2332** No CCI edits apply to this code.
**D2335** No CCI edits apply to this code.
**D2390** No CCI edits apply to this code.
**D2391** No CCI edits apply to this code.
**D2392** No CCI edits apply to this code.
**D2393** No CCI edits apply to this code.
**D2394** No CCI edits apply to this code.
**D2410** No CCI edits apply to this code.
**D2420** No CCI edits apply to this code.
**D2430** No CCI edits apply to this code.
**D2510** No CCI edits apply to this code.
**D2520** No CCI edits apply to this code.
**D2530** No CCI edits apply to this code.
**D2542** No CCI edits apply to this code.
**D2543** No CCI edits apply to this code.
**D2544** No CCI edits apply to this code.
**D2610** No CCI edits apply to this code.
**D2620** No CCI edits apply to this code.
**D2630** No CCI edits apply to this code.
**D2642** No CCI edits apply to this code.
**D2643** No CCI edits apply to this code.
**D2644** No CCI edits apply to this code.
**D2650** No CCI edits apply to this code.
**D2651** No CCI edits apply to this code.
**D2652** No CCI edits apply to this code.
**D2662** No CCI edits apply to this code.
**D2663** No CCI edits apply to this code.
**D2664** No CCI edits apply to this code.
**D2710** No CCI edits apply to this code.
**D2712** No CCI edits apply to this code.
**D2720** No CCI edits apply to this code.
**D2721** No CCI edits apply to this code.
**D2722** No CCI edits apply to this code.
**D2740** No CCI edits apply to this code.
**D2750** No CCI edits apply to this code.
**D2751** No CCI edits apply to this code.
**D2752** No CCI edits apply to this code.
**D2753** No CCI edits apply to this code.
**D2780** No CCI edits apply to this code.
**D2781** No CCI edits apply to this code.
**D2782** No CCI edits apply to this code.
**D2783** No CCI edits apply to this code.
**D2790** No CCI edits apply to this code.
**D2791** No CCI edits apply to this code.
**D2792** No CCI edits apply to this code.
**D2794** No CCI edits apply to this code.
**D2799** No CCI edits apply to this code.
**D2910** No CCI edits apply to this code.
**D2915** No CCI edits apply to this code.
**D2920** No CCI edits apply to this code.
**D2921** No CCI edits apply to this code.
**D2928** No CCI edits apply to this code.
**D2929** No CCI edits apply to this code.
**D2930** No CCI edits apply to this code.
**D2931** No CCI edits apply to this code.
**D2932** No CCI edits apply to this code.
**D2933** No CCI edits apply to this code.
**D2934** No CCI edits apply to this code.
**D2940** No CCI edits apply to this code.
**D2941** No CCI edits apply to this code.
**D2950** No CCI edits apply to this code.
**D2951** No CCI edits apply to this code.
**D2952** No CCI edits apply to this code.
**D2953** No CCI edits apply to this code.
**D2954** No CCI edits apply to this code.
**D2955** No CCI edits apply to this code.

**D2957** No CCI edits apply to this code.
**D2960** No CCI edits apply to this code.
**D2961** No CCI edits apply to this code.
**D2962** No CCI edits apply to this code.
**D2971** No CCI edits apply to this code.
**D2975** No CCI edits apply to this code.
**D2980** No CCI edits apply to this code.
**D2981** No CCI edits apply to this code.
**D2982** No CCI edits apply to this code.
**D2983** No CCI edits apply to this code.
**D2990** No CCI edits apply to this code.
**D3110** No CCI edits apply to this code.
**D3120** No CCI edits apply to this code.
**D3220** No CCI edits apply to this code.
**D3221** No CCI edits apply to this code.
**D3222** No CCI edits apply to this code.
**D3230** No CCI edits apply to this code.
**D3240** No CCI edits apply to this code.
**D3310** No CCI edits apply to this code.
**D3320** No CCI edits apply to this code.
**D3330** No CCI edits apply to this code.
**D3331** No CCI edits apply to this code.
**D3332** No CCI edits apply to this code.
**D3333** No CCI edits apply to this code.
**D3346** No CCI edits apply to this code.
**D3347** No CCI edits apply to this code.
**D3348** No CCI edits apply to this code.
**D3351** No CCI edits apply to this code.
**D3352** No CCI edits apply to this code.
**D3353** No CCI edits apply to this code.
**D3355** No CCI edits apply to this code.
**D3356** No CCI edits apply to this code.
**D3357** No CCI edits apply to this code.
**D3410** No CCI edits apply to this code.
**D3421** No CCI edits apply to this code.
**D3425** No CCI edits apply to this code.
**D3426** No CCI edits apply to this code.
**D3430** No CCI edits apply to this code.
**D3450** No CCI edits apply to this code.
**D3460** No CCI edits apply to this code.
**D3470** No CCI edits apply to this code.
**D3471** No CCI edits apply to this code.
**D3472** No CCI edits apply to this code.
**D3473** No CCI edits apply to this code.
**D3501** No CCI edits apply to this code.
**D3502** No CCI edits apply to this code.
**D3503** No CCI edits apply to this code.
**D3910** No CCI edits apply to this code.
**D3911** No CCI edits apply to this code.
**D3920** No CCI edits apply to this code.
**D3921** No CCI edits apply to this code.
**D3950** No CCI edits apply to this code.
**D4210** No CCI edits apply to this code.
**D4211** No CCI edits apply to this code.
**D4212** No CCI edits apply to this code.
**D4230** No CCI edits apply to this code.
**D4231** No CCI edits apply to this code.
**D4240** No CCI edits apply to this code.
**D4241** No CCI edits apply to this code.
**D4245** No CCI edits apply to this code.
**D4249** No CCI edits apply to this code.
**D4260** No CCI edits apply to this code.
**D4261** No CCI edits apply to this code.
**D4263** No CCI edits apply to this code.
**D4264** No CCI edits apply to this code.
**D4265** No CCI edits apply to this code.
**D4266** No CCI edits apply to this code.
**D4267** No CCI edits apply to this code.
**D4268** No CCI edits apply to this code.
**D4270** No CCI edits apply to this code.
**D4273** No CCI edits apply to this code.
**D4274** No CCI edits apply to this code.
**D4275** No CCI edits apply to this code.
**D4276** No CCI edits apply to this code.
**D4277** No CCI edits apply to this code.
**D4278** No CCI edits apply to this code.
**D4283** No CCI edits apply to this code.
**D4285** No CCI edits apply to this code.
**D4322** No CCI edits apply to this code.
**D4323** No CCI edits apply to this code.
**D4341** No CCI edits apply to this code.
**D4342** No CCI edits apply to this code.
**D4346** No CCI edits apply to this code.
**D4355** No CCI edits apply to this code.
**D4381** No CCI edits apply to this code.
**D4910** No CCI edits apply to this code.
**D4920** No CCI edits apply to this code.
**D4921** No CCI edits apply to this code.
**D5110** No CCI edits apply to this code.
**D5120** No CCI edits apply to this code.
**D5130** No CCI edits apply to this code.
**D5140** No CCI edits apply to this code.
**D5211** No CCI edits apply to this code.
**D5212** No CCI edits apply to this code.
**D5213** No CCI edits apply to this code.
**D5214** No CCI edits apply to this code.

**D5221** No CCI edits apply to this code.
**D5222** No CCI edits apply to this code.
**D5223** No CCI edits apply to this code.
**D5224** No CCI edits apply to this code.
**D5225** No CCI edits apply to this code.
**D5226** No CCI edits apply to this code.
**D5227** No CCI edits apply to this code.
**D5228** No CCI edits apply to this code.
**D5282** No CCI edits apply to this code.
**D5283** No CCI edits apply to this code.
**D5284** No CCI edits apply to this code.
**D5286** No CCI edits apply to this code.
**D5410** No CCI edits apply to this code.
**D5411** No CCI edits apply to this code.
**D5421** No CCI edits apply to this code.
**D5422** No CCI edits apply to this code.
**D5511** No CCI edits apply to this code.
**D5512** No CCI edits apply to this code.
**D5520** No CCI edits apply to this code.
**D5611** No CCI edits apply to this code.
**D5612** No CCI edits apply to this code.
**D5621** No CCI edits apply to this code.
**D5622** No CCI edits apply to this code.
**D5630** No CCI edits apply to this code.
**D5640** No CCI edits apply to this code.
**D5650** No CCI edits apply to this code.
**D5660** No CCI edits apply to this code.
**D5670** No CCI edits apply to this code.
**D5671** No CCI edits apply to this code.
**D5710** No CCI edits apply to this code.
**D5711** No CCI edits apply to this code.
**D5720** No CCI edits apply to this code.
**D5721** No CCI edits apply to this code.
**D5725** No CCI edits apply to this code.
**D5730** No CCI edits apply to this code.
**D5731** No CCI edits apply to this code.
**D5740** No CCI edits apply to this code.
**D5741** No CCI edits apply to this code.
**D5750** No CCI edits apply to this code.
**D5751** No CCI edits apply to this code.
**D5760** No CCI edits apply to this code.
**D5761** No CCI edits apply to this code.
**D5765** No CCI edits apply to this code.
**D5810** No CCI edits apply to this code.
**D5811** No CCI edits apply to this code.
**D5820** No CCI edits apply to this code.
**D5821** No CCI edits apply to this code.
**D5850** No CCI edits apply to this code.
**D5851** No CCI edits apply to this code.
**D5862** No CCI edits apply to this code.
**D5863** No CCI edits apply to this code.
**D5864** No CCI edits apply to this code.
**D5865** No CCI edits apply to this code.
**D5866** No CCI edits apply to this code.
**D5867** No CCI edits apply to this code.
**D5876** No CCI edits apply to this code.
**D5931** No CCI edits apply to this code.
**D5932** No CCI edits apply to this code.
**D5936** No CCI edits apply to this code.
**D5937** No CCI edits apply to this code.
**D5952** No CCI edits apply to this code.
**D5953** No CCI edits apply to this code.
**D5954** No CCI edits apply to this code.
**D5955** No CCI edits apply to this code.
**D5958** No CCI edits apply to this code.
**D5959** No CCI edits apply to this code.
**D5960** No CCI edits apply to this code.
**D5982** No CCI edits apply to this code.
**D5986** No CCI edits apply to this code.
**D5987** No CCI edits apply to this code.
**D5988** No CCI edits apply to this code.
**D5991** No CCI edits apply to this code.
**D5992** No CCI edits apply to this code.
**D5993** No CCI edits apply to this code.
**D5995** No CCI edits apply to this code.
**D5996** No CCI edits apply to this code.
**D6010** No CCI edits apply to this code.
**D6012** No CCI edits apply to this code.
**D6013** No CCI edits apply to this code.
**D6040** No CCI edits apply to this code.
**D6050** No CCI edits apply to this code.
**D6051** No CCI edits apply to this code.
**D6055** No CCI edits apply to this code.
**D6056** No CCI edits apply to this code.
**D6057** No CCI edits apply to this code.
**D6058** No CCI edits apply to this code.
**D6059** No CCI edits apply to this code.
**D6060** No CCI edits apply to this code.
**D6061** No CCI edits apply to this code.
**D6062** No CCI edits apply to this code.
**D6063** No CCI edits apply to this code.
**D6064** No CCI edits apply to this code.
**D6065** No CCI edits apply to this code.
**D6066** No CCI edits apply to this code.
**D6067** No CCI edits apply to this code.
**D6068** No CCI edits apply to this code.

**D6069** No CCI edits apply to this code.
**D6070** No CCI edits apply to this code.
**D6071** No CCI edits apply to this code.
**D6072** No CCI edits apply to this code.
**D6073** No CCI edits apply to this code.
**D6074** No CCI edits apply to this code.
**D6075** No CCI edits apply to this code.
**D6076** No CCI edits apply to this code.
**D6077** No CCI edits apply to this code.
**D6080** No CCI edits apply to this code.
**D6081** No CCI edits apply to this code.
**D6082** No CCI edits apply to this code.
**D6083** No CCI edits apply to this code.
**D6084** No CCI edits apply to this code.
**D6085** No CCI edits apply to this code.
**D6086** No CCI edits apply to this code.
**D6087** No CCI edits apply to this code.
**D6088** No CCI edits apply to this code.
**D6090** No CCI edits apply to this code.
**D6091** No CCI edits apply to this code.
**D6092** No CCI edits apply to this code.
**D6093** No CCI edits apply to this code.
**D6094** No CCI edits apply to this code.
**D6095** No CCI edits apply to this code.
**D6096** No CCI edits apply to this code.
**D6097** No CCI edits apply to this code.
**D6098** No CCI edits apply to this code.
**D6099** No CCI edits apply to this code.
**D6100** No CCI edits apply to this code.
**D6101** No CCI edits apply to this code.
**D6102** No CCI edits apply to this code.
**D6103** No CCI edits apply to this code.
**D6104** No CCI edits apply to this code.
**D6110** No CCI edits apply to this code.
**D6111** No CCI edits apply to this code.
**D6112** No CCI edits apply to this code.
**D6113** No CCI edits apply to this code.
**D6114** No CCI edits apply to this code.
**D6115** No CCI edits apply to this code.
**D6116** No CCI edits apply to this code.
**D6117** No CCI edits apply to this code.
**D6118** No CCI edits apply to this code.
**D6119** No CCI edits apply to this code.
**D6120** No CCI edits apply to this code.
**D6121** No CCI edits apply to this code.
**D6122** No CCI edits apply to this code.
**D6123** No CCI edits apply to this code.
**D6190** No CCI edits apply to this code.
**D6191** No CCI edits apply to this code.
**D6192** No CCI edits apply to this code.
**D6194** No CCI edits apply to this code.
**D6195** No CCI edits apply to this code.
**D6198** No CCI edits apply to this code.
**D6205** No CCI edits apply to this code.
**D6210** No CCI edits apply to this code.
**D6211** No CCI edits apply to this code.
**D6212** No CCI edits apply to this code.
**D6214** No CCI edits apply to this code.
**D6240** No CCI edits apply to this code.
**D6241** No CCI edits apply to this code.
**D6242** No CCI edits apply to this code.
**D6243** No CCI edits apply to this code.
**D6245** No CCI edits apply to this code.
**D6250** No CCI edits apply to this code.
**D6251** No CCI edits apply to this code.
**D6252** No CCI edits apply to this code.
**D6253** No CCI edits apply to this code.
**D6545** No CCI edits apply to this code.
**D6548** No CCI edits apply to this code.
**D6549** No CCI edits apply to this code.
**D6600** No CCI edits apply to this code.
**D6601** No CCI edits apply to this code.
**D6602** No CCI edits apply to this code.
**D6603** No CCI edits apply to this code.
**D6604** No CCI edits apply to this code.
**D6605** No CCI edits apply to this code.
**D6606** No CCI edits apply to this code.
**D6607** No CCI edits apply to this code.
**D6608** No CCI edits apply to this code.
**D6609** No CCI edits apply to this code.
**D6610** No CCI edits apply to this code.
**D6611** No CCI edits apply to this code.
**D6612** No CCI edits apply to this code.
**D6613** No CCI edits apply to this code.
**D6614** No CCI edits apply to this code.
**D6615** No CCI edits apply to this code.
**D6624** No CCI edits apply to this code.
**D6634** No CCI edits apply to this code.
**D6710** No CCI edits apply to this code.
**D6720** No CCI edits apply to this code.
**D6721** No CCI edits apply to this code.
**D6722** No CCI edits apply to this code.
**D6740** No CCI edits apply to this code.
**D6750** No CCI edits apply to this code.
**D6751** No CCI edits apply to this code.
**D6752** No CCI edits apply to this code.

**D6753** No CCI edits apply to this code.
**D6780** No CCI edits apply to this code.
**D6781** No CCI edits apply to this code.
**D6782** No CCI edits apply to this code.
**D6783** No CCI edits apply to this code.
**D6784** No CCI edits apply to this code.
**D6790** No CCI edits apply to this code.
**D6791** No CCI edits apply to this code.
**D6792** No CCI edits apply to this code.
**D6793** No CCI edits apply to this code.
**D6794** No CCI edits apply to this code.
**D6920** No CCI edits apply to this code.
**D6930** No CCI edits apply to this code.
**D6940** No CCI edits apply to this code.
**D6950** No CCI edits apply to this code.
**D6980** No CCI edits apply to this code.
**D6985** No CCI edits apply to this code.
**D7111** No CCI edits apply to this code.
**D7140** No CCI edits apply to this code.
**D7210** No CCI edits apply to this code.
**D7220** No CCI edits apply to this code.
**D7230** No CCI edits apply to this code.
**D7240** No CCI edits apply to this code.
**D7241** No CCI edits apply to this code.
**D7250** No CCI edits apply to this code.
**D7251** No CCI edits apply to this code.
**D7260** No CCI edits apply to this code.
**D7261** No CCI edits apply to this code.
**D7270** No CCI edits apply to this code.
**D7272** No CCI edits apply to this code.
**D7280** No CCI edits apply to this code.
**D7282** No CCI edits apply to this code.
**D7283** No CCI edits apply to this code.
**D7285** No CCI edits apply to this code.
**D7286** No CCI edits apply to this code.
**D7287** No CCI edits apply to this code.
**D7288** No CCI edits apply to this code.
**D7290** No CCI edits apply to this code.
**D7291** No CCI edits apply to this code.
**D7292** No CCI edits apply to this code.
**D7293** No CCI edits apply to this code.
**D7294** No CCI edits apply to this code.
**D7296** No CCI edits apply to this code.
**D7297** No CCI edits apply to this code.
**D7298** No CCI edits apply to this code.
**D7299** No CCI edits apply to this code.
**D7300** No CCI edits apply to this code.
**D7310** No CCI edits apply to this code.
**D7311** No CCI edits apply to this code.
**D7320** No CCI edits apply to this code.
**D7321** No CCI edits apply to this code.
**D7340** No CCI edits apply to this code.
**D7350** No CCI edits apply to this code.
**D7410** No CCI edits apply to this code.
**D7411** No CCI edits apply to this code.
**D7412** No CCI edits apply to this code.
**D7413** No CCI edits apply to this code.
**D7414** No CCI edits apply to this code.
**D7415** No CCI edits apply to this code.
**D7440** No CCI edits apply to this code.
**D7441** No CCI edits apply to this code.
**D7450** No CCI edits apply to this code.
**D7451** No CCI edits apply to this code.
**D7460** No CCI edits apply to this code.
**D7461** No CCI edits apply to this code.
**D7465** No CCI edits apply to this code.
**D7471** No CCI edits apply to this code.
**D7472** No CCI edits apply to this code.
**D7473** No CCI edits apply to this code.
**D7485** No CCI edits apply to this code.
**D7490** No CCI edits apply to this code.
**D7510** No CCI edits apply to this code.
**D7511** No CCI edits apply to this code.
**D7520** No CCI edits apply to this code.
**D7521** No CCI edits apply to this code.
**D7530** No CCI edits apply to this code.
**D7540** No CCI edits apply to this code.
**D7550** No CCI edits apply to this code.
**D7560** No CCI edits apply to this code.
**D7840** No CCI edits apply to this code.
**D7880** No CCI edits apply to this code.
**D7881** No CCI edits apply to this code.
**D7899** No CCI edits apply to this code.
**D7910** No CCI edits apply to this code.
**D7911** No CCI edits apply to this code.
**D7912** No CCI edits apply to this code.
**D7920** No CCI edits apply to this code.
**D7921** No CCI edits apply to this code.
**D7922** No CCI edits apply to this code.
**D7941** No CCI edits apply to this code.
**D7943** No CCI edits apply to this code.
**D7944** No CCI edits apply to this code.
**D7945** No CCI edits apply to this code.
**D7953** No CCI edits apply to this code.
**D7955** No CCI edits apply to this code.
**D7961** No CCI edits apply to this code.

**D7962** No CCI edits apply to this code.
**D7970** No CCI edits apply to this code.
**D7971** No CCI edits apply to this code.
**D7972** No CCI edits apply to this code.
**D7979** No CCI edits apply to this code.
**D7981** No CCI edits apply to this code.
**D7982** No CCI edits apply to this code.
**D7983** No CCI edits apply to this code.
**D7990** No CCI edits apply to this code.
**D7991** No CCI edits apply to this code.
**D7993** No CCI edits apply to this code.
**D7994** No CCI edits apply to this code.
**D7995** No CCI edits apply to this code.
**D7996** No CCI edits apply to this code.
**D7997** No CCI edits apply to this code.
**D7998** No CCI edits apply to this code.
**D8010** No CCI edits apply to this code.
**D8020** No CCI edits apply to this code.
**D8030** No CCI edits apply to this code.
**D8040** No CCI edits apply to this code.
**D8070** No CCI edits apply to this code.
**D8080** No CCI edits apply to this code.
**D8090** No CCI edits apply to this code.
**D8210** No CCI edits apply to this code.
**D8220** No CCI edits apply to this code.
**D8660** No CCI edits apply to this code.
**D8670** No CCI edits apply to this code.
**D8680** No CCI edits apply to this code.
**D8681** No CCI edits apply to this code.
**D8695** No CCI edits apply to this code.
**D8696** No CCI edits apply to this code.
**D8697** No CCI edits apply to this code.
**D8698** No CCI edits apply to this code.
**D8699** No CCI edits apply to this code.
**D8701** No CCI edits apply to this code.
**D8702** No CCI edits apply to this code.
**D8703** No CCI edits apply to this code.
**D8704** No CCI edits apply to this code.
**D9110** No CCI edits apply to this code.
**D9120** No CCI edits apply to this code.
**D9130** No CCI edits apply to this code.
**D9210** No CCI edits apply to this code.
**D9211** No CCI edits apply to this code.
**D9212** No CCI edits apply to this code.
**D9215** No CCI edits apply to this code.
**D9219** No CCI edits apply to this code.
**D9222** No CCI edits apply to this code.
**D9223** No CCI edits apply to this code.
**D9230** No CCI edits apply to this code.
**D9239** No CCI edits apply to this code.
**D9243** No CCI edits apply to this code.
**D9248** No CCI edits apply to this code.
**D9310** No CCI edits apply to this code.
**D9311** No CCI edits apply to this code.
**D9410** No CCI edits apply to this code.
**D9420** No CCI edits apply to this code.
**D9430** No CCI edits apply to this code.
**D9440** No CCI edits apply to this code.
**D9450** No CCI edits apply to this code.
**D9610** No CCI edits apply to this code.
**D9612** No CCI edits apply to this code.
**D9613** No CCI edits apply to this code.
**D9910** No CCI edits apply to this code.
**D9911** No CCI edits apply to this code.
**D9912** No CCI edits apply to this code.
**D9920** No CCI edits apply to this code.
**D9930** No CCI edits apply to this code.
**D9932** No CCI edits apply to this code.
**D9933** No CCI edits apply to this code.
**D9934** No CCI edits apply to this code.
**D9935** No CCI edits apply to this code.
**D9941** No CCI edits apply to this code.
**D9942** No CCI edits apply to this code.
**D9943** No CCI edits apply to this code.
**D9944** No CCI edits apply to this code.
**D9945** No CCI edits apply to this code.
**D9946** No CCI edits apply to this code.
**D9947** No CCI edits apply to this code.
**D9948** No CCI edits apply to this code.
**D9949** No CCI edits apply to this code.
**D9950** No CCI edits apply to this code.
**D9951** No CCI edits apply to this code.
**D9952** No CCI edits apply to this code.
**D9961** No CCI edits apply to this code.
**D9970** No CCI edits apply to this code.
**D9971** No CCI edits apply to this code.
**D9972** No CCI edits apply to this code.
**D9973** No CCI edits apply to this code.
**D9974** No CCI edits apply to this code.
**D9986** No CCI edits apply to this code.
**D9987** No CCI edits apply to this code.
**D9990** No CCI edits apply to this code.
**D9991** No CCI edits apply to this code.
**D9992** No CCI edits apply to this code.
**D9993** No CCI edits apply to this code.
**D9994** No CCI edits apply to this code.

**D9995** No CCI edits apply to this code.

**D9996** No CCI edits apply to this code.

# Dental Code Index


## A

- **Abscess, incision and drainage**, D7510-D7521
- **Abutments**
  - for implants, D6051, D6056-D6057
  - retainers for resin bonded "Maryland bridge", D6545-D6549
- **Accession of brush biopsy sample**, D0486
- **Accession of tissue**, D0472-D0474
- **Adjunctive services**, D0431, D9110-D9613, D9910-D9974, D9986-D9997
- **Adjustment**
  - complete denture
    - mandibular, D5411
    - maxillary, D5410
  - maxillofacial prosthetic appliance, D5992
  - occlusal, D9951-D9952
  - partial denture
    - mandibular, D5422
    - maxillary, D5421
  - retainer, D8681
- **Allograft**
  - maxillofacial, D7955
  - soft dental tissue, D4275-D4285
- **Alveoloplasty**
  - with extraction(s), D7310-D7311
  - without extractions, D7320-D7321
- **Amalgam, restoration**, D2140-D2161
- **Ambulatory surgical center call**, D9420
- **Analgesia**, D9210-D9248
- **Analysis**
  - saliva sample, D0418
- **Anesthesia**, D9210-D9248
  - block
    - regional, D9211
    - trigeminal, D9212
  - deep or general, each 15 minutes, D9223
  - evaluation, deep or general, D9219
  - intravenous moderate sedation, each 15 minutes, D9243
  - local
    - in conjunction with surgical procedures, D9215
    - not in conjunction with surgical procedures, D9210
  - nitrous oxide inhalation, D9230
  - nonintravenous moderate sedation, D9248
- **Antibody testing**, D0605
- **Antigen testing**, D0604
- **Antimicrobial delivery device**
  - crevicular tissue, D4381
- **Apexification, dental**, D3351-D3353
- **Apexogenesis**, D3222
- **Apicoectomy, dental**, D3410-D3426
- **Appliance**
  - orthodontic
    - fixed, D8220
    - removable, D8210
    - removal, D7997
  - removal by different provider, D7997
  - sleep apnea, custom, D9947-D9949
- **Application**
  - fluoride, D1206-D1208
- **Appointment**
  - canceled, D9987
  - missed, D9986
- **Assessment**
  - saliva, D0419
- **Autologous blood concentrate**, D7921

## B

- **Barrier, intraorifice**, D3911
- **Behavior management, dental care**, D9942-D9946
- **Biologic dressing, intra-socket**, D7922
- **Biologic materials, dental**, D4265
- **Biological dressing, intrasocket**, D7922
- **Biopsy**
  - hard tissue, dental, D7285
  - soft tissue, dental, D7286
  - transepithelial brush, D7288
- **Bitewings**, D0270-D0277
- **Bleaching, dental**
  - external, per arch, D9972
  - external, per tooth, D9973
  - internal, per tooth, D9974
- **Blood glucose testing**, D0412
  - HbA1c, D0411
- **Bone**
  - replacement graft, D7953
  - tissue excision, D7471-D7490
- **Bridge**
  - crowns, D6710-D6794
  - implant/abutment supported, D6068-D6077, D6098-D6099, D6120-D6123, D6194-D6195
  - inlay/onlay, D6600-D6634
  - pediatric, D6985
  - pontics, D6205-D6253
  - recementation, D6930
  - repair, D6980
  - resin bonded, D6545-D6549
  - sectioning, D9120
- **Bruxism appliance**, D9942-D9946

## C

- **Caries**
  - application of inhibiting medication, D1354-D1355
  - assessment, risk, D0601-D0603
- **Carrier**
  - fluoride gel, D5986
  - medicament, periodontal, D5995-D5996
  - pharmaceutical
    - periodontal, D1355
    - vesiculobolus, D5991
- **Case**
  - management, D9991-D9994, D9997
    - special needs, D9997
  - presentation, D9450
- **Cast**
  - diagnostic, D0470
  - post and core, D2952-D2953
- **CAT scan, cone beam**
  - image and interpreation, D0364-D0368
  - image only, D0380-D0384
  - interpretation and report, D0391
  - post-processing imaging, D0393-D0394
- **Change in tooth structure, diagnostic**, D0600
- **Cleaning, removable denture**
  - full, D9932-D9933
  - partial, D9934-D9935
- **Closure**
  - oroantral fistula, D7260
  - sinus perforation, D7261
- **Collection**
  - autologous blood, D7921
  - for culture and sensitivity
    - microorganisms, D0415
    - viral, D0416
  - genetic sample, D0422
  - saliva samples, D0417
- **Combined connective tissue and pedicle graft, dental**, D4276
- **Complications, postoperative**, D9930
- **Composite, resin based**, D2330-D2394
- **Condylectomy**, D7840
- **Connector bar**
  - dental implant, supported, D6055
  - fixed partial denture, D6920
- **Conscious sedation, dental**, D9230-D9248
- **Consultation**
  - slides prepared elsewhere, D0484
  - with prep of slides, D0485
- **Coping**, D2975
- **Core buildup, including pins**, D2950
- **Coronavirus testing**, D0604-D0606
- **Coronectomy, intentional**, D7251
- **Coronoidectomy,**, D7991
- **Corticotomy**, D7296-D7297
- **Counseling, disease prevention**, D1310-D1321
- **Crevicular tissue**
  - antimicrobial delivery device, D4381
- **Crown**
  - abutment supported, D6058-D6064, D6094, D6097
    - implant supported prosthetics, D6065-D6067
    - retainer for FPD, D6068-D6077, D6098-D6099, D6120-D6123, D6194-D6195, D6710-D6792, D6794
  - additional construction, partial denture framework, D2971
  - as retainer for FPD, D6068-D6077, D6194, D6710-D6792, D6794
  - base metal, D2721, D2751, D2781, D2791
  - composite resin, D2390
  - high noble metal, D2720, D2780, D2790
  - implant supported, D6065-D6067, D6082-D6084, D6086-D6088
  - indirect resin based composite, D6710
  - individual restoration, D2710-D2794
  - interim, D2799, D6793
  - lengthening, D4249
  - noble metal, D2722, D2752, D2782, D2792
  - other single tooth restoration, D2710-D2799
    - coping, D2975
    - core buildup, D2950
    - pin retention, D2951
    - post and core, D2952-D2954
    - post removal, D2955-D2957
    - protective, D2940
    - reattach tooth fragment, D2921
    - recement/rebond, D2910-D2920
    - repair, D2980-D2983
    - resin, D2932
      - infiltration of lesion, D2990
    - stainless steel, D2930-D2931, D2933-D2934
    - veneer, D2960-D2962
  - porcelain/ceramic, D2710-D2752, D2783
  - prefabricated, D2928-D2933
  - recementation, D2920
  - repair, D2980
  - resin with metal, D2720-D2722
  - resin-based composite, D2710-D2712
  - retainer, D6710-D6793
  - stainless steel, D2934
  - titanium, D2794, D6794
- **Culture and sensitivity**, D0414-D0415
- **Culture, viral**, D0416
- **Curettage**, D4240-D4241, D4341-D4342
- **Cyst**
  - destruction, soft tissue lesions, D7465
  - excision, intra-osseous leisons, D7440-D7461
  - excision, soft tissue lesions, D7410-D7415
- **Cytologic**
  - sample collection, D7287
  - smears, D0480

## D

- **Debridement**
  - endodontic, D3221
  - periodontal, D4355
    - implant
      - peri, D6101-D6102
      - single, D6081
- **Decalcification procedure**, D0475
- **Decoronation erupted tooth**, D3921
- **Dentures**
  - complete, D5110-D5120
    - adjustment, D5410-D5422
    - immediate, D5130-D5140
    - implant/abutment supported, D6110-D6111, D6114-D6115
    - interim, D5810-D5811
    - rebase, D5710, D5720
    - reline
      - direct, D5730-D5731
      - indirect, D5750-D5751
    - repair, D5511-D5520
- **Dentures** — *continued*
  - interim
    - implant/abutment supported, D6118-D6119
  - overdenture, D5863-D5866
  - partial
    - implant/abutment supported, D6068-D6077, D6098-D6099, D6120-D6123, D6194-D6195
    - interim, D5820-D5821
    - lower, D5212, D5214, D5222, D5224, D5226-D5227
    - pontics, fixed, D6205-D6253
    - rebase, D5711, D5721-D5725
    - reline
      - direct, D5740-D5741
      - indirect, D5760-D5761
    - removal, D5282-D5286
    - repair, D5611-D5671
    - retainers, fixed, D6545-D6794
    - sectioning, fixed, D9120
    - upper, D5211, D5213, D5221, D5223, D5225, D5228
  - rebase, hybrid prosthesis, D5725
  - soft liner for removable denture, D5765
- **Desensitizing medicine**, D9910
- **Desensitizing resin**, D9911
- **Destruction of lesion**, D7465
- **Device placement**
  - eruption impacted tooth aid, D7283
  - temporary anchorage, D7294
- **Diagnostic services**, D0120-D0250, D0270-D0394, D0411-D0423, D0431-D0502
  - casts, models, D0470
  - radiology services, D0210-D0250, D0270-D0391
- **Dietary planning, dental nutrition**, D1310
- **Discoloration removal**, D9970
  - bleaching, D9972-D9974
- **Dressing change, periodontal**
  - unscheduled, D4920
- **Dressing, intrasocket biological**, D7922
- **Drugs** — *see* Table of Drugs
  - parenteral administration
    - single drug, D9610
    - two or more drugs, D9612
  - sustained release infiltration
    - for pain control, D9613
- **Dry socket, localized osteitis**, D9930

## E

- **Electron microscopy - diagnostic**, D0481
- **Emergency**
  - treatment, D0140, D9110
- **Enamel microabrasion**, D9970
- **Enameloplasty**, D9971
- **Endodontic procedures**, D3110-D3426, D3430, D3450-D3950
  - apexification/recalcification, D3351-D3353
  - apiocoectomy, periradicular, D3410-D3426, D3430, D3450-D3470
    - endosseous implant, D3460
    - filling, retrograde, D3430
    - intentional implantation, D3470
    - root amputation, D3450
  - decoronation/submergence erupted tooth, D3921
  - hemisection, D3920
  - intraorifice barrier, D3911
  - isolation with rubber dam, D3910
  - preparation, canal, D3950
  - pulp capping, D3110-D3120
  - pulpotomy, D3220-D3222
  - regeneration, D3355-D3357
  - resorbable filling, D3230-D3240
  - retreatment, D3346-D3348
  - root resorption
    - surgical repair, D3471-D3473
  - surgical exposure root surface, D3501-D3503
  - therapy, tooth
    - anterior, D3310

**Endodontic procedures** — *continued*
therapy, tooth — *continued*
bicuspid, D3320
incomplete, D3332
molar, D3330
perforation defect, D3333
root canal obstruction, D3331
**Equilibration, dental**, D9951-D9952
**Eruption, tooth**
device placement for impacted tooth, D7283
exposure, unerupted tooth, D7280
surgical mobilization, D7282
**Evaluation**
dental, D0120-D0180
**Evaluation**, D0120-D0180
fo pre-orthodontic treatment, D8660
**Examination**
brush biopsy sample, D0486
exfoliative smears, D0480
oral, D0120-D0160, D8660
tissue, gross and microscopic, D0472-D0474
**Excision**
hyperplastic tissue, D7970
lesion
benign, D7410-D7412
malignant, D7413-D7441
pericoronal gingiva, D7971
salivary gland, D7981
**Exostosis (tuberosity) removal**
lateral, D7471
osseous tuberosity, D7485
reduction of fibrous tuberosity, D7972
torus
mandibularis, D7473
palatinus, D7472
**Exposure**
anatomical crown, D4230-D4231
unerupted tooth, D7280
**Extractions**, D7111-D7140
surgical, D7210-D7250
**Extraoral films**, D0250, D0310-D0391

## F

**Facial bone radiographic survey**, D0250
2D oral/facial, D0350
**Fiberotomy, dental, transeptal**, D7291
**Fibroma excision**, D7410-D7412
**Film/radiograph**, D0210-D0250, D0270-D0391
radiographic, dental, D0210-D0250, D0270-D0340
**Fissurotomy**, D9971
**Fistula**
oroantral, D7260
salivary, D7983
**Fixation device, not fracture related**, D7998
**Fixed partial dentures (bridges), retainers**
crowns, D6710-D6794
implant/abutment support, D6068-D6077, D6194
inlay/onlay, D6600-D6634
pediatric, D6985
pontics, D6205-D6253
recementation, D6930
repair, D6980
resin bonded, D6545-D6549
sectioning, D9120
**Flap, gingival**, D4240-D4241
apically positioned, D4245
**Flexible base partial denture**, D5225-D5226
**Flipper, dental prosthesis**, D5820-D5821
**Fluoride**
custom tray/gel carrier, D5986
topical, D1206
varnish, D1206
**Foreign body removal**, D7530-D7540
**Frenectomy/frenotomy (frenulectomy)**, D7961-D7962
**Full mouth series films**, D0210

## G

**Genetic testing**, D0422-D0423
**Gingiva/gingival**
flap, D4240-D4241
gingivectomy, gingivoplasty, D4210-D4212
**Gingiva/gingival** — *continued*
irrigation, D4921
periocoronal removal, D7971
**Gingivectomy/gingivoplasty**, D4210-D4212
**Glass ionomer (resin restoration)**, D2330-D2394
**Gold foil**, D2410-D2430
**Graft**
bone replacement, D4263-D4264, D6103-D6104, D7953
connective tissue, D4273, D4275, D4283-D4285
autogenous, D4273, D4283
nonautogenous, D4275, D4285
with pedicle, D4276
maxillofacial soft/hard tissue, D7955
skin, D7920
soft tissue, D4270-D4273
free, D4277-D4278
with pedicle, D4270
synthetic, D7955
**Guided tissue regeneration, dental**, D4266-D4267

## H

**HbA1c testing**, D0411
**Hemisection**, D3920
**Hospital/ambulatory surgery call**, D9420
**House/nursing home call**, D9410
**Hygiene instruction, oral**, D1330
**Hyperplastic tissue excision**, D7970

## I

**I&D**
extraoral, D7520-D7521
intraoral, D7510-D7511
**Images**
capture and interpretation, D0210-D0250, D0270-D0371
image only, D0380-D0386
interpretation only, D0391
post processing, D0393-D0394
**Immediate dentures**, D5130-D5140, D5221-D5224
**Immunofluorescence**
direct, D0482
indirect, D0483
**Impacted tooth, removal**, D7220-D7241
**Impaction**
device placement, D7283
removal, D7220-D7241
**Implant procedures**
abutments, D6051, D6056-D6057
bone graft, D6103-D6104
chin, D7995
craniofacial, D7993
endodontic, D3460
endosteal/endosseous, D6010
eposteal/subperiosteal, D6040
facial, D7995
index, film/surgical, D6190
interim, D6012
maintenance, D6080
mandible, D7996
maxillofacial, D5931-D5932, D5936-D5937
mini, D6013
other implant service, D6080-D6198
peri-implant
bone graft for repair, D6103
debridement, D6101-D6102
removal, D6100
broken retaining screw, D6096
interim component, D6198
repair, D6090-D6091, D6095
scaling and debridement, D6081
supported prosthetics, D6051-D6077
supported retainer, D6098-D6123, D6195
transosteal/transosseous, D6050
zygomatic, D7994
**Implant**
craniofacial, D7993
mandible, D7996
zygomatic, D7994
**Implantation/reimplantation, tooth**
accidental, D7270
**Implantation/reimplantation, tooth** — *continued*
intentional reimplantation, D3470
**In-situ tissue hybridization**, D0479
**Infiltration therapeutic drug**, D9613
**Infiltration, sustained release**
for pain control, D9613
**Inhalation analgesia**, D9230
**Inlay, dental**
fixed partial denture retainers
metallic, D6545-D6615
porcelain/ceramic, D6548-D6609
metallic, D2510-D2530
porcelain/ceramic, D2610-D2630
recement inlay, D2910
resin-based composite, D2650-D2652
titanium, D6624
**Intentional replantation**, D3470
**Interim**
abutment, D6051
complete denture, D5810-D5811
implant crown, D6085
partial denture, D5820-D5821
pontic, D6253
retainer crown (FPD), D6793
single crown, D2799
**Internal root repair**
perforation defect, D3333
**Interpretation, diagnostic image**
from other practitioner, D0391
**Intra-socket biological dressing**, D7922
**Intraoral radiographs**, D0210-D0240, D0270-D0277
**Intraorifice barrier**, D3911
**Intravenous sedation/analgesia**, D9243
**Irrigation, gingival**, D4921

## L

**Labial veneer/laminate**, D2960-D2962
**Laboratory services**, D0415-D0423, D0431-D0709
**Lateral exostosis, removal**, D7471
**Lesions**, D7410-D7465
destruction, D7465
surgical excision
odontogenic cyst/tumor, benign, D7450-D7461
soft tissue
benign, D7410-D7412
malignant, D7413-D7441
**Liner, soft**, D5765
**Localized osteitis, dry socket**, D9930

## M

**Maintenance maxillofacial prosthesis**, D5993
**Malocclusion correction**, D8010-D8704
**Mandibular partial denture**, D5212, D5214, D5226
immediate, D5222, D5224, D5228
**Maryland bridge (resin-bonded fixed prosthesis)**
pontic, D6210-D6252
retainer/abutment, D6545-D6549
**Maxillary partial denture**, D5211, D5213, D5225
immediate, D5221, D5223, D5227
**Maxillofacial defect, repair**, D7955
**Maxillofacial prosthetics**, D5931-D5932, D5936-D5937, D5952-D5982, D5986-D5996
adjustment and maintenance, D5992-D5993
commissure, D5988
fluoride, D5986
obturator, D5931-D5932, D5936
palatal, D5954-D5959
speech, D5952-D5953, D5960
surgical
splint, D5988
tent, D5982
trismus, D5937
**Medicinal carrier, topical**, D1355, D5991
**Mesial/distal wedge, single tooth**, D4274
**Microabrasion, enamel**, D9970
**Minimal sedation**, D9248
**Missed appointment**, D9986
**Mobilization erupted/malpositioned tooth**, D7282
**Moderate (conscious) sedation**, D9243-D9248
**Mouthguard, athletic**, D9941
**MRI (Magnetic Resonance Imaging)**, D0369, D0385
**Mucosal abnormalities, adjunctive**, D0431

## N

**Neoplasms**, D7410-D7465
**Nightguard**, D9942-D9946
**Nitrous oxide, analgesia**, D9230
**Nonintravenous conscious sedation**, D9248
**Nonodontogenic cyst removal**, D7460-D7461
**Nursing home visit**, D9410
**Nutrition, counseling**, D1310

## O

**Obturator prosthesis**
definitive, D5932
interim, D5936
surgical, D5931
**Occlusal**
adjustment, D9951-D9952
guard
adjustment, D9943
hard
full arch, D9944
partial arch, D9946
reline/repair, D9942
soft, full arch, D9945
image, D0240
orthotic device, D7880
adjustment, D7881
**Occlusion/analysis**, D9950
**Odontogenic cyst, removal**, D7450-D7451
**Odontoplasty (enameloplasty)**, D9971
**Office visit**, D0120-D0180, D9430-D9440
after hours, D9440
observation, D9430
**Onlay**
fixed partial denture retainer, metallic, D6610-D6615, D6634
metallic, D2542-D2544
porcelain/ceramic, D2642-D2644
resin-based composite, D2662, D2664
titanium, D6634
**Operculectomy**, D7971
**Oral and maxillofacial surgery**, D7111-D7294, D7296-D7560, D7840, D7880-D7922, D7941-D7945, D7953-D7962, D7970-D7979, D7981-D7998
**Oral**
disease
test for detection, D0431
test for susceptibility, D0423
test for vitality, D0460
examination, D0120-D0180
hygiene instruction, D1330
pathology
accession of tissue, D0472-D0474, D0480, D0486
bacteriologic studies, D0415
consultation on slides, D0484-D0485
cytology, D0480
decalcification, D0475
electron microscopy, D0481
hybridization, tissue, D0479
immunofluorescence, D0482-D0483
other oral pathology procedures, D0502
stains
immunofluorescence, D0482-D0483
special, D0476-D0477
**Oroantral fistula closure**, D7260
**Orthodontics**
comprehensive, D8070-D8090
limited, D8010-D8040
minor, D8210-D8220
other examination or treatment, D8660-D8670
periodic treatment visit, D8670
retainer
adjustment, D8681

**Orthodontics** — *continued*
retainer — *continued*
recementing, D8698-D8699
repair, D8701-D8702
replacement, D8703-D8704
**Orthotic appliance**, D7880
**Osseous surgery, graft**, D4260-D4264
**Ostectomy**, D7550
**Osteitis, localized (dry socket)**, D9930
**Osteotomy**
mandibular, D7941-D7943, D7945
segmented/subapical, D7944
**Overdenture**
complete
mandibular, D5863
maxillary, D5865
partial
mandibular, D5864
maxillary, D5866
supported by implant
fixed, D6114-D6117
removable, D6110-D6113

## P

**Palliative treatment, emergency**, D9110
**Panoramic x-ray**, D0330, D0701
**Partial dentures**
implant/abutment supported, D6112-D6113, D6116-D6117
interim, D5820-D5821
lower, D5212, D5214, D5222, D5224, D5226-D5227
pontics, fixed, D6205-D6253
rebase, D5711, D5721-D5725
reline, D5740-D5741, D5760-D5761
repair, D5611-D5671
retainers, fixed, D6545-D6794
sectioning, fixed, D9120
upper, D5211, D5213, D5221, D5223, D5225, D5228
**Patient assessment**, D0191
**Perforation defect, repair**, D3333
**Periapical service**, D3410-D3426, D3430, D3450-D3470
x-rays, D0220-D0230
**Pericoronal excision, gingival**, D7971
**Periodontal medicament carrier**, D5995-D5996
**Periodontics**, D4210-D4921
biologic materials, D4265
crown exposure, D4230-D4285
crown lengthening, D4249
debridement, full mouth, D4355
dressing change, unscheduled, D4920
evaluation, D0180
flap
apically positioned, D4245
gingival, D4240-D4241
gingivectomy/gingivoplasty, D4210-D4212
graft
bone, D4263-D4264
connective tissue, D4273, D4275
autogenous, D4273, D4283
nonautogenous, D4275, D4285
with pedicle graft, D4276
soft tissue, pedicle, D4270
free, D4277-D4278
irrigation, gingival, D4921
maintenance, D4910
osseous, with flap and closure, D4260-D4261
scaling and root planing, D4341-D4346
splinting, D4322-D4323
surgical revision, D4268
tissue regeneration, guided, D4266-D4267
wedge, mesial/distal, D4274
**Periradicular/apicoectomy**, D3410-D3426
**Phamacologicals**, D9610
parenteral administration
single drug, D9610
two or more drugs, D9612
**Photographs, diagnostic**, D0350-D0351
**Pin retention, per tooth**, D2951
**Pit and fissure sealant**, D1351
**Placement**
eposteal implant, D6040
fixation device, D7998
**Placement** — *continued*
interim implant body, D6012
intra-socket biologic dressing, D7922
mini implant, D6013
temporary anchorage device, D7292-D7294
transosteal implant, D6050
**Plasma rich protein, autologous**, D7921
**Pontic**, D6205-D6253
indirect resin based composite, D6205
interim, D6253
metal, D6210-D6243, D6250-D6252
resin, D6250-D6252
titanium, D6214
**Post and core**, D2952-D2954, D2957
**Post removal**, D2955
**Precision attachment**, D5862, D6950
**Prefabricated crown**, D2928-D2934
**Prefabricated post and core**, D2954
each additional (same tooth), D2957
**Preparation**
genetic sample, D0422
saliva samples, D0417
**Preventive**, D1110-D1558
application caries arresting medication, D1354-D1355
counseling
high-risk behavior, D1321
hygiene, D1330
nutrition, D1310
tobacco, D1320
fluoride application, D1206-D1208
prophylaxis, D1110-D1120
resin restoration, D1352
sealant, per tooth, D1351, D1353
space maintenance, D1510-D1558
**Prophylaxis**, D1110-D1120
**Prosthesis**
adjustment and maintenance, D5992-D5993
commissure, D5988
dental, fixed, D6205-D6985
dental, removable, D5110-D5867, D5876
fluoride, D5986
obturator, D5931-D5932, D5936
palatal, D5954-D5959
speech, D5952-D5953, D5960
surgical
splint, D5988
tent, D5982
trismus, D5937
**Prosthodontic procedures**
fixed, D6205-D6985
implant-supported, D6094, D6110-D6117, D6194
maxillofacial, D5931-D5932, D5936-D5937, D5952-D5982, D5986-D5996
pediatric partial denture, D6985
removable, D5110-D5867, D5876, D5931-D5932, D5936-D5937, D5952-D5982, D5986-D5996
**Pulp cap**, D3110-D3120
**Pulp capping**, D3110-D3120
**Pulp regeneration**, D3355-D3357
**Pulp sedation**, D2940
**Pulp vitality test**, D0460
**Pulpal debridement**, D3221
**Pulpal therapy, on primary teeth**, D3230-D3240
**Pulpotomy**
partial, for apexogenesis, D3222

## R

**Radiograph**, D0210-D0250, D0270-D0394
implant index, D6190
**Reattachment, tooth fragment**, D2921
**Recalcification (apexification)**, D3351-D3353
**Recement**
crown, D2920, D6092
implant, D6093
crown, D6092
inlay/onlay, D2910
maintainer, space, D1516-D1558
post and core, cast or prefabricated, D2915
retainers, D8698-D8699
veneer, D2910
**Reduction fibrous tuberosity**, D7972
**Reimplantation, dental**
accidentally evulsed, D7270
intentional, D3470
**Removal**
anchorage device, temporary, D7298-D7300
appliance, D7997
bone fragment, D9930
coronectomy (partial tooth removal), D7251
cyst/tumor, D7450-D7461
foreign body, D7530-D7540
impacted tooth, D7220-D7241
implant, D6100
interim component, D6198
lateral exostosis, D7471
post, D2955
pulp, D3220, D3222
residual tooth root, D7250
retaining screw, D6096
tooth, surgical, D7111-D7251
torus, D7472-D7473
**Repair**
crown, D2980
denture
fixed partial, D6980
removable
complete, D5511-D5520
partial, D5611-D5671
fixed retainer, D8701-D8702
implant attachment, D6091
inlay/only, D2981-D2982
maxillofacial soft/hard tissue defect, D7955
occlusal guard, D9942
orthodontic
appliance, D8696-D8697
retainer, fixed, D8701-D8702
precision/semi-precision attachment, D5867, D6091
root resorption, D3471-D3473
sealant, D1353
traumatic wounds, D7910
veneer, D2983
**Replacement**
broken/lost retainer, D8703-D8704
broken/missing tooth
complete, D5520
partial, D5640, D5670-D5671
graft, bone, D4263-D4264, D7953
implant/abutment prosthesis, D6091
precision/semi-precision attachment, D5867, D6091
**Resin dental restoration**
direct
anterior, D2330-D2335
crown, D2390
posterior, D2391-D2394
veneers, D2960
indirect
abutment, fixed partial denture, D6710
crown, D2710
inlay/onlay, D2650-D2664
pontic, D6205
three-quarter crown, D2712
veneers, D2961-D2962
**Restorations**
amalgam, D2140-D2161
gold foil, D2410-D2430
inlay/onlay, D2510-D2664, D2981-D2982, D6600-D6634
protective, D2940
resin
composite, D2330-D2394
infiltration, D2990
therapeutic, interim, D2941
**Restorative services**, D2140-D2941, D2950-D2990
**Retainers**
crowns, D6710-D6794
implant/abutment supported, D6068-D6077, D6098-D6099, D6120-D6123, D6194-D6195
inlay/onlay, D6600-D6634
orthodontic, D8680
pediatric, D6985
pontics, D6205-D6253
**Retainers** — *continued*
recementation, D6930
repair, D6980
resin bonded, D6545-D6549
sectioning, D9120
**Retreatment, endodontic**, D3346-D3348
**Retrograde filling**, D3430
**Revision, tooth (surgical)**, D4268
**Root**
canal, therapy, D3310-D3353
incomplete, D3332
obstruction, D3331
planing and scaling, D4341
removal, D7140, D7250
resection/amputation, D3450
resorption, repair, D3471-D3473
surgical exposure root surface, D3501-D3503
**Rubber dam, tooth isolation**, D3910

## S

**Saliva**
analysis, D0418-D0419
assessment by measurement, D0419
collection and preparation, D0417
**Salivary gland**
excision or fistula closure, D7983
**Scaling**
debridement, single implant, D6081
gingival inflammation, D4346
with planing, D4341-D4342
**Screening, patient**, D0190
pre-visit, D9912
**Sealant**
application, per tooth, D1351
repair, D1353
**Sectioning**
denture, fixed partial, D9120
**Sedation**
deep, D9222-D9223
evaluation for, D9219
intravenous, conscious, D9239-D9243
moderate, D9243
non-intravenous, D9248
**Sedative filling**, D2940
**Semi-precision attachment abutment**, D6091
replacement, D5867
**Sequestrectomy**, D7550
**Sialodochoplasty**, D7982
**Sialography**, D0310, D0371
**Sinus lift**
closure of perforation, D7261
**Sinusotomy, in dentistry**, D7560
**Skin graft**, D7920
**Sleep apnea appliance, custom**, D9947-D9949
**Space maintainer**, D1516-D1558
**Speech aid**
adult, D5953
pediatric, D5952
**Splinting, dental**
commissure, D5987
extra-coronal, D4323
intra-coronal, D4322
surgical, D5988
**Stabilization evulsed/displace tooth**, D7270
**Stainless steel crown**, D2930-D2931, D2933-D2934
**Stains**
immunohistochemical, D0478
microorganisms, D0476
not for microorganisms, D0477
**Stayplate for partial denture**, D5820-D5821
**Stent**
periodontal/columellar, D5982
**Stress breaker**, D6940
**Submergence erupted tooth**, D3921
**Supra crestal fibrotomy**, D7291
**Surgery**
oral, D7111-D7294, D7296-D7560, D7840, D7880-D7922, D7941-D7945, D7953-D7962, D7970-D7979, D7981-D7998
**Surgical**
repositioning, teeth, D7290
**Suturing**, D7910-D7912
complicated, D7911-D7912

**Suturing** — *continued*
small, D7910

## T

**Teledenistry**, D9995-D9996
**Temporomandibular joint (TMJ)**, D7840, D7880-D7899
condylectomy, D7840
occlusal device, D7880-D7881
radiographs, D0320-D0321
therapy, D9130
treatment, D7840, D7880-D7899
**Testing**
Antibody, D0605
Antigen, D0604
**Tests, in office**
blood glucose, D0412
HbA1c, D0411
**Thumb sucking device**, D8210-D8220
**Tissue**
conditioning, D5850-D5851
excision of hyperplastic, D7970
**Tobacco counseling**, D1320
**Tomographic radiograph, dental**, D0322
**Tongue thrusting device**, D8210-D8220
**Tooth, natural**
exposure, unerupted tooth, D7280
extraction, D7111-D7250
impacted, removal, D7220-D7241
intentional reimplantation, D3470
pulp vitality test, D0460
reimplantation, evulsed tooth, D7270
surgical exposure, D7280
surgical repositioning, D7290
transplantation, D7272
**Topical medicament carrier**, D5991
**Torus, removal of**
mandibularis, D7473
palatinus, D7472
**Tracheotomy, emergency**, D7990
**Transplant, tooth**, D7272
**Transseptal fiberotomy**, D7291
**Trigeminal division block (anesthesia)**, D9212
**Trismus appliance**, D5937
**Tuberosity reduction**
fibrous, D7972
osseous, D7485
**Tumor, removal**, D7440-D7465

## U

**Ultrasound**, D0370, D0386
**Unerupted tooth exposure**, D7280

## V

**Vaccination Adminstration**, D1701-D1707
**Veneers**, D2960-D2962
**Vestibuloplasty**, D7340-D7350
**Viral culture**, D0416

## W

**Wax up (diagnostic cast)**, D9950
**Wedge, mesial/distal**, D4274
**Whitening (bleaching)**
external, per arch, D9972
external, per tooth, D9973
internal, per tooth, D9974
**Wound repair (suture)**, D7910-D7912

## X

**X-ray**, D0210-D0250, D0270-D0394
image capture only
2-D cephalometric, D0702
2-D oral/facial photographic, D0703
3-D photographic, D0704
extraoral posterior, D0705
intraoral, D0706-D0709
panoramic, D0701
implant index, D6190

# CPT Index


## A

- **Abscess**
  - Mouth
    - Floor of Mouth
      - Extraoral, 41015-41018
      - Intraoral, 41000-41009
  - Tongue, 41000-41009
- **Advanced Life Support**
  - Emergency Department Services, 99281-99285
- **Alveoloplasty**, 41874
- **Application**
  - Topical Fluoride Varnish, 99188

## B

- **Biopsy**
  - Mouth, 40808

## C

- **Cyst**
  - Excision
    - Mouth
      - Lingual, 41000
      - Masticator Space, 41009, 41018
      - Sublingual, 41005-41006, 41015
      - Submandibular, 41008, 41017
      - Submental, 41007, 41016
  - Incision and Drainage
    - Mouth
      - Lingual, 41000
      - Masticator Space, 41009, 41018
      - Sublingual, 41005-41006
      - Submandibular, 41008, 41017
      - Submental, 41007, 41016
  - Mouth
    - Lingual, 41000
    - Masticator Space, 41009, 41018
    - Sublingual, 41005-41006
    - Submandibular, 41008, 41017
    - Submental, 41007, 41016
  - Tongue
    - Incision and Drainage, 41000-41009

## D

- **Dehiscence**
  - Suture
    - Skin and Subcutaneous Tissue
      - Simple, 12020
        - with Packing, 12021
      - Superficial, 12020
        - with Packing, 12021
  - Wound
    - Skin and Subcutaneous Tissue
      - Simple, 12020
        - with Packing, 12021
      - Superficial, 12020
        - with Packing, 12021
- **Discharge Services**
  - Hospital, 99238-99239
- **Drainage**
  - Abscess
    - Mouth
      - Lingual, 41000
      - Masticator Space, 41009, 41018
      - Sublingual, 41005-41006, 41015
      - Submandibular Space, 41008, 41017
      - Submental Space, 41007, 41016
    - Tongue
      - Incision and Drainage, 41000-41006, 41015-41018
  - Cyst
    - Mouth
      - Lingual, 41000
      - Masticator Space, 41009, 41018
      - Sublingual, 41005-41006, 41015
      - Submandibular Space, 41008, 41017
      - Submental Space, 41007, 41016

**Drainage** — *continued*

  - Hematoma
    - Mouth
      - Lingual, 41000
      - Masticator Space, 41009, 41018
      - Sublingual, 41005-41006, 41015
      - Submandibular Space, 41008, 41017
      - Submental Space, 41007, 41016

## E

- **ED**, 99281-99285
- **Emergency Department Services**, 99281-99285
- **ER**, 99281-99285
- **Established Patient**
  - Emergency Department Services, 99281-99285
  - Hospital Inpatient Services, 99221-99223, 99231-99233, 99238-99239
  - Office Visit, 99211-99215
  - Outpatient Visit, 99211-99215
- **Evaluation and Management**
  - Emergency Department, 99281-99285
  - Hospital, 99221-99223, 99231-99233
  - Hospital Discharge, 99238-99239
  - Hospital Services
    - Initial, 99221-99223, 99231-99233
    - Subsequent, 99231
  - Office and Other Outpatient, 99202-99215
- **Excision**
  - Gingiva, 41820
  - Gums, 41820
    - Operculum, 41821
  - Lesion
    - Gums, 41822-41823, 41828
    - Mouth, 40810-40812
  - Lip
    - Frenum, 40819
  - Mandibular, Exostosis, 21031
  - Maxilla
    - Exostosis, 21032
  - Maxillary Torus Palatinus, 21032
  - Mucosa
    - Gums, 41828
  - Tongue
    - Frenum, 41115
  - Torus Mandibularis, 21031

## F

- **Fluoride Varnish Application**, 99188
- **Foreign Body**
  - Removal
    - Mouth, 40804-40805
- **Frenectomy**, 40819, 41115
- **Frenoplasty**, 41520
- **Frenotomy**, 40806, 41010
- **Frenulectomy**, 40819
- **Frenuloplasty**, 41520
- **Frenum**
  - Lip
    - Incision, 40806
- **Frenumectomy**, 40819

## G

- **Gingivectomy**, 41820
- **Gingivoplasty**, 41872
- **Graft**
  - Gum Mucosa, 41870
- **Gums**
  - Excision
    - Gingiva, 41820
    - Operculum, 41821
  - Graft
    - Mucosa, 41870
  - Lesion
    - Excision, 41822-41823, 41828
  - Mucosa
    - Excision, 41828
  - Reconstruction
    - Alveolus, 41874

**Gums** — *continued*

  - Reconstruction — *continued*
    - Gingiva, 41872

## H

- **Head**
  - Excision, 21031-21032
- **Hematoma**
  - Mouth, 41005-41009, 41015-41018
  - Tongue, 41000-41006, 41015
- **Hospital Services**
  - Inpatient Services
    - Discharge Services, 99238-99239
    - Initial Care New or Established Patient, 99221-99223
    - Initial Hospital Care, 99221-99223
    - Subsequent Hospital Care, 99231-99233

## I

- **Incision and Drainage**
  - Abscess
    - Mouth, 41005-41009, 41015-41018
    - Tongue, 41000-41006, 41015
  - Cyst
    - Mouth, 41005-41009, 41015-41018
    - Tongue, 41000-41006, 41015
  - Hematoma
    - Mouth, 41005-41009, 41015-41018
    - Tongue, 41000-41006, 41015
- **Incision**
  - Lip
    - Frenum, 40806
  - Temporomandibular Joint, 21031-21032
  - Tongue
    - Frenum, 41010
- **Integumentary System**
  - Repair
    - Simple, 12020-12021

## L

- **Lesion**
  - Gums
    - Excision, 41822-41823, 41828
  - Mouth
    - Excision, 40810-40812
    - Vestibule
      - Repair, 40830
- **Lip**
  - Excision
    - Frenum, 40819
  - Incision
    - Frenum, 40806

## M

- **Mandible**
  - Torus Mandibularis
    - Excision, 21031
- **Maxilla**
  - Excision, 21032
- **Maxillary Torus Palatinus**
  - Tumor Excision, 21032
- **Mouth**
  - Abscess
    - Incision and Drainage, 41005-41009, 41015-41018
  - Biopsy, 40808
  - Cyst
    - Incision and Drainage, 41005-41009, 41015-41018
  - Excision
    - Frenum, 40819
  - Hematoma
    - Incision and Drainage, 41005-41009, 41015-41018
  - Lesion
    - Excision, 40810-40812
    - Vestibule of
      - Repair, 40830

**Mouth** — *continued*

  - Reconstruction, 40840-40845
  - Removal
    - Foreign Body, 40804-40805
  - Repair
    - Laceration, 40830-40831
  - Vestibule
    - Excision
      - Destruction, 40808-40812, 40819
    - Incision, 40804-40806
    - Removal
      - Foreign Body, 40804
    - Repair, 40830-40845
- **Mucosa**
  - Excision of Lesion
    - Alveolar, Hyperplastic, 41828
    - Vestibule of Mouth, 40810-40812
  - Periodontal Grafting, 41870

## N

- **New Patient**
  - Emergency Department Services, 99281-99285
  - Hospital Inpatient Services, 99221-99223, 99231-99233, 99238-99239
  - Initial Office Visit, 99202-99205
  - Outpatient Visit, 99211-99215

## O

- **Office and/or Other Outpatient Visits**
  - Established Patient, 99211-99215
  - New Patient, 99202-99205
  - Office Visit
    - Established Patient, 99211-99215
    - New Patient, 99202-99205
  - Outpatient Visit
    - Established Patient, 99211-99215
    - New Patient, 99202-99205
- **Operculectomy**, 41821
- **Outpatient Visit**, 99202-99215

## P

- **Physical Examination**
  - Office and/or Other Outpatient Services, 99202-99215

## R

- **Reconstruction**
  - Gums
    - Alveolus, 41874
    - Gingiva, 41872
  - Mouth, 40840-40845
  - Tongue
    - Frenum, 41520
- **Removal**
  - Foreign Bodies
    - Mouth, 40804-40805
- **Repair**
  - Mouth
    - Laceration, 40830-40831
    - Vestibule of, 40830-40845
  - Simple, Integumentary System, 12020-12021
  - Skin
    - Wound
      - Simple, 12020-12021
  - Wound
    - Simple, 12020-12021
  - Wound Dehiscence
    - Skin and Subcutaneous Tissue
      - Simple, 12020-12021

## S

- **Stomatoplasty**
  - Vestibule, 40840-40845
- **Subcutaneous Tissue**
  - Repair
    - Simple, 12020-12021

**Suture**
Wound
Skin
Simple, 12020-12021
**System, Body**
Digestive, 40804-40812, 40819, 40830-40845, 41000-41018, 41115, 41520, 41820-41823, 41828, 41870-41874
Integumentary, 12020-12021
Musculoskeletal, 21031-21032

## T

**Tongue**
Abscess
Incision and Drainage, 41000-41006, 41015
Cyst
Incision and Drainage, 41000-41006, 41015
**Tongue** — *continued*
Excision
Frenum, 41115
Hematoma
Incision and Drainage, 41000-41006, 41015
Incision
Frenum, 41010
Reconstruction
Frenum, 41520
**Torus Mandibularis**
Tumor Excision, 21031
**Tumor**
Maxillary Torus Palatinus, 21032
Torus Mandibularis, 21031

## V

**Vestibule of Mouth**
Biopsy, 40808
**Vestibule of Mouth** — *continued*
Excision
Lesion, 40810-40812
**Vestibuloplasty**, 40840-40845

## W

**Wound**
Dehiscence
Repair
Skin and Subcutaneous Tissue
Simple, 12020
with Packing, 12021
Superficial, 12020
with Packing, 12021
Suture
Skin and Subcutaneous Tissue
Simple, 12020
with Packing, 12021
Superficial, 12020
with Packing, 12021
**Wound** — *continued*
Repair
Skin
Simple, 12020-12021
Secondary
Skin and Subcutaneous Tissue
Simple, 12020
Simple with Packing, 12021
Superficial, 12020
with Packing, 12021

## Z

**Z-Plasty**, 41520

# Medicare Official Regulatory Information



## The CMS Online Manual System

The Centers for Medicare and Medicaid Services (CMS) restructured its paper-based manual system as a web-based system on October 1, 2003. Called the CMS Online Manual System, it combines all of the various program instructions into internet-only manuals (IOM), which are used by all CMS programs and contractors. Complete versions of all of the manuals can be found at http://www.cms.gov/manuals.

The provider reimbursement manuals (Pub. 15-1, Pub. 15-2) and the *State Medicaid Manual* (Pub. 45) are exceptions to the IOM system and are still active paper-based manuals.

Effective with implementation of the IOMs, the former method of publishing program memoranda (PM) to communicate program instructions was replaced by the following four templates:

- One-time notification
- Manual revisions
- Business requirements
- Confidential requirements

The Office of Strategic Operations and Regulatory Affairs (OSORA), Division of Issuances, will continue to communicate advanced program instructions to the regions and contractor community every Friday as it currently does. These instructions will also contain a transmittal sheet to identify changes pertaining to a specific manual, requirement, or notification.

The web-based system has been organized by functional area (e.g., eligibility, entitlement, claims processing, benefit policy, program integrity) in an effort to eliminate redundancy within the manuals, simplify updating, and make CMS program instructions available more quickly. The web-based system contains the functional areas included below:

| | |
|---|---|
| Pub. 100 | Introduction |
| Pub. 100-01 | Medicare General Information, Eligibility and Entitlement Manual |
| Pub. 100-02 | Medicare Benefit Policy Manual |
| Pub. 100-03 | Medicare National Coverage Determinations (NDC) Manual |
| Pub. 100-04 | Medicare Claims Processing Manual |
| Pub. 100-05 | Medicare Secondary Payer Manual |
| Pub. 100-06 | Medicare Financial Management Manual |
| Pub. 100-07 | State Operations Manual |
| Pub. 100-08 | Medicare Program Integrity Manual |
| Pub. 100-09 | Medicare Contractor Beneficiary and Provider Communications Manual |
| Pub. 100-10 | Quality Improvement Organization Manual |
| Pub. 100-11 | Programs of All-Inclusive Care for the Elderly (PACE) Manual |
| Pub. 100-12 | State Medicaid Manual (under development) |
| Pub. 100-13 | Medicaid State Children's Health Insurance Program (under development) |
| Pub. 100-14 | Medicare ESRD Network Organizations Manual |
| Pub. 100-15 | Medicaid Integrity Program (MIP) |
| Pub. 100-16 | Medicare Managed Care Manual |
| Pub. 100-17 | CMS/Business Partners Systems Security Manual |
| Pub. 100-18 | Medicare Prescription Drug Benefit Manual |
| Pub. 100-19 | Demonstrations |
| Pub. 100-20 | One-Time Notification |
| Pub. 100-21 | Reserved |
| Pub. 100-22 | Medicare Quality Reporting Incentive Programs Manual |
| Pub. 100-23 | Payment Error Rate Measurement (Under Development) |
| Pub. 100-24 | State Buy-In Manual |
| Pub. 100-25 | Information Security Acceptable Risk Safeguards Manual |

A brief description of the Medicare manuals primarily used for this publication follows.

### National Coverage Determinations Manual

Pub. 100-03, the *National Coverage Determinations* (NCD) *Manual*, is organized according to categories such as diagnostic services, supplies, and medical procedures. The table of contents lists each category and subject within that category. A revision transmittal sheet will identify any new material and recap the changes as well as provide an effective date for the change and any background information. At any time, one can refer to a transmittal indicated on the page of the manual to view this information.

By the time it is complete, the book will contain two chapters. Chapter 1 includes a description of national coverage determinations that have been made by CMS. When available, chapter 2 will contain a list of HCPCS codes related to each coverage determination. To make the manual easier to use, it is organized in accordance with CPT category sequences. Where there is no national coverage determination that affects a particular CPT category, the category is listed as reserved in the table of contents.

### Medicare Benefit Policy Manual

Pub. 100-02, the *Medicare Benefit Policy Manual* contains Medicare general coverage instructions that are not national coverage determinations. As a general rule, in the past these instructions have been found in chapter II of the *Medicare Carriers Manual*, the *Medicare Intermediary Manual*, other provider manuals, and program memoranda. New instructions will be published in this manual. As new transmittals are included they will be identified.

On the CMS website, a crosswalk from the new manual to the source manual is provided with each chapter and may be accessed from the chapter table of contents. In addition, the crosswalk for each section is shown immediately under the section heading.

The list below is the contents for the *Medicare Benefit Policy Manual*:

| Chapter | Title |
|---|---|
| 1 | Inpatient Hospital Services Covered Under Part A |
| 2 | Inpatient Psychiatric Hospital Services |
| 3 | Duration of Covered Inpatient Services |
| 4 | Inpatient Psychiatric Benefit Days Reduction and Lifetime Limitation |
| 5 | Lifetime Reserve Days |
| 6 | Hospital Services Covered Under Part B |
| 7 | Home Health Services |
| 8 | Coverage of Extended Care (SNF) Services Under Hospital Insurance |
| 9 | Coverage of Hospice Services Under Hospital Insurance |
| 10 | Ambulance Services |
| 11 | End Stage Renal Disease (ESRD) |
| 12 | Comprehensive Outpatient Rehabilitation Facility (CORF) Coverage |
| 13 | Rural Health Clinic (RHC) and Federally Qualified Health Center (FQHC) Services |
| 14 | Medical Devices |
| 15 | Covered Medical and Other Health Services |
| 16 | General Exclusions from Coverage |

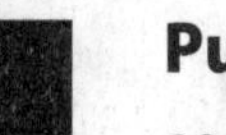



# Pub. 100 References

## 100-01, 5, 70.2

***Dentists***

(Rev. 1, 09-11-02)

A dentist qualifies as a physician if he/she is a doctor of dental surgery or of dental medicine who is legally authorized to practice dentistry by the State in which he/she performs such function and who is acting within the scope of his/her license when he/she performs such functions. Such services include any otherwise covered service that may legally and alternatively be performed by doctors of medicine, osteopathy and dentistry; e.g., dental examinations to detect infections prior to certain surgical procedures, treatment of oral infections and interpretations of diagnostic X-ray examinations in connection with covered services. Because the general exclusion of payment for dental services has not been withdrawn, payment for the services of dentists is also limited to those procedures which are not primarily provided for the care, treatment, removal, or replacement of teeth or structures directly supporting the teeth. The coverage of any given dental service is not affected by the professional designation of the physician rendering the service; i.e., an excluded dental service remains excluded and a covered dental service is still covered whether furnished by a dentist or a doctor of medicine or osteopathy.

## 100-02, 1, 70

***Inpatient Services in Connection With Dental Services***

(Rev. 1, 10-01-03) A3-3101.7, HO-210.7

When a patient is hospitalized for a dental procedure and the dentist's service is covered under Part B, the inpatient hospital services furnished are covered under Part A. For example, both the professional services of the dentist and the inpatient hospital expenses are covered when the dentist reduces a jaw fracture of an inpatient at a participating hospital. In addition, hospital inpatient services, which are necessary because of the patient's underlying medical condition and clinical status or the severity of a noncovered dental procedure, are covered.

When the hospital services are covered, all ancillary services such as x-rays, administration of anesthesia, use of the operating room, etc., are covered.

Regardless of whether the inpatient hospital services are covered, the medical services of physicians furnished in connection with noncovered dental services are not covered. The services of an anesthesiologist, radiologist, or pathologist whose services are performed in connection with the care, treatment, filling, removal, or replacement of teeth or structures directly supporting teeth are not covered.

## 100-03, 260.6

***Dental Examination Prior to Kidney Transplantation***

(Rev. 1, 10-03-03)

CIM 50-26

Despite the "dental services exclusion" in §1862(a)(12) of the Act (see the Medicare Benefit Policy Manual, Chapter 16, "General Exclusions From Coverage," §140;), an oral or dental examination performed on an inpatient basis as part of a comprehensive workup prior to renal transplant surgery is a covered service. This is because the purpose of the examination is not for the care of the teeth or structures directly supporting the teeth. Rather, the examination is for the identification, prior to a complex surgical procedure, of existing medical problems where the increased possibility of infection would not only reduce the chances for successful surgery but would also expose the patient to additional risks in undergoing such surgery.

Such a dental or oral examination would be covered under Part A of the program if performed by a dentist on the hospital's staff, or under Part B if performed by a physician. (When performing a dental or oral examination, a dentist is not recognized as a physician under §1861(r) of the Act.) (See the Medicare General Information, Eligibility, and Entitlement Manual, Chapter 5, "Definitions," §70.2, and the Medicare Benefit Policy Manual, Chapter 15, "Covered Medical and Other Health Services," §150.)

## 100-04, 4, 20.5

***Clarification of HCPCS Code to Revenue Code Reporting***

(Rev. 1487, Issued: 04-08-08, Effective: 04-01-08, Implementation: 04-07-08)

Generally, CMS does not instruct hospitals on the assignment of HCPCS codes to revenue codes for services provided under OPPS since hospitals' assignment of cost vary. Where explicit instructions are not provided, providers should report their charges under the revenue code that will result in the charges being assigned to the same cost center to which the cost of those services are assigned in the cost report.